Application of Brain Oscillations in Neuropsychiatric Diseases

Selected papers from "Brain Oscillations in Cognitive Impairment and Neurotransmitters" Conference, Istanbul, Turkey, 29 April–1 May 2011

Application of Brain Oscillations in Neuropsychiatric Diseases

Selected papers from "Brain Oscillations in Cognitive Impairment and Neurotransmitters" conference, Istanbul, Turkey, 29 April–1 May 2011

EDITED BY

E. BAŞAR
*Brain Dynamics, Cognition and Complex Systems Research Center,
Istanbul Kultur University, Istanbul 34156, Turkey*

C. BAŞAR-EROĞLU
Institute of Psychology and Cognition Research, University of Bremen, D-28359 Bremen, Germany

A. ÖZERDEM
Department of Psychiatry, Dokuz Eylül University Medical School, Narlidere, 35340 Izmir, Turkey

P.M. ROSSINI
Department of Neurology, Catholic University, 00186 Rome, Italy

G.G. YENER
*Department of Neurology, Dokuz Eylül University Medical School,
Balçova, Izmir 35340, Turkey*

SUPPLEMENTS TO CLINICAL NEUROPHYSIOLOGY
VOLUME 62
2013

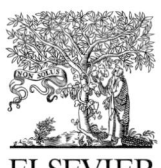

ELSEVIER

ELSEVIER B.V.	ELSEVIER Inc.	ELSEVIER Ltd.	ELSEVIER Ltd
Radarweg 29	525 B Street, Suite 1900	The Boulevard, Langford Lane	84 Theobalds Road
1043 NX Amsterdam	San Diego, CA 92101-4495	Kidlington, Oxford OX5 1GB	London WC1X 8RR
The Netherlands	USA	UK	UK

First edition 2013

Library of Congress Cataloging in Publication Data
A catalog record is available from the Library of Congress.

British Library Cataloguing in Publication Data
A catalogue record is available from the British Library.

ISBN-13: 978-0-7020-5307-8 (HB)
ISBN: 978-0-7020-5561-4 (PB)
ISBN: 978-0-7020-5562-1 (Eonly)
ISSN (Series): 1567-424X

∞ The paper used in this publication meets the requirements of ANSI/NISO Z39.48-1992 (Permanence of Paper).
Printed in The Netherlands.

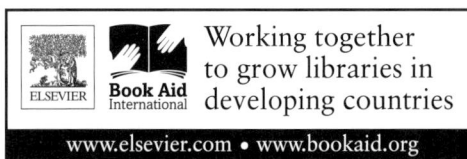

Preface

Application of brain oscillations to neuropsychiatric diseases: a new land?

More than 80 years have passed since Hans Berger recorded the first human electroencephalograms (EEGs) in the 1920s and more than 60 years since the publication of the first *"Supplement of Clinical Neurophysiology"* in 1950.

Berger's first description of EEG caused great excitement within the field of neuroscience during the late 1920s and early 1930s. The use of electroencephalography peaked in the 1940s and, thereafter, such studies reached a plateau in the 1960s (Mountcastle, 1992). With the subsequent introduction of CT scan and MRI, the use of EEG became progressively less attractive to most experimental neuroscientists.

According to Mountcastle (1998), a sudden paradigm change occurred: the understanding that our percepts are generated by the integration of brain activity triggered by sensory/cognitive stimuli with the activation of the neural images of past or current experience. The brain mechanisms involved in perception can now be studied directly, and with the appropriate time discrimination, by measuring ongoing changes in the electrical activity of the human brain using a large number of EEG recording sites on the scalp (Mountcastle, 1998), or the use of multiple microelectrodes implanted in primates. Furthermore, according to Mountcastle (1998), the paradigm change of using brain oscillations has become one of the most important conceptual and analytical tools for the understanding of cognitive processes. Mountcastle proposed that a major goal for neuroscience is to devise ways to study and analyze the activity of distributed systems in waking brains, particularly in human brains.

The great interest in investigating oscillatory brain dynamics (including evoked and/or event-related oscillations) for understanding cognitive impairment started around 10 years ago. In recent years, great attention has been focused on the evaluation of quantitative EEG (qEEG) and/or event-related potentials (ERPs) as clinical markers of the early stages of Alzheimer disease (AD; Rossini et al., 2007; Rossini, 2009). Regarding the classification of these subjects at an individual level, most studies showed moderate accuracy (70–80%) in the classification of EEG markers relative to normal and AD subjects. This means that the analysis of resting state EEG markers is promising for large-scale, low-cost, fully non-invasive screening of elderly subjects at risk of AD (Vecchio et al., this volume).

Başar and Güntekin (2008) reviewed the progress in event-related oscillations in schizophrenia, MCI, bipolar disorders, and Alzheimer's disease. Following the enormous progress made in the previous 4 years, an international conference workshop was organized in Istanbul (28th April–1st May 2011), sponsored by the Istanbul Kultur University, under the umbrella of the International Federation of Clinical Neurophysiology.

The present *Volume 62* of *Supplements to Clinical Neurophysiology* contains reviews, original contributions and concept papers delivered by participants of that 2011 conference. Following the conference, additional papers were also included from other significant contributors to the research field. The work collected in this supplement covers *EEG, evoked oscillations* and *event-related oscillations* in four different types of disorder. The application of medication is explained in some studies. Transcranial magnetic stimulation (TMS) as a research tool in pathology is also covered, as a framework for further investigation of brain oscillations in neuropsychiatric diseases. We are not aware of any other special issue or book addressing the applications of brain oscillations in cognitive diseases from such a broad range of perspectives. The relevant book by Simone Lovestone (2009) does not include electrophysiological markers.

A cardinal theme of the conference and of the present *Volume 62* of *Supplements to Clinical Neurophysiology* is the following:

After discussing the electrophysiological details of schizophrenia, Alzheimer's disease, bipolar disorders, MCI, ADHD, etc., can we develop an ensemble of neurophysiologic biomarkers for these disorders, and what should we be doing to translate those valuable parameters into clinical practice?

In order to analyze this major question, a panel discussion at the end of the conference led to fruitful thoughts on achieving important syntheses related to brain oscillations in neuropsychiatric diseases. The contributions of Claudio Babiloni and Giovanni Frisoni, in particular, added significant value to this workshop. This panel discussion, which could be considered as one of the core outputs of the conference, has been edited by G.G. Yener and E. Başar. The panel reflects emerging features that may be useful in the future development of biomarkers. These will be assigned as ensembles of EEG markers, combining spontaneous EEG, sensory evoked oscillations, event-related oscillations, and sensory and event-related coherences. Essential progress will most probably incorporate insights from all of these areas. The rich information and strong inter-disciplinary progress documented in the present volume provides hope for a quantum leap, within the next 5–6 years, in our understanding of brain oscillations in neuropsychiatric diseases. The present *Volume 62* may be most useful in manifesting the strong recent trend to develop biomarkers for brain oscillations in at least four to five neuropsychiatric diseases discussed in this volume.

Erol Başar
Canan Başar-Eroğlu
Ayşegül Özerdem
Paolo Maria Rossini
Görsev Gülmen Yener

References

Başar, E. and Güntekin, B. (2008) A review of brain oscillations in cognitive disorders and the role of neurotransmitters. *Brain Res.*, 1235: 172–193.
Lovestone, S. (2009) Biomarkers in brain disease. *Ann. NY Acad. Sci.*, 1180: vii.
Mountcastle, V.B. (1992) Preface. In: E. Başar and T.H. Bullock (Eds.), *Induced Rhythms in the Brain*. Birkhäuser, Boston, MA, pp. 217–231.
Mountcastle, V.B. (1998) *Perceptual Neuroscience: The Cerebral Cortex*. Harvard Univ. Press, Cambridge, MA.
Rossini, P.M. (2009) Implications of brain plasticity to brain–machine interfaces operation a potential paradox? *Int. Rev. Neurobiol.*, 86: 81–90.
Rossini, P.M., Rossi, S., Babiloni, C. and Polich, J. (2007) Clinical neurophysiology of aging brain: from normal aging to neurodegeneration. *Prog. Neurobiol.*, 83: 375–400.
Vecchio, F., Babiloni, C., Lizio, R., De Vico, F.F., Blinowska, K., Verrienti, G., Frisoni, G.B. and Rossini, P.M. (2013) Resting state cortical EEG rhythms in Alzheimer's disease: towards EEG markers for clinical applications. A review. In: *Suppl. to Clinical Neurophysiology*, this volume.
Yener, G.G. and Başar, E. (2013) Brain oscillations as biomarkers in neuropsychiatric disorders: following an interactive panel discussion and synopsis. In: *Suppl. to Clinical Neurophysiology*, this volume.

Acknowledgments

The organization of the "Biomarkers in Neuropsychiatry" conference, held in April 29th–May 1st 2011 in Istanbul and the achievement of the present *Volume 62* of *Supplements to Clinical Neurophysiology* (Elsevier) has been possible due to steady encouragement and generous financial support of the Istanbul Kultur University.

Special thanks to Dr. Bahar Akıngüç Günver (Chairman of the Board of Trustees), Civil Engineer Fahamettin Akıngüç (Honorary Chairman of the Board of Trustees) and Prof. Dr. Dursun Koçer (Rector of the University) who have strongly supported this endeavor.

The secretarial achievement, preparation of the manuscripts and communication have been accomplished by Melis Diktaş, Elif Tülay, and Bilge Turp Gölbaşı.

We express our special thanks to all these people. Without their help this work could not have been accomplished.

List of Contributors

Atagün, M.İ.   Bakirkoy Research and Training Hospital for Psychiatry and Neurology, 34145 Istanbul, Turkey.

Babiloni, C.   Department of Biomedical Sciences, University of Foggia, Viale Pinto 7, 71100 Foggia, Italy.

Baglieri, A.   IRCCS Centro Neurolesi Bonino-Pulejo, 98124 Messina, Italy.

Bagnato, S.   Neurorehabilitation and Neurophysiology Unit, Rehabilitation Department, Fondazione Istituto "San Raffaele – G. Giglio", 90015 Cefalù (PA), Italy.

Barry, R.J.   Brain & Behaviour Research Institute and School of Psychology, University of Wollongong, Northfields Avenue, Wollongong, NSW 2522, Australia.

Başar, E.   Brain Dynamics, Cognition and Complex Systems Research Center, Istanbul Kultur University, Istanbul 34156, Turkey.

Başar-Eroğlu, C.   Institute of Psychology and Cognition Research, University of Bremen, Grazer Strasse 4, D-28359 Bremen, Germany.

Bender, S.   Child and Adolescent Psychiatry, Section for Clinical Neurophysiology and Multimodal Neuroimaging, Technical University of Dresden, D-01307 Dresden, Germany.

Blinowska, K.   Department of Biomedical Physics, Warsaw University, 00-927 Warsaw, Poland.

Boccagni, C.   Neurorehabilitation and Neurophysiology Unit, Rehabilitation Department, Fondazione Istituto "San Raffaele – G. Giglio", 90015 Cefalù (PA), Italy.

Bonetti, M.   Service of Neuroradiology, Istituto Clinico Città di Brescia, 25125 Brescia, Italy.

Bramanti, P.   IRCCS Centro Neurolesi Bonino-Pulejo, 98124 Messina, Italy.

Clarke, A.R.   Brain & Behaviour Research Institute and School of Psychology, University of Wollongong, Northfields Avenue, Wollongong, NSW 2522, Australia.

De Vico Fallani, F. IRCCS "Fondazione Santa Lucia", 00142 Rome, Italy.

Ferreri, F. Department of Neurology, University Campus Bio-Medico, 00100 Rome, Italy, and Department of Clinical Neurophysiology, Kuopio University Hospital, University of Eastern Finland, 70100 Kuopio, Finland.

Fingelkurts, Alexander A. BM-Science – Brain and Mind Technologies Research Center, P.O. Box 77, FI-02601 Espoo, Finland.

Fingelkurts, Andrew A. BM-Science – Brain and Mind Technologies Research Center, P.O. Box 77, FI-02601 Espoo, Finland.

Ford, J.M. Department of Psychiatry, San Francisco Veterans Administration Medical Center, Bldg. 8, Room 9B, 116D, 4150 Clement Street, San Francisco, CA 94121, USA.

Frisoni, G.B. Laboratory of Epidemiology, Neuroimaging and Telemedicine, IRCCS Centro San Giovanni di Dio-Fatebenefratelli, Via Pilastroni 1, 25125 Brescia, Italy.

Galardi, G. Neurorehabilitation and Neurophysiology Unit, Rehabilitation Department, Fondazione Istituto "San Raffaele – G. Giglio", 90015 Cefalù (PA), Italy.

Güntekin, B. Brain Dynamics, Cognition and Complex Systems Research Center, Istanbul Kultur University, Istanbul 34156, Turkey.

Hetrick, W.P. Department of Psychological and Brain Sciences, Indiana University, 1101 East 10th Street, Bloomington, IN 47405, USA.

Hoffman, R.E. Department of Psychiatry, Yale University, 300 George Street, New Haven, CT 06511, USA.

Kanba, S. Department of Neuropsychiatry, Graduate School of Medical Sciences, Kyushu University, 3-1-1 Maidashi, Higashiku, Fukuoka 812-8582, Japan.

Koch, M. Department of Neuropharmacology, Brain Research Institute, University of Bremen – FB 2, PO Box 330440, D-28334 Bremen, Germany.

Kolev, V. Institute of Neurobiology, Bulgarian Academy of Sciences, Acad. G. Bonchev Str., Bl.23, 1113 Sofia, Bulgaria.

Krishnan, G.P. Department of Cell Biology and Neuroscience, University of California Riverside, Riverside, CA 92521, USA.

Lizio, R.   IRCCS San Raffaele Pisana, 00163 Rome, Italy.

Marino, S.   IRCCS Centro Neurolesi Bonino-Pulejo, 98124 Messina, Italy.

Mathalon, D.H.   Mental Health Service, San Francisco Veterans Administration Medical Center, Bldg. 8, Room 9B, 116D, 4150 Clement Street, San Francisco, CA 94121, USA.

Mathes, B.   Institute of Psychology and Cognition Research, University of Bremen, Grazer Strasse 4, D-28359 Bremen, Germany.

McCarley, R.W.   Boston Veterans Affairs Healthcare System, Brockton Division, Brockton, MA 02301, USA.

McGlashan, T.H. Department of Psychiatry, Yale University, 300 George Street, New Haven, CT 06511, USA.

Morzorati, S.L. Department of Psychiatry, Larue D. Carter Memorial Hospital, Indianapolis, IN 46222, USA.

O'Donnell, B.F. Department of Psychological and Brain Sciences, Indiana University, 1101 East 10th Street, Bloomington, IN 47405, USA.

Onitsuka, T.   Department of Neuropsychiatry, Graduate School of Medical Sciences, Kyushu University, 3-1-1 Maidashi, Higashiku, Fukuoka 812-8582, Japan.

Oribe, N.   Department of Neuropsychiatry, Graduate School of Medical Sciences, Kyushu University, 3-1-1 Maidashi, Higashiku, Fukuoka 812-8582, Japan.

Özerdem, A.   Department of Psychiatry, Dokuz Eylül University Medical School, Narlidere, 35340 Izmir, Turkey.

Perez, V.B.   Department of Psychiatry, San Francisco Veterans Administration Medical Center, Bldg. 8, Room 9B, 116D, 4150 Clement Street, San Francisco, CA 94121, USA.

Pievani, M.   Laboratory of Epidemiology, Neuroimaging and Telemedicine, IRCCS Centro San Giovanni di Dio Fatebenefratelli, The National Center for Research and Care of Alzheimer's and Mental Diseases, 25125 Brescia, Italy.

Prestia, A.   Laboratory of Epidemiology, Neuroimaging and Telemedicine, IRCCS Centro San Giovanni di Dio Fatebenefratelli, The National Center for Research and Care of Alzheimer's and Mental Diseases, 25125 Brescia, Italy.

Rass, O.   Department of Psychological and Brain Sciences, Indiana University, 1101 East 10th Street, Bloomington, IN 47405, USA.

Rasser, P.E.   Schizophrenia Research Institute, Darlinghurst, Sydney, NSW 2010, and Priority Centre for Brain and Mental Health Research, University of Newcastle, Newcastle, NSW 2300, Australia.

Roach, B.J.   Department of Psychiatry, San Francisco Veterans Administration Medical Center, Bldg. 8, Room 9B, 116D, 4150 Clement Street, San Francisco, CA 94121, USA.

Rossini, P.M.   Department of Neurology, Policlinic A. Gemelli, Catholic University, Largo Agostino Gemelli 8, 00186 Rome, Italy.

Rothenberger, A.   Child and Adolescent Psychiatry, University of Göttingen, D-37075 Göttingen, Germany.

Salisbury, D.F.   Cognitive Neuroscience Laboratory, McLean Hospital, 115 Mill Street, NBG21, Belmont, MA 02478, USA.

Schmiedt-Fehr, C.   Institute of Psychology and Cognition Research, University of Bremen, Grazer Strasse 4, D-28359 Bremen, Germany.

Sharma, A.   Section for Experimental Psychopathology and Neurophysiology, Department of General Psychiatry, Center for Psychosocial Medicine, University of Heidelberg, Vossstrasse 4, D-69115, Germany.

Srihari, V.H.   Department of Psychiatry, Yale University, 300 George Street, New Haven, CT 06511, USA.

Taylor, G.W.   Cognitive Neuroscience Laboratory, McLean Hospital, 115 Mill Street, NBG21, Belmont, MA 02478, USA.

Thompson, P.M.   Laboratory of Neuro Imaging, UCLA School of Medicine, Los Angeles, CA 90095-7334, USA.

Vecchio, F.   A.Fa.R., Dipartimento di Neuroscienze, Ospedale Fatebenefratelli, Isola Tiberina, 00186 Rome, Italy.

Verrienti, G.   Department of Neurology, University "Campus Biomedico", 00128 Rome, Italy.

Vohs, J.L.   Department of Psychiatry, Indiana University School of Medicine, and Larue D. Carter Memorial Hospital, Indianapolis, IN 46222, USA.

Weisbrod, M.   Psychiatric Department, SRH Klinikum Karlsbad-Langensteinbach, D-76307 Karlsbad, Germany.

Woods, S.W.   Department of Psychiatry, Yale University, 300 George Street, New Haven, CT 06511, USA.

Yener, G.G.   Department of Neurology, Dokuz Eylül University Medical School, Balçova, Izmir 35340, Turkey.

Yordanova, J.   Institute of Neurobiology, Bulgarian Academy of Sciences, Acad. G. Bonchev Str., Bl.23, 1113 Sofia, Bulgaria.

Contents

Application of Brain Oscillations in Neuropsychiatric Diseases
(Supplements to Clinical Neurophysiology, Vol. 62)
Editors: E. Başar, C. Başar-Eroğlu, A. Özerdem, P.M. Rossini, G.G. Yener

Chapter 1

Neurophysiological techniques in the study of the excitability, connectivity, and plasticity of the human brain

Paolo Maria Rossini[a,b,*] and Florinda Ferreri[c,d]

[a]*Department of Neurology, Catholic University, 00186 Rome, Italy*
[b]*IRCCS S. Raffaele Pisana, Rome, and Casa di Cura S. Raffaele, 03043 Cassino, Italy*
[c]*Department of Neurology, University Campus Bio-Medico, 00100 Rome, Italy*
[d]*Department of Clinical Neurophysiology, Kuopio University Hospital, University of Eastern Finland,*
70100 Kuopio, Finland

ABSTRACT

There is increasing evidence to support the concept that brain plasticity involves distinct functional and structural components, each requiring several cellular mechanisms operating at different time scales, synaptic loci, and developmental phases within an extremely complex framework. However, the precise relationship between functional and structural components of brain plasticity/connectivity phenomena is still unclear and its explanation represents a major challenge within modern neuroscience. The key feature of neurophysiological techniques described in this review paper is their pivotal role in tracking temporal dynamics and inner hierarchies of brain functional and effective connectivities, possibly clarifying some crucial issues underlying brain plasticity. Taken together, the findings presented in this review open an intriguing new field in neuroscience investigation and are important for the adoption of neurophysiological techniques as a tool for basic research and, in future, even for clinical diagnostics purposes.

KEYWORDS

Brain excitability; Brain connectivity; Brain plasticity; Electroencephalography; Magnetoencephalography; Transcranial magnetic stimulation; EEG–TMS co-registration

1.1. Introduction

A growing body of evidence from animal models and from neuroimaging and neurophysiological studies in humans provides confirmation of plastic changes and adaptation in the central nervous system throughout life, in order to cope with

experiences and inputs from the surrounding as well as from the "interior" environments (Pascual-Leone et al., 1998, 1999, 2005; Hallett, 1999; Rossini et al., 2003; Siebner and Rothwell, 2003; Ziemann et al., 2008). This capacity, termed neuroplasticity, encompasses the possibility of synapses, neurons, neuronal circuits, and networks in the brain being able to modify, adapt, and respond to the continuous flow of information, sensory stimulation, development as well as to instances of damage or dysfunction, allowing short-term to long-lasting changes in their

---
Correspondence to: Prof. P.M. Rossini, Department of Neurology, Catholic University, Largo Agostino Gemelli 8, 00186 Rome, Italy.
E-mail: paolomaria.rossini@afar.it

connections and behavior (Pascual-Leone et al., 1998, 1999; Rossini et al., 2003; Rossini and Dal Forno, 2004; Pascual-Leone et al., 2005).

Neuroplasticity has been extensively studied in recent years, not only because it supports several brain functions including cognitive processes but also because of its implications in neuropsychiatric disorders. Plastic neuronal wiring occurs principally during the period of development when neurons in the brain grow branches and structure synapses and also prune pre-existing but useless synapses and connections; as the brain starts to process sensory information, some of these synapses/connections strengthen, some weaken and others, if unutilized, are eliminated. However, such mechanisms also function during the lifespan under different circumstances — although less than during maturation — underlying the acquisition of new skills, learning, memory, adaptation to new contexts, and recovery of function after nervous system injury, when the brain attempts to compensate for lost activity, leading not only to useful but also to aberrant reorganization (Rossini et al., 2010a,b, 2011). On the one hand, adult neural networks show modularity and accomplish specific functions, on the other, they maintain the capacity to diverge from their usual functions and to rearrange themselves. That is, while the developing nervous system seems more proficient in plastic modifications, dynamic neuronal rewiring can also be recognized in the adult nervous system. The neocortex is a significant region for plasticity, since it accomplishes sensory, motor, and cognitive tasks with strong learning components (Feldman, 2009).

Researchers have achieved many significant advances toward full comprehension of the molecular underpinnings of these essential plasticity processes and toward the characterization of the learning rules that regulate their induction (Buonomano and Merzenich, 1998; Buonomano, 1999). Since the 1970s, neuroplasticity has gained extensive recognition throughout the scientific community as an essential property of the brain. Plastic changes in synapses, neurons, neuronal

circuits, and networks have been directly studied following progress in modern molecular, electrophysiological, and imaging techniques that allow study at the cellular level.

1.2. Principles of brain excitability, connectivity, and plasticity

Most studies of neural plasticity focus on *functional plasticity,* particularly on Hebbian-like long-term synaptic potentiation and depression (respectively LTP and LTD; Hebb, 1949; for reviews, see Malenka and Bear, 2004; Massey and Bashir, 2007; Raymond, 2007). In functional plasticity, synapses and synaptic strengths are considered as changeable amplification factors within a hardwired network structure (Butz et al., 2009). However, functional plasticity manifests through synaptic (Bliss and Collingridge, 1993; Malenka and Bear, 2004) and also nonsynaptic modifications (Hansel et al., 2001; Debanne, 2009). The former case involves modifications in synaptic transmission characteristics, while in the latter there is a modulation of the voltage-gated ion channels and passive "leak" channels hosted in neuronal membranes, able to change the neuronal intrinsic excitability homeostasis. Recent studies tend to integrate these mechanisms at least in part, supporting the idea that homeostatic excitability mechanisms are invoked to ensure that neurons constantly operate within a dynamic range of physiological activity (Burrone and Murthy, 2003), possibly acting to regularize overall neuronal activity after synapse-specific Hebbian LTP and LTD (Turrigiano and Nelson, 2004).

Conversely to functional plasticity, *structural plasticity* alters neural anatomy, modifying synaptic connectivity patterns, synapse numbers and extension, axonal and dendritic branching patterns, axonal fiber densities, and even numbers of neurons. Many structural plasticity mechanisms have been identified (Kim and Linden, 2007; Sjöström et al., 2008). Sudden structural changes (hours to days) occur constantly at the level of spines and synapses; spine formation and retraction are coupled with synapse formation and elimination (Kleim et al., 1996; Florence et al., 1998; Trachtenberg et al., 2002; Holtmaat et al., 2005). Consequently, rapid synapse formation and elimination may contribute to rapid experience-dependent plasticity. In contrast, large-scale structural changes, that are slow as they proceed over several days or weeks, involve macroscopic axonal projections, including thalamocortical and horizontal axonal projections and sometimes dendrites (for reviews, see Fox and Wong, 2005; Broser et al., 2008).

It is evident that the structural plasticity concept strongly implies the brain connectivity concept; however, when used in reference to the brain, the term connectivity alludes to many different but related aspects of brain organization (Horwitz and Poeppel, 2002). In general terms, connectivity can be examined on several spatial and temporal scales and at several levels of complexity (Sporns, 2011).

In space, this scale ranges from the axonal wiring within and between cortical layers to the connections between distant brain regions based on large fibers or functional coupling (Sporns et al., 2004; Sporns, 2011).

In time, this scale extends from functional connectivity, based on the existence of dynamic synapses with an instantaneous spiking pattern, to the genetically determined macroscopic structure of the brain, which can be modified only on a timescale of several generations (Friston et al., 2003).

In terms of complexity, these levels consist of individual synaptic connections relating single neurons at the microscale, networks connecting neuronal assemblies in local circuits at the mesoscale, as well as large-scale inter-regional brain connections or functional coupling at the macroscale (Sporns et al., 2004; Sporns, 2011). Particularly at the microscale, the basic element is the individual neuron and the spatial resolution required for investigation is in the order of micrometers. Although recent developments offer new methods to track neural connectivity at the cellular level, tract tracing agents/markers and electronic microscopy remain the

preferred techniques (Sporns, 2011). The mesoscale corresponds to a spatial resolution of hundreds of micrometers, the basic element being represented by neuronal assemblies/populations with local circuits (i.e., cortical columns) connecting hundreds-to-thousands of individual neurons. The macroscale requires a spatial resolution of several millimeters or even centimeters and includes brain regions and large-scale inter-regional connections (Sporns, 2011).

The availability of measurements of connectivity at these different scales is determined by existing measurement (structural, electrophysiological, or metabolic imaging) and analysis methods. Brain theories suggesting great significance of cortico-cortical connectivities were proposed by pioneers such as Jackson (1874–1958) and Wernicke (1874–1977) but were revitalized more recently by the studies of Geschwind (1965a,b) and Lev and Sperry (1970). Modern network theories include the historical mathematical problem of "The Seven Bridges of Königsberg," concerning the possibility of crossing serially and individually seven bridges connecting two islands in the Pregel river (Euler, 1736) which is considered the foundation of the "graph theory"; more recently, randomized graphs determined the equal probability of connectivity amongst nodes of a given network (Erdős and Rényi, 1960). In the real world, networks characterized by high clustering coefficient with low distribution power are frequently encountered; they represent a scenario described by Stanley Milgram, termed the "small world phenomenon" (Milgram, 1967). Technological advances progressively allowed researchers to approach, verify, and implement some of these pioneer hypotheses in vivo, and the online investigation of information processing based on brain connectivity in healthy subjects will soon become a reality. For example, experimental data suggest that cerebral functional networks follow the power's law, where a large proportion of nodes have very few connections and a small proportion of nodes have many connections, plus small world network characteristics (He et al., 2009).

Currently, these measurements and methods still do not offer complete information but at least permit some conclusions and may be sufficient to speculate on detailed hypothesis (Friston et al., 2003). Meanwhile, an increasing proportion of studies are focused on brain connectivity dysfunctions to better understand pathophysiologic mechanisms (and sometimes mechanisms of recovery) in neuropsychiatric disorders (e.g., see Stam, 2005; Dal Forno et al., 2006; Squitti et al., 2007; He et al., 2009; Ferreri et al., 2011c; Guerra et al., 2011). On these bases, three main types of connectivity can be recognized: anatomical, functional, and effective connectivity (Friston et al., 2003; Sporns, 2011).

The human brain structure comprises innumerable neurons that form an intricate network of innumerable connections as a formidable substrate for information processing; the *anatomical connectivity* concept refers to a network of synaptic connections linking sets of neurons or neuronal elements, along with their biophysical attributes such as synaptic strength or effectiveness (Sporns et al., 2004; Sporns, 2011). As the physical substrate at which all neural information processes take place, it defines the "functional connectivity space," providing possible biological constraints for theories of neural interactions (Lee et al., 2003). That is, because the structural/anatomical input/output connections of a given brain region are the main constraints for its functional properties, structural brain connectivity does not rigidly determine neural interactions but acts as a dynamic support that reduces the dimensionality of the neural space (Sporns et al., 2004; Sporns, 2011). Meanwhile, functional interactions (increasing or decreasing) contribute to modifying the underlying structural/anatomical substrate by reorganizing the synaptic connections. In the human brain, the connectome concept is strongly based on the identification of which neuronal populations can interact with each other and on the directness and strength of their connections as well as of their temporal dynamics (Sporns et al., 2004; Sporns, 2011).

When considering the countless brain dynamic states — which vary instantaneously and continuously on the basis of changing sensory inputs from internal and external environments (Sporns, 2011) — in the light of the evidence described above, it is clear that they are likely supported by functionally distributed but integrated brain networks. These networks are therefore the basis of conscious and highly sophisticated cognitive activities, including learning and memory; for higher functions, including memory, planning, and abstract reasoning, these dynamically connecting adjacent and/or remote cortical neuronal assemblies interact with each other via cortico-cortical connections. The principles behind this evidence are segregation and integration (Tononi et al., 1994). Segregation concerns the existence of specialized neurons structured into distinct neuronal assemblies and grouped together to form segregated cortical areas. The complementary principle, integration, refers to the coordinated activation of distributed neuronal assemblies, enabling the development of coherent states. In human nervous systems, brain anatomical connections are both specific and variable. Specificity originates from the precise organization of individual synaptic connections between morphologically and physiologically diverse neuronal types, in the arrangement of axonal arborizations and long-range connectivity between separate cell nuclei or brain regions (Sporns et al., 2004; Sporns, 2011); variability originates from the changeable configuration of processes of single neurons, as well as in the size, organization, and interconnection of large-scale structures; variability can be evaluated between corresponding structures in brains of individuals of the same species or within the brain of the same individual over time. It may seem evident that the function of a network is crucially related to the organization of its structural interconnections and that anatomical variability is therefore one of the primary sources of functional variability (Sporns et al., 2004; Sporns, 2011). Diffusion-weighted imaging techniques such as diffusion tensor magnetic imaging (DTI) have inadequate spatial resolution, being difficult to distinguish between crossing and closely running parallel fibers but are helpful as whole brain in vivo markers of temporal changes in fiber tract anatomy, and have provided a preliminary large-scale map of human anatomical connectivity (Sporns et al., 2004; Sporns, 2011).

Functional connectivity mainly represents a statistical concept based upon patterned deviation from statistical independence between defined neuronal units, often spatially remote from each other. Eventual statistical interdependence can be measured on the basis of correlation or covariance or phase-locking. In contrast to anatomical connectivity, this type is strictly time-dependent. In this light, functional connectivity is defined as the "temporal correlations between spatially remote neurophysiological events" (Friston et al., 2003). Physiological recordings with multiple electrodes have revealed that distant neurons can synchronize their firing, and neuroimaging studies have extensively reported the co-activation of distant brain regions under different experimental conditions, setting the foundations for novel approaches to understand brain function. That is, networks of segregated but interacting processes govern neural dynamics on top of the processing of the specialized regions (Tononi et al., 1994). It should be noted that functional connectivity does not make any explicit reference to specific directional effects or to an underlying structural model (Sporns et al., 2004; Sporns, 2011) and is often calculated between all elements of a system, regardless of whether these elements are connected by direct structural links.

Finally, *effective connectivity* describes the causative interrelations between two neuronal systems (Sporns et al., 2004; Sporns, 2011). It is defined as "the influence that one neural system exerts over another, either directly or indirectly" (Friston et al., 2003) and requires causal or noncausal models, in which regions and connections of interest are circumstantiated and constrained by means of neuroanatomical, neurophysiological, and functional neuroimaging data (Lee et al., 2003). Several techniques have been used to study effective connectivity, of which functional magnetic resonance imaging (fMRI), electroencephalography (EEG), transcranial magnetic stimulation (TMS), and magnetoencephalography (MEG) are the most widely used (see below).

1.3. Neurophysiological techniques in the study of brain excitability, connectivity, and plasticity

The neurophysiological techniques described here are not involved in depicting structural connectivity; however, they play a pivotal role in tracking functional and effective connectivities, mainly when their temporal dynamics and inner hierarchies must be investigated. This is due to their high temporal discrimination, which is in the order of milliseconds and therefore faster than any other technique based on flow/metabolism/energy consumption parameters (in the order of seconds or minutes). Moreover, because "temporal correlations between neurophysiological events in spatially remote neural systems (functional connectivity) may or may not be caused by the influence of one neural system over another (effective connectivity)," two possible methods of inferring effective connectivity (temporal precedence and perturbational studies) can be considered (for review, see Lee et al., 2003). That is, in principle, causal effects can be inferred either through systematic perturbations of the system or through time series analysis, because causes precede effects in time. In the context of fMRI, temporal precedence at the neuronal networks level may be masked by hemodynamic activity, due to temporal smoothing intrinsic in the coupling between synaptic activity and hemodynamic changes (Bestmann et al., 2008). Even EEG and MEG studies, which provide a temporal resolution in the order of milliseconds, may not provide a totally adequate solution, since temporal precedence is not unequivocally related to causality. However, time-series causality analysis methods, such as Granger causality or transfer entropy, of these types of data appear to resolve this issue. Granger causality, for example, has been used for both EEG and fMRI time series and has provided valuable information about direct interactions between neural networks during cognitive tasks. Moreover, covariance modeling recently permitted the recognition of noteworthy differences in effective connectivity between a given set of brain regions working in different cognitive tasks, thus explaining the time- and task-dependent nature of these patterns (Brovelli et al., 2004). The other means of inferring causality involves the principle of perturbing the system; the majority of functional neuroimaging experiments contemplate experimental manipulations of neural activation (i.e., perturbations) in the form of visual, auditory, or psychological stimuli. There are two significant advantages of using perturbation studies; first, the manipulation is under explicit experimental control and can therefore be placed precisely in time and space; second, it is possible to specifically modify neural activity in selective cortical areas and to measure the result that this alteration has on the activity and interactions between the nonperturbed areas (for a review, see Lee et al., 2003).

In this context, the combination of TMS with functional neuroimaging (Siebner et al., 2009; Ziemann, 2011) is of particular interest. There are several advantages of such a combination: first, TMS allows the use of discrete perturbations of brain networks while they are engaged in the performance of specific tasks; second, TMS is independent of behavior and so any modification observed in neural activity is not influenced by the subject's ability to perform a task or by the strategy used; finally, and perhaps of more interest, the combination can be used to modify the activity of one brain area and observe the effects on activity in other areas, either in response to further TMS or during behavioral paradigms. Amongst the various methods of functional neuroimaging available, high-density EEG (hd-EEG) (see below) is particularly important for its millisecond-scale temporal resolution compared to other TMS-imaging approaches. Its high temporal resolution renders the EEG method a perfect complement to the transient perturbations caused by TMS in the brain's processing modes. TMS–EEG conveys precise information about the temporal order of activations of distant cortical areas with high signal-to-noise ratio and at relatively low cost.

1.3.1. EEG and MEG

EEG and MEG are noninvasive techniques that detect brain electrophysiological signals with the temporal resolution of 1 ms or better (Başar, 2006; Tecchio et al., 2007). For both techniques, the origin of the signal is mainly the effect of the postsynaptic currents associated with synchronous neuronal firing in the cortical mantle. However, the EEG signal is distorted in space and time by passage through the conductivity discontinuities of cerebrospinal fluid, meninges, skull, and scalp and requires contact between the recording electrodes and the scalp; the MEG signal is transparent to these discontinuities in the first approximation of a spherical head, and its recording system is brought near the head and the sensors are not in contact with the scalp (no time-consuming scalp preparation or application of several electrodes with good electrode/skin contacts). EEG detects the difference in electrical potentials measured from the scalp and is, therefore, a reference-dependent measure and is similarly sensitive to cerebral sources orientated both radially and tangentially to the head surface, whereas MEG is almost selectively sensitive to the latter and is a *reference-free* recording system (Romani et al., 2005). This renders MEG and EEG complementary techniques with otherwise similar excellent temporal resolution. Spatial resolution, however, may be poor and essentially depends on the number of recording sites. While hd-EEG or MEG can achieve spatial resolution close to a few millimeters, the spatial resolution of standard EEG recordings ranges between one and several centimeters depending on the number of electrodes. EEG can be recorded using a variety of different electrode configurations, ranging from a few electrodes (readiness potentials, somatosensory evoked potentials, etc.) to hd-EEG using 64 or up to 256 channels, depending on the purpose of the study. EEG recordings can reveal temporal and spatial information about externally triggered event-related potentials (ERPs) or spontaneous brain activity. Event-related cortical activity can be quantified by measuring the latencies and amplitudes of distinct ERP components.

Spontaneous EEG is usually recorded over longer time periods to assess states of vigilance or consciousness such as wakefulness and sleep. EEG analysis of oscillatory activity is often restricted to distinct frequency bands that are linked to specific neuronal processes. As the small signals (microvolt and femtotesla for EEG and MEG, respectively) rapidly decay over distance, activity in deeper cortical or even subcortical structures can at best be indirectly inferred by source localization methods (inverse problem). In the case of EEG, there is additional spatial smoothing caused by the tissue compartments between the electrodes and the cortex (skin, muscles, skull, meninges, blood vessels, etc.). In the case of MEG, signals reflect the spatial and temporal production of a dipolar source modeled as an equivalent current dipole (ECD). This method provides three-dimensional localization of dipolar field distributions over the scalp with a time resolution of milliseconds (Tecchio et al., 2007). Hence, MEG signals can directly estimate the number of active neural pools and provide accurate measures of the intracellular currents within a limited shallow (deeper regions are poorly probed since the MEG signals decay with the cube of the distance) brain region below the recording sensor without influence from volume conduction. ECD spatial properties not only indicate the location of neural sources but also their orientation and strength. This occurs because restriction or enlargement of the brain area activated by impulse arrival is usually secondary to dynamic phenomena regulating the number of recruited synapses such as use-dependent modulation of

synaptic efficacy, changes of excitatory/inhibitory input from adjacent/remote brain areas, or from sensory flow (Rossini et al., 1994b; Tecchio et al., 2007).

Co-registration of MEG with structural and fMRI provides insight into the anatomo-physiological substrate of the examined function. Specific cutting-edge findings include insight into the mechanisms of blood oxygenation level-dependent (BOLD) contrast, higher resolution and improved sensitivity in evaluating hemodynamic contrast, and new paradigms and methods for analyzing and generating data (for a review, see Bandettini, 2009). BOLD changes have helped to confine dipole source estimations, allowing forward solutions that delineate precise timing (within the limits of hemodynamic temporal resolution) between remote brain regions (for a review, see Bandettini, 2009). However, MEG recordings cannot be made simultaneously with MRI acquisition, whereas EEG recordings can now be acquired at the same time. In terms of utility, EEG studies have the remarkable advantage of being carried out simultaneously with fMRI studies, allowing the evaluation of repeatable effects in patients (Lemieux et al., 2008) and healthy volunteers (Horovitz et al., 2008; Mantini et al., 2010).

Moreover, in humans, EEG and MEG methods can also usefully evaluate the transient synchronization of neuronal firing, due to their intrinsic proprieties. This has been proposed as one of most significant mechanisms underlying brain functional connectivity, as it determines functional linkages of separate and widely distributed neuronal assemblies that govern, for example, the sensory processing within a unique and functionally coherent group (Uhlhaas and Singer, 2006). Due to the distributed networks underlying sensory systems, sensory processing requires a high degree of integration of information flow from several different and often remote brain areas; such intramodal integration must also be enriched by intermodal integrations combining several visual, acoustic, olfactive, and tactile inputs (Uhlhaas and Singer, 2006). This process is orchestrated by attentive mechanisms that organize the individual sensory elements in a context-dependent hierarchical order (Engel et al., 2001); finally, if the whole sensorimotor system is considered, a dynamic "binding" and "unbinding" between sensory and motor cortical functions is also necessary (Roelfsema et al., 1997). EEG and MEG are applied to the study of connectivity, moving from the concept that synchronization of rhythmic oscillations is analogous to the previously described binding/unbinding phenomena of individual or groups of neurons firing in experimental models; these synchronization mechanisms are also linked with cognitive functions (Uhlhaas and Singer, 2006; Määttä et al., 2010). Specific methods have been developed to identify transient functional coupling of distributed neuronal assemblies via EEG and MEG recordings; some can evaluate synchrony independently from the amplitude of the signals (the shorter the connectivity between neurons, the higher the signal amplitude) and differ from measurements of coherence, which determine the covariance of signal amplitude recorded at different sites for different EEG and MEG frequency bands (Andrew and Pfurtscheller, 1996; Vecchio et al., 2007, 2010). On one hand, experimental studies have shown that a brief distance synchronization usually involves high-frequency bands in the γ-range, while longer distance synchronizations more often manifest themselves in the β- or even θ- (4–8 Hz) and α- (8–12 Hz) ranges (Schnitzler and Gross, 2005); and that synchronization of neuronal firing within the high-frequency bands (β- and γ-) is mainly mediated by cortico-cortical connections, while subcortical structures — namely, thalamic relays — dominate in synchronizing slower frequencies (α-, θ-, and δ-; Steriade et al., 1993). Coherence of rhythmic EEG oscillations also represents a quantitative measure for the degree of functional connectivity between different brain areas, from which the EEG or the MEG signal is simultaneously picked up. It is expressed by synchrony or coupling of signals at different electrodes within a given frequency band (Stam et al., 2007; He et al., 2009).

Recently, EEG and TMS co-registration studies have been employed successfully with this purpose (see below).

1.3.2. Transcranial magnetic stimulation

TMS is a noninvasive and painless method to stimulate excitable tissues with an electric current induced by an external time-varying magnetic field (Rossini et al., 1994a; Kobayashi and Pascual-Leone, 2003; Rossini and Rossi, 2007). However, it has potential for more sophisticated uses when declined in different paradigms and applied together with several kinds of neuroimaging techniques, such as EEG or fMRI (Siebner et al., 2009; Ziemann, 2011). Both electric and magnetic stimulation methods excite the biological membranes with electric current: the former is done directly, whereas the latter is achieved via an electric current which is induced within the volume conductor by a time-varying magnetic field. Following the revolutionary works of D'Arsonval (1896) and Thompson (1910), demonstrating for the first time the possibility of stimulating the retina by means of magnetic fields, it took some time before the magnetic method was used again. It was not until 1985, 5 years after the first presentation of the transcranial electrical stimulation by Merton and Morton (1980), that Barker et al., presented the TMS at the London Congress of the International Federation of Clinical Neurophysiology. They then demonstrated that the stimulation of the human motor cortex and peripheral nerves could be performed using a brief but strong external time-varying magnetic field applied through a wire coil. After stimulation of the corticospinal tract, a motor twitch, termed motor evoked potential (MEP), can be recorded by surface electrodes from the connected muscles in an awake and collaborative subject without causing distress or pain (Rossini et al., 1987a,b, 1994a; Rothwell et al., 1991; Rothwell, 1993). Even though the magnetic pulses are considered capable of stimulating neural tissues through the cortically induced electric field depolarizing cell membranes

(Barker et al., 1985), it is essential to acknowledge that the real recruited pathways are not completely known. However, they incorporate the fastest conducting fibers, presumably including the pyramidal tracts (Rossini et al., 1987a,b; Sanger et al., 2001).

Examination of the physical and physiological bases of TMS is beyond the scope of the present chapter and interested readers are referred to specialized papers (see Rossi et al., 2009; Rossini et al., 2010a,b).

Since the publication of pioneering works on motor conduction (Rossini et al., 1987a,b; Rothwell et al., 1987, 1991; Hallett, 2011), several other application areas of TMS have emerged (Ferreri et al., 2003, 2006, 2011b; Ziemann, 2004; Hallett, 2011). The main technological innovations in recent years are repetitive stimulators and coils for focal stimulation (Hasey, 1999). A train of pulses appears to be capable of producing more prolonged time changes in neuronal activity than those produced by a single pulse. In particular, repetitive TMS produces longer-lasting effects which continue past the period of stimulation, increasing or decreasing the excitability of the corticospinal tract on the basis on the intensity of stimulation, coil orientation, and frequency. The mechanism of these effects is not obvious, but it is generally believed to reflect modifications in synaptic efficacy akin to LTP and LTD (Basso et al., 2006; Esser et al., 2006; Fitzgerald et al., 2006). Commercially available devices can generate magnetic fields of intensity greatly exceeding the threshold for the depolarization of neurons, at least in M1, and advances in coil design have led to stimulators capable of activating a small enough region of the cortex to allow mapping of cortical functioning with a degree of precision rivaling that achieved using direct electrode stimulation of the brain (Hasey, 1999).

1.3.2.1. Magnetic resonance imaging-guided stereotactic TMS

As previously mentioned, stimulus intensity and coil dimension, shape, position, and orientation relative to the head determine the volume of brain tissue that is excited by TMS pulses. In theory, the reproducibility of phenomena following brain stimulation, both within and between subjects, is based on the ability to stimulate the same brain regions with the same intensity at different times (Ilmoniemi and Kičić, 2010). Precise targeting of definite brain locations requires a common reference system within a three-axis space to achieve full correspondence between the location and orientation of the coil at the scalp, the stimulus intensity, and the brain volume that is stimulated. This is fundamental, particularly when highly focused stimulation is desired using small coils. The simplest way to report coil positioning order to specify the stimulated region is based on scalp anatomical landmarks according to the standardized 10–20 EEG electrode placement system. There are some known correspondences between the electrode locations and the underlying cerebral structures, although these are somewhat inconsistent due to intersubject anatomical variability (Homan et al., 1987). Namely, individual variability in brain anatomy and the functional reorganization that often accompanies brain pathologies add imprecision to navigational systems based solely on scalp landmarks.

Magnetic resonance imaging (MRI)-based stereotactic navigational techniques have been developed by several laboratories in recent years and commercial products have recently become available for MRI-guided TMS. The level of accuracy provided by these navigational techniques makes it possible to utilize TMS as a reliable tool for presurgical mapping of eloquent cortical areas (Krings et al., 2001). The navigational techniques basically calculate the transformation required between a coordinate system based on skull or scalp landmarks and one defined in terms of brain anatomy based on MRI. As soon as this transformation is identified, it is possible to compute and display the volume of brain tissue that would receive the stimulation according to the position and orientation of the coil relative to the head. This clearly reduces the inaccuracy arising from the inconsistent relationship between scalp structure and underlying brain anatomy (Gugino et al., 2001).

1.3.3. EEG–TMS co-registration

In addition to what has been briefly presented above, TMS potentiality has far more sophisticated uses if applied together with different types of neuroimaging techniques (Siebner et al., 2009; Rothwell, 2011; Ziemann, 2011). Although MEPs are routinely used in research and sometimes in clinical settings to study motor cortex excitability, a proper evaluation should clearly differentiate between the indices of the overall excitability and connectivity of the corticospinal system (corticospinal excitability), and those directly and specifically reflecting the excitability and connectivity of the motor cortex (cortical excitability). Indeed, the problem with EMG in general, and with MEPs in particular, is that they are affected by a combination of cortical, subcortical, and spinal cord mechanisms that usually coincide in time, making their separation very difficult. The amplitudes and latencies of MEPs result from a combination of excitatory and inhibitory events occurring in a complex synaptic network at different neural levels along the motor pathway (Rossini et al., 1987a; Rothwell et al., 1987; Hallett, 2007, 2011; Rossini and Rossi, 2007) and the relative contribution of these events is far from fully elucidated (Rothwell, 2011). Therefore, any conclusions based exclusively on MEP recordings, that concern the involvement of M1 in a given process or cortical pathologies generally, are likely to be uncertain. Recently, a technical device has been introduced that allows the recording EEG responses to different TMS paradigms with millisecond resolution, likely without spinal and muscular influences. This means that, in combination with EEG, TMS is developing into a brain research method in which stimulation can be precisely directed to a chosen brain area and the simultaneously recorded scalp potentials

are processed into source images of the TMS-evoked neuronal activation (Komssi et al., 2004) enabling a noninvasive, finally direct method to study cortical excitability, connectivity, and plasticity (Ilmoniemi et al., 1997).

The first published attempt to measure TMS-evoked brain responses was made in 1989 by Cracco et al. (1989); in their setup, one scalp electrode was employed to record responses to TMS at homologous cortical area contralateral to the stimulation site and it was possible to record cortico-cortically mediated activity with an onset latency of 9–12 ms (for a review, see Komssi and Kähkönen, 2006). However, this initial attempt was significantly hampered by technical limitations. It was necessary to resolve these technical issues to obtain multichannel EEG recordings at the same time as TMS: one way to manage the stimulus artifact was to employ a sample-and-hold circuit that was able to lock the EEG signal for some milliseconds immediately post TMS, as previously recommended by electrical stimulation experiments (Freeman, 1971). This avoided saturation of the recording amplifiers by the magnetic stimuli and allowed, for the first time, the recording of multichannel EEG activity in response to TMS (Ilmoniemi et al., 1997; Virtanen et al., 1999). The spread of TMS-evoked brain activity was then followed between brain areas, beginning from a few milliseconds post stimulus. Subsequently, some novel TMS-compatible EEG amplifiers have been built: one with 64 channels and a sample-and-hold circuit, another with 128 channels and a slow-rate limiter, and finally TMS-compatible EEG equipment that works in very high time-varying magnetic fields without saturation and does not use particular devices to pin the amplifier output to a constant level during and after stimulation (BrainAmp MRplus, BrainProducts GmbH, Munich, Germany; Bonato et al., 2006; Ferreri et al., 2011a).

Recently, TMS–EEG studies have started to explain the physiology of the TMS-evoked EEG responses in order to expand our understanding of the activation mechanisms of TMS; moreover, they have established the potentiality of TMS–EEG as a tool for basic neurophysiological research and probably for diagnostic purposes.

The electric currents induced in the brain by TMS can depolarize cell membranes so that voltage-sensitive ion channels are opened and action potentials are initiated. Subsequent synaptic activations are directly reflected in the EEG (Ilmoniemi et al., 1997), which records a linear projection of the postsynaptic current distribution on the lead fields of its measurement channels. EEG is not particularly sensitive to action potentials (see above) because of their symmetric current distribution and short duration, so it is believed that postsynaptic currents cause most of the EEG signals. If the conductivity organization of the head is considered, the EEG signals can be used to situate and calculate these synaptic current distributions and to formulate inferences on local excitability and area-to-area functional connectivity in the nervous system (Komssi et al., 2002, 2004, 2007; Massimini et al., 2005; Huber et al., 2008). The initial TMS-evoked response, although difficult to evaluate due to artifact contamination, appears to stem from the activation of the target area, whereas later deflections are somewhat related to activity triggered by axonall-propagated signals. The way in which the signals are transmitted is strongly determined by the state of the firing of diffused neuromodulatory systems of the brain (Kähkönen et al., 2001; Massimini et al., 2005) and also depends on local activation at the time of stimulus delivery (Ilmoniemi and Kičić, 2010).

Attempts to understand the TMS-evoked activity that is elicited at sites remote from the TMS target can benefit from knowledge of the anatomical connectivity of the brain as seen, for example, by DTI studies (Ilmoniemi and Kičić, 2010). In contrast to the high variability of MEPs, TMS-evoked EEG averaged responses are consistently reproducible under the same experimental conditions and the delivery and targeting of TMS is well controlled and stable from pulse to pulse. Several components of the EEG response to single-pulse TMS in the motor cortex have been recognized (for a review, see Komssi and Kähkönen, 2006; Ilmoniemi and Kičić, 2010). In particular, single-pulse TMS is able to evoke EEG activity lasting up to 300 ms, which is composed at the vertex of a succession of deflections of negative polarity peaking at roughly 7, 18, 44, 100, and 280 ms, alternating with positive polarity peaks at roughly 13, 30, 60, and 190 ms post TMS (Ilmoniemi et al., 1997; Paus et al., 2001b; Komssi et al., 2002, 2004, 2007; Nikulin et al., 2003; Kähkönen et al., 2004, 2005; Bonato et al., 2006; Kähkönen and Wilenius, 2007; Daskalakis et al., 2008; Farzan et al., 2009; Lioumis et al., 2009; Ferreri et al., 2011a). However, these components are not an invariable pattern since, in addition to inter-individual differences, the responses are influenced by the exact coil location (Komssi et al., 2002) and orientation; by the state of the cortex (Nikulin et al., 2003); by the TMS paradigm used; and by the alertness of the subject (Massimini et al., 2005). In addition to standard evoked responses, TMS may also generate oscillatory activity (Paus et al., 2001a; Fuggetta et al., 2005; Rosanova et al., 2009; Ferreri et al., 2012) or perturb ongoing rhythms (Rosanova et al., 2009), eliciting event-related synchronization or desynchronization (Pfurtscheller and Lopes da Silva, 1999) or more complex phenomena (Ilmoniemi and Kičić, 2010).

The standard purpose of a topographic plot of TMS-evoked EEG responses is to detect both local and remote effects of TMS, that is, to evaluate both local excitability of the stimulated patch of the cortex and the distribution of TMS-evoked activity in broader cortical networks. Normally, the overall response amplitudes are highest beneath the coil and weaken with increasing distance from the stimulation point. Locally, within one hemisphere, increased EEG activity can be observed in a number of neighboring electrodes, signifying the spread of TMS-evoked activity to anatomically interconnected cortical areas (Ilmoniemi et al., 1997; Paus et al., 2001a). An important characteristic of TMS-evoked EEG topography is that even though just one brain hemisphere is stimulated, bilateral EEG responses are evoked. TMS-evoked activity spreads ipsilaterally from the stimulated site via association fibers, contralaterally via transcallosal fibers and to subcortical structures via projection fibers (Ilmoniemi et al., 1997; Komssi et al., 2002, 2004; Ilmoniemi and Kičić, 2010; Ferreri et al., 2011a). Therefore, EEG wavelets, as a measurement of cortical activity after the TMS pulse, provide the opportunity to evaluate cortico-cortical interactions by applying TMS to one area and following responses in distant but interconnected areas. Moreover, it also gives the opportunity to study how activity in one area influences ongoing activity in other areas (Ilmoniemi and Kičić, 2010). Finally, similar to cortical studies (Krnjevic et al., 1966; Rosenthal et al., 1967), in addition to activating the large excitatory Betz cells, which are present in great numbers in the motor cortex, TMS also activates the inhibitory interneurons. Their postsynaptic effects are considered to be represented as the TMS-evoked N44 and N100 components (Nikulin et al., 2003; Bender et al., 2005; Bonato et al., 2006; Ferreri et al., 2011a), as it has been demonstrated that inhibitory processes in deeper cortical layers can generate preferentially surface-negative potentials (Caspers et al., 1980). An important challenge in evaluating TMS and EEG–TMS results from the fact that the induced neuronal activation is nonunequivocally physiological. Moreover, the effects of brain stimulation extend from the target site ortho- and antidromically within the neuronal networks (Ilmoniemi and Kičić, 2010) and, likewise, the stimulated area is affected by interconnected areas. As area-to-area modulation is frequently inhibitory, corticospinal excitability (as expressed by the size of the descending volley evoked by a cortical stimulus) does not necessarily increase with the general level of cortical activity. Furthermore, areas where normal operation could be disrupted are not restricted to the stimulated spot but are distributed along the neuronal network involved (Ilmoniemi and Kičić, 2010).

There is growing evidence, mostly from stimulation of cortical areas other than the M1, that the effect of TMS on EEG response is not determined solely by the properties of the stimulus but also by the initial state of the activated brain region. This was preliminarily established following examination of EEG-based prestimulus spectrogram characteristics to test the hypothesis that fluctuations in neuronal activity have a functional significance and may explain the variability in neuronal or behavioral responses to physically identical stimuli such as TMS (Ilmoniemi and Kičić, 2010). Besides evaluation of the general state of the brain (Kähkönen et al., 2001; Massimini et al., 2005), concurrent TMS and EEG have the potential to suggest insight into how brain areas interact during sensory processing (Bikmullina et al., 2009), cognition (Bonnard et al., 2009), or motor control (Nikulin et al., 2003; Ferreri et al., 2011a). In particular, recent studies (Ferreri et al., 2011a; Veniero et al., 2011) permitted detailed characterization of the neuronal circuits underlying human M1 excitability and effective connectivity and investigated whether EEG measures of short intracortical inhibition and facilitation (respectively SICI and ICF), as induced by paired pulse TMS paradigm according to Kujirai et al. (1993), are related to the same mechanisms underlying EMG measures of SICI and ICF (Ferreri et al., 2011a). Numerous recent findings suggest promising applications of this technique to directly evaluate whether and where within the cortex, these LTP or LTD plasticity phenomena can be induced under several different paradigms (Esser et al., 2006). Finally, based on the significant interest in the functional role of oscillatory brain activity in specific frequency bands and in specific cortical areas (Van der Werf and Paus, 2006; Rosanova et al., 2009), the use of TMS–EEG in this field is particularly promising (Thut and Miniussi, 2009). Moreover, the detection of natural frequencies using TMS–EEG may also have diagnostic potential and clinical applications, as it opens up possibilities of mapping the natural frequency of different cortical areas in various neuropsychiatric conditions such as depression, schizophrenia, epilepsy, dementia, or disorders of consciousness

(Rosanova et al., 2009). Since natural frequencies reveal significant circuit properties, TMS-evoked EEG may dramatically expand the opportunities provided by peripherally evoked MEPs. Whereas TMS–MEP utility is substantially restricted to motor areas, TMS–EEG can access any cortical region (primary and associative) in any category of patients, and may offer a clear-cut and flexible way to evaluate and monitor the state of corticothalamic circuits.

1.4. Conclusion

In conclusion, there is increasing evidence to support the concept that brain plasticity involves distinct functional and structural components, each requiring multiple cellular mechanisms working at distinct synaptic loci, time scales, and developmental stages within an extremely complex framework (Feldman and Brecht, 2005; Feldman, 2009). However, the precise relationship between functional and structural components of brain plasticity/connectivity phenomena is still unclear and its explanation represents a major challenge within modern neuroscience (Tononi et al., 1994; Sporns et al., 2004; Sporns, 2011). For example, it is not obvious which definite functional components, if any, influence which types or sites of rapid structural components; or whether chemical signaling is a proximal driver (Feldman, 2009). In the past 10 years, these concepts have also been introduced in clinical settings by means of techniques that have revealed a continuous plasticity/connectivity modulation driven by many physiological and pathological conditions, as well as many similarities and differences across cortical areas. The key feature of neurophysiological techniques described here is their pivotal role in tracking temporal dynamics and inner hierarchies of brain functional and effective connectivities; raising the possibility of clarifying some crucial issues underlying brain plasticity and potentially allowing its modulation, contingent on improved knowledge of its basic mechanisms

and awareness of the constrains (Platz and Rothwell, 2010). This approach may have a tremendous impact in a variety of neuropsychiatric disorders whose pathophysiologies have been closely linked to the integrated function of multiple cortical areas.

References

Andrew, C. and Pfurtscheller, G. (1996) Event-related coherence as a tool for studying dynamic interaction of brain regions. *Electroencephalogr. Clin. Neurophysiol.*, 98(2): 144–148.

Bandettini, P.A. (2009) What's new in neuroimaging methods (review)? *Ann. N.Y. Acad. Sci.*, 1156: 260–293.

Barker, A.T., Jalinous, R. and Freeston, I.L. (1985) Non-invasive magnetic stimulation of human motor cortex. *Lancet*, 1: 1106–1107.

Başar, E. (2006) The theory of the whole-brain work. *Int. J. Psychophysiol.*, 60(2): 133–138.

Basso, D., Lotze, M., Vitale, L., Ferreri, F., Bisiacchi, P., Olivetti Belardinelli, M., Rossini, P.M. and Birbaumer. (2006) The role of prefrontal cortex in visuo-spatial planning: A repetitive TMS study. *Exp. Brain Res.*, 171(3): 411–415.

Bender, S., Basseler, K., Sebastian, I., Resch, F., Kammer, T., Oelkers-Ax, R. and Weisbrod, M. (2005) Electroencephalographic response to transcranial magnetic stimulation in children: evidence for giant inhibitory potentials. *Ann. Neurol.*, 58: 58–67.

Bestmann, S., Ruff, C.C., Blankenburg, F., Weiskopf, N., Driver, J. and Rothwell, J.C. (2008) Mapping causal interregional influences with concurrent TMS-fMRI. *Exp. Brain Res.*, 191: 383–402.

Bikmullina, R., Kičić, D., Carlson, S. and Nikulin, V.V. (2009) Electrophysiological correlates of short-latency afferent inhibition: a combined EEG and TMS study. *Exp. Brain Res.*, 194: 517–526.

Bliss, T.V. and Collingridge, G.L. (1993) A synaptic model of memory: long-term potentiation in the hippocampus. *Nature (Lond.)*, 361: 31–39.

Bonato, C., Miniussi, C. and Rossini, P.M. (2006) Transcranial magnetic stimulation and cortical evoked potentials: a TMS/EEG co-registration study. *Clin. Neurophysiol.*, 117: 1699–1707.

Bonnard, M., Spieser, L., Meziane, H.B., De Graaf, J.B. and Pailhous, J. (2009) Prior intention can locally tune inhibitory processes in the primary motor cortex: direct evidence from combined TMS-EEG. *Eur. J. Neurosci.*, 30: 913–923.

Broser, P., Grinevich, V., Osten, P., Sakmann, B. and Wallace, D.J. (2008) Critical period plasticity of axonal arbors of layer 2/3 pyramidal neurons in rat somatosensory cortex: layer-specific reduction of projections into deprived cortical columns. *Cereb. Cortex*, 18: 1588–1603.

Brovelli, A., Ding, M., Ledberg, A., Chen, Y., Nakamura, R. and Bressler, S.L. (2004) Beta oscillations in a large-scale

14

sensorimotor cortical network: directional influences revealed by Granger causality. *Proc. Natl. Acad. Sci. USA*, 101: 9849–9854.

Buonomano, D.V. (1999) Distinct functional types of associative long-term potentiation in neocortical and hippocampal pyramidal neurons. *J. Neurosci.*, 19: 6748–6754.

Buonomano, D.V. and Merzenich, M.M. (1998) Cortical plasticity: from synapses to maps. *Annu. Rev. Neurosci.*, 21: 149–186.

Burrone, J. and Murthy, V.N. (2003) Synaptic gain control and homeostasis. *Curr. Opin. Neurobiol.*, 13: 560–567.

Butz, M., Worgotter, F. and Van Ooyen, A. (2009) Activity-dependent structural plasticity. *Brain Res. Rev.*, 60: 287–305.

Caspers, H., Speckmann, E.J. and Lehmenkuhler, A. (1980) Electrogenesis of cortical DC potentials. *Prog. Brain Res.*, 54: 3–15.

Cracco, R.Q., Amassian, V.E., Maccabee, P.J. and Cracco, J.B. (1989) Comparison of human transcallosal responses evoked by magnetic coil and electrical stimulation. *Electroencephalogr. Clin. Neurophysiol.*, 74: 417–424.

Dal Forno, G., Chiovenda, P., Bressi, F., Ferreri, F., Grossi, E., Brandt, J., Rossini, P.M. and Pasqualetti, P. (2006) Use of an Italian version of the telephone interview for cognitive status in Alzheimer's disease. *Int. J. Geriatr. Psychiatry*, 21(2): 126–133.

D'Arsonval, J.A. (1896) Dispositifs pour la mesure des courants alternatifs de toutes fréquences. *C. R. Soc. Biol. (Paris)*, 2: 450–451.

Daskalakis, Z.J., Farzan, F., Barr, M.S., Maller, J.J., Chen, R. and Fitzgerald, P.B. (2008) Long-interval cortical inhibition from the dorsolateral prefrontal cortex: a TMS-EEG study. *Neuropsychopharmacology*, 33: 2860–2869.

Debanne, D. (2009) Plasticity of neuronal excitability in vivo. *J. Physiol. (Lond.)*, 587: 3057–3058.

Engel, A.K., Fries, P. and Singer, W. (2001) Dynamic predictions: oscillations and synchrony in top-down processing. *Nat. Rev. Neurosci.*, 2(10): 704–716.

Erdős, P. and Rényi, A. (1960) The evolution of random graphs. *Magyar Tud. Akad. Mat. Kutató Int. Közl.*, 5: 17–61.

Esser, S.K., Huber, R., Massimini, M., Peterson, M.J., Ferrarelli, F. and Tononi, G. (2006) A direct demonstration of cortical LTP in humans: a combined TMS/EEG study. *Brain Res. Bull.*, 69: 86–94.

Euler, L. (1736) Solutio problematis ad geometriam situs pertinentis. *Comment. Acad. Sci. Univ. Petrop.*, 8: 128–140. (Reprinted in *Opera Omnia Series Prima*, 1766, Vol. 7: pp. 1–10.).

Farzan, F., Barr, M.S., Wong, W., Chen, R., Fitzgerald, P.B. and Daskalakis, Z.J. (2009) Suppression of gamma-oscillations in the dorsolateral prefrontal cortex following long interval cortical inhibition: a TMS-EEG study. *Neuropsychopharmacology*, 34: 1543–1551.

Feldman, D.E. (2009) Synaptic mechanisms for plasticity in neocortex. *Annu. Rev. Neurosci.*, 32: 33–55.

Feldman, D.E. and Brecht, M. (2005) Map plasticity in somatosensory cortex. *Science*, 310: 810–815.

Ferreri, F., Pauri, F., Pasqualetti, P., Fini, R., Dal Forno, G. and Rossini, P.M. (2003) Motor cortex excitability in Alzheimer's disease: a transcranial magnetic stimulation study. *Ann. Neurol.*, 53: 102–108.

Ferreri, F., Curcio, G., Pasqualetti, P., De Gennaro, L., Fini, R. and Rossini, P.M. (2006) Mobile phone emissions and human brain excitability. *Ann. Neurol.*, 60: 188–196.

Ferreri, F., Pasqualetti, P., Määttä, S., Ponzo, D., Ferrarelli, F., Tononi, G., Mervaala, E., Miniussi, C. and Rossini, P.M. (2011a) Human brain connectivity during single and paired pulse transcranial magnetic stimulation. *Neuroimage*, 54: 90–102.

Ferreri, F., Pasqualetti, P., Määttä, S., Ponzo, D., Guerra, A., Bressi, F., Chiovenda, P., Del Duca, M., Giambattistelli, F., Ursini, F., Tombini, M., Vernieri, F. and Rossini, P.M. (2011b) Motor cortex excitability in Alzheimer's disease: a transcranial magnetic stimulation follow-up study. *Neurosci. Lett.*, 492: 94–98.

Ferreri, F., Määttä, S., Vecchio, F., Curcio, G. and Ferrarelli, F. (2011c) Clinical neurophysiology in Alzheimer's disease. *Int. J. Alzheimer's Dis.*, 1: 134–157.

Ferreri, F., Ponzo, D., Hukkanen, T., Mervaala, E., Könönen, M., Pasqualetti, P., Vecchio, F., Rossini, P.M. and Määttä, S. (2012) Human brain cortical correlates of short-latency afferent inhibition: a combined EEG-TMS study. *J. Neurophysiol.*, 108(1): 314–323.

Fitzgerald, P.B., Benitez, J., Daskalakis, J.Z., De Castella, A. and Kulkarni, J. (2006) The treatment of recurring auditory hallucinations in schizophrenia with rTMS. *World J. Biol. Psychiatry*, 7: 119–122.

Florence, S.L., Taub, H.B. and Kaas, J.H. (1998) Large-scale sprouting of cortical connections after peripheral injury in adult macaque monkeys. *Science*, 282: 1117–1121.

Fox, K. and Wong, R.O. (2005) A comparison of experience-dependent plasticity in the visual and somatosensory systems. *Neuron*, 48: 465–477.

Freeman, J.A. (1971) An electronic stimulus artifact suppressor. *Electroencephalogr. Clin. Neurophysiol.*, 31: 170–172.

Friston, K.J., Harrison, L. and Penny, W. (2003) Dynamic causal modelling. *Neuroimage*, 19: 1273–1302.

Fuggetta, G., Fiaschi, A. and Manganotti, P. (2005) Modulation of cortical oscillatory activities induced by varying single-pulse transcranial magnetic stimulation intensity over the left primary motor area: a combined EEG and TMS study. *Neuroimage*, 27: 896–908.

Geschwind, N. (1965a) Disconnexion syndromes in animals and man. Part I. *Brain*, 88(2): 237–294.

Geschwind, N. (1965b) Disconnexion syndromes in animals and man. Part II. *Brain*, 88(3): 585–644.

Guerra, A., Assenza, F., Bressi, F., Scrascia, F., Del Duca, M., Ursini, F., Vollaro, S., Trotta, L., Tombini, M., Chisari, C. and Ferreri, F. (2011) Transcranial magnetic stimulation studies in Alzheimer's disease. *Int. J. Alzheimer's Dis.*, 2011: 263–817.

Gugino, L.D., Romero, J.R., Aglio, L., Titone, D., Ramirez, M., Pascual-Leone, A., Grimson, E., Weisenfeld, N., Kikinis, R. and Shenton, M.E. (2001) Transcranial magnetic stimulation coregistered with MRI: a comparison of a guided versus blind stimulation technique and its effect on evoked compound muscle action potentials. *Clin. Neurophysiol.*, 112: 1781–1792.

Hallett, M. (1999) Motor cortex plasticity. *Electroencephalogr. Clin. Neurophysiol. Suppl.*, 50: 85–91.

Hallett, M. (2007) Transcranial magnetic stimulation: a primer. *Neuron*, 55: 187–199.

Hallett, M. (2011) Neurophysiology of dystonia: the role of inhibition. *Neurobiol. Dis.*, 42: 177–184.

Hansel, C., Linden, D.J. and D'Angelo, E. (2001) Beyond parallel fiber LTD: the diversity of synaptic and non-synaptic plasticity in the cerebellum. *Nat. Neurosci.*, 4: 467–475.

Hasey, G.M. (1999) Transcranial magnetic stimulation: using a law of physics to treat psychopathology. *J. Psychiatry Neurosci.*, 24: 97–101.

He, Y., Chen, Z., Gong, G. and Evans, A. (2009) Neuronal networks in Alzheimer's disease. *Neuroscientist*, 15(4): 333–350.

Hebb, D.O. (1949) Temperament in chimpanzees; method of analysis. *J. Comp. Physiol. Psychol.*, 42: 192–206.

Holtmaat, A.J., Trachtenberg, J.T., Wilbrecht, L., Shepherd, G.M., Zhang, X., Knott, G.W. and Svoboda, K (2005) Transient and persistent dendritic spines in the neocortex in vivo. *Neuron*, 45: 279–291.

Homan, R.W., Herman, J. and Purdy, P. (1987) Cerebral location of international 10–20 system electrode placement. *Electroencephalogr. Clin. Neurophysiol.*, 66: 376–382.

Horovitz, S.G., Fukunaga, M., De Zwart, J.A., Van Gelderen, P., Fulton, S.C., Balkin, T.J. and Duyn, J.H. (2008) Low frequency BOLD fluctuations during resting wakefulness and light sleep: a simultaneous EEG-fMRI study. *Hum. Brain Mapp.*, 29(6): 671–682.

Horwitz, B. and Poeppel, D. (2002) How can EEG/MEG and fMRI/PET data be combined? *Hum. Brain Mapp.*, 17(1): 1–3.

Huber, R., Määttä, S., Esser, S.K., Sarasso, S., Ferrarelli, F., Watson, A., Ferreri, F., Peterson, M.J. and Tononi, G. (2008) Measures of cortical plasticity after transcranial paired associative stimulation predict changes in electroencephalogram slow-wave activity during subsequent sleep. *J. Neurosci.*, 28: 7911–7918.

Ilmoniemi, R.J. and Kičić, D. (2010) Methodology for combined TMS and EEG. *Brain Topogr.*, 22: 233–248.

Ilmoniemi, R.J., Virtanen, J., Ruohonen, J., Karhu, J., Aronen, H.J., Näätänen, R. and Katila, T. (1997) Neuronal responses to magnetic stimulation reveal cortical reactivity and connectivity. *Neuroreport*, 8: 3537–3540.

Kähkönen, S. and Wilenius, J. (2007) Effects of alcohol on TMS-evoked N100 responses. *J. Neurosci. Meth.*, 166: 104–108.

Kähkönen, S., Kesäniemi, M., Nikouline, V.V., Karhu, J., Ollikainen, M., Holi, M. and Ilmoniemi, R.J. (2001) Ethanol modulates cortical activity: direct evidence with combined TMS and EEG. *Neuroimage*, 14: 322–328.

Kähkönen, S., Wilenius, J., Komssi, S. and Ilmoniemi, R.J. (2004) Distinct differences in cortical reactivity of motor and prefrontal cortices to magnetic stimulation. *Clin. Neurophysiol.*, 115: 583–588.

Kähkönen, S., Komssi, S., Wilenius, J. and Ilmoniemi, R.J. (2005) Prefrontal transcranial magnetic stimulation produces intensity-dependent EEG responses in humans. *Neuroimage*, 24: 955–960.

Kim, S.J. and Linden, D.J. (2007) Ubiquitous plasticity and memory storage. *Neuron*, 56: 582–592.

Kleim, J.A., Lussnig, E., Schwarz, E.R., Comery, T.A. and Greenough, W.T. (1996) Synaptogenesis and Fos expression in the motor cortex of the adult rat after motor skill learning. *J. Neurosci.*, 16: 4529–4535.

Kobayashi, M. and Pascual-Leone, A. (2003) Transcranial magnetic stimulation in neurology. *Lancet Neurol.*, 2: 145–156.

Komssi, S. and Kähkönen, S. (2006) The novelty value of the combined use of electroencephalography and transcranial magnetic stimulation for neuroscience research. *Brain Res. Rev.*, 52: 183–192.

Komssi, S., Aronen, H.J., Huttunen, J., Kesäniemi, M., Soinne, L., Nikouline, V.V., Ollikainen, M., Roine, R.O., Karhu, J., Savolainen, S. and Ilmoniemi, R.J. (2002) Ipsi- and contralateral EEG reactions to transcranial magnetic stimulation. *Clin. Neurophysiol.*, 113: 175–184.

Komssi, S., Kähkönen, S. and Ilmoniemi, R.J. (2004) The effect of stimulus intensity on brain responses evoked by transcranial magnetic stimulation. *Hum. Brain Mapp.*, 21: 154–164.

Komssi, S., Savolainen, P., Heiskala, J. and Kähkönen, S. (2007) Excitation threshold of the motor cortex estimated with transcranial magnetic stimulation electroencephalography. *Neuroreport*, 18: 13–16.

Krings, T., Reinges, M.H., Foltys, H., Cosgrove, G.R. and Thron, A. (2001) Multimodality neuroimaging: research and clinical applications. *Neurol. Clin. Neurophysiol.*, 2001: 2–11.

Krnjevic, K., Randic, M. and Straughan, D.W. (1966) Nature of a cortical inhibitory process. *J. Physiol. (Lond.)*, 184: 49–77.

Kujirai, T., Caramia, M.D., Rothwell, J.C., Day, B.L., Thompson, P.D., Ferbert, A., Wroe, S., Asselman, P. and Marsden, C.D. (1993) Corticocortical inhibition in human motor cortex. *J. Physiol. (Lond.)*, 471: 501–519.

Lee, L., Harrison, L.M. and Mechelli, A. (2003) A report of the functional connectivity workshop, Düsseldorf 2002. *Neuroimage*, 19. 457–465.

Lemieux, L., Laufs, H., Carmichael, D., Paul, J.S., Walker, M.C. and Duncan, J.S. (2008) Noncanonical spike-related BOLD responses in focal epilepsy. *Hum. Brain Mapp.*, 29(3): 29–45.

Lev, J. and Sperry, R.W. (1970) Crossed temperature discrimination following section of forebrain neocortical commissures. *Cortex*, 6(4): 349–361.

Lioumis, P., Kičić, D., Savolainen, P., Mäkelä, J.P. and Kähkönen, S. (2009) Reproducibility of TMS-evoked EEG responses. *Hum. Brain Mapp.*, 30: 1387–1396.

Määttä, S., Landsness, E., Sarasso, S., Ferrarelli, F., Ferreri, F., Ghilardi, M.F. and Tononi, G. (2010) The effects of morning training on night sleep: a behavioral and EEG study. *Brain Res. Bull.*, 82(1–2): 118–123.

Malenka, R.C. and Bear, M.F. (2004) LTP and LTD: an embarrassment of riches. *Neuron*, 44: 5–21.

Mantini, D., Marzetti, L., Corbetta, M., Romani, G.L. and Del Gratta, C. (2010) Multimodal integration of fMRI and EEG data for high spatial and temporal resolution analysis of brain networks. *Brain Topogr.*, 23(2): 150–158.

Massey, P.V. and Bashir, Z.I. (2007) Long-term depression: multiple forms and implications for brain function. *Trends Neurosci.*, 30: 176–184.

16

Massimini, M., Ferrarelli, F., Huber, R., Esser, S.K., Singh, H. and Tononi, G. (2005) Breakdown of cortical effective connectivity during sleep. *Science*, 309: 2228–2232.

Merton, P.A. and Morton, H.B. (1980) Stimulation of the cerebral cortex in the intact human subject. *Nature (Lond.)*, 285: 227.

Milgram, N.A. (1967) In defense of intelligence. *Ment. Retard.*, 5(6): 31–32.

Nikulin, V.V., Kičić, D., Kähkönen, S. and Ilmoniemi, R.J. (2003) Modulation of electroencephalographic responses to transcranial magnetic stimulation: evidence for changes in cortical excitability related to movement. *Eur. J. Neurosci.*, 18: 1206–1212.

Pascual-Leone, A., Tormos, J.M., Keenan, J., Tarazona, F., Canete, C. and Catala, M.D. (1998) Study and modulation of human cortical excitability with transcranial magnetic stimulation. *J. Clin. Neurophysiol.*, 15: 333–343.

Pascual-Leone, A., Tarazona, F. and Catala, M.D. (1999) Applications of transcranial magnetic stimulation in studies on motor learning. *Electroencephalogr. Clin. Neurophysiol. Suppl.*, 51: 157–161.

Pascual-Leone, A., Amedi, A., Fregni, F. and Merabet, L.B. (2005) The plastic human brain cortex. *Annu. Rev. Neurosci.*, 28: 377–401.

Paus, T., Castro-Alamancos, M.A. and Petrides, M. (2001a) Cortico-cortical connectivity of the human mid-dorsolateral frontal cortex and its modulation by repetitive transcranial magnetic stimulation. *Eur. J. Neurosci.*, 14: 1405–1411.

Paus, T., Sipila, P.K. and Strafella, A.P. (2001b) Synchronization of neuronal activity in the human primary motor cortex by transcranial magnetic stimulation: an EEG study. *J. Neurophysiol.*, 86: 1983–1990.

Pfurtscheller, G. and Lopes da Silva, F.H. (1999) Event-related EEG/MEG synchronization and desynchronization: basic principles. *Clin. Neurophysiol.*, 110: 1842–1857.

Platz, T. and Rothwell, J.C. (2010) Brain stimulation and brain repair — rTMS: from animal experiment to clinical trials — what do we know? *Restor. Neurol. Neurosci.*, 28: 387–398.

Raymond, C.R. (2007) LTP forms 1, 2 and 3: different mechanisms for the "long" in long-term potentiation. *Trends Neurosci.*, 30: 167–175.

Roelfsema, P.R., Engel, A.K., König, P. and Singer, W. (1997) Visuomotor integration is associated with zero time-lag synchronization among cortical areas. *Nature (Lond.)*, 385 (6612): 157–161.

Romani, G.L., Brunetti, M., Ferretti, A., Pizzella, V., Torquati, K. and Del Gratta, C. (2005) Functional imaging with MEG and fMRI. *Proc. IEEE Eng. Med. Biol. Soc.*, 4: 4183–4186.

Rosanova, M., Casali, A., Bellina, V., Resta, F., Mariotti, M. and Massimini, M. (2009) Natural frequencies of human corticothalamic circuits. *J. Neurosci.*, 29: 7679–7685.

Rosenthal, J., Waller, H.J. and Amassian, V.E. (1967) An analysis of the activation of motor cortical neurons by surface stimulation. *J. Neurophysiol.*, 30: 844–858.

Rossi, S., Hallett, M., Rossini, P.M., Pascual-Leone, A. and Safety of TMS Consensus Group. (2009) Safety, ethical considerations, and application guidelines for the use of transcranial magnetic stimulation in clinical practice and research. *Clin. Neurophysiol.*, 120(12): 2008–2039.

Rossini, P.M. and Dal Forno, G. (2004) Neuronal post-stroke plasticity in the adult. *Restor. Neurol. Neurosci.*, 22: 193–206.

Rossini, P.M. and Rossi, S. (2007) Transcranial magnetic stimulation: diagnostic, therapeutic, and research potential. *Neurology*, 68: 484–488.

Rossini, P.M., Caramia, M. and Zarola, F. (1987a) Central motor tract propagation in man: studies with non-invasive, unifocal, scalp stimulation. *Brain Res.*, 415: 211–225.

Rossini, P.M., Gigli, G.L., Marciani, M.G., Zarola, F. and Caramia, M. (1987b) Non-invasive evaluation of input–output characteristics of sensorimotor cerebral areas in healthy humans. *Electroencephalogr. Clin. Neurophysiol.*, 68: 88–100.

Rossini, P.M., Barker, A.T., Berardelli, A., Caramia, M.D., Caruso, G., Cracco, R.Q., Dimitrijevic, M.R., Hallett, M., Katayama, Y., Lücking, C.H., et al. (1994a) Non-invasive electrical and magnetic stimulation of the brain, spinal cord and roots: basic principles and procedures for routine clinical application. Report of an IFCN committee. *Electroencephalogr. Clin. Neurophysiol.*, 91: 79–92.

Rossini, P.M., Martino, G., Narici, L., Pasquarelli, A., Peresson, M., Pizzella, V., Tecchio, F., Torrioli, G. and Romani, G.L. (1994b) Short-term brain 'plasticity' in humans: transient finger representation changes in sensory cortex: somatotopy following ischemic anesthesia. *Brain Res.*, 642: 169–177.

Rossini, P.M., Calautti, C., Pauri, F. and Baron, J.C. (2003) Post-stroke plastic reorganisation in the adult brain. *Lancet Neurol.*, 2: 493–502.

Rossini, P.M., Micera, S., Benvenuto, A., Carpaneto, J., Cavallo, G., Citi, L., Cipriani, C., Denaro, L., Denaro, V., Di Pino, G., Ferreri, F., Guglielmelli, E., Hoffmann, K.P., Raspopovic, S., Rigosa, J., Rossini, L., Tombini, M. and Dario, P. (2010a) Double nerve intraneural interface implant on a human amputee for robotic hand control. *Clin. Neurophysiol.*, 121: 777–783.

Rossini, P.M., Rossini, L. and Ferreri, F. (2010b) Brain–behavior relations: transcranial magnetic stimulation: a review. *IEEE Eng. Med. Biol. Magn.*, 29(1): 84–95.

Rossini, P.M., Rigosa, J., Micera, S., Assenza, G., Rossini, L. and Ferreri, F. (2011) Stump nerve signals during transcranial magnetic motor cortex stimulation recorded in an amputee via longitudinal intrafascicular electrodes. *Exp. Brain Res.*, 210(1): 1–11.

Rothwell, J.C. (1993) Evoked potentials, magnetic stimulation studies, and event-related potentials. *Curr. Opin. Neurol.*, 6: 715–723.

Rothwell, J.C. (2011) Using transcranial magnetic stimulation methods to probe connectivity between motor areas of the brain. *Hum. Mov. Sci.*, 30(5): 906–915.

Rothwell, J.C., Thompson, P.D., Day, B.L., Dick, J.P., Kachi, T., Cowan, J.M. and Marsden, C.D. (1987) Motor cortex stimulation in intact man. 1. General characteristics of EMG responses in different muscles. *Brain*, 110(5): 1173–1190.

Rothwell, J.C., Thompson, P.D., Day, B.L., Boyd, S. and Marsden, C.D. (1991) Stimulation of the human motor cortex through the scalp. *Exp. Physiol.*, 76(2): 159–200.

Sanger, T.D., Garg, R.R. and Chen, R. (2001) Interactions between two different inhibitory systems in the human motor cortex. *J. Physiol. (Lond.)*, 530: 307–317.

Schnitzler, A. and Gross, J. (2005) Functional connectivity analysis in magnetoencephalography. *Int. Rev. Neurobiol.*, 68: 173–195.

Siebner, H.R. and Rothwell, J. (2003) Transcranial magnetic stimulation: new insights into representational cortical plasticity. *Exp. Brain Res.*, 148: 1–16.

Siebner, H.R., Bergmann, T.O., Bestmann, S., Massimini, M., Johansen-Berg, H., Mochizuki, H., Bohning, D.E., Boorman, E.D., Groppa, S., Miniussi, C., Pascual-Leone, A., Huber, R., Taylor, P.C., Ilmoniemi, R.J., De Gennaro, L., Strafella, A.P., Kähkönen, S., Kloppel, S., Frisoni, G.B. and George, M.S. (2009) Consensus paper: combining transcranial stimulation with neuroimaging. *Brain Stimul.*, 2: 58–80.

Sjöström, P.J., Rancz, E.A., Roth, A. and Hausser, M. (2008) Dendritic excitability and synaptic plasticity. *Physiol. Rev.*, 88: 769–840.

Sporns, O. (2011) The non-random brain: efficiency, economy, and complex dynamics. *Front. Comput. Neurosci.*, 5: 5.

Sporns, O., Chialvo, D.R., Kaiser, M. and Hilgetag, C. (2004) Organization, development and function of complex brain networks. *Trends Cogn. Sci.*, 8: 418–425.

Squitti, R., Ventriglia, M., Barbati, G., Cassetta, E., Ferreri, F., Dal Forno, G., Ramires, S., Zappasodi, F. and Rossini, P.M. (2007) 'Free' copper in serum of Alzheimer's disease patients correlates with markers of liver function. *J. Neural Transm.*, 114(12): 1589–1594.

Stam, C.J. (2005) Nonlinear dynamical analysis of EEG and MEG: review of an emerging field. *Clin. Neurophysiol.*, 116(10): 266–301.

Stam, C.J., Nolte, G. and Daffertshofer, A. (2007) Phase lag index: assessment of functional connectivity from multichannel EEG and MEG with diminished bias from common sources. *Hum. Brain Mapp.*, 28(11): 1178–1193.

Steriade, M., McCormick, D.A. and Sejnowski, T.J. (1993) Thalamocortical oscillations in the sleeping and aroused brain. *Science*, 262: 679–685.

Tecchio, F., Porcaro, C., Barbati, G. and Zappasodi, F. (2007) Functional source separation and hand cortical representation for a brain–computer interface feature extraction. *J. Physiol. (Lond.)*, 580(3): 703–721.

Thompson, S.P. (1910) A physiological effect of an alternating magnetic field. *Proc. R. Soc. Biol.*, 82: 396–398.

Thut, G. and Miniussi, C. (2009) New insights into rhythmic brain activity from TMS-EEG studies. *Trends Cogn. Sci.*, 13: 182–189.

Tononi, G., Sporns, O. and Edelman, G.M. (1994) A measure for brain complexity: relating functional segregation and integration in the nervous system. *Proc. Natl. Acad. Sci. USA*, 91: 5033–5037.

Trachtenberg, J.T., Chen, B.E., Knott, G.W., Feng, G., Sanes, J.R., Welker, E. and Svoboda, K. (2002) Long-term in vivo imaging of experience-dependent synaptic plasticity in adult cortex. *Nature (Lond.)*, 420: 788–794.

Turrigiano, G.G. and Nelson, S.B. (2004) Homeostatic plasticity in the developing nervous system. *Nat. Rev. Neurosci.*, 5: 97–107.

Uhlhaas, P.J. and Singer, W. (2006) Neural synchrony in brain disorders: relevance for cognitive dysfunctions and pathophysiology. *Neuron*, 52(1): 155–168.

Van der Werf, Y.D. and Paus, T. (2006) The neural response to transcranial magnetic stimulation of the human motor cortex. I. Intracortical and cortico-cortical contributions. *Exp. Brain Res.*, 175: 231–245.

Vecchio, F., Babiloni, C., Ferreri, F., Curcio, G., Fini, R., Del Percio, C. and Rossini, P.M. (2007) Mobile phone emission modulates interhemispheric functional coupling of EEG alpha rhythms. *Eur. J. Neurosci.*, 25(6): 1908–1913.

Vecchio, F., Babiloni, C., Ferreri, F., Buffo, P., Cibelli, G., Curcio, G., Van Dijkman, S., Melgari, J.M., Giambattistelli, F. and Rossini, P.M. (2010) Mobile phone emission modulates inter-hemispheric functional coupling of EEG alpha rhythms in elderly compared to young subjects. *Clin. Neurophysiol.*, 121(2): 163–171.

Veniero, D., Brignani, D., Thut, G. and Miniussi, C. (2011) Alpha-generation as basic response-signature to transcranial magnetic stimulation (TMS) targeting the human resting motor cortex: a TMS/EEG co-registration study. *Psychophysiology*, 48(10): 1381–1389.

Virtanen, J., Ruohonen, J., Näätänen, R. and Ilmoniemi, R.J. (1999) Instrumentation for the measurement of electric brain responses to transcranial magnetic stimulation. *Med. Biol. Eng. Comput.*, 37: 322–326.

Ziemann, U. (2004) LTP-like plasticity in human motor cortex. *Suppl. Clin. Neurophysiol.*, 57: 702–707.

Ziemann, U. (2011) Transcranial magnetic stimulation at the interface with other techniques: a powerful tool for studying the human cortex. *Neuroscientist*, 17: 368–381.

Ziemann, U., Paulus, W., Nitsche, M.A., Pascual-Leone, A., Byblow, W.D., Berardelli, A., Siebner, H.R., Classen, J., Cohen, L.G. and Rothwell, J.C. (2008) Consensus: motor cortex plasticity protocols. *Brain Stimul.*, 1: 164–182.

Chapter 2

Brain's alpha, beta, gamma, delta, and theta oscillations in neuropsychiatric diseases: proposal for biomarker strategies

Erol Başar[a,*], Canan Başar-Eroğlu[b], Bahar Güntekin[a]
and Görsev Gülmen Yener[a,c,d,e]

[a]*Brain Dynamics, Cognition and Complex Systems Research Center, Istanbul Kultur University, Istanbul 34156, Turkey*
[b]*Institute of Psychology and Cognition Research, University of Bremen, D-28359 Bremen, Germany*
[c]*Brain Dynamics Multidisciplinary Research Center, Dokuz Eylül University, Izmir 35340, Turkey*
[d]*Department of Neurosciences, Dokuz Eylül University, Izmir 35340, Turkey*
[e]*Department of Neurology, Dokuz Eylül University Medical School, Izmir 35340, Turkey*

ABSTRACT

Brain oscillations have gained tremendous importance in neuroscience during recent decades as functional building blocks of sensory–cognitive processes. Research also shows that event-related oscillations (EROs) in "alpha," "beta," "gamma," "delta," and "theta" frequency windows are highly modified in pathological brains, especially in patients with cognitive impairment. The strategies and methods applied in the present report reflect the innate organization of the brain: "*the whole brain work.*" The present paper is an account of methods such as evoked/event-related spectra, evoked/ERDs, coherence analysis, and phase-locking. The report does not aim to cover all strategies related to the systems theory applied in brain research literature. However, the essential methods and concepts are applied in several examples from Alzheimer's disease (AD), schizophrenia, and bipolar disorder (BD), and such examples lead to fundamental statements in the search for neurophysiological biomarkers in cognitive impairment.

An overview of the results clearly demonstrates that it is obligatory to apply the method of oscillations in *multiple electroencephalogram frequency windows* in search of functional biomarkers and to detect the effects of drug applications. Again, according to the summary of results in AD patients and BD patients, multiple oscillations and selectively distributed recordings must be analyzed and should include multiple locations. *Selective connectivity between selectively distributed neural networks* has to be computed by means of *spatial coherence*. Therefore, by designing a strategy for diagnostics, the differential diagnostics, and application of (preventive) drugs, neurophysiological information should be analyzed within a framework including multiple methods and multiple frequency bands. The *application of drugs/neurotransmitters* gains a new impact with the analysis of oscillations and coherences. A more clear and differentiated analysis of drug effects can be attained in comparison to the application of the conventional wide-band evoked potential and event-related potential applications.

─────────────
Correspondence to: Prof. Erol Başar, Brain Dynamics, Cognition and Complex Systems Research Center, Istanbul Kultur University, Istanbul 34156, Turkey.
Tel.: +90 212 498 43 92; Fax: +90 212 498 45 46;
E-mail: e.basar@iku.edu.tr

20

The interpretation of results in AD, schizophrenia, and BD (patients mostly with damaged cognitive neural networks) becomes most efficient by joint analysis of results on oscillatory responses and coherences obtained by means of *cognitive tasks*. In these diseases, strong cognitive impairment is observed; the use of spectra therefore allows cognitive deficits to be seen more clearly upon application of stimulation involving a cognitive task.

The report concludes by presenting highlights for neurophysiological explorations in diagnostics, drug application, and progressive monitoring of such diseases.

KEYWORDS

Electroencephalography (evoked, oscillations); Event-related (systems theory, power spectrum, time–frequency analysis); Phase-locking (delta, theta, alpha, beta, gamma, coherence); Alzheimer's disease; Bipolar disorder; Schizophrenia (lithium, acetylcholine)

2.1. Introduction

Brain oscillations as functional building blocks in sensory–cognitive processes have gained tremendous importance in the recent decades. Research also shows that event-related oscillations (EROs) are highly modified in pathological brains, especially in patients with cognitive impairment. The major aim of the present study is to show that, in pathological states of brain, multiple brain oscillations in the "whole cortex" are altered. The identification of clinical biomarkers requires large spectra of mathematical parameters and multiple strategies. The oscillatory changes in *multiple frequency windows* and the whole cortex should be taken into consideration by analyzing relevant changes in the amplitude of *function-related oscillations*, together with *multiple connectivity deficits*. At the end of the paper, we will present highlights for neurophysiological explorations in diagnostics, drug application, and progressive monitoring of diseases.

The present report will present some methods, concepts, and strategies of use in analyzing brain oscillations in neuropsychiatric diseases. It provides a general overview of the methods reported in the present volume and does not aim to cover all strategies related to systems theory that are applied across the brain research literature. The strategies and methods applied are examples reflecting the innate organization of the brain: *"the whole brain work."*

The report also includes a critical view providing an orientation for readers with an interest in reviewing the results emerging from reports contained in the present volume. The presented analyses will serve as proposals and do not constitute a systematic review. The review should be considered rather as a workshop, showing the utility of the applied analyses. The examples provide a summary of statistically significant and previously published results. We have chosen examples from our research groups, as the data can easily be displayed.

Our research group has published a series of papers related to methods of brain oscillations over a period of more than 40 years; accordingly, we aim to describe core ideas for using methods of electroencephalogram *(EEG)/ERO* analysis (see also Başar et al., 1975a–c, 2001a; Başar, 1980, 2011; Güntekin and Başar, 2010).

We also have to emphasize that there are important functional and interpretational differences between EEG, evoked oscillations, and EROs.

In the analysis of spontaneous EEG, only sporadic changes of amplitudes from hidden sources are measured. Sensory evoked oscillations reflect the property of sensory networks activated by a simple sensory stimulation. Event-related (or cognitive) oscillations manifest modification of sensory and cognitive networks triggered by a cognitive task (see Fig. 1).

It is evident that, by performing and comparing all types of analyses, a large number of permutations are possible, thus giving rise to a wider spectrum of interpretations related to the *differentiation of diseases*, *progress of diseases*, and modifications upon *application of medication*. The final

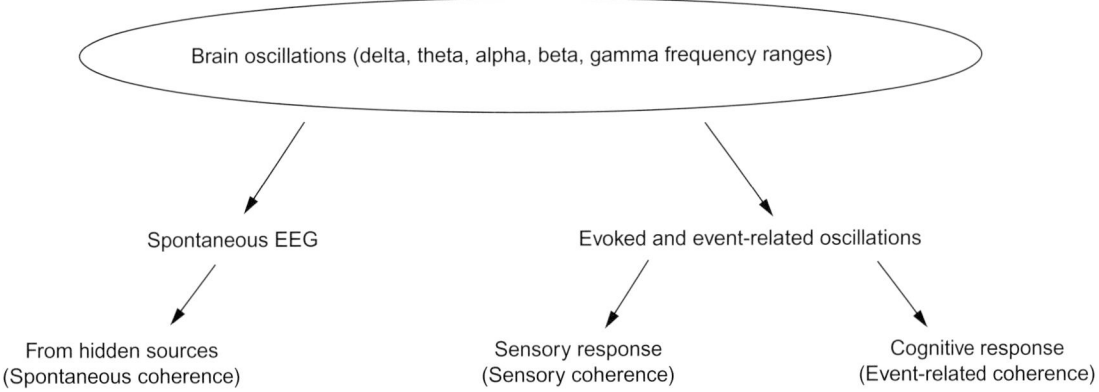

Fig. 1. A schematic presentation of differentiation in search of biomarkers related to brain oscillations.

aim of the present report, as presented in the last section, is therefore to indicate that a valid analysis of brain electrical potentials in search of bio-markers can be achieved only by successive application of analysis tools and should not be reduced to the search to a given frequency range or to a given stimulus modality.

It is also fundamental to note that comparison of results obtained upon application of sensory signals and cognitive inputs is extremely important: in diseases as Alzheimer's disease (AD), schizophrenia, mild cognitive impairment (MCI), and bipolar disorder (BD), patients show cognitive deficits depending on the state of illness, ages, and also cultural differences. Accordingly, cognitive deficits can be demonstrated only after comparing results upon sensory and cognitive signals (see papers by Başar-Eroğlu et al., Özerdem et al., 2013, this volume and Yener and Başar (a)).

The methods outlined in Table 1 can be applied step-by-step or in a random sequence; some of the methods can be omitted, depending on the application possibilities in patients. This also depends on the research priorities of different laboratories. Therefore, we do not aim to demonstrate all possible applications; we will give only a few examples. Several useful applications are presented in this volume (see Başar-Eroğlu et al., Özerdem et al., Vecchio et al., Yener and Başar (a)).

2.2. Why application of several methods and strategies is important in search of biomarkers

Fig. 2 illustrates new approaches and strategies in functional neuroscience. The usefulness of an *"ensemble of methods"* should be emphasized, since the application of single methods has severe shortcomings for understanding integrative brain functions. The methods range from indirect means of measuring changes in cerebral blood flow in local regions of the human cortex (functional magnetic resonance imaging (fMRI)), or changes in the electrical activity of the human brain with EEG recording with multiple electrodes, to the use of chronically implanted multiple electrodes in primates. According to Mountcastle (1998), measurement using large populations of neurons is presently the most useful experimental paradigm used in perception experiments. However, fMRI has the disadvantage of low temporal resolution and long distance measurements cannot yet be performed with multiple microelectrodes. Therefore, measurements of *macro-activity* (EEG/event-related potentials (ERP) and magnetoencephalography) seem to be the most appropriate method to measure the dynamic properties of memory and of integrative brain function.

Since neuroscientists have come to the general conclusion that large numbers of different brain regions must cooperate in any brain function, the

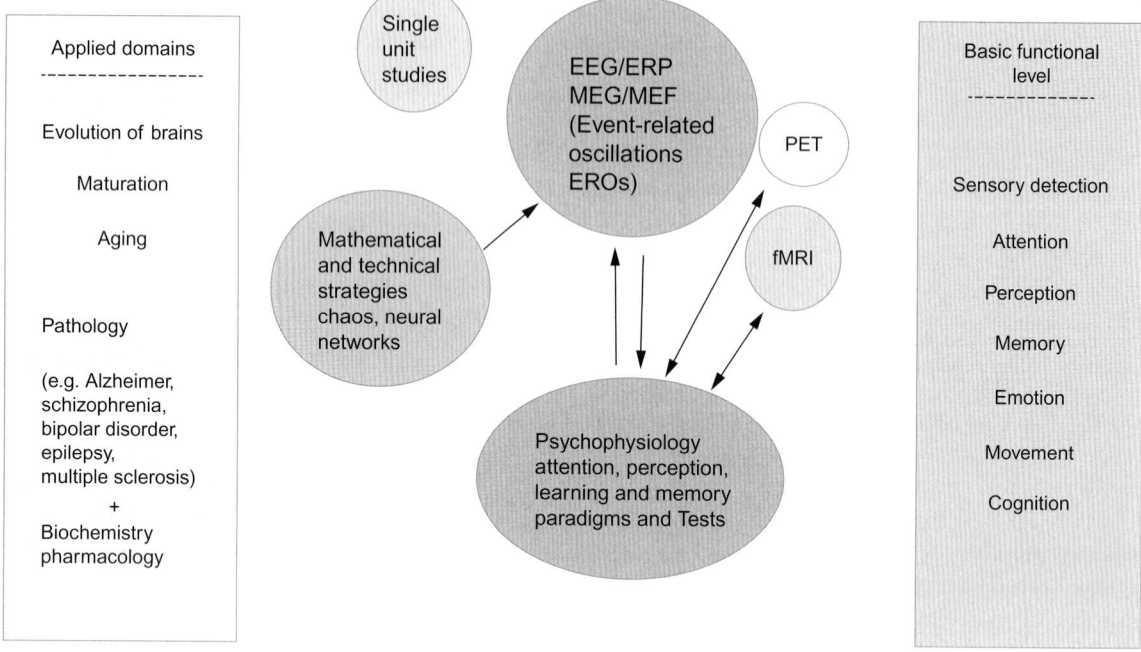

Fig. 2.   New approaches and strategies in functional neuroscience (modified from Başar, 2004). (For color figures, please refer to the color figures in last section of the book.)

analysis of relationships between different regions of the brain is becoming increasingly important.

In the following section, we will briefly discuss the outcomes of methods and strategies shown in Fig. 1. The expression *strategy* refers here to the combined application of several methods, in parallel or sequentially.

(1) Studies at the single-cell level have been of great importance in elucidating the basic physiological mechanisms of communication between cells (Eccles, 1973; Mountcastle, 1998). However, the importance of these studies for understanding integrative brain functions is questionable since, during the integrative processes, the whole brain is involved, as Adey et al. (1960) and Adey (1966, 1989) merely underlined, and the new trends in neuroscience clearly emphasize (see also Freeman, 1999).

(2) Positron emission tomography is an invasive procedure applied to patients. It has a large

temporal resolution in the range of half an hour and offers no possibility for dynamic measurements at the level of microseconds.

(3) The methods incorporating analyses of EEG/ERPs (and especially EROs) and fMRI provide further excellent strategies to illuminate brain functions, since they cover dynamic changes in the brain and the morphological structure. The MEG and study of magnetic evoked fields (MEFs) greatly increase the spatial resolution in comparison to EEG and ERP. Accordingly, these methods are likely to provide excellent results in future applications.

(4) The new strategies are interwoven with the use of relevant mathematical and psychophysiological strategies. These are:

(i) Mathematical and systems theoretical approaches including, in recent decades: (a) the concepts of *chaos, entropy*; (b) modeling with *neural networks*, interpretation of *frequency domain approach*, new approaches utilizing wavelet analysis and spatial and temporal coherences.

(ii) Psychological strategies with the use of behavioral paradigms and application of neuropsychological tests (Karakaş et al., 2002, 2003).

(iii) An important strategy, not included in Fig. 2, is recording with chronically implanted intracranial electrodes in the animal brain.

In order to achieve relevant progress in functional neuroscience, it became fundamental to apply several methods together (Freeman, 1999). However, the application of all strategies in every laboratory is not yet possible. Fig. 2 further illustrates the levels of basic central nervous system (CNS) functions (right side) and the applied domains (left side). Functions such as *sensory detection, movement,* and *memory* can be successfully analyzed by using individual methods or strategies from several research domains, such as *evolution, aging, pathology,* and *pharmacology* (use of drugs or pharmacological agents in pathological states). The application of combined strategies in all these fields has led to new horizons for understanding the integrative functions of the brain, especially of memory function. The role of memory in the human mind and behavior cannot be overemphasized, since very few aspects of higher nervous function could operate successfully without some memory contribution; perception, recognition, language, planning, problem solving, and decision-making all rely on memory (Damasio and Damasio, 1994).

2.3. Some established rules in the application of oscillatory dynamics

The functional significance of oscillatory neural activity begins to emerge from the analysis of responses to well-defined events *(ERO that is phase- or time-locked to a sensory or cognitive event)*. Among other approaches, it is possible to investigate such oscillations by frequency domain analysis of ERP, based on the following hypothesis:

The EEG consists of the activity of an ensemble of generators producing rhythmic activity in several frequency ranges. These oscillators are usually active in a random way. However, by application of sensory stimulation, these generators are coupled and act together in a coherent way. This synchronization and enhancement of EEG activity gives rise to "evoked" or "induced" rhythms. Evoked potentials (EPs), representing ensembles of neural population responses, were considered to be a result of the transition from a disordered to an ordered state. The compound ERP manifests a superposition of evoked oscillations in the EEG frequencies, ranging from delta to gamma ("natural frequencies of the brain" such as delta (0.5–3.5 Hz), theta (4–7 Hz), alpha (8–13 Hz), beta (15–28 Hz), and gamma (30–70 Hz). (See publications by Başar, 1980; Klimesch et al., 1997; Yordanova and Kolev, 1998; see also reports in Başar and Bullock, 1992; Gurtubay et al., 2004; Buszáki, 2006.)

There are several strategies available for measuring cognitive changes, including spontaneous EEG, sensory evoked oscillation, and EROs. The term "sensory evoked" implies responses elicited upon a simple sensory stimulation, whereas "event-related" indicates responses elicited upon a cognitive task, generally an oddball paradigm. Further selective connectivity deficit in sensory or cognitive networks is reflected by coherence measurements. When a simple sensory stimulus is used, a sensory network becomes activated and "sensory evoked coherence" can be measured between brain regions, whereas an oddball task initiates activation in both a sensory network and an additional cognitive network, and then "event-related coherence" can be measured.

In the following, some rules and concepts are presented:

(1) Intrinsic oscillatory activity of single neurons forms the basis of the natural frequencies of neural assemblies. Oscillatory activity of the neural assemblies of the brain consists of the *alpha, beta, gamma, theta,* and *delta* frequencies. These frequencies are the natural frequencies and thus the real responses of the brain (Başar et al., 2001a–c).

(2) Morphologically different neurons or neural networks are excitable upon sensory–cognitive stimulation in the same frequency range of EEG oscillations; the type of neuronal assembly does not play a major role in the frequency tuning of oscillatory networks. Research has shown that neural populations in the cerebral *cortex, hippocampus*, and *cerebellum* are all tuned to the very same frequency ranges, although these structures have completely different neural organizations (Eckhorn et al., 1988; Llinás, 1988; Singer, 1989; Steriade et al., 1992; Başar, 1998, 1999). It is therefore suggested that brain networks in the whole brain communicate by means of the same set of frequency codes of EEG oscillations.

(3) The brain has *response susceptibilities*. These susceptibilities mostly originate from its intrinsic rhythmic activity, i.e., its spontaneous activity (Başar, 1980, 1983a,b; Narici et al., 1990; Başar et al., 1992). A brain system responds to external or internal stimuli with those rhythms or frequency components that are among its intrinsic (natural) rhythms. Accordingly, if a given frequency range does not exist in its spontaneous activity, it will also be absent in the evoked activity. Conversely, if activity in a given frequency range does not exist in the evoked activity, it will also be absent in the spontaneous activity. However, in the presence of high pre-stimulus activity, aftercoming post-stimulus activity enhancement will not be adequate for eliciting a significant response upon a stimulus application.

(4) There is an inverse relationship between EEG and ERPs. The amplitude of the EEG thus serves as a control parameter for responsiveness of the brain, which can be obtained in the form of EPs or ERPs (Jansen et al., 1993; Rahn and Başar, 1993; Başar, 1998; Barry et al., 2003; Başar et al., 2003).

(5) This characteristic and the concept of response susceptibility led to the conclusion that the oscillatory activity that forms the EEG governs the most general transfer functions in the brain (Başar, 1990).

(6) Oscillatory neural tissues that are selectively distributed in the whole brain are activated upon sensory–cognitive input. The oscillatory activity of neural tissues may be described through a number of response parameters. Different tasks, and the functions that they elicit, are represented by different configurations of parameters. Due to this characteristic, the same frequency range is used in the brain to perform not just one but *multiple functions*. The response parameters of the oscillatory activity are as follows: enhancement (amplitude), delay (latency), blocking or desynchronization, phase-locking, phase changes, prolongation (duration), degree of coherence between different oscillations, degree of entropy (Pfurtscheller, 1997, 2001; Neuper and Pfurtscheller, 1998a,b; Başar et al., 1999a,b; Miltner et al., 1999; Pfurtscheller et al., 1999, 2006; Schürmann et al., 2000; Kocsis et al., 2001; Rosso et al., 2001, 2002; Başar, 2004).

(7) The number of oscillations and the ensemble of parameters that are obtained under a given condition increase as the complexity of the stimulus increases, or as the recognition of the stimulus becomes more difficult (Başar, 1980, 1999; Başar et al., 2000, 2001a).

(8) Each function is represented in the brain by the superposition of the oscillations in various frequency ranges. The values of the oscillations vary across a number of response parameters. The comparative polarity and phase angle of different oscillations are decisive in producing function-specific configurations. Neuronal assemblies do not obey the *all-or-none* rule that the single neurons obey (Karakaş et al., 2000a,b; Klimesch et al., 2000a,b; Chen and Herrmann, 2001).

(9) The *superposition principle* indicates synergy between the alpha, beta, gamma, theta, and delta oscillations during the performance of

sensory–cognitive tasks. Thus, according to the superposition principle, integrative brain function operates through the combined action of multiple oscillations.

ESSENTIAL FEATURES OF THE "WHOLE BRAIN" WORK IN INTEGRATIVE BRAIN FUNCTION AS CONSEQUENCE OF THE ABOVE RULES

According to Başar (2006, 2011) all structures of the brain work in concert during sensory–cognitive processes. This overall coordination of oscillatory processes is based on a type of super-synergy, which comprises an ensemble of at least six mechanisms working in parallel upon sensory–cognitive input. It is proposed that the coexistence and cooperative action of these interwoven and interacting sub-mechanisms shape the integrative brain functions.

The sub-mechanisms and/or related processes are as follows:

1. The "superposition" is the parallel activation of electrical activity in alpha, beta, gamma, theta, and delta bands during integrative functional processes of the brain (Başar et al., 1999a,b; Karakaş et al., 2000a,b; Klimesch et al., 2000b; Chen and Herrmann, 2001).

2. The parallel activation of oscillations in gamma, beta, alpha, theta, and delta responses upon exogenous or endogenous inputs is selectively distributed oscillations in the brain. These responses are manifested with the occurrence of multiple parameters such as *phase-locking enhancement*, *delay*, *blocking (desynchronization)*, and *prolongation* (Başar, 1980, 1999; Başar et al., 1999a,b, 2000, 2001a,b). The ensemble of oscillations and amplitude of oscillations and coherence values between different brain areas usually increase as the complexity of the stimulation increases or the recognition of the stimulus becomes more difficult.

3. Temporal and spatial changes of entropy in the brain (Quiroga et al., 1999; Yordanova et al., 2002).

4. Temporal coherence between cells in cortical columns contributes to the simple binding mechanism (Eckhorn et al., 1988; Gray and Singer, 1989).

5. Varying degrees of spatial coherence occur over long distances as parallel processing (Başar, 1980, 1983a,b; Miltner et al., 1999; Schürmann et al., 2000; Kocsis et al., 2001).

6. Inverse relationship between EEG and ERPs: EEG is a control parameter for responsiveness of the brain.

2.4. Ensemble of systems theory methods

2.4.1. Systems theory methods

In order to analyze the dynamics of brain oscillatory processes, several mathematical methods are applied. Table 1 summarizes the methods included in the "systems theory" of brain-state analysis.

More refined methods were also incorporated in order to analyze evoked brain activity, including the combined EEG–EP analysis, and wavelet analysis methods (Başar et al., 1999c, 2001a; Demiralp et al., 1999; Quiroga et al., 2001a, b). Our group first applied the system theory methods to brain waves by using the conventional methods. Later, our group has also applied new methods such as *wavelet entropy* (Quiroga et al., 1999; Rosso et al., 2001). In addition to the systems theory methods, newly emerging methods of analyzing EROs include studies of nonlinearities and the incorporation of the concept of chaos, which aim to further increase understanding of the properties of the system.

Among the applications described in the following sections, spectral signal analysis constitutes one of the most important and most commonly used analytical tools for the evaluation of neurophysiological signals. It is not only amplitude and phase that are of interest, but there are also a variety of measures derived from them, including important coupling measures such as coherence or phase synchrony. Başar et al. (1999c), Demiralp et al. (1999), and Başar (2011) compared wavelet transform techniques and conventional Fourier analysis in the human and cat brains and showed the

TABLE 1

THE ENSEMBLE OF SYSTEMS THEORY METHODS

(a) Power spectral density of the spontaneous EEG
(b) *Evoked spectra* (FFT analysis of the sensory evoked potential (elicited by simple light, tone signal, etc.))
(c) Event-related spectra (FFT analysis of an ERP, for example, target or non-target signal during an oddball paradigm).
(d) Phase-locking, phase synchrony
(e) Cross correlation
(f) Cross spectrum
(g) EEG coherence
(h) Evoked coherence
(i) Event-related coherence

---

equivalence of these techniques. A most fundamental comparison of various spectral techniques was performed by Bruns (2004), comparing the three classical spectral analysis approaches: Fourier, Hilbert, and wavelet transform. Although recently there seems to be increasing acceptance of the notion that Hilbert- or wavelet-based analyses might be superior to Fourier-based analyses, Bruns (2004) demonstrated that the three techniques are formally (i.e., mathematically) equivalent when using the class of wavelets that is typically applied in spectral analyses. Moreover, spectral amplitude serves as an example that Fourier, Hilbert, and wavelet analysis also yield equivalent results in practical applications to neuronal signals.

2.4.2. Some fundamental remarks

The functional significance of oscillatory neural activity begins to emerge from the analysis of responses to well-defined events *(ERO that is phase- or time-locked to sensory and cognitive event)* (Başar, 1980, 1998).

Time-locked and/or phase-locked methods show that the responses of a specific frequency after stimulation can be identified by computing the amplitude frequency characteristics (AFCs)

of the averaged ERPs (Başar, 1980; Röschke et al., 1995; Yordanova and Kolev, 1997), or the event-related and evoked power spectra. The AFCs and event-related power spectra describe the brain system's transfer properties, e.g., excitability and susceptibility to respond, by revealing resonant as well as salient frequencies. Therefore, it does not simply represent the spectral power density characterizing the transient signal in the frequency domain but also the predicted behavior of the system (brain) if sinusoidal modulated input signals of defined frequencies were applied as stimulation. Since it reflects the amplification in a given frequency channel, the AFC is expressed in relative units. Hence, the presence of a peak in the AFC or post-stimulus spectra reveals the *resonant frequencies* interpreted as the preferred oscillations of the system during the response to a stimulus. In order to calculate the AFCs, the ERPs were first averaged and then transformed to the frequency domain by means of one-sided Fourier transform (Laplace transform, see Solodovnikov, 1960; Başar, 1980), as shown in Fig. 3. Further, Fig. 3 illustrates the proposed ensemble of systems theory analysis methods in search of neurophysiological markers in healthy subjects and neuropsychiatric patients. A core stage in this ensemble of methods is the recording of electrical potentials, known as EP and ERPs in the

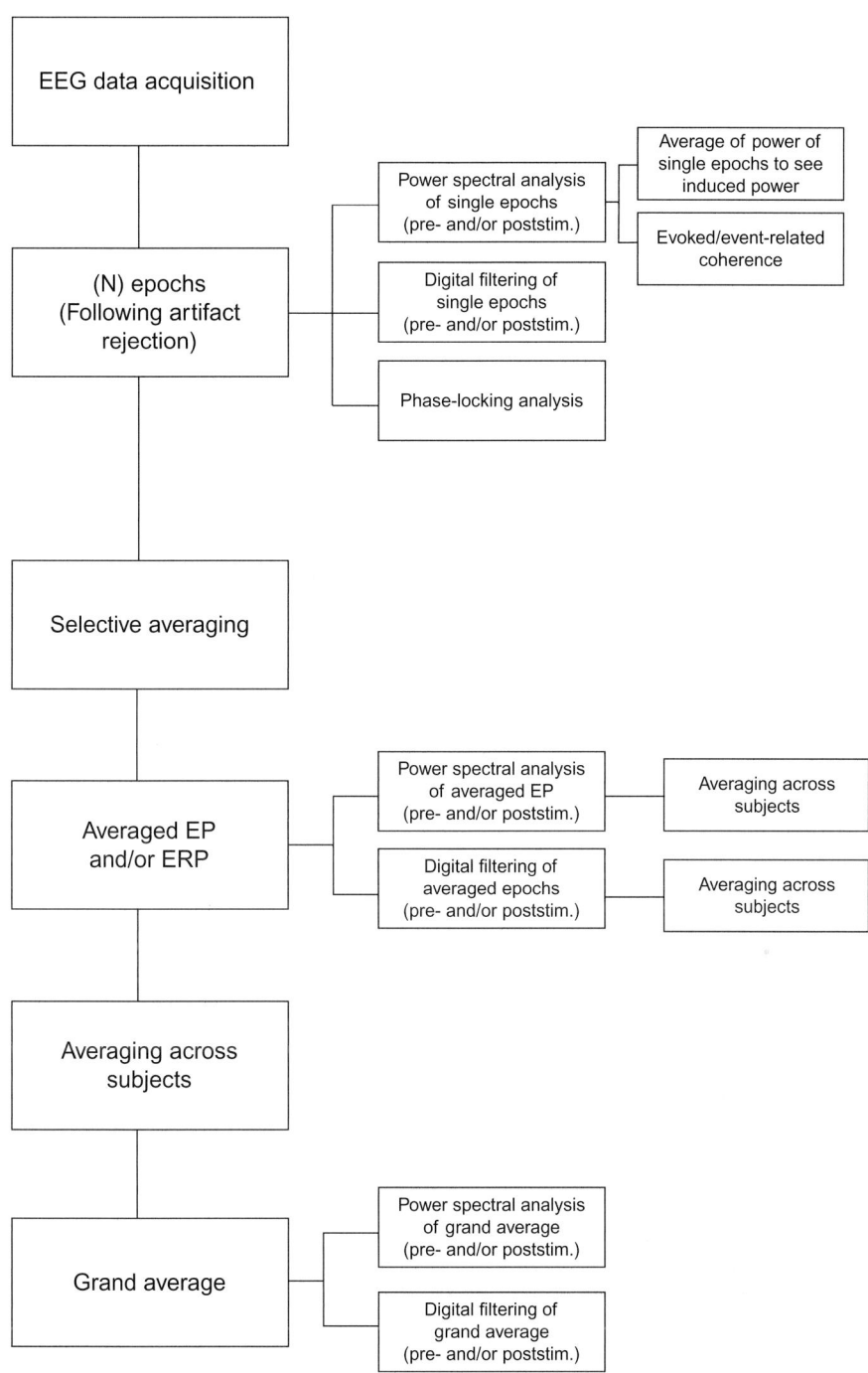

Fig. 3. Combined time and frequency domain analysis of EEG–EP epochs (modified from Schürmann and Başar, 1994; Başar et al., 2000).

28

conventional nomenclature of electrophysiology analysis. However, brain oscillations upon application of stimulation have been now a relevant progress in the analysis. First of all, in order to perform Fourier analysis of brain responses, an averaging procedure is applied to data from healthy subjects and patients. Following artifact rejection, selective averaging is performed. The averaged potentials (EP and/or ERP) are then analyzed with FFT and, according to the cut-off frequencies of evoked power spectra, digital filtering is applied to single epochs. A grand average is also applied by performing averaging across subjects. Another option is power-spectral analysis of grand average, in which adaptive digital filtering of grand average is performed.

2.5. Changes in EEG and ERO by means of some examples

2.5.1. Power spectral analysis of spontaneous EEG

Power spectral analysis of EEG spontaneous activity is one of the most successfully applied methods in the search for biomarkers (see Vecchio et al., 2013, this volume). Fig. 4 represents the grand averages of power spectra of 18 healthy (indicated by black line) and 18 bipolar euthymic subjects (red line) in the alpha frequency range for the eyes-closed spontaneous EEG recording session for occipital locations (O_1, O_z, and O_2). As seen from Fig. 4, within the alpha frequency range, the power spectrum of healthy subjects reaches up to 4.8 μV^2 for O_1, 4 μV^2 for O_z, and 4.5 μV^2 for O_2 electrodes, while that of euthymic subjects reaches up to 1 μV^2 for all occipital electrodes.

Event-related spectra of bipolar patients in the alpha frequency range are also drastically reduced, as recently shown by Başar et al. (2012b). Only the prominent decrease of alpha power illustrated in Fig. 4 could possibly serve as a neurophysiological marker in BD. Additionally, the disappearance of event-related theta power in BD may also be a relevant change; this will be explained in the next sections.

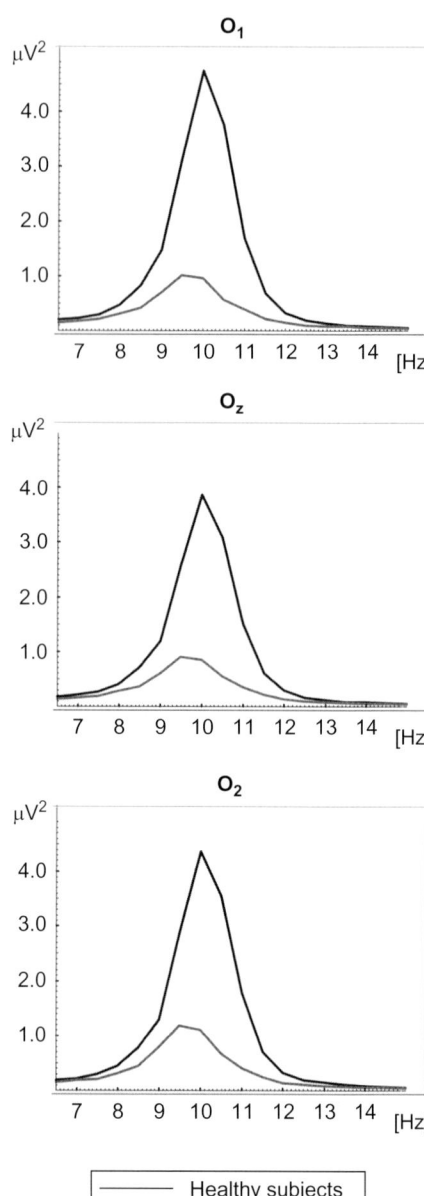

Fig. 4. Mean eyes-closed power values for occipital electrodes (modified from Başar et al., 2012b). (For color figures, please refer to the color figures in last section of the book.)

2.5.2. Analysis of evoked and event-related spectra

As seen in Fig. 5, in the grand average of post-stimulus power spectrum upon stimulation of

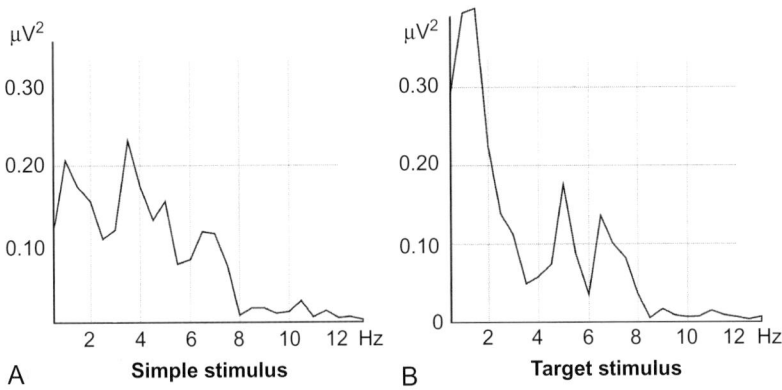

Fig. 5. Grand average of power spectra of auditory evoked (A) and event-related responses (B) over left frontal (F$_3$) location. Target stimuli (B) create increased amplitudes than simple sensory stimuli (A) in the delta frequency range in healthy subjects.

target stimuli, two different theta frequency peaks were detected in the healthy control group, in the 0.5–15 Hz frequency range for both slow theta (4–6 Hz) and fast theta (6–8 Hz). Adaptive digital filtering was applied to these identified frequency ranges. Adaptive filtering of the response provides a major advantage that subsystems of the system might be selectively removed to obtain isolation. Isolation of the filters separately may lead to choosing the amplitude and frequency characteristics of the filters. Ideal filters may be applied without phase shifts. In addition, the method also allows the definition of filters with exact characteristics and regulating them adequately according to the amplitude characteristics of the system (for further information, see Başar, 2004). Doppelmayr et al. (1998) and Dumont et al. (1999) also suggested that narrow-band filtered analyses may be more informative for obtaining task specific parameters of the responses.

Accordingly, each subject's averaged evoked and ERPs were digitally filtered in slow theta (4–6 Hz) and fast theta (6–8 Hz) frequency ranges. The maximum peak-to-peak amplitudes for each subject's averaged slow theta (4–6 Hz) and fast theta (6–8 Hz) responses were analyzed; that is, the largest peak-to-peak value in these frequency ranges in terms of μVs found in the time window between 0 and 500 ms.

The event-related (target) response shows a highly increased delta response (1.5 Hz) in comparison to sensory evoked delta. It is of further interest that two different responses are recorded upon simple auditory versus target stimuli in healthy subjects: slow theta (4 Hz) and fast theta (7 Hz).

It is important to note that the delta response to sensory stimulation is not high as event-related delta response. Changes are markedly higher upon cognitive load. This is most possibly because in healthy subjects and patients, the sensory–cognitive stimulation activates a larger number of neural populations in comparison to the effect of pure sensory stimulation. Further, it is important to analyze the changes in two different windows: the selection of digital filters in the conventional 4–7 Hz filter limits could lead to crucial information lost in this example.

2.5.3. Differentiated changes of theta responses in BD

Evoked and event-related slow and fast theta oscillations in response to auditory stimuli were studied in 22 euthymic, drug-free patients with BD.

Slow (4–6 Hz) and fast (6–8 Hz) theta responses behaved differently during oddball paradigm in

30

patients with BD. Fast theta responses (6–8 Hz) almost disappeared in euthymic BD patients (Atagün et al., 2011).

Application of digital filters in the analysis of neuropsychiatry patients requires refinement with the use of adaptive filters selected according to the cut-off frequency in power spectra rather than predefined filters in the conventional frequency ranges. Sometimes a peak is missed or shifted to other frequencies in patients; this is also especially the case following drug applications.

2.5.4. AD and MCI delta responses: frequency shift, amplitude decreases, and delays

In order to compare cognitive responses between healthy subjects and AD patients, a further study used a two-tone auditory oddball task. We confined our attention to the delta frequency range, as this frequency band shows major reduction in AD patients. Fig. 7 shows a comparative analysis of event-related power spectra computed by means of FFT applied to oddball target tones. Healthy subjects show a maximum around 2 Hz,

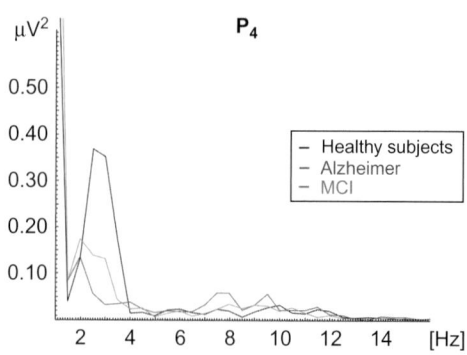

Healthy, Alzheimer, MCI
Auditory target power spectrum
(N=13)

Fig. 7. Event-related spectral analysis of healthy control subjects, mild cognitive impairment (MCI), and Alzheimer's disease (AD). (For color figures, please refer to the color figures in last section of the book.)

whereas in MCI and AD subjects the frequency of the response is decreased to approximately 1 Hz. These results can be immediately interpreted as a frequency slowing in MCI and AD patients during cognitive performance in comparison to healthy subjects.

According to the cut-off frequency (0.5–2.2 Hz) of the target responses, the transient target responses were analyzed in frontal and parietal locations with adaptive digital filters.

Fig. 8 illustrates adaptively filtered frontal and parietal EROs of healthy, MCI, and AD subjects in the delta frequency range. In all locations, delta responses of healthy subjects show peak-to-peak response amplitudes around 4–5 μV, whereas delta responses of MCI subjects have only the half value, at around 2 μV. Frontal and parietal delta responses of AD patients were extremely low. A delay in peak delta ERO response and a gradual decrease in amplitude of delta ERO response across healthy control subjects, MCI, and AD patients can be noted. This delay is much more pronounced in parietal locations.

A decrease in delta response is also observed in euthymic bipolar patients (Fig. 6) and in schizophrenia in measurements upon inputs with cognitive task.

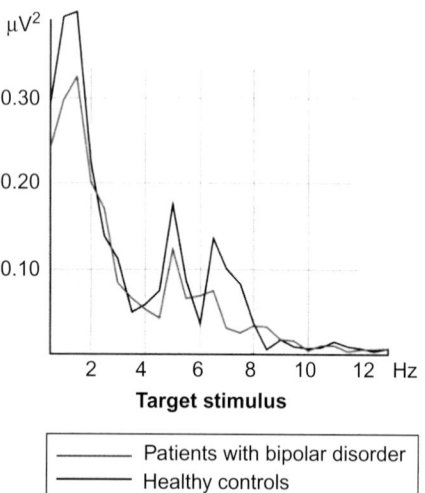

Fig. 6. Grand average of power spectra of auditory event-related responses over left frontal (F₃) location in bipolar disorder subjects and healthy controls upon auditory oddball stimulation (modified from Özerdem et al., 2013, this volume). (For color figures, please refer to the color figures in last section of the book.)

Auditory event-related delta (0.5–2.2 Hz) responses (*N*=13)

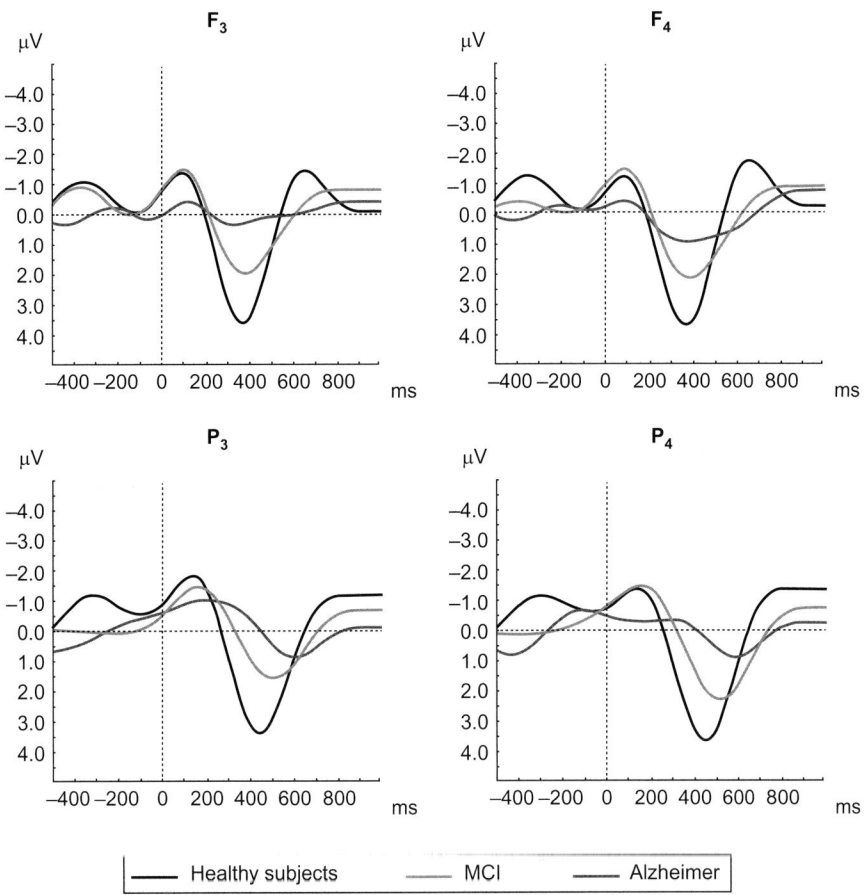

Fig. 8. MCI and AD continuity is prominent in auditory event-related delta oscillatory activity. Results show grad-ually decreasing delta amplitude and increasing delta peak latency among healthy elderly subjects, MCI, and mild-stage Alzheimer subjects (MCI: mild cognitive impairment, AD: Alzheimer's disease). (For color figures, please refer to the color figures in last section of the book.)

For AD, there are specific biomarker methods related to structural changes in the CNS. Those methods are described by Lovestone (2009), Vecchio et al. (2013, this volume), and Yener and Başar (2013a, this volume).

2.6. Selective connectivity deficit

There are several connections between different structures of the brain. The connectivity that can be measured by means of coherence function in

healthy subjects is well defined, whereas patients in whom some given brain substructures are ana-tomically or physiologically disrupted display def-icit in selective connectivity.

An important brain mechanism underlying cog-nitive processes is the exchange of information between brain areas (Güntekin et al., 2008; Başar et al., 2010). The oscillatory analyses of isolated brain areas alone are not sufficient to explain all aspects of information processing within the brain. Therefore, for a description of neurophysio-logical mechanisms underlying cognitive deficits

32

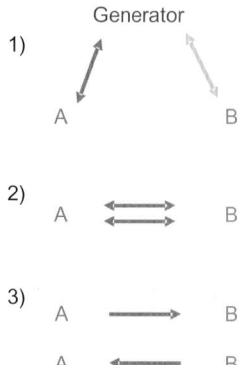

Fig. 9. A description of possible underlying mechanism of coherence between two structures (see text). (For color figures, please refer to the color figures in last section of the book.)

of neuropsychiatric diseases, connectivity dynamics between different brain areas must be investigated (Sharma et al., 2013, this volume; Yener and Başar, 2013a,b, this volume).

According to Bullock et al. (2003), increased coherence between two structures, namely A and B, can be caused by the following processes: (1) structures A and B are driven by the same generator; (2) structures A and B can mutually drive each other; (3) one of the structures, A or B, drives the other (Fig. 9).

In the following section, two examples of the selective connectivity deficit in AD and BD patients will be presented.

2.6.1. Decrease of event-related coherence in Alzheimer patients

Several research groups have already published a number of studies related to analysis of oscillatory dynamics in MCI and AD patients. Jelic et al. (2000), Babiloni et al. (2006, 2007, 2009), and Rossini et al. (2006) published core results on spontaneous EEG coherence in MCI patients. Hogan et al. (2003), Zheng-yan (2005), Yener et al. (2007, 2008, 2009), Güntekin et al. (2008), Dauwels et al. (2009), and Başar et al. (2010) published results on evoked/event-related coherence in AD patients. At this point, it is vital to

emphasize that there are important functional differences between "*EEG coherence*," "*evoked coherence*," and "*event-related coherence*." In the EEG analysis, only sporadically occurring coherences from hidden sources can be measured. Sensory evoked coherences reflect the property of sensory networks activated by a sensory stimulation. Event-related (or cognitive) coherences manifest coherent activity of sensory and cognitive networks triggered by a cognitive task. Accordingly, the cognitive response coherences comprise activation of a greater number of neural networks that are most possibly not activated, or less activated, in the EEG and sensory evoked coherences. Therefore, event-related coherence merits special attention. Particularly in AD patients with strong cognitive impairment, it is relevant to analyze whether medical treatment (drug application) selectively acts upon sensory and cognitive networks manifested in topologically different areas and in different frequency windows. Such an observation may provide, in future, a deeper understanding of the physiology of distributed functional networks and, in turn, the possibility of determination of biomarkers for medical treatment.

Başar et al. (2010) compared visual sensory evoked and event-related coherences of patients with Alzheimer-type dementia (AD). A total of 38 mild, probable AD subjects (19 untreated, 19 treated with cholinesterase inhibitors) were compared with a group of 19 healthy controls. The sensory evoked coherence and event-related target coherences were analyzed for all frequency ranges for long-range intra-hemispheric (F_3-P_3, F_4-P_4, F_3-T_5, F_4-T_6, F_3-O_1, F_4-O_2) electrode pairs. The healthy control group showed significantly higher values of event-related coherence in "*delta*," "*theta*," and "*alpha*" bands in comparison to the de novo and medicated AD groups upon application of target stimuli. In contrast, almost no changes in event-related coherences were observed in beta and gamma frequency bands. Furthermore, almost no differences were recorded between healthy and AD groups upon application of simple light stimuli. Besides this, coherence values upon application of target stimuli were higher than sensory evoked coherence in all groups and in all frequency bands ($p < 0.01$). These results give the hints for the preserved visual-sensory network in contrast to damaged visual cognitive network in mild AD.

Fig. 10 illustrates the histogram of mean Z values for delta frequency range upon application of "simple light" stimuli for all electrode pairs. Fig. 11 provides a histogram of mean Z values for delta frequency range upon application of "target" stimuli for all electrode pairs. In both figures, red bars represent the mean Z values for healthy subjects, whereas green bars represent untreated AD subjects, and blue bars represent treated AD subjects. Fig. 11 shows that the healthy subjects had higher delta response coherence compared to both untreated and treated AD subjects upon application of target stimuli for all electrode pairs. The mean Z value of healthy subjects is 40–50% higher than AD patients in most of the electrode pairs upon application of "target" stimuli. Fig. 10 shows that the evoked delta coherence

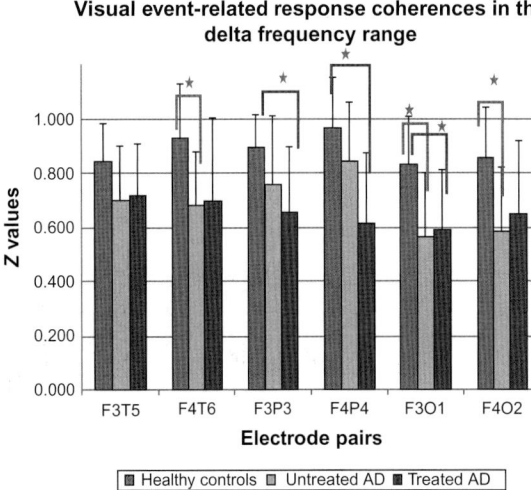

Fig. 11. Mean Z values of healthy control, treated AD, and untreated AD subjects for delta frequency range upon target stimuli. "*" sign represents $p < 0.01$ (modified from Başar et al., 2010). (For color figures, please refer to the color figures in last section of the book.)

upon "simple light" is not as high and almost no difference was recorded between healthy controls and AD subjects except for slightly lower F_3-O_1 delta sensory evoked coherence in AD.

Fig. 12 shows no difference in mean Z values for theta frequency range upon application of "simple light" stimuli for all electrode pairs between healthy controls and AD subjects. Fig. 13 shows mean Z values for theta frequency range upon application of "target" stimuli for all electrode pairs. Both figures show the mean Z values for healthy subjects (red bars), untreated AD subjects (green bars), and treated AD subjects (blue bars). Fig. 13 shows that the healthy subjects had higher theta response coherence compared to both untreated and treated AD subjects upon application of target stimuli for all electrode pairs. The mean Z value of healthy subjects is 30–40% higher than AD patients in most of the electrode pairs upon application of "target" stimuli. As Fig. 12 illustrates, the mean Z values upon application of simple light are between 0.3 and 0.48, while upon application of "target stimuli" the mean Z values increase to 0.9. Comparison of Figs 12 and 13

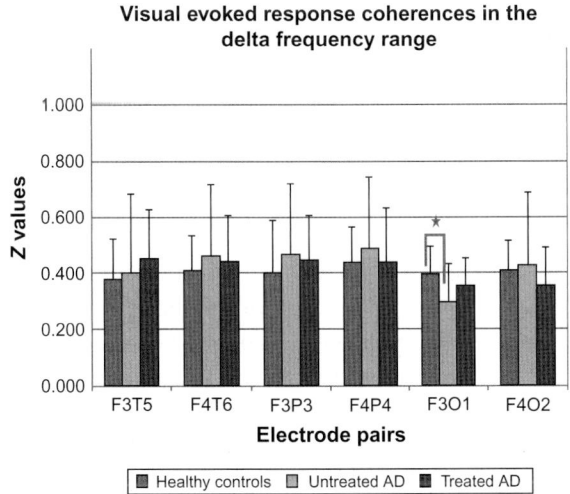

Fig. 10. Mean Z values of healthy control, treated AD, and untreated AD subjects for delta frequency range upon simple light stimuli. "*" sign represents $p < 0.01$ (modified from Başar et al., 2010). (For color figures, please refer to the color figures in last section of the book.)

34

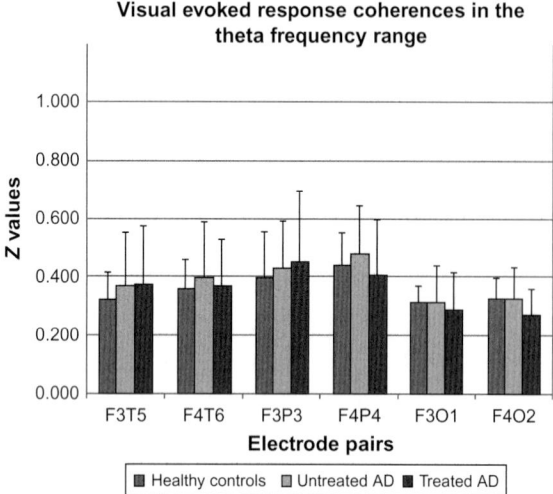

Visual evoked response coherences in the theta frequency range

Z values

Electrode pairs

■ Healthy controls ☐ Untreated AD ■ Treated AD

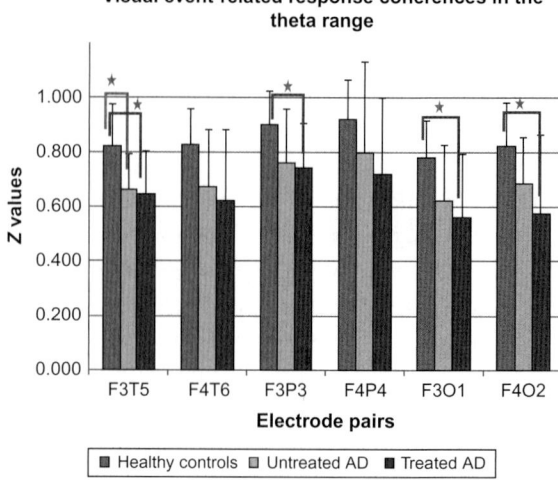

Visual event-related response coherences in the theta range

Z values

Electrode pairs

■ Healthy controls ☐ Untreated AD ■ Treated AD

Fig. 12. Mean Z values of healthy control, treated AD, and untreated AD subjects for theta frequency range upon simple light stimuli (modified from Başar et al., 2010). (For color figures, please refer to the color figures in last section of the book.)

Fig. 13. Mean Z values of healthy control, treated AD, and untreated AD subjects for theta frequency range upon target stimuli. "*" sign represents $p < 0.01$ (modified from Başar et al., 2010). (For color figures, please refer to the color figures in last section of the book.)

shows that the sensory evoked theta coherence upon "simple light" is not as high as event-related coherence and no difference was recorded between healthy controls and AD subjects.

The results show evidence for the existence of separate sensory and cognitive networks that are activated either on sensory or cognitive stimulation. The cognitive networks of AD patients were highly impaired in comparison to networks activated by sensory stimulation. Accordingly, analysis of coherences upon cognitive load may serve, in future, as a biomarker in diagnostics of AD patients (see also Yener and Başar, 2013a, this volume).

2.6.2. Decrease of event-related gamma coherence in euthymic bipolar patients

Özerdem et al. (2011) studied the cortico-cortical connectivity by examining sensory evoked coherence and event-related coherence values for the gamma frequency band during simple light stimulation and visual oddball paradigm in euthymic

drug-free patients. The study group consisted of 20 drug-free euthymic bipolar patients and 20 sex- and age-matched healthy controls. Groups were compared for the coherence values of the left (F_3-T_3, F_3-TP_7, F_3-P_3, F_3-O_1) and right (F_4-T_4, F_4-TP_8, F_4-P_4, F_4-O_2) intra-hemispheric electrode pairs and showed significantly diminished bilateral long-distance gamma coherence between frontal and temporal as well as between frontal and temporo-parietal regions compared to healthy controls.

However, no significant reduction in sensory evoked coherence was recorded in the patient group compared to the healthy controls. The decrease in event-related coherence differed topologically and ranged between 29% (right fronto-temporal location) and 44% (left fronto-temporo-parietal location). Fig. 14A and B depicts the grand average of visual event-related coherence in gamma frequency (28–48 Hz) band in response to target stimuli between the right (F_4-T_8) and left (F_3-T_7) fronto-temporal electrode pairs in euthymic bipolar patients ($n = 20$) compared with healthy controls ($n = 20$) (Özerdem et al., 2011).

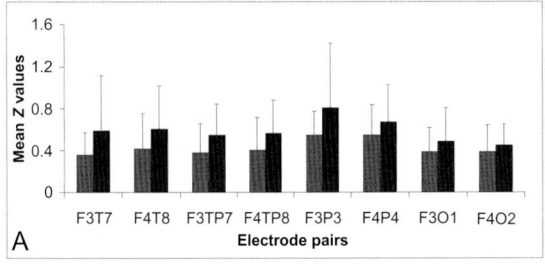

Event-related gamma (28–48 Hz) coherence in response to simple sensory stimuli

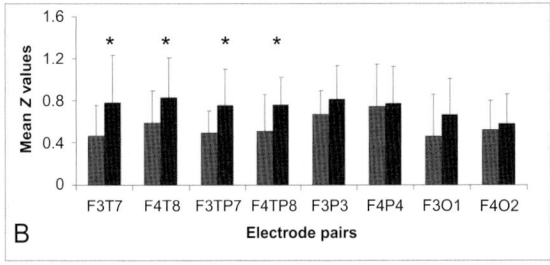

Event-related gamma (28–48 Hz) coherence in response to target stimuli

■ Euthymic bipolar patients
■ Healthy controls

Fig. 14. Mean Z values for sensory evoked (A) and target (B) coherence in response to visual stimuli at all electrode pairs. "*" sign represents $p < 0.05$ (modified from Özerdem et al., 2011). (For color figures, please refer to the color figures in last section of the book.)

Oscillatory responses to both target and non-target stimuli are manifestations of working memory (WM) processes. Therefore, the coherence decrease in response to both types of stimuli indicates inadequate connectivity between different parts of the brain during a cognitive process, in comparison to pure sensory signal processing.

2.7. Event-related delta, theta, and gamma oscillations in schizophrenia patients during N-back working memory tasks

A more differentiated visual event-related response paradigm in comparison to a simple oddball paradigm was applied to healthy subjects and schizophrenia patients by Schmiedt et al. (2005)

and Başar-Eroğlu et al. (2007). The authors used the paradigm derived from classic N-back tasks under varying WM load. It consisted of three tasks: a simple choice reaction task (serving as a control), easy WM task (1-back), and hard WM (2-back) task.

Fig. 15 shows grand-average ERPs and the corresponding event-related gamma oscillations during the three tasks in patients and controls. In healthy subjects, the gamma amplitude increased gradually from control task to hard WM task. The event-related gamma activity significantly differed between tasks, indicating higher gamma amplitude values during the hard WM task compared to the control task. The ERPs were not filtered in the delta frequency range. However, the strong contribution of delta component to the ERPs is easily seen. The WM tasks usually trigger large delta responses in healthy subjects. Such large delta responses are not observed in schizophrenia patients upon WM tasks. The reduced theta responses in all three tasks and at all locations in patients were also reported (Schmiedt et al., 2005). In contrast, the gamma activity was higher in schizophrenia patients than in healthy subjects and remained constant regardless of task demand.

These results show increases of evoked and induced gamma, since enhanced gamma activities can be observed in both pre- and poststimulus time windows. This modulation of gamma activity seems to be related to increased cognitive load (Fig. 16, lower panel). The results in healthy subjects further suggest a task-related allocation of attentional processes with increased WM load. In contrast, the patients did not show a modulation of gamma activity with varying task demands. Accordingly, these results could be interpreted as a consequence of impairment in focused attention. Another possible interpretation is that higher gamma activity in patients could be related to cortical hyper-excitability, as suggested by Eichhammer et al. (2004) and Spencer et al. (2004).

Most studies on auditory steady-state evoked gamma responses showed reduced gamma response

36

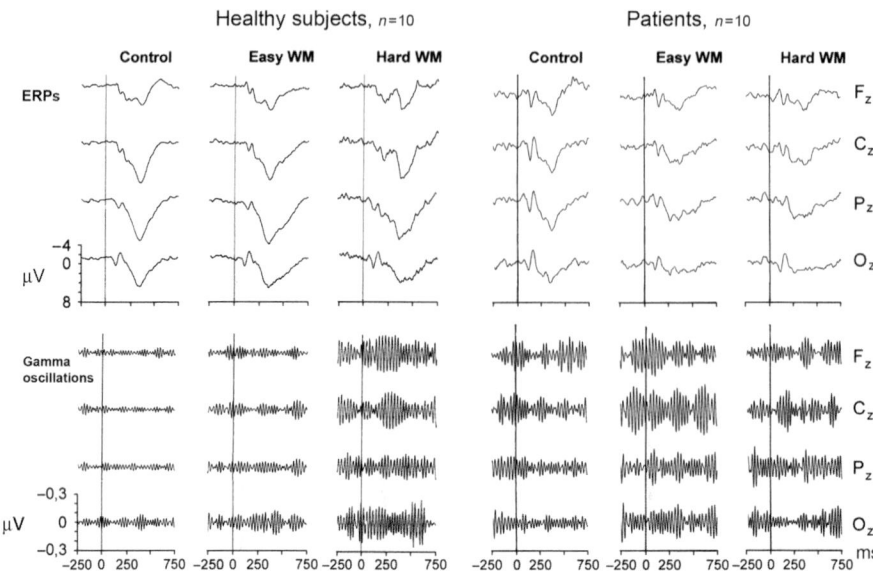

Fig. 15. Grand-average event-related oscillations (ERPs) in healthy controls (left upper panel) and in schizophrenia patients (right upper panel) during N-back tasks under varying working memory (WM) demands. $T = 0$ represents the stimulus onset. Lower panel shows grand-average gamma activities corresponding to the upper panel (modified from Başar-Eroğlu et al., 2007).

oscillations in schizophrenia patients compared to healthy controls. To our knowledge, there is only one study in which previous findings of reduced steady-state gamma band synchronization in schizophrenic patients were not directly replicated (Hong et al., 2004). On the other hand, event-related gamma responses in schizophrenia patients in comparison to healthy subjects show contradictory results in cognitive paradigms. In auditory oddball paradigms, previous authors mostly evaluated event-related gamma responses in two different time windows (early and late time window). Some studies showed that early evoked gamma band responses did not show significant group differences. However, schizophrenic patients showed reduced evoked gamma band responses in late latency range stimuli (Haig et al., 2000; Gallinat et al., 2004). Other studies (Lee et al., 2001; Slewa-Younan et al., 2004; Symond et al., 2005; Lenz et al., 2010) reported that schizophrenia subjects showed lower early-gamma phase synchrony compared to healthy subjects. Some recent studies reported increased

gamma response in schizophrenic subjects compared to healthy controls upon application of an auditory paradigm. Başar-Eroğlu et al. (2011) reported that passive listening to stimuli was related to increased single-trial gamma power at frontal sites. Flynn et al. (2008) reported that, in first-episode patients, gamma phase synchrony was generally increased during auditory oddball task processing, especially over left centro-temporal sites in the 800 ms post-stimulus time window. Further research is needed to make robust conclusions on gamma response in auditory oddball paradigm in schizophrenia.

2.8. Analysis of drug/neurotransmitter application

The following two examples show how drug applications significantly influence event-related (and/or evoked) brain oscillations.

A special responsiveness of the frontal lobe in the theta frequency range has been demonstrated in a time prediction task in humans (Başar-Eroğlu

Pre-stimulus gamma RMS-values

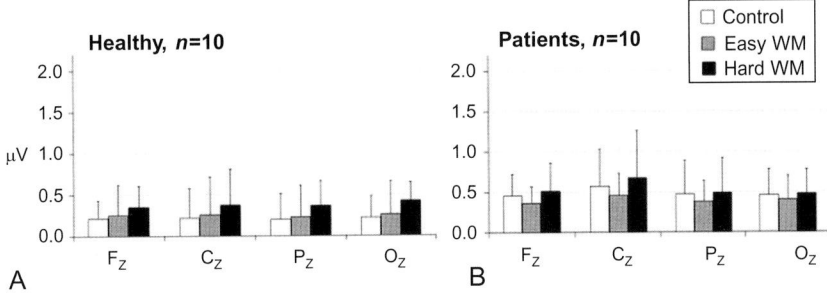

Post-stimulus gamma max. amplitude

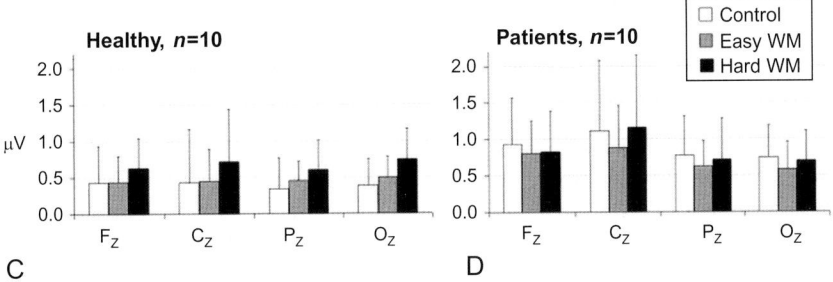

Fig. 16.   Upper panel represents pre-stimulus RMS gamma values in healthy subjects and in schizophrenia patients in the three tasks. Lower panel shows post-stimulus maximal gamma amplitudes (modified from Başar-Eroğlu et al., 2007).

et al., 1992) and in a paradigm with regular omitted stimuli in cats (Demiralp et al., 1994). In these studies, the theta responsiveness in frontal lobes was interpreted as an indication of the function of the hippocampal–fronto-parietal system during cognitive processes.

2.8.1. Application of cholinergic drugs in AD patients

Phase-locked and non-phase-locked activity. Non-phase-locked activities contain evoked oscillations that are not rigidly time locked to the moment of stimulus delivery. These are, for example, induced alpha, beta, gamma, etc., oscillations that may relate to specific aspects of information processing. In the framework of the additive model of EPs, non-phase-locked activity includes the background EEG. For analysis of only non-phase-locked or both phase-locked and non-phase-locked EEG responses, specific approaches have been used. Phase-locked activity is suggested to include all types of event-related brain potentials. For quantification of the phase-locked activity, the averaging procedure is usually applied, whereby the phase-locked responses are enhanced and the non-phase-locked ones are attenuated.

Yener et al. (2007) investigated the phase locking of visual event-related theta oscillations in frontal locations in two groups of AD and elderly controls. It was hypothesized that the non-treated AD would show weaker phase locking of theta oscillations than both controls and the AD group treated with acetylcholine esterase inhibitors (AChEIs). The results indicated that, at the F_3 location, the non-treated AD patients had a weaker theta response than both the control and treated AD groups. This result was related to the reduced phase locking in this group (Figs. 17 and 18). Moreover,

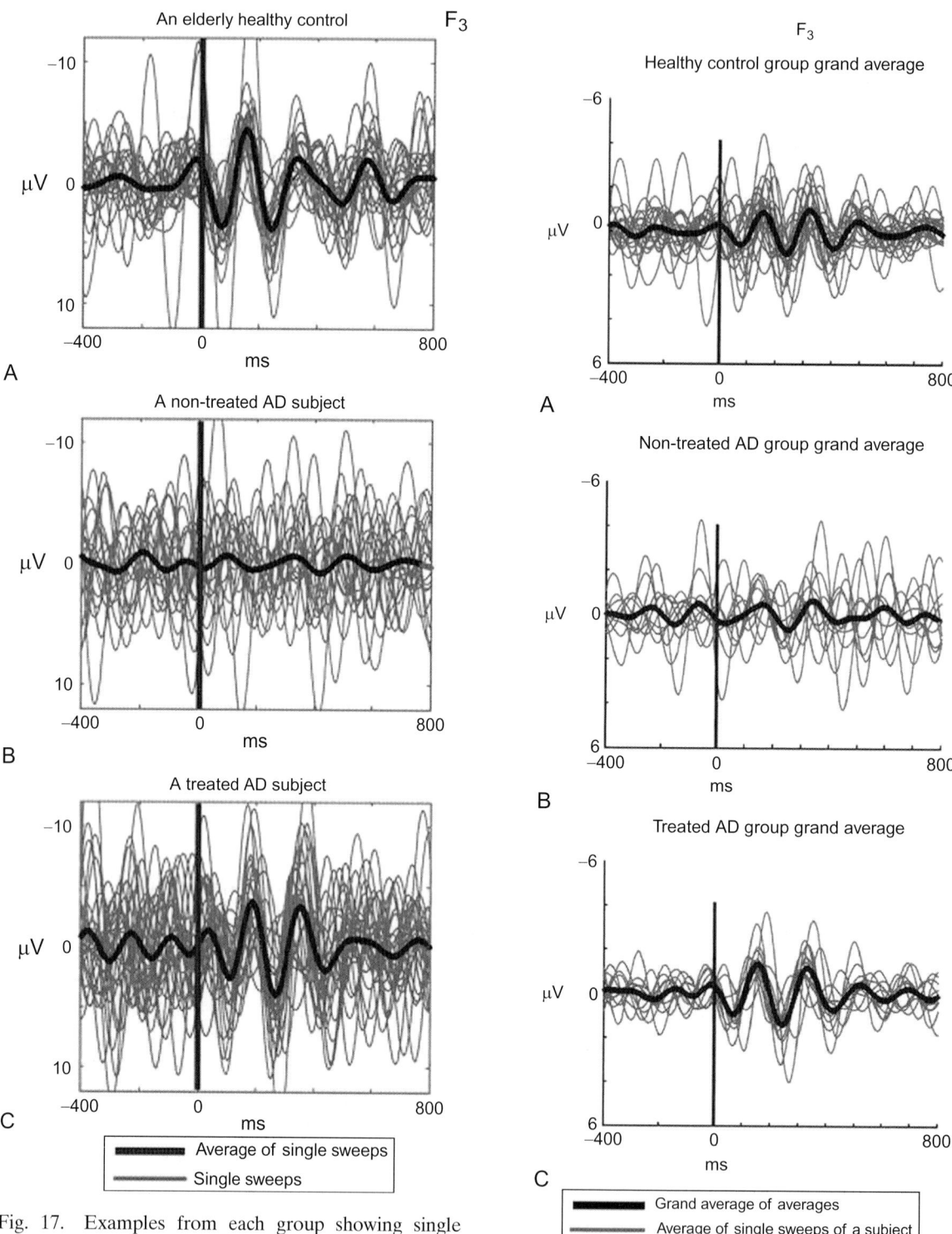

Fig. 17. Examples from each group showing single sweeps to the target stimuli elicited by a classical visual oddball paradigm recorded from F_3 scalp electrode. The thick black line indicates the average of single sweeps, and the thin gray lines show each single sweep for the subject. (A) An elderly healthy control. (B) A non-treated Alzheimer subject. (C) A treated (cholinesterase inhibitor) Alzheimer subject (modified from Yener et al., 2007).

Fig. 18. Decreased visual event-related theta phase locking in AD. The thick black line represents the grand-average response of each group to the target stimuli elicited by a classical visual oddball paradigm and the thin gray and thin lines show averages of single sweeps from each subject (modified from Yener et al., 2007).

cholinergically treated AD group and healthy control did not differ from each other.

There are several methods to analyze the changes in phase locking (for further reading, see Tallon-Baudry et al., 1996; Yordanova and Kolev, 1997, 1998; Herrmann et al., 1999; Ergen et al., 2008; Vinck et al., 2011).

2.8.2. Application of lithium in BD patients

In a study by Özerdem et al. (2013, this volume) both drug-free euthymic patients and patients on lithium monotherapy had higher beta responses compared to healthy controls. However, the responses from the lithium-treated patients were significantly higher than both drug-free patients and healthy controls. Fig. 19 depicts grand averages of event-related beta responses in left (F_3) and right (F_4) frontal electrode sites in (from top to bottom) healthy controls, euthymic drug-free patients, and patients under lithium monotherapy.

Lithium is known to have a neuroprotective effect through changes in the activity of pro- and anti-apoptotic proteins (Machado-Vieira et al., 2009). This finding is important from the point of view that these are lithium-responsive patients and this lithium sensitivity of beta responses may be of crucial importance in tracking treatment response in patients with BD.

2.9. How to present ensembles of neurophysiological markers describing cognitive deficits and connectivity deficits

EEG analysis only measures sporadically occurring coherences from hidden sources. Sensory evoked coherences reflect the degree of connectivity (links) between sensory networks activated only by a sensory stimulation. Event-related (or cognitive) coherences manifest coherent activity of sensory–cognitive networks triggered by a cognitive task. Accordingly, the cognitive response coherences comprise activation of a greater number of neural networks that are most possibly not activated or less activated in the EEG or in pure sensory evoked coherences (see papers by Yener and Başar, 2013a,b, this volume). Therefore, *event-related coherences* and EROs merit special attention for analysis of results from patients with cognitive impairment. In particular, in AD patients with strong cognitive impairment, it is relevant to analyze whether medical treatment (drug application) selectively acts upon sensory and cognitive networks manifested in topologically different places and in different frequency windows. Such an observation may serve to increase understanding in physiology of distributed functional networks and, in turn, the possibility of determining markers for medical treatment.

Although each individual oscillatory finding presented in different diseases in the present report can serve as a candidate biomarker, we recommend that these electrophysiological markers should not be used separately. Instead, a constellation of these electrophysiological markers should be considered as being more appropriate for diagnostic and response-tracking purposes in cognitive deficits. This approach can provide a more solid basis for application of oscillatory assessments and a substantial reduction in potential errors when assessing diagnosis and medication response. Table 2 describes the possibilities to apply methods of oscillatory analysis in post-stimulus responses and the ensemble of significant results. Table 3 provides a similar overview of biomarkers in BD. In these tables, sub-frequency (i.e., alpha 1, alpha 2, theta 1, theta 2) groups are not yet included. We expect that at least four or five additional candidate biomarkers may be discovered in future studies applying these methods. Table 4 provides a similar overview of candidate biomarkers in schizophrenia upon application of auditory sensory and auditory oddball paradigms. For more detailed information see Başar and Güntekin (2013, this volume). Spontaneous EEG alpha activity was found to be lower in schizophrenia by several groups (Itil et al., 1972, 1974; Iacono, 1982; Miyauchi et al., 1990; Sponheim et al., 1994, 2000; Alfimova and Uvarova, 2008).

40

Visual event-related beta responses grand averages
target
Healthy subjects

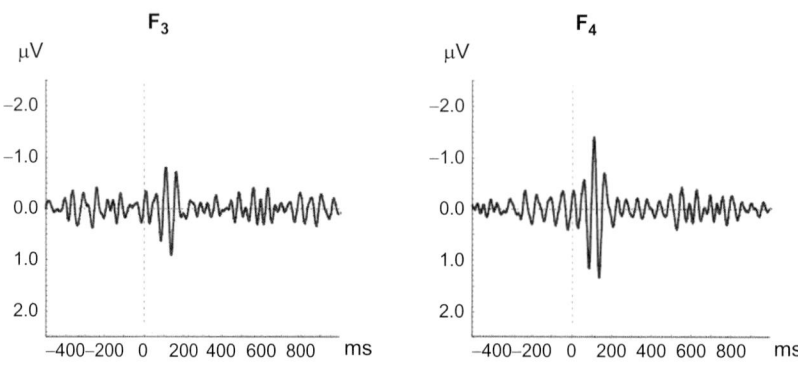

Drug-free euthymic patients

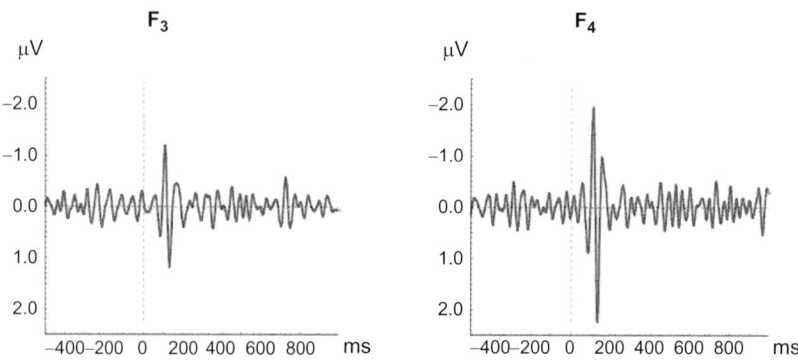

Lithium-treated euthymic patients

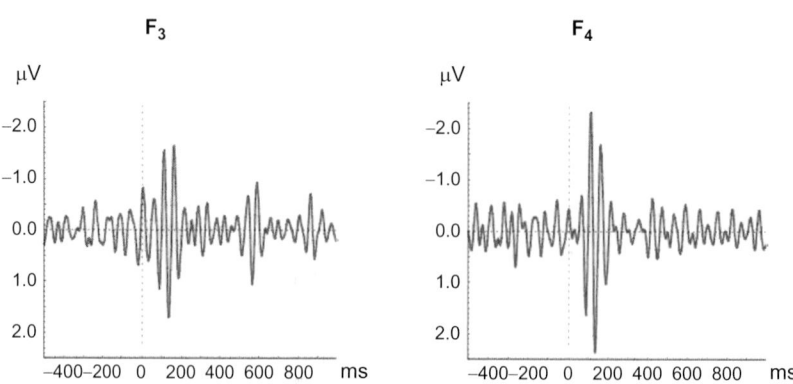

Fig. 19. Grand averages of event-related beta responses in left (F₃) and right (F₄) frontal electrode sites in (from top to bottom) healthy controls, euthymic drug-free patients, and in euthymic patients under lithium monotherapy (modified from Özerdem et al., 2013, this volume). (For color figures, please refer to the color figures in last section of the book.)

TABLE 2

OVERVIEW OF STUDIES ON ELECTROPHYSIOLOGICAL BIOMARKER CANDIDATES IN MCI OR AD

Frequency	Power spectrum			Evoked oscillations	Event-related oscillations	Phase locking	Coherence	Evoked coherence	Event-related coherence
	Spontaneous EEG	Evoked power	Event-related power				EEG coherence		
Delta	↑	↑ ↔	↓↓	↔ (Yener et al., 2009, visual sensory)	↓ (Yener et al., 2008, visual oddball; Yener et al., 2012, auditory oddball)		↑ Delta coherence in progressive MCI (Rossini et al., 2006)	↔ (Except F$_3$O$_1$ delta decrease) (Başar et al., 2010, visual oddball)	↓ (Güntekin et al., 2008, visual oddball; Başar et al., 2010)
Theta	↑		↓	↑ (Yener et al., 2009, visual sensory)	↔ (Yener et al., 2008, visual oddball)	↓↑ (Yener et al., 2007, visual oddball)		↔ (Başar et al., 2010, visual oddball)	↓ (Güntekin et al., 2008, visual oddball; Başar et al., 2010)
Alpha	↓			↔ (Yener et al., 2009, visual sensory)	↔ (Yener et al., 2008, visual oddball)		↓ α1 Coherence in MCI (Babiloni et al., 2010). ↓ α Coherence in AD (Jelic et al., 2000; Knott et al., 2000; Adler et al., 2003)	↔ (Başar et al., 2010, visual oddball)	↓↑ (Güntekin et al., 2008, visual oddball; Başar et al., 2010)
Beta	↓			↔ (Yener et al., 2009, visual sensory)	↔ (Yener et al., 2008, visual oddball)			↔ (Başar et al., 2010, visual oddball)	↔ (Güntekin et al., 2008, visual oddball; Başar et al., 2010)
Gamma				↔ (Yener et al., 2009, visual sensory)	↔ (Yener et al., 2008, visual oddball)		↑ Gamma coherence in progressive MCI (Rossini et al., 2006)	↔ (Başar et al., 2010, visual oddball)	↔ (Güntekin et al., 2008, visual oddball; Başar et al., 2010)

Blue arrows represent the difference between unmedicated AD patients and healthy controls; red arrows represent the medicated AD patients. Empty cells remain to be analyzed. (For interpretation of the references to color in this table legend, the reader is referred to the color plates in the last section of this book.)

TABLE 3

OVERVIEW OF STUDIES ON ELECTROPHYSIOLOGICAL BIOMARKER CANDIDATES IN BIPOLAR DISORDERS

Frequency	Power spectrum			Evoked oscillations	Event-related oscillations	Phase locking	Coherence		
	EEG	Evoked power	Event-related power				EEG coherence	Evoked coherence	Event-related coherence
Delta									
Fast theta			↓ Atagün et al., 2011, auditory oddball						
Alpha	↓ Clementz et al., 1994; Başar et al., 2012b				↓ Özerdem et al., 2008, manic BD, visual oddball				
Beta	↑↑ Başar et al., 2012a				↑ Özerdem et al., 2008, manic BD visual oddball				
Gamma								↔ Özerdem et al., 2010, visual sensory	↓ Özerdem et al., 2010, visual oddball

Blue arrows represent unmedicated bipolar manic and euthymic patients. Green arrows show bipolar patients medicated with lithium. Empty cells have not yet been analyzed. (For interpretation of the references to color in this table legend, the reader is referred to the color plates last section of this book.)

TABLE 4

OVERVIEW OF STUDIES ON ELECTROPHYSIOLOGICAL BIOMARKER CANDIDATES IN SCHIZOPHRENIA

Frequency	Power spectrum			Filtered evoked oscillations	Filtered event-related oscillations	Phase locking	Coherence		
	EEG	Evoked power	Event-related power				EEG coherence	Evoked coherence	Event-related coherence
Delta						↓ Ford et al. 2008; Doege et al., 2010(a)			
Theta						↓ Ford et al. 2008; Doege et al., 2010(a)			
Alpha	↓								↓ Koh et al. 2011 (inter-trial phase coherence)
Beta									
Gamma	↔ Gallinat et al., 2004; Spencer et al., 2008		↓ Lee et al., 2001; Gallinat et al., 2004; Hall et al., 2011 ↑ Başar-Eroğlu et al., 2011, single trail evoked power		↓ Haig et al., 2000	↓ Slewa-Youman et al., 2004; Symond et al. 2005 (decreased frontal. Lee et al., 2003; Roach and Mathalon, 2008) ↑ increased posterior syncrony (Lee et al., 2003)			

(For interpretation of the reference to color in this table legend, the reader is referred to the color plates last section of this book.)

Similar summaries of spontaneous EEG activity must also be included in order to present a complete overview of the oscillatory manifestation of the disease under study. We also mention that Tables 2–4 serve as examples; similar tables should also be prepared for other diseases.

There are many results combining various analysis methods in all EEG frequency windows that are relevant to the search for biomarkers. These tables describe at least 45 combinations, indicating the potential discovery and/or comparative analysis of at least 5–10 biomarkers for each pathology.

2.10. Highlights for neurophysiological explorations in diagnostics, drug application, and progressive monitoring of diseases

In the following parts, we bring together strategies, methods, and their short results in order to provide a synopsis and proposals for efficient analysis of cognitive impairment.

(1) The procedure of EEG (and/or MEG) oscillations allows measurement of brain dynamics related to changes in perception, memory, learning, and attention within a very short time window of 0–500 ms. With applications of the brain imaging methods illustrated in Fig. 2, or with the application of structural biomarkers described by Yener and Başar (2013a,b, this volume), it is not possible to compare function-related alterations (especially cognitive functions) between healthy subjects and patients.

(2) EEG/MEG procedures are inexpensive and noninvasive.

(3) The importance of analyzing spontaneous EEG is explained, with numerous examples, by Vecchio et al., Yener and Başar (a), Başar and Güntekin (all 2013, this volume).

2.10.1. Multiple oscillations

The present report clearly demonstrates that it is obligatory to apply the method of oscillations in multiple EEG frequency windows in the search for functional biomarkers and to detect the effects of drug applications (see Tables 2–4).

2.10.2. Selectively distributed oscillatory networks

Again, according to the summary of results for AD, schizophrenia, and BD patients in Tables 2–4, recordings should be analyzed for multiple oscillations and at selectively distributed sites, rather than at one location.

2.10.3. Selective connectivity

Selective connectivity between selectively distributed neural networks has to be computed by means of spatial coherence. It is necessary to compare EROs (triggered by stimulations including a cognitive load) with sensory evoked oscillations (see Tables 2–4). These results show that, in AD and bipolar groups, EROs show more prominent changes in comparison to simple sensory evoked oscillations. Moreover, event-related spatial coherences in AD and bipolar patients also show considerably more differentiation than simple sensory evoked coherences.

2.10.4. Importance of temporal coherence

It is suggested that such integrative brain functions combine the actions of multiple oscillations and are a necessity for temporal coherence of perceptions and actions (Başar, 2006). The basis for these mechanisms lies in the resonance properties of cortical networks, i.e., the tendency to engage in oscillatory activity (e.g., Başar et al., 2001a,b; Buszáki and Draguhn, 2004; Başar, 2008).

2.10.5. Phase locking

Phase-locked activity is suggested to include all types of event-related brain potentials. The averaging procedure is usually applied to quantify the phase-locked activity, whereby the phase-locked responses are enhanced and non-phase-locked ones are attenuated. An example of phase-locking deficits in AD patients and the restoration of phase locking is demonstrated in Section 8 and Figs. 17 and 18.

Frequency shift and delay can be also indicators of cognitive impairment as, explained in Fig. 8, indicating reduced delta frequency response.

It is recommended to standardize the causality of pre-stimulus activity for considering ERD as a cognitive biomarker (see Appendix).

Steady-state responses (SSRs) may be used as markers; however, they are less efficient since patients cannot be analyzed upon a cognitive load. A study by Capilla et al. (2011) provides evidence that visual SSRs can be explained as a superposition of transient ERPs: these findings have critical implications in the current understanding of brain oscillations. Contrary to the idea that neural networks can be tuned to a wide range of frequencies, the findings of these authors rather suggest that the oscillatory response of a given neural network is constrained within its natural frequency range.

Most analyses of cognitive impairment are in the gamma frequency band, especially in schizophrenia. Steady-state responses, which do not encompass a cognitive paradigm, elicit decreased gamma responses, whereas oddball paradigm evokes greatly variable gamma responses.

Cognitive tasks with progressively increasing difficulty open the way to interpreting various brain functions or insights into differentiated cognitive deficits, as shown in Fig. 15.

(a) The superposition of decreased delta activity and enhanced gamma activity in schizophrenic patients indicates the necessity of analyzing multiple oscillations in tasks with progressive increase of difficulty. Further, application of different tasks enables the interpretation of multiple functions, such as increased attention and short-term memory.

(b) Through the use of tasks with progressive increase of difficulty, it was possible to indicate that the oscillatory components (here gamma) are not decreased in diseases, and that enhancements are also observed as the increase of spontaneous delta (Vecchio et al., 2013, this volume).

(c) Similarly, the work of Karakaş et al. (2000b) notably applied easy and difficult oddball tasks to healthy subjects. This application can be useful in measuring differentiability during progression of diseases, for example, to analyze the progression between MCI and AD.

(1) *Beta increases* are observed in BD patients, accompanied by a major decrease of alpha. The increase of beta in BD indicates, again, that enhancements can be also observed in diseases.

(2) *Application of drugs/neurotransmitters* gains new implications with the analysis of oscillations and coherences. Better differentiated analysis of drug effects can be achieved by conventional wide-band EP and ERP applications (see Section 8).

(3) *The efficiency of assemblies of neurophysiological markers* in describing diseases and biomarkers is clearly emphasized in Tables 2–4. According to Giovanni Frisoni, Michael Koch, and Dean Salisbury, in the panel described by Yener and Başar (2013b, this volume), neurophysiological markers are not only useful for diagnosis of a specific disease but also for tracking the disease, differential diagnosis, monitoring the effects of drug therapy, and identifying subtypes.

Therefore, in designing a strategy for diagnostics, differential diagnostics, application of (preventive) drugs, and neurophysiological information should be analyzed within a framework incorporating multiple methods and multiple frequency bands, as shown in Tables 2 and 3.

The interpretation of results in AD, schizophrenia, and BD becomes most efficient by joint analysis of results on oscillatory responses and coherences obtained by means of *cognitive tasks*.

Finally, we can conclude that the highlight for exploration of brain oscillations as biomarkers in pathology is based on two important fundaments:

(a) The innate interwoven, multifold mechanisms that constitute "whole brain work" (see Section 2) are highly affected and modulated by diseases. Accordingly, methods for identifying biomarkers should be tailored according to relevant changes within the ensemble of innate mechanisms and should not rely only on single, specific mechanisms.

(b) It is evident that such strategies must be derived from observation of pathological changes such as frequency shifts, delays, abolishment or changes of some oscillatory responses, and deficits of connectivity. These pathological changes are often structural and also due to changes in biochemical pathways or changes in release of neurotransmitters. Therefore, the use of neurophysiological markers is also useful in monitoring drug application and drug development.

(c) It is also almost imperative to compute *evoked* or *event-related power spectra* before deciding on the application of adaptive digital filters. Depending on the type of cognitive tasks, event-related spectra can show modification in frequency windows of ERO. Most critical is the choice of frequency windows in cognitive impairment. Patients can show highly altered frequency windows or frequency shifts. The choice of rigid filters in conventional EEG bands can lead to errors.

In this final part of the chapter, the outlined strategies, methods, and conclusions are based on experiences from our research group, related to AD, BD, and schizophrenia. Although the results and conclusions of our group were presented in a wide spectrum, we want to emphasize that research groups should tailor further frameworks to present ensemble of results leading to biomarkers. The present paper is intended to emphasize that the search for biomarkers is complicated; therefore, such work must encompass all possible combinations derived from the applications of multiple oscillatory frequencies by means of multiple methods. The search for biomarkers is certainly not limited to the content presented above and it is hoped that, other groups could further develop this type of analysis.

2.11. Appendix

Can event-related desynchronization be considered as a cognitive marker?

2.11.1. Further remarks related to the role of alpha in cognitive processes

The theories presented by Squire (1992), Baddeley et al. (1995), Fuster (1995, 1997), and Goldman-Rakic (1996) clearly explain the role of inborn phyletic memory (iconic, echoic) and, also, that memory states are not separable from basic brain functions. Besides remembering, memory functioning also comprehends processes of sensation, perception, and learning. Accordingly, memory theories manifested in brain oscillations could not be considered as pure top-down processes; bottom-up processes do occur in parallel or as serial processing. Sensory alpha responses in human have been described by several authors, starting with Başar (1972, 1980), Spekreijse and Van der Tweel (1972), and Başar et al. (1975a–c). In terms of the most fundamental findings, Dudkin et al. (1978) and Dinse et al. (1997) described visual evoked oscillations at the cellular level; the 10-Hz responses demonstrated by these authors were triggered by pure light signals and did not include cognitive tasks. The association of alpha activity with working memory was described by Başar and Stampfer (1985). More comprehensive and detailed studies of brain oscillations and memory were presented, in a long series of papers, by the Klimesch group, emphasizing differences between good and bad memory performers.

Recently, Klimesch et al. (2007) launched a hypothesis related to the "inhibition timing in alpha oscillations," which suggested that the event-related alpha response can be described solely in terms of suppression or event-related synchronization.

However, the alpha sensory and event-related responses were first described by Adrian (1941) and Bishop et al. (1953), who measured alpha responses upon pure sensory stimulation. In contrast, Klimesch et al. (1993, 1997) and Klimesch (1996) claimed that the vast majority of experiments correlates alpha with cognitive performance. These authors also indicate that, under certain conditions, alpha responds reliably, with an increase in amplitudes (event-related synchronization or ERS).

Several authors supported the hypothesis of Klimesch and co-workers. However, there are also fundamental critics of the inhibition theory. Knyazev et al. (2006) explained the essential shortcomings as follows: "The idea of inhibitory function for alpha synchronization is appealing but it raises some doubts. First, it is not clear how the same mechanism might be linked with perceptual activation, as in the case of phase-locked evoked alpha oscillations described by Başar (1998, 1999), and perceptual inhibition (as proposed for event-related alpha synchronization, ERS). Further, if ERS served a function of selective attention (e.g., inhibition of non-task-relevant perception), one would expect that relatively small cortical areas within a task-relevant zone would show ERD, whereas larger cortical areas, which are not related to the task processing, would show ERS; actually the opposite applies. Alpha ERD is usually more pronounced and widespread during first presentations of a signal or a task is stronger during more complex tasks compared to the relatively simple ones (Neubauer et al., 1999). All these observations are difficult to reconcile with the idea of lateral inhibition as a function of ERS."

Knyazev et al. (2006) further indicated the relevance of background activity: Extensive studies by Brandt and Jansen (1991), Başar (1998, 1999), Barry et al. (2000), and other authors accumulated considerable evidence that different reactions of EEG bands could be observed, depending on background activity. According to the concept demonstrated by several authors, the ongoing EEG determines (controls) evoked activity.

Compared to the abundance of experiments dealing with alpha power measurements, relatively few studies focused on task-related shifts in alpha frequency. The experiments by Osaka (1984) showed that, only for difficult but not for easy tasks, alpha frequency increases selectively in the hemisphere that is dominant for a particular task.

The review by Ward (2003) summarized the recent evidence that synchronous neural oscillations reveal much about the origin and nature of cognitive processes such as memory, attention, and consciousness, and that memory processes are most closely related to theta and gamma rhythms, whereas attention seems closely associated with alpha and gamma rhythms. These conclusions are not in accordance with the fundamental views of Fuster (1995, 1997), Baddeley (1996), Desimone (1996), and Goldman-Rakic (1996), who demonstrated that processes of memory and attention are inseparable. This discordance is also evident in the "time inhibition hypothesis" (Klimesch et al., 2007), that omitted the important relationship between pre-stimulus activity and ERO in that model. As already stated by Rémond and Lesèvre (1967) and Walter (1950), there are several mechanisms underlying the spontaneous alpha activity and evoked/event-related alpha oscillations; according to Rémond and Lesèvre (1967), the phase angle of the alpha oscillations at the time of the stimulus plays a crucial role in the generation of evoked alpha response.

We have started a new pilot study (as yet unpublished), analyzing the qualitative and quantitative behavior of alpha activity and alpha responsiveness. Besides the phase angle described by Rémond and Lesèvre (1967), five different types of alpha process were detected in pre-stimulus alpha and post-stimulus alpha sweeps in the analysis of 17 subjects (-500 ms pre-stimulus/ $+500$ ms post-stimulus alpha).

In all subjects we have encountered five different groups in the pre-stimulus–post-stimulus epochs:
(1) EEG–EP sweeps showing alpha phase locking and enhancement.
(2) EEG–EP sweeps showing alpha blocking and no phase locking following stimulation.
(3) EEG–EP sweeps showing only phase locking upon stimulus onset.

48

Evoked potential visual alpha (8–13Hz) blocked sweeps (*N*=1)

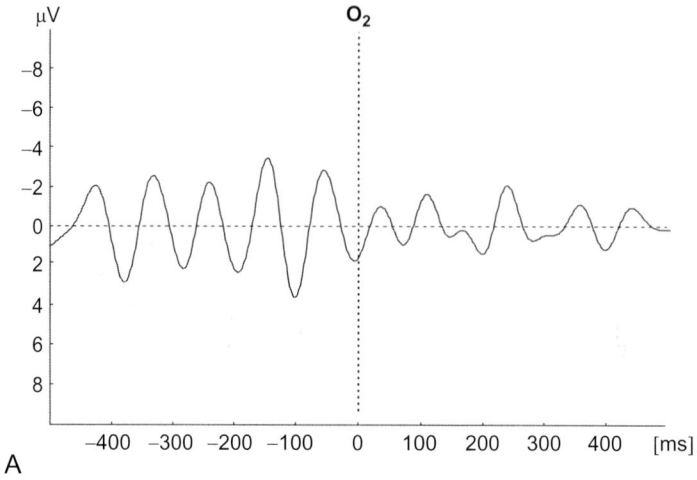

A

Evoked potential visual alpha (8–13Hz) enhanced sweeps (*N*=1)

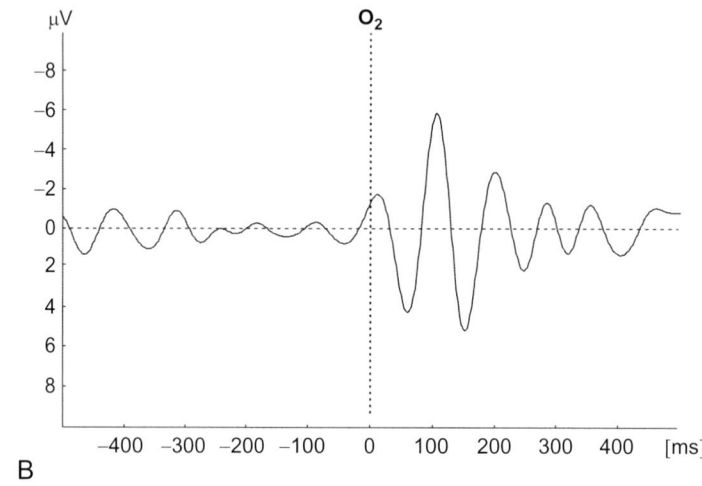

B

Fig. A1.   Alpha blocking (A) and enhanced alpha (B) in a single subject.

(4) EEG–EP sweeps showing no enhancement and no phase locking.
(5) EEG–EP sweeps showing time locking (induced responses).

According to the above grouping of single EEG–ERP records, we have performed averaging of selected EEG–EP ensembles for each subject and further grand average of 17 subjects.

Fig. A1 shows two selective ensembles for a typical subject in which alpha blocking (A) and alpha enhancement (B) have been recorded. It is clearly seen that pre-stimulus alpha activity is high in the case of alpha blocking (ERD), whereas enhanced (ERS) is recorded only when the post-stimulus alpha activity is low.

The grand average from 17 subjects in Fig. A2 confirms the results of a typical single subject. The evaluation of five different types of responsiveness is currently in progress. The existence of these five different alpha responsiveness processes

Evoked potential visual alpha (8–13Hz) blocked sweeps (N=17)

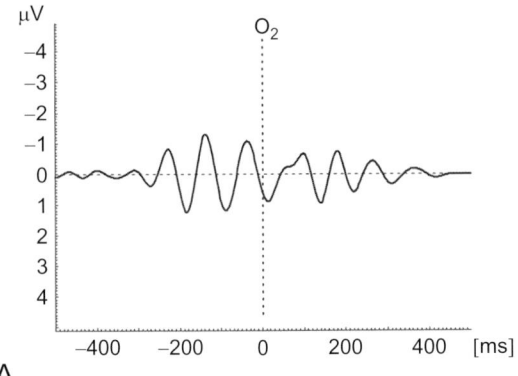

A

Evoked potential visual alpha (8–13Hz) enhanced sweeps (N=17)

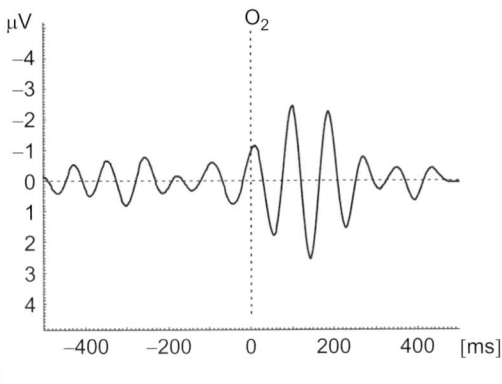

B

Fig. A2. Alpha blocking (A) and enhanced alpha (B) in a grand average of 17 subjects.

is encountered in all subjects. However, the distribution shows significant variability between subjects. A comprehensive analysis of this matter will be presented in a future publication.

According to the results of this appendix, it is recommended to standardize the causality of pre-stimulus activity before considering ERD as cognitive biomarker.

Abbreviations

ACh = acetylcholine
AChEI = acetylcholine esterase inhibitor
AD = Alzheimer's disease
AFC = amplitude frequency characteristic
BD = bipolar disorder
CNS = central nervous system
EEG = electroencephalography
EROs = event-related oscillations
ERPs = event-related potentials
FFT = Fast Fourier Transform
fMRI = functional magnetic resonance imaging
MCI = mild cognitive impairment
MEG = magnetoencephalography
MEF = magnetic evoked field
MRI = magnetic resonance imaging
PET = positron emission tomography
PLF = phase-locking factor
TMS = transcranial magnetic stimulation
WM = working memory

Acknowledgments

The authors are thankful to Elif Tülay and Pınar Kurt for arranging the reference list and overall error finding throughout.

References

Adey, W.R. (1966) Neurophysiological correlates of information transaction and storage in brain tissue. In: E. Stellar and J.M. Sprague (Eds.), *Progress in Physiological Psychology*. Academic Press, New York, pp. 1–43.

Adey, W.R. (1989) Cell membranes, electromagnetic fields, and intercellular communication. In: E. Başar and T.H. Bullock (Eds.), *Brain Dynamics: Progress and Perspectives*. Springer, Berlin, pp. 26–42.

Adey, W.R., Dunlop, C.W. and Hendrix, C.E. (1960) Hippocampal slow waves. Distribution and phase relationships in the course of approach learning. *Arch. Neurol. (Chic.)*, 3: 74–90.

Adler, G., Brassen, S. and Jajcevic, A. (2003) EEG coherence in Alzheimer's dementia. *J. Neural. Transm.*, 110: 1051–1058.

Adrian, E.D. (1941) Afferent discharges to the cerebral cortex from peripheral sense organs. *J. Physiol. (Lond.)*, 100: 159–191.

Alfimova, M.V. and Uvarova, L.G. (2008) Changes in EEG spectral power on perception of neutral and emotional words in patients with schizophrenia, their relatives, and healthy subjects from the general population. *Neurosci. Behav. Physiol.*, 38: 533–540.

Atagün, İ., Özerdemm, A., Güntekin, B. and Başar, E. (2011) Evoked and event related theta oscillations are decreased in drug-free euthymic bipolar patients. In: *Society of Biological*

Psychiatry, 66th Annual Meeting, 12–14 May 2011. Hyatt Regency, San Francisco, CA, Abstract Book, p.: 97S.

Babiloni, C., Visser, P.J., Frisoni, G., De Deyn, P.P., Bresciani, L., Jelic, V., Nagels, G., Rodriguez, G., Rossini, P.M., Vecchio, F., Colombo, D., Verhey, F., Wahlund, L.O. and Nobili, F. (1996) Cortical sources of resting EEG rhythms in mild cognitive impairment and subjective memory complaint. *Neurobiol. Aging*, 31: 1787–1798.

Babiloni, C., Frisoni, G., Steriade, M., Bresciani, L., Binetti, G., Del Percio, C., Geroldi, C., Miniussi, C., Nobili, F., Rodriguez, G., Zappasodi, F., Carfagna, T. and Rossini, P.M. (2006) Frontal white matter volume and delta EEG sources negatively correlate in awake subjects with mild cognitive impairment and Alzheimer's disease. *Clin. Neurophysiol.*, 117(5): 1113–1129.

Babiloni, C., Cassetta, E., Binetti, G., Tombini, M., Del Percio, C., Ferreri, F., Ferri, R., Frisoni, G., Lanuzza, B., Nobili, F., Parisi, L., Rodriguez, G., Frigerio, L., Gurzì, M., Prestia, A., Vernieri, F., Eusebi, F. and Rossini, P.M. (2007) Resting EEG sources correlate with attentional span in mild cognitive impairment and Alzheimer's disease. *Eur. J. Neurosci.*, 25(12): 3742–3757.

Babiloni, C., Ferri, R., Binetti, G., Vecchio, F., Frisoni, G.B., Lanuzza, B., Miniussi, C., Nobili, F., Rodriguez, G., Rundo, F., Cassarino, A., Infarinato, F., Cassetta, E., Salinari, S., Eusebi, F. and Rossini, P.M. (2009) Directionality of EEG synchronization in Alzheimer's disease subjects. *Neurobiol. Aging*, 30(1): 93–102.

Babiloni, C., Visser, P.J., Frisoni, G., De Deyn, P.P., Bresciani, L., Jelic, V., Nagels, G., Rodriguez, G., Rossini, P.M., Vecchio, F., Colombo, D., Verhey, F., Wahlund, L.O. and Nobili, F. (2010) Cortical sources of resting EEG rhythms in mild cognitive impairment and subjective memory complaint. *Neurobiol. Aging*, 31: 1787–1798.

Baddeley, A. (1996) The fractionation of working memory. *Proc. Natl. Acad. Sci. USA*, 93: 13468–13472.

Baddeley, A., Wilson, B.A. and Watts, F.N. (1995) *Handbook of Memory Disorders.* Wiley, New York.

Barry, R.J., Kirkaikul, S. and Hodder, D. (2000) EEG alpha activity and the ERP to target stimuli in an auditory oddball paradigm. *Int. J. Psychophysiol.*, 39: 39–50.

Barry, R.J., De Pascalis, V., Hodder, D., Clarke, A.R. and Johnstone, S.J. (2003) Preferred EEG brain states at stimulus onset in a fixed interstimulus interval auditory oddball task and their effects on ERP components. *Int. J. Psychophysiol.*, 47(3): 187–198.

Başar, E. (1972) A study of the time and frequency characteristics of the potentials evoked in the acoustical cortex. *Kybernetik*, 10: 61–66.

Başar, E. (1980) *EEG–Brain Dynamics. Relation between EEG and Brain Evoked Potentials.* Elsevier, Amsterdam.

Başar, E. (1983a) Toward a physical approach to integrative physiology. I. Brain dynamics and physical causality. *Am. J. Physiol.*, 14: R510–R533.

Başar, E. (1983b) Synergetics of neuronal populations. A survey on experiments. In: E. Başar, H. Flohr, H. Haken and A. Mandell (Eds.), *Synergetics of the Brain.* Springer, Berlin, pp. 183–200.

Başar, E. (1990) *Chaos in Brain Function.* Springer, Berlin.

Başar, E. (1998) *Brain Oscillations I. Principles and Approaches.* Springer, Heidelberg.

Başar, E. (1999) *Brain Function and Oscillations. II. Integrative Brain Function. Neurophysiology and Cognitive Processes.* Springer, Heidelberg.

Başar, E. (2004) *Memory and Brain Dynamics: Oscillations Integrating Attention, Perception Learning and Memory.* CRC Press, Boca Raton, FL.

Başar, E. (2006) The theory of the whole-brain work. *Int. J. Psychophysiol.*, 60(2): 133–138.

Başar, E. (2008) Oscillations in "brain–body–mind": a holistic view including the autonomous system. *Brain Res.*, 1235: 2–11.

Başar, E. (2011) *Brain–Body–Mind in the Nebulous Cartesian System: A Holistic Approach by Oscillations.* Springer, Heidelberg.

Başar, E. and Bullock, T.H. (1992) *Induced Rhythms in the Brain.* Birkhäuser, Boston, MA.

Başar, E. and Güntekin, B. (2013) Review of delta, theta, alpha, beta and gamma response oscillations in neuropsychiatric disorders. *Suppl. Clin. Neurophysiol.*, Vol. 62, Ch. 2, this volume.

Başar, E. and Stampfer, H.G. (1985) Important associations among EEG-dynamics, event-related potentials, short-term memory and learning. *Int. J. Neurosci.*, 26(3–4): 161–180.

Başar, E., Gönder, A., Özesmi, C. and Ungan, P. (1975a) Dynamics of brain rhythmic and evoked potentials I. Some computational methods for the analysis of electrical signals from the brain. *Biol. Cybern.*, 20: 137–143.

Başar, E., Gönder, A., Özesmi, C. and Ungan, P. (1975b) Dynamics of brain rhythmic and evoked potentials. II. Studies in the auditory pathway, reticular formation, and hippocampus during the waking stage. *Biol. Cybern.*, 20: 145–160.

Başar, E., Gönder, A., Özesmi, C. and Ungan, P. (1975c) Dynamics of brain rhythmic and evoked potentials. III. Studies in the auditory pathway, reticular formation, and hippocampus during sleep. *Biol. Cybern.*, 20: 161–169.

Başar, E., Dössel, O., Fuchs, M., Rahn, E., Saermark, K. and Schürmann, M. (1992) Evoked alpha responses from frontal-temporal areas in multichannel SQUID systems. In: *Proceedings of IEEE Symposium on Neuroscience and Technology*, Lyon, pp. 28–33.

Başar, E., Başar-Eroğlu, C., Karakaş, S. and Schürmann, M. (1999a) Are cognitive processes manifested in event-related gamma, alpha, theta and delta oscillations in the EEG? *Neurosci. Lett.*, 15: 165–168.

Başar, E., Başar-Eroğlu, C., Karakaş, S. and Schürmann, M. (1999b) Oscillatory brain theory: a new trend in neuroscience. The role of oscillatory processes in sensory and cognitive functions. *IEEE Eng. Med. Biol.*, 18(3): 56–66.

Başar, E., Demiralp, T., Schürmann, M., Başar-Eroğlu, C. and Ademoğlu, A. (1999c) Oscillatory brain dynamics, wavelet analysis and cognition. *Brain Lang.*, 66: 146–183.

Başar, E., Başar-Eroğlu, C., Karakaş, S. and Schürmann, M. (2000) Brain oscillations in perception and memory. *Int. J. Psychophysiol.*, 35(2–3): 95–124.

Başar, E., Başar-Eroğlu, C., Karakaş, S. and Schürmann, M. (2001a) Gamma, alpha, delta, and theta oscillations govern cognitive processes. *Int. J. Psychophysiol.*, 39(2–3): 241–248.

Başar, E., Özgören, M. and Karakaş, S. (2001b) A brain theory based on neural assemblies and superbinding. In: H. Reuter, P. Schwab and K.D. Gniech (Eds.), *Wahrnehmen und Erkennen*. PABST Science Publishers, Lengerich, pp. 11–24.

Başar, E., Schürmann, M. and Sakowitz, O. (2001c) The selectively distributed theta system: functions. *Int. J. Psychophysiol.*, 39: 197–212.

Başar, E., Özgören, M., Başar-Eroğlu, C. and Karakas, S. (2003) Superbinding: spatio-temporal oscillatory dynamics. *Theory Biosci.*, 121: 370–385.

Başar, E., Güntekin, B., Tülay, E. and Yener, G.G. (2010) Evoked and event-related coherence of Alzheimer patients manifest differentiation of sensory-cognitive networks. *Brain Res.*, 1357: 79–90.

Başar, E., Tülay, E., Özerdem, A., Atagün, I. and Güntekin, B. (2012a) Decrease of alpha/beta ratio in EEG activity in drug free euthymic bipolar patients. In: *Society of Biological Psychiatry, 67th Annual Meeting, 3–5 May, 2012*. Philadelphia, PA.

Başar, E., Güntekin, B., Atagün, I., Turp-Gölbaşı, B., Tülay, E. and Özerdem, A. (2012b) Brain's alpha activity is highly reduced in euthymic bipolar disorder patients. *Cogn. Neurodyn.*, 6: 11–20.

Başar-Eroğlu, C., Başar, E., Demiralp, T. and Schürmann, M. (1992) P300-response: possible psychophysiological correlates in delta and theta frequency channels. A review. *Int. J. Psychophysiol.*, 13(2): 161–179.

Başar-Eroğlu, C., Brand, A., Hildebrandt, H., Karolina Kedzior, K., Mathes, B. and Schmiedt, C. (2007) Working memory related gamma oscillations in schizophrenia patients. *Int. J. Psychophysiol.*, 64(1): 39–45.

Başar-Eroğlu, C., Mathes, B., Brand, A. and Schmiedt-Fehr, C. (2011) Occipital γ response to auditory stimulation in patients with schizophrenia. *Int. J. Psychophysiol.*, 79(1): 3–8.

Bishop, P.O., Jeremy, D. and McLeod, J.G. (1953) Phenomenon of repetitive firing in lateral geniculate of cat. *J. Neurophysiol.*, 16: 443–447.

Brandt, M.E. and Jansen, B.H. (1991) The relationship between prestimulus alpha amplitude and visual evoked potential amplitude. *Int. J. Neurosci.*, 61: 261–268.

Bruns, A. (2004) Fourier-, Hilbert- and wavelet-based signal analysis: are they really different approaches? *J. Neurosci. Meth.*, 137: 321–332.

Bullock, T.H., McClune, M.C. and Enright, J.T. (2003) Are the electroencephalograms mainly rhythmic? Assessment of periodicity in wide-band time series. *Neuroscience*, 121(1): 233–252.

Buszáki, G. (2006) *Rhythms of the Brain*. Oxford University Press, New York.

Buszáki, G. and Draguhn, A. (2004) Neuronal oscillations in cortical networks. *Science*, 304(5679): 1926–1929.

Capilla, A., Pazo-Alvarez, P., Darriba, A., Campo, P. and Gross, J. (2011) Steady-state visual evoked potentials can be explained by temporal superposition of transient event-related responses. *PLoS One*, 6(1): e14543.

Chen, A.C. and Herrmann, C.S. (2001) Perception of pain coincides with the spatial expansion of electroencephalographic dynamics in human subjects. *Neurosci. Lett.*, 297: 183–186.

Clementz, B.A., Sponheim, S.R. and Iacono, W.G. (1994) Resting EEG in first-episode schizophrenia patients, bipolar psychosis patients and their first degree relatives. *Psychophysiology*, 31: 486–494.

Damasio, A.R. and Damasio, H. (1994) Cortical systems for retrieval of concrete knowledge: the convergence zone framework. In: C. Koch and J.L. Davis (Eds.), *Large-Scale Neuronal Theories of the Brain*. MIT Press, Cambridge, MA, pp. 61–74.

Dauwels, J., Vialatte, F., Latchoumane, C., Jeong, J. and Cichocki, A. (2009) EEG synchrony analysis for early diagnosis of Alzheimer's disease: a study with several synchrony measures and EEG data sets. *Proc. IEEE Eng. Med. Biol. Soc.*, 2009: 2224–2227.

Demiralp, T., Başar-Eroğlu, C., Rahn, E. and Başar, E. (1994) Event-related theta rhythms in cat hippocampus and prefrontal cortex during an omitted stimulus paradigm. *Int. J. Psychophysiol.*, 18: 35–48.

Demiralp, T., Ademoglu, A., Schurmann, M., Başar-Eroğlu, C. and Başar, E. (1999) Detection of P300 in single trials by the wavelet transform (WT). *Brain Lang.*, 66: 108–128.

Desimone, R. (1996) Neural mechanisms for visual memory and their role in attention. *Proc. Natl. Acad. Sci. USA*, 26: 13494–13499.

Dinse, H.R., Krüger, K., Akhavan, A.C., Spengler, F., Schöner, G. and Schreiner, C.E. (1997) Low-frequency oscillations of visual, auditory and somatosensory cortical neurons evoked by sensory stimulation. *Int. J. Psychophysiol.*, 26: 205–227.

Doege, K., Jansen, M., Mallikarjun, P., Liddle, E.B. and Liddle, P.F. (2010a) How much does phase resetting contribute to event-related EEG abnormalities in schizophrenia? *Neurosci. Lett.*, 481(1): 1–5.

Doppelmayr, M., Klimesch, W., Pachinger, T. and Ripper, B. (1998) Individual differences in brain dynamics: important implications for the calculation of event-related band power measures. *Biol. Cybern.*, 79: 49–57.

Dudkin, K.N., Glezer, V.D., Gauselman, V.E. and Panin, A.I. (1978) Types of receptive fields in the lateral geniculate body and their functional model. *Biol. Cybern.*, 29: 37–47.

Dumont, M., Macchi, M.M., Carrier, J., Lafrance, C. and Hebert, M. (1999) Time course of narrow frequency bands in the waking EEG during sleep deprivation. *NeuroReport*, 10(2): 403–437.

Eccles, J.C. (1973) *The Understanding of the Brain*. McGraw Hill, New York.

Eckhorn, R., Bauer, R., Jordan, R., Brosch, W., Kruse, M., Munk, M. and Reitboeck, H.J. (1988) Coherent oscillations: a mechanism of feature linking in the visual cortex. *Biol. Cybern.*, 60: 121–130.

Eichhammer, P., Wiegand, R., Kharraz, A., Langguth, B., Binder, H. and Hajak, G. (2004) Cortical excitability in neuroleptic-naive first-episode schizophrenic patients. *Schizophr. Res.*, 67(2–3): 253–259.

Ergen, M., Marbach, S., Brand, A., Başar-Eroğlu, C. and Demiralp, T. (2008) P3 and delta band responses in visual oddball paradigm in schizophrenia. *Neurosci. Lett.*, 440(3): 304–308.

Flynn, G., Alexander, D., Harris, A., Whitford, T., Wong, W., Galletly, C., Silverstein, S., Gordon, E. and Williams, L.M.

52

(2008) Increased absolute magnitude of gamma synchrony in first-episode psychosis. *Schizophr. Res.*, 105(1–3): 262–271.

Ford, J.M., Roach, B.J., Hoffman, R.S. and Mathalon, D.H. (2008) The dependence of P300 amplitude on gamma synchrony breaks down in schizophrenia. *Brain Res.*, 1235: 133–142.

Freeman, W.J. (1999) Foreword. In: E. Başar (Ed.), *Brain Function and Oscillations. II. Integrative Brain Function. Neurophysiology and Cognitive Processes.* Springer, Berlin.

Fuster, J.M. (1995) *Memory in the Cerebral Cortex: An Empirical Approach to Neural Networks in the Human and Non-human Primate.* MIT Press, Cambridge, MA.

Fuster, J.M. (1997) Network memory. *Trends Neurosci.*, 20: 451–459.

Gallinat, J., Winterer, G., Herrmann, C.S. and Senkowski, D. (2004) Reduced oscillatory gamma-band responses in unmedicated schizophrenic patients indicate impaired frontal network processing. *Clin. Neurophysiol.*, 115(8): 1863–1874.

Goldman-Rakic, P.S. (1996) Regional and cellular fractionation of working memory. *Proc. Natl. Acad. Sci. USA*, 93: 13473–13480.

Gray, C.M. and Singer, W. (1989) Stimulus-specific neuronal oscillations in orientation columns of cat visual cortex. *Proc. Natl. Acad. Sci. USA*, 86: 1698–1702.

Gurtubay, I.G., Alegre, M., Labarga, A., Malanda, A. and Artieda, J. (2004) Gamma band responses to target and non-target auditory stimuli in humans. *Neurosci. Lett.*, 367(1): 6–9.

Güntekin, B. and Başar, E. (2010) A new interpretation of P300 responses upon analysis of coherences. *Cogn. Neurodyn.*, 4: 107–118.

Güntekin, B., Saatçi, E. and Yener, G. (2008) Decrease of evoked delta, theta and alpha coherence in Alzheimer patients during a visual oddball paradigm. *Brain Res.*, 1235: 109–116.

Haig, A.R., Gordon, E., De Pascalis, V., Meares, R.A., Bahramali, H. and Harris, A. (2000) Gamma activity in schizophrenia: evidence of impaired network binding? *Clin. Neurophysiol.*, 111(8): 1461–1468.

Hall, M.H., Taylor, G., Sham, P., Schulze, K., Rijsdijk, F., Picchioni, M., Toulopoulou, T., Ettinger, U., Bramon, E., Murray, R.M. and Salisbury, D.F. (2011) The early auditory gamma-band response is heritable and a putative endophenotype of schizophrenia. *Schizophr. Bull.*, 37: 778–787.

Herrmann, C.S., Mecklinger, A. and Pfeifer, E. (1999) Gamma responses and ERPs in a visual classification task. *Clin. Neurophysiol.*, 110(4): 636–642.

Hogan, M.J., Swanwick, G.R., Kaiser, J., Rowan, M. and Lawlor, B. (2003) Memory-related EEG power and coherence reductions in mild Alzheimer's disease. *Int. J. Psychophysiol.*, 49: 147–163.

Hong, L.E., Summerfelt, A., McMahon, R., Adami, H., Francis, G., Elliott, A., Buchanan, R.W. and Thaker, G.K. (2004) Evoked gamma band synchronization and the liability for schizophrenia. *Schizophr. Res.*, 70(2–3): 293–302.

Iacono, W.G. (1982) Bilateral electrodemal habituation–dishabituation and resting EEG in remitted schizophrenics. *J. Nerv. Ment. Dis.*, 170: 91–101.

Itil, T.M., Saletu, B. and Davis, S. (1972) EEG findings in chronic schizophrenics based on digital computer period analysis and analog power spectra. *Biol. Psychiatry*, 5: 1–13.

Itil, T.M., Saletu, B., Davis, S. and Allen, M. (1974) Stability studies in schizophrenics and normals using computer-analyzed EEG. *Biol. Psychiatry*, 8: 321–335.

Jansen, B.H., Zouridakis, G. and Brandt, M.E. (1993) A neurophysiologically based mathematical model of flash visual evoked potentials. *Biol. Cybern.*, 68(3): 275–283.

Jelic, V., Johansson, S.E., Almkvist, O., Shigeta, M., Julin, P., Nordberg, A., Winblad, B. and Wahlund, L.O. (2000) Quantitative electroencephalography in mild cognitive impairment: longitudinal changes and possible prediction of Alzheimer's disease. *Neurobiol. Aging*, 21(4): 533–540.

Karakaş, S., Erzengin, O.U. and Başar, E. (2000a) The genesis of human event related responses explained through the theory of oscillatory neural assemblies. *Neurosci. Lett.*, 285: 45–48.

Karakaş, S., Erzengin, O. and Başar, E. (2000b) A new strategy involving multiple cognitive paradigms demonstrates that ERP components are determined by the superposition of oscillatory responses. *Clin. Neurophysiol.*, 111: 1719–1732.

Karakaş, S., Karakaş, H. and Erzengin, O.U. (2002) Early sensory gamma represents the integration of bottom-up and top-down processing. *Int. J. Psychophysiol.*, 45: 39.

Karakaş, S., Bekçi, B. and Erzengin, O.U. (2003) Early gamma response in human neuroelectric activity is correlated with neuropsychological test scores. *Neurosci. Lett.*, 340(1): 37–40.

Klimesch, W. (1996) Memory processes, brain oscillations and EEG synchronization. *Int. J. Psychophysiol.*, 24(1–2): 61–100.

Klimesch, W., Schimke, H. and Pfurtscheller, G. (1993) Alpha frequency, cognitive load, and memory performance. *Brain Topogr.*, 5: 241–251.

Klimesch, W., Doppelmayr, M., Pachinger, T. and Ripper, B. (1997) Brain oscillations and human memory performance: EEG correlates in the upper alpha and theta bands. *Neurosci. Lett.*, 238: 9–12.

Klimesch, W., Doppelmayr, M., Röhm, D., Pöllhuber, D. and Stadler, W. (2000a) Simultaneous desynchronization and synchronization of different alpha responses in the human electroencephalograph: a neglected paradox? *Neurosci. Lett.*, 284: 97–100.

Klimesch, W., Doppelmayr, M., Schwaiger, J., Winkler, T. and Gruber, W. (2000b) Theta oscillations and the ERP old/new effect: independent phenomena? *Clin. Neurophysiol.*, 111: 781–793.

Klimesch, W., Sauseng, P., Hanslmayr, S., Gruber, W. and Freunberger, R. (2007) Event-related phase reorganization may explain evoked neural dynamics. *Neurosci. Biobehav. Rev.*, 31(7): 1003–1016.

Knott, V., Mohr, E., Mahoney, C. and Ilivitsky, V. (2000) Electroencephalographic coherence in Alzheimer's disease: comparisons with a control group and population norms. *J. Geriatr. Psychiatry Neurol.*, 13: 1–8.

Knyazev, G.G., Savostyanov, A.N. and Levin, E.A. (2006) Alpha synchronization and anxiety: implications for inhibition vs. alertness hypotheses. *Int. J. Psychophysiol.*, 59: 151–158.

Kocsis, B., Viana di Prisco, G. and Vertes, R.P. (2001) Theta synchronization in the limbic system: the role of Gudden's tegmental nuclei. *Eur. J. Neurosci.*, 13: 381–388.

Koh, Y., Shin, K.S., Kim, J.S., Choi, J.S., Kang, D.H., Jang, J.H., Cho, K.H., O'Donnell, B.F., Chung, C.K. and Kwon, J.S. (2011) An MEG study of alpha modulation in patients with schizophrenia and in subjects at high risk of developing psychosis. *Schizophr. Res.*, 126(1–3): 36–42.

Lee, Y.J., Zhu, Y.S., Xu, Y.H., Shen, M.F., Tong, S.B. and Thakor, N.V. (2001) The nonlinear dynamical analysis of the EEG in schizophrenia with temporal and spatial embedding dimension. *J. Med. Eng. Technol.*, 25(2): 79–83.

Lee, K.H., Williams, L.M., Haig, A. and Gordon, E. (2003) "Gamma (40 Hz) phase synchronicity" and symptom dimensions in schizophrenia. *Cogn. Neuropsychiatry*, 81: 57–71.

Lenz, D., Fischer, S., Schadow, J., Bogerts, B. and Herrmann, C.S. (2010) Altered evoked γ-band responses as a neurophysiological marker of schizophrenia? *Int. J. Psychophysiol.*, 79(1): 25–31.

Llinás, R.R. (1988) The intrinsic electrophysiological properties of mammalian neurons: insights into central nervous system function. *Science*, 242(4886): 1654–1664.

Lovestone, S. (2009) Biomarkers in brain disease. *Ann. NY Acad. Sci.*, 1180: 1–124.

Machado-Vieira, R., Manji, H.K. and Zarate, C.A., Jr. (2009) The role of lithium in the treatment of bipolar disorder: convergent evidence for neurotrophic effects as a unifying hypothesis. *Bipolar Disord.*, 11 (Suppl. 2): 92–109.

Miltner, W., Braun, C., Arnold, M., Witte, H. and Taub, E. (1999) Coherence of gamma-band EEG activity as a basis for associative learning. *Nature*, 397: 434–436.

Miyauchi, T., Tanaka, K., Hagimoto, H., Miura, T., Kishimoto, H. and Matsushita, M. (1990) Computerised EEG in schizophrenic patients. *Biol. Psychiatry*, 28: 488–494.

Mountcastle, V.B. (1998) *Perceptual Neuroscience: The Cerebral Cortex.* Harvard University Press, Cambridge, MA.

Narici, L., Pizzella, V., Romani, G.L., Torrioli, G., Traversa, R. and Rossini, P.M. (1990) Evoked alpha and mu rhythms in humans: a neuromagnetic study. *Brain Res.*, 520: 222–231.

Neubauer, A.C., Sange, G. and Pfurtscheller, G. (1999) Psychometric intelligence and event-related desynchronization during performance of a letter matching task. In: G. Pfurtscheller and F.H. Lopes da Silva (Eds.), *Event-Related Desynchronization and Related Oscillatory EEG Phenomena of the Awake Brain. Handbook of EEG and Clinical Neurophysiology (Revised Series)*, Vol. 6. Elsevier, Amsterdam, pp. 219–231.

Neuper, C. and Pfurtscheller, G. (1998a) Event-related desynchronization (ERD) and synchronization (ERS) of rolandic EEG rhythms during motor behavior. *Int. J. Psychophysiol.*, 30(1–2): 7–8.

Neuper, C. and Pfurtscheller, G. (1998b) 134 ERD/ERS based brain computer interface (BCI): effects of motor imagery on sensorimotor rhythms. *Int. J. Psychophysiol.*, 30(1–2): 53–54.

Osaka, M. (1984) Peak alpha frequency of EEG during a mental task: task difficulty and hemispheric differences. *Psychophysiology*, 21: 101–105.

Özerdem, A., Güntekin, B., Tunca, Z. and Başar, E. (2008) Brain oscillatory responses in patients with bipolar disorder manic episode before and after valproate treatment. *Brain Res.*, 1235: 98–108.

Özerdem, A., Güntekin, B., Saatçi, E., Tunca, Z. and Başar, E. (2010) Disturbance in long distance gamma coherence in bipolar disorder. *Prog. Neuropsychopharmacol. Biol. Psychiatry*, 16, 34(6): 861–865.

Özerdem, A., Güntekin, B., Atagün, I., Turp, B. and Başar, E. (2011) Reduced long distance gamma (28–48 Hz) coherence in euthymic patients with bipolar disorder. *J. Affect. Dis.*, 132: 325–332.

Özerdem, A., Güntekin, B., Atagün, I. and Başar, E. (2013) Brain oscillations in bipolar disorder in search of new biomarkers, this volume.

Pfurtscheller, G. (1997) EEG event-related desynchronization (ERD) and synchronization (ERS). *Electroencephalogr. Clin. Neurophysiol.*, 103(1): 26.

Pfurtscheller, G. (2001) Functional brain imaging based on ERD/ERS. *Vision Res.*, 41(10–11): 1257–1260.

Pfurtscheller, G., Neuper, C., Ramoser, H. and Müller-Gerking, J. (1999) Visually guided motor activates sensorimotor areas in humans. *Neurosci. Lett.*, 269(3): 153–156.

Pfurtscheller, G., Brunner, C., Schlogl, A. and Lopes da Silva, F.H. (2006) Mu rhythm, (de)synchronization and EEG single-trial classification of different motor imagery tasks. *Neuroimage*, 31(1): 153–159.

Quiroga, R.Q., Rosso, O.A. and Başar, E. (1999) Wavelet entropy: a measure of order in evoked potentials. *Electroencephalogr. Clin. Neurophysiol.*, 49: 299–303.

Quiroga, R.Q., Rosso, O.A., Basar, E. and Schürmann, M. (2001a) Wavelet entropy in eventrelated potentials: a new method shows ordering of EEG oscillations. *Biol. Cybern.*, 84: 291–299.

Quiroga, R.Q., Sakowitz, O.W., Basar, E. and Schürmann, M. (2001b) Wavelet transform in the analysis of the frequency composition of evoked potentials. *Brain Res. Protoc.*, 8: 16–24.

Rahn, E. and Başar, E. (1993) Prestimulus EEG activity strongly influences the auditory evoked vertex responses: a new method for selective averaging. *Int. J. Neurosci.*, 69: 207–220.

Rémond, A. and Lesèvre, N. (1967) Variations in average visual evoked potential as a function of the alpha rhythm phase ("autostimulation"). *Electroencephalogr. Clin. Neurophysiol.*, Suppl. 26: 42–52.

Roach, B.J. and Mathalon, D.H. (2008) Event-related EEG time-frequency analysis: an overview of measures and an analysis of early gamma band phase locking in schizophrenia. *Schizophr. Bull.*, 34(5): 907–926.

Röschke, J., Mann, K., Riemann, D., Frank, C. and Fell, J. (1995) Sequential analysis of the brain's transfer properties during consecutive REM episodes. *Electroencephalogr. Clin. Neurophysiol.*, 96: 390–397.

Rossini, P.M., Del Percio, C., Pasqualetti, P., Cassetta, E., Binetti, G., Dal Forno, G., Ferreri, F., Frisoni, G., Chiovenda, P., Miniussi, C., Parisi, L., Tombini, M., Vecchio, F. and Babiloni, C. (2006) Conversion from mild cognitive impairment to Alzheimer's disease is predicted by sources and coherence of brain electroencephalography rhythms. *Neuroscience*, 143(3): 793–803.

Rosso, O.A., Blanco, S., Yordanova, J., Kolev, V., Figliola, A., Schürmann, M. and Başar, E. (2001) Wavelet entropy: a new tool for analysis of short time brain electrical signals. *J. Neurosci. Meth.*, 105: 65–75.

Rosso, O.A., Martin, M.T. and Plastino, A. (2002) Brain electrical activity analysis using wavelet-based informational tools. *Physica Statist. Mech. Applic.*, 15: 587–608.

Schmiedt, C., Brand, A., Hildebrandt, H. and Başar-Eroğlu, C. (2005) Event-related theta oscillations during working memory tasks in patients with schizophrenia and healthy controls. *Cogn. Brain Res.*, 25(3): 936–947.

Schürmann, M. and Başar, E. (1994) Topography of alpha and theta oscillatory responses upon auditory and visual stimuli in humans. *Biol. Cybern.*, 72(2): 161–174.

Schürmann, M., Demiralp, T., Başar, E. and Başar-Eroğlu, C. (2000) Electroencephalogram alpha (8–15 Hz), responses to visual stimuli in cat cortex, thalamus, and hippocampus: a distributed alpha network? *Neurosci. Lett.*, 292: 175–178.

Sharma, A., Weisbrod, M. and Bender, S. (2013) Connectivity and local activity within the fronto-posterior brain network in schizophrenia, this volume.

Singer, W. (1989) The brain: a self-organizing system. In: K.A. Klivington (Ed.), *The Science of Mind*. MIT Press, Cambridge, MA, pp. 174–179.

Slewa-Younan, S., Gordon, E., Harris, A.W., Haig, A.R., Brown, K.J., Flor-Henry, P. and Williams, L.M. (2004) Sex differences in functional connectivity in first-episode and chronic schizophrenia patients. *Am. J. Psychiatry*, 161(9): 1595–1602.

Solodovnikov, V.V. (1960) *Introduction to the Statistical Dynamics of Automatic Control Systems*. Dover Press, New York.

Spekreijse, H. and Van der Tweel, L.H. (1972) System analysis of linear and nonlinear processes in electrophysiology of the visual system. *I. Proc. K. Ned. Akad. Wet. C.*, 75(2): 92–105.

Spencer, K.M., Nestor, P.G., Perlmutter, R., Niznikiewicz, M.A., Klump, M.C., Frumin, M., Shenton, M.E. and McCarley, R.W. (2004) Neural synchrony indexes disordered perception and cognition in schizophrenia. *Proc. Natl. Acad. Sci. USA*, 101 (49): 17288–17293.

Spencer, K.M., Niznikiewicz, M.A., Shenton, M.E. and McCarley, R.W. (2008) Sensory-evoked gamma oscillations in chronic schizophrenia. *Biol. Psychiatry*, 63(8): 744–747.

Sponheim, S.R., Clementz, B.A., Iacono, W.G. and Beiserm, M. (1994) Resting EEG in first-episode and chronic schizophrenia. *Psychophysiology*, 31: 37–43.

Sponheim, S.R., Clementz, B.A., Iacono, W.G. and Beiser, M. (2000) Clinical and biological concomitans of resting state EEG power abnormalities in schizophrenia. *Biol. Psychiatry*, 48: 1088–1097.

Squire, L.R. (1992) Declarative and non-declarative memory: multiple brain systems supporting learning and memory. *J. Cogn. Neurosci.*, 4: 232–243.

Steriade, M., Corró Dossi, R. and Pare, D. (1992) Mesopontine cholinergic system suppress slow rhythms and induce fast oscillations in thalamocortical circuits. In: E. Başar and T.H. Bullock (Eds.), *Induced Rhythm in the Brain*. Birkhäuser, Boston, MA, pp. 251–268.

Symond, M.P., Harris, A.W., Gordon, E. and Williams, L.M. (2005) "Gamma synchrony" in first-episode schizophrenia: a disorder of temporal connectivity? *Am. J. Psychiatry*, 162 (3): 459–465.

Tallon-Baudry, C., Bertrand, O., Delpuech, C. and Pernier, J. (1996) Stimulus specificity of phase-locked and non-phase-locked 40 Hz visual responses in human. *J. Neurosci.*, 6 (13): 4240–4249.

Vecchio, F., Babiloni, C., Lizio, R., De Vico, F.F., Blinowska, K., Verrienti, G., Frisoni, G.B. and Rossini, P.M. (2013) Resting state cortical EEG rhythms in Alzheimer's disease: towards EEG markers for clinical applications. A review. *Suppl. Clin. Neurophysiol.*, this volume.

Vinck, M., Battaglia, F.P., Womelsdorf, T. and Pennartz, C. (2011) Improved measures of phase-coupling between spikes and the local field potential. *J. Comput. Neurosci.*, Epub: doi:1.1007/s10827-011-0374-4.

Walter, W.G. (1950) Normal rhythms: their development, distribution and significance. In: D. Hill and G. Parr (Eds.), *Electroencephalograpy*. McDonald, London.

Ward, L.M. (2003) Synchronous neural oscillations and cognitive processes. *Trends Cogn. Sci.*, 7(12): 553–559.

Yener, G. and Başar, E. (2013a) A review in the search of an electrophysiologic biomarker: brain oscillatory responses in Alzheimer's disease. *Suppl. Clin. Neurophysiol.*, this volume.

Yener, G. and Başar, E. (2013b) Brain oscillations as biomarkers in neuropsychiatric disorders: following an interactive panel discussion and synopsis. *Suppl. Clin. Neurophysiol.*, this volume.

Yener, G.G., Güntekin, B., Öniz, A. and Başar, E. (2007) Increased frontal phase-locking of event-related theta oscillations in Alzheimer patients treated with cholinesterase inhibitors. *Int. J. Psychophysiol.*, 64(1): 46–52.

Yener, G., Güntekin, B. and Başar, E. (2008) Event related delta oscillatory responses of Alzheimer patients. *Eur. J. Neurol.*, 15(6): 540–547.

Yener, G., Güntekin, B., Tülay, E. and Başar, E. (2009) A comparative analysis of sensory visual evoked oscillations with visual cognitive event related oscillations in Alzheimer's disease. *Neurosci. Lett.*, 462: 193–197.

Yener, G.G., Güntekin, B., Orken, D.N., Tülay, E., Forta, H. and Basar, E. (2012) Auditory delta event-related oscillatory responses are decreased in Alzheimer's disease. *Behav. Neurol.*, 25(1): 3–11.

Yordanova, J. and Kolev, V. (1997) Developmental changes in the event-related EEG theta response and P300. *Electroencephalogr. Clin. Neurophysiol.*, 104: 418–430.

Yordanova, J. and Kolev, V. (1998) Event-related alpha oscillations are functionally associated with P300 during information processing. *NeuroReport*, 9(14): 3159–3164.

Yordanova, J., Kolev, V., Rosso, O.A., Schürmann, M., Sakowitz, O.W., Özgören, M. and Başar, E. (2002) Wavelet entropy analysis of event-related potentials indicates modality-independent theta dominance. *J. Neurosci. Meth.*, 117: 99.

Zheng-yan, J. (2005) Abnormal cortical functional connections in Alzheimer's disease: analysis of inter- and intra-hemispheric EEG coherence. *J. Zhejiang Univ. SCI*, 6B(4): 259–264.

Application of Brain Oscillations in Neuropsychiatric Diseases
(Supplements to Clinical Neurophysiology, Vol. 62)
Editors: E. Başar, C. Başar-Eroğlu, A. Özerdem, P.M. Rossini, G.G. Yener

Chapter 3

Preferred pre-stimulus EEG states affect cognitive event-related potentials

Robert J. Barry*

Brain & Behaviour Research Institute and School of Psychology, University of Wollongong, Northfields Avenue, Wollongong, NSW 2522, Australia

ABSTRACT

Current views of the genesis of the event-related potential (ERP) emphasize the contribution of ongoing oscillations — the ongoing electroencephalogram (EEG) is recognized as much more than "background noise" to be removed by response averaging to find the ERP. Early work from Başar's group noted that repetitive stimuli led to selective phase re-ordering of activity in the delta and alpha bands, such that enhanced brain negativity occurred at the time of the regular stimulus. Other work related negativity in alpha activity at stimulus onset to improved reaction times and ERP enhancements. These findings led us to begin a program of brain dynamics studies exploring pre-stimulus EEG phase states, their preferential occurrence in paradigms with regularly presented stimuli, and their relation to ERP outcomes. In particular, with very narrow EEG bands, we have repeatedly found that certain phase states preferentially occur at stimulus onset, implying ongoing phase re-ordering driven by stimulus occurrence. Effects are weakened with slightly varying inter-stimulus intervals, but still occur reliably. Further, these preferential phase states are functionally effective in relation to the ERP correlates of efficient stimulus processing. Preferential phase occurrence and their effects were originally reported in auditory oddball tasks, using narrow EEG bands derived by digital filtering. A recent study is presented illustrating generalization of the phenomenon in the auditory Go/NoGo task, using narrow bands derived by FFT techniques. Our current work is extending this research in normal children (to provide a comparative context for research in children with AD/HD), and well functioning elderly (to provide a context for future work in relation to Alzheimer's disease).

KEYWORDS

Brain dynamics; Event-related potentials; Orthogonal phase effects; Phase synchronization; Auditory Go/NoGo task; Cognitive processing

Correspondence to: Dr. Robert J. Barry, Brain & Behaviour Research Institute and School of Psychology, University of Wollongong, Northfields Avenue, Wollongong, NSW 2522, Australia.
Tel./fax: +61 2 4221 4421;
E-mail: robert_barry@uow.edu.au

3.1. Introduction

It is widely recognized today that the efficient processing of stimuli in cognitive paradigms depends on the ongoing electroencephalogram (EEG) and the dynamic brain processes it reflects (Başar, 1980; Makeig et al., 2004). For example, Barry (2009) illustrated the importance of phase re-setting of ongoing EEG oscillations in the genesis and selective determination of event-related

56

potentials (ERPs) in the auditory Go/NoGo task. An interesting line of brain-dynamics research, relevant particularly to the phase-resetting model of the ERP, began with a pioneering study by Başar and Stampfer (1985). They reported that stimuli presented at regular intervals led to phase re-ordering in the delta and alpha frequency bands of the ongoing EEG, producing a "preferred phase angle", associated with enhanced cortical negativity at stimulus onset. Other early work had noted that stimuli presented at negative alpha peaks produced faster reactions (Callaway and Yeager, 1960; Trimble and Potts, 1975), as well as enhanced ERPs (Rémond and Lesèvre, 1967). To us, this suggested that Başar and Stampfer's (1985) preferential phase occurrence could be of fundamental importance in perceptual and cognitive functioning. We found that other evidence of such dynamic phase adjustment had also been reported (Başar et al., 1984; Rockstroh et al., 1989; Pleydell-Pearce, 1994). Hence we began a program of research exploring this phenomenon. This chapter outlines the published findings from that program, providing detail to explain its developmental changes over the years. Our most recent published study (Barry et al., 2010) is described here in some detail in order to framework our current perspectives on this phenomenon.

Working with comparative phase angles and their effects in the EEG is relatively difficult, so Barry et al. (2003) introduced two more-intuitive physical dimensions based on the phase divisions defined in Fig. 1. What we termed cortical *negativity*/positivity compares effects of (A+B) versus (C+D), thus accommodating the phase effects described above. A second dimension, *negative*/positive *driving*, compares (A+D) versus (B+C), and reflects changes in the first (cortical *negativity*) variable — as it increases (phases A, D) or decreases (phases B, C). This dimension accommodates other ERP effects reported when stimuli were presented at the positive-going zero crossing of alpha activity (e.g., Rémond and Lesèvre, 1967; Jansen and Brandt, 1991). In this paper, we use italics to label

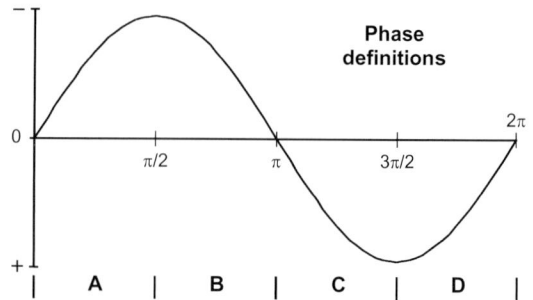

Fig. 1. An illustration defining the narrow-band EEG phases. Phases (A+B) define cortical *negativity*, (A+D) define *negative driving*, and (A+C) define *waxing*. For each pair defining a dimension (e.g., A+B), the other two phases (e.g., C+D) define the other extreme of that dimension. These three orthogonal dimensions are easier to conceptualize and work with than differences in traditional phase measures (degrees or radians).

one extreme of each of these orthogonal EEG phase dimensions and use this shorthand to aid communication and save space. Barry et al. (2003) used an active auditory task with a fixed inter-stimulus interval (ISI), requiring a button-press to targets. We employed narrow 1-Hz filtered EEG bands from 1 to 13 Hz to estimate phases at Cz. We found that these were dynamically adjusted so that "preferred brain states" occurred at stimulus onset. As broadly expected from the pioneering Başar and Stampfer (1985) study, some of these defined phase states (e.g., *negativity* cf. positivity) at different frequencies occurred at up to twice the rate expected by chance. Barry et al. (2003) also reported that the preferred states facilitated cortical processing, apparent in large effects in the broadband ERPs.

With four divisions of phase activity, numerous sets of three orthogonal (statistically independent) comparisons between the means can be constructed. An alpha phase study by Barry et al. (2004) continued use of the two comparisons described above and introduced the only possible third mutually independent phase contrast, which compared effects of EEG *waxing* (A+C) versus waning (B+D) at stimulus onset. This third phase dimension can be conceptualized simply in terms of EEG amplitude — *waxing* refers to amplitudes increasing, and waning to amplitudes decreasing. Barry et al. (2004) reported that preferred alpha states associated with *waxing* at stimulus onset occurred 33% more than waning phases. These were associated with increased alpha amplitude and frequency, and shorter N1 and P2 latencies.

The observed ERP effects initially reported by Barry et al. (2003) were not bound by the traditional delta, theta, or alpha EEG bands, suggesting the importance of continuing with our narrow-band approach in further more-focussed research. Hence, we began a series of studies of phase effects using data from an auditory oddball paradigm with deviants differing from the standards in terms of intensity. Because of the need to have large numbers of responses for subdivision into four phase ranges, these investigated effects associated with the standard rather than deviant stimuli. In Barry et al. (2006) we reported a study of ERPs obtained in passive conditions, comparing two groups of subjects with interchanged standard/deviant intensities. This paradigm was broadly similar to that used by Barry et al. (2003), but rather than using a fixed ISI, we varied it randomly in a range between 1000 and 1300 ms. As expected, this variability reduced, but did not eliminate, the occurrence of preferred brain states, which occurred 16–34% more often than expected by chance. The observed preferential states were functionally effective, producing evidence of more efficient processing of the standard stimuli in the passive oddball paradigm. Amplitude and latency effects were noted in the N1, P2, N2, P3, and the late slow wave. That is, ERP correlates of stimulus processing were substantially impacted by preferential narrow-band EEG phase states at stimulus onset, even with a slightly varying ISI.

We next sought to extend beyond the passive oddball, and explored the impact of task demands (Barry et al., 2007). This study used data from the passive low-intensity standards group of Barry et al. (2006) and data from a similar group of subjects presented with the same auditory sequence, but who were required to press a button in response to deviants. This task change from passive to active produced different preparatory processes in the two groups, different preferred brain states, and ERP differences to the standard stimuli investigated. Preferred brain states again occurred ~20% more than expected by chance, and these were associated with ERP evidence of more efficient processing.

We then sought to extend and integrate these oddball results by adding further subjects to complete a full factorial design over stimulus intensity and response requirements. A fourth group (high intensity standards in the active task paradigm) was added to the three groups in the previous oddball studies (high and low intensity standards in a passive task (Barry et al., 2006) and low intensity standards in active and passive tasks (Barry et al., 2007)). This design allowed us to explore these effects with more power (associated with the increased N), and examine the interaction between the standard stimulus intensity and active/passive task requirements. Thus, Barry et al. (2009) confirmed the occurrence of preferred narrow-band EEG phase-defined brain states in an auditory oddball paradigm, finding clear phase effects in all the ERP components measured. The nature of these effects confirmed the functional efficiency of the preferred brain states in enhancing stimulus processing. There was little evidence of variation in the occurrence of these brain states between the four groups, suggesting that the preferred brain states are reflexive, largely driven by the timing of stimulus occurrence.

3.2. FFT band separation

The studies reviewed above had examined phase effects at Cz in the alpha band, or in narrow 1-Hz bands, derived from the recorded wide-band EEG using digital filters. One disadvantage of signal filtering is the smearing of the signal voltages in the time domain. The left panels of Fig. 2 illustrate filter time-smearing for two simulated signals. The top panel shows a simulated alpha burst, while a simulated alpha phase reset is shown at the bottom, both before and after narrow-band 1-Hz digital filtering centered at 10 Hz. Although amplitude increases/

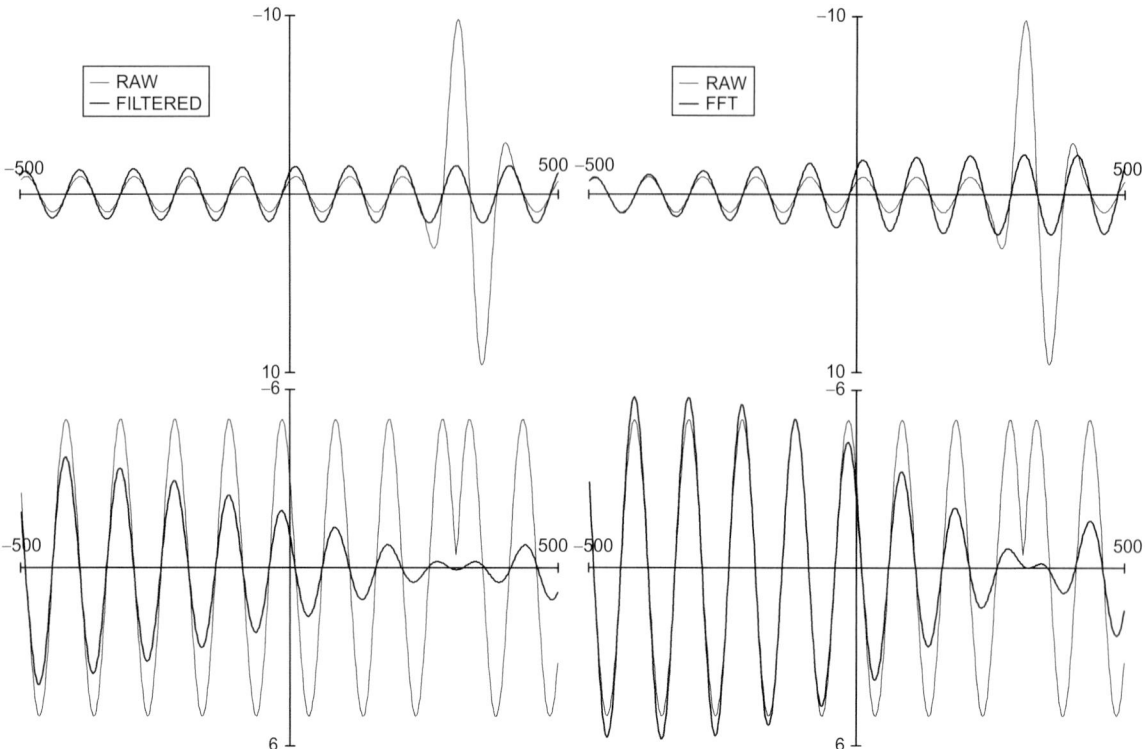

Fig. 2. Left: effect of filtering a 10-Hz sinusoidal signal containing a simulated "alpha burst" (top panel) or "phase reset" (bottom panel) in the time range of the P3. Note that both the raw and filtered signals are exactly in phase. Although amplitude changes are smeared over time in the filtered signal, the filtered signals show relative amplitude changes in the post-stimulus period corresponding to the changes in the raw signals: an increase (top) or decrease (bottom). Right: corresponding signals before and after separation into a narrow 10-Hz band using FFT. FFT decomposition retains better temporal fidelity than filtering. Note: signals were embedded in 5 s of data before filtering and FFT separation to avoid epoch-end effects. Vertical scales are in μV; horizontal scales are in ms from stimulus onset.

decreases associated with the two events are still dominant in the post-stimulus epoch, substantial smearing of the signal is apparent in the time domain. This occurs with all filters and is directly proportional to the sharpness of the filter. However, apart from this "smearing" problem, it is important to note that the signal's phase at stimulus onset is unchanged by filtering (see Barry et al., 2006).

As an alternative approach, we then explored the use of FFT decomposition. The right panels of Fig. 2 show the same alpha burst and phase reset simulations before frequency separation by FFT, and after recombination into a 1-Hz narrow band centered at 10 Hz via the inverse FFT. The major time characteristics of the signals are better preserved than with

filtering — there is less smearing apparent. Again, note the invariance of phase at stimulus onset before and after narrow-band decomposition.

In this new procedure, the whole block of EEG recorded from Cz was treated as one epoch. In the study where this was first applied, the block was 171 s in duration. For each subject, this block was decomposed by FFT. Then, frequencies within ± 0.5 Hz of each narrow band's center frequency were selected and recombined into bands of 1-Hz width, centered from 1 to 13 Hz, using separate inverse FFTs. This is equivalent to realizing a series of ideal acausal filters. As an example of this high-resolution separation, the frequency spectrum of a white noise sample, derived from epochs of the same size as our real EEG blocks, is shown in Fig. 3. The 171 frequencies/Hz obtained have been grouped into 19 sets of 9 frequencies for plotting (with a resolution of 1/19 Hz: black line). From this distribution, sets of 171 frequencies were grouped into 1-Hz bands (from 1 to 13 Hz) using the inverse FFT. These bands were each submitted to FFT to obtain the frequency profile of each narrow band. These are plotted in Fig. 3 as gray lines. For the 1-Hz band, each of the 19 points plotted per Hz is indicated by a black circle, to demonstrate the zero levels outside the band. It can be seen that the sum of these "filter characteristics" exactly matches the FFT of the original white noise data used to form the 1-Hz bands — the gray lines completely cover the black line, except at the edge of each band, where the grouped data are shared between adjacent bands. Note that there is no suggestion of "ringing" in the data.

There is another potential problem with narrow-band decomposition: as frequency resolution is increased, time resolution necessarily decreases. A very narrow filter reduces time resolution so that data at any particular time may predict what comes

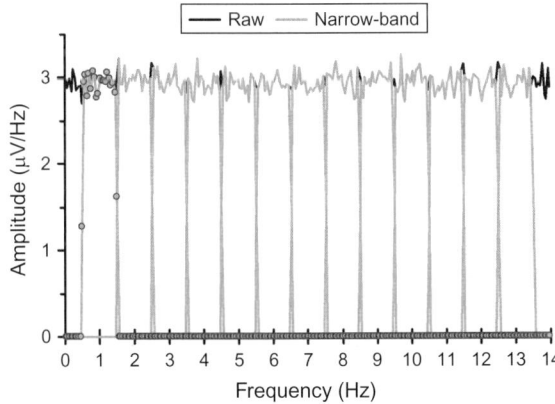

Fig. 3. The frequency spectrum of a white noise sample (black line), and its FFT separation into 13 bands of 1-Hz bandwidth (gray lines). Data were clumped into 19 points/Hz for plotting. The separation is exact, with complete data overlap except at the band edges, where the clumped data point is shared by adjacent bands. The 1-Hz band data points are shown as black circles to indicate the zero amplitudes beyond the pass band.

before and after. However, each 1-Hz band derived by our FFT approach contains 171 frequency components, and we expected this spread of frequencies to counter the problem of "prediction." This was tested by Barry et al. (2010) by comparing prediction between pre-stimulus and post-stimulus epochs in raw wide-band and summed narrow-band data streams. Results indicated that no substantial problem of prediction was likely in the FFT separation method.

3.3. Phase effects in a Go/NoGo paradigm

Using such an FFT decomposition to form narrow EEG bands, Barry et al. (2010) examined the existence of preferred brain states in an equiprobable auditory Go/NoGo paradigm with fixed ISIs. The advantage of moving to this paradigm was that it included equal numbers of Go and NoGo stimuli, with well-defined different ERPs. Because the exploration of phase effects in each of 13-1-Hz narrow bands is laborious, we restricted our efforts to the N1 and P3 peaks. N1 was not expected to differ between Go and NoGo stimuli, but we expected the different stimulus types to elicit different P3s. The NoGo stimulus is associated with a more anterior P3 than the Go stimulus, and these different responses have been identified as the P3a and P3b, respectively (Barry and Rushby, 2006).

The major focus of this study was whether comparable phase-related effects were apparent when such a different procedure was used to derive the 1-Hz narrow bands, and in a different paradigm. We explored frequency effects in the pre-stimulus phase occurrences for both Go and NoGo stimuli. As the occurrence of each stimulus type was random, effects were not expected to differ between them. These preferred phase impacts on the Go and NoGo ERP components were expected to differ, reflecting their functional efficiency in the paradigm.

Each subject received two blocks of an auditory Go/NoGo task, each containing 150 tones of 50-ms duration, with 5-ms rise/fall times, presented at 60-dB SPL with a fixed SOA of 1100 ms. Half the tones were 1000 Hz and half were 1500 Hz, presented in random order. Participants were required to button-press to one of the tones, with the target frequency balanced between subjects.

Continuous EEG from 24 participants was recorded from 17 scalp sites using an electrode cap with tin electrodes, referenced to linked ears. Data were continuously sampled at 512 Hz. The phase at stimulus onset for each 1-Hz EEG band, for each Go and NoGo stimulus, was determined using a 1-cycle sinusoidal wavelet and separated into four subdivisions (labeled A, B, C, and D), corresponding to the four phase ranges $0–\pi/2$, $\pi/2–\pi$, $\pi–3\pi/2$, and $3\pi/2–2\pi$, shown in Fig. 1. These four phases were used to sub-average both the narrow-band and wide-band EEG activity at each of the nine central sites (F3, Fz, F4, C3, Cz, C4, P3, Pz, and P4) into ERPs for Go and NoGo stimuli (note that all sites were sorted according to phase at stimulus onset occurring at Cz). ERP parameters were examined as a function of phase separately for Go and NoGo stimuli.

The mean ERPs obtained for each stimulus are shown in Fig. 4 at each of the analysis sites. A large fronto-central N1 with a peak latency of approx. 100 ms and a large P3 near 350 ms are apparent. The latter shows the expected parietal Go P3b and anteriorization of the NoGo P3a (Barry and Rushby, 2006).

Fig. 5 is a three-dimensional plot generated in the freely available EEGLAB toolbox (Delorme and Makeig, 2004), showing the preferential occurrence of EEG phases at stimulus onset for a representative subject. It displays amplitude as a function of time for each Go trial. Fig. 5A shows raw EEG at Cz for all trials accepted, in their order of stimulus presentation; the mean across-trials ERP is shown below. Fig. 5B shows the corresponding 4-Hz FFT-derived data stream, with trials ordered in terms of the phase at stimulus onset, obtained using a 1-cycle 4-Hz sinusoidal wavelet and ranking on its phase centered at stimulus onset (corresponding mean across-trials ERP is shown below). Note the non-linear distribution of the positive peak near stimulus onset across

trials in these sorted data. Phases A, B, C, and D at stimulus onset are indicated, showing the preferential occurrence of phases A and D (*negative driving*) at 4 Hz in this subject. Fig. 5C shows the mean 4-Hz ERPs derived from each of these phase ranges. The phases at time 0 can be compared with the phases defined in Fig. 1, showing the validity of our phase separation. Fig. 5D shows the raw data from Fig. 5A with trials in the same order as in Fig. 5B. The mean ERPs at each phase in Fig. 5E, derived from the data in Fig. 5D, show that N1 activity is particularly prominent in phase D, and P3 is most evident in phase B.

Across subjects, preferred brain states were apparent in that *negativity* occurred significantly more often than positivity at 1, 2, 10, and 11 Hz, and less often at 4 and 5 Hz. These and main effects of *negativity* vs. positivity are shown in the top panel of Table 1. *Negative driving* occurred significantly more often than positive driving phases at 2, 3, and 13 Hz, and less often at 1, 6, 7, and 9 Hz (see middle panel of Table 1 for these and other main effects of *negative driving* vs. positive driving). *Waxing* occurred significantly more often than waning phases at 2 Hz, and less often at 1 Hz (see bottom panel of Table 1 for all main effects of *waxing* vs. waning). The preferred phases occurred 5–38% more often than the non-preferred phases, but did not differ between Go and NoGo stimuli.

Go N1 amplitudes in *negativity* compared with positivity phases were somewhat smaller at 1 and 5 Hz, significantly smaller at 2, 3, 4, and 6 Hz, and larger at 9 and 10 Hz. Amplitudes for Go N1 in *negative driving* compared with positive driving phases were larger at 1, 2, 3, 4, and 5 Hz, and smaller at 7, 8, and 9 Hz. Go N1 latency in *negativity* compared with positivity phases was reduced somewhat at 2 and 4 Hz, and significantly reduced at 3, 11, 12, and 13 Hz, but increased at 6, 7, 8, and 9 Hz. In *negative driving* compared with positive driving phases, Go N1 latencies were significantly decreased at 5 and 6 Hz, and increased at 8, 9, 10, and 11 Hz. In *waxing* compared with waning phases, there was a significant decrease in Go N1 latency at 10 Hz.

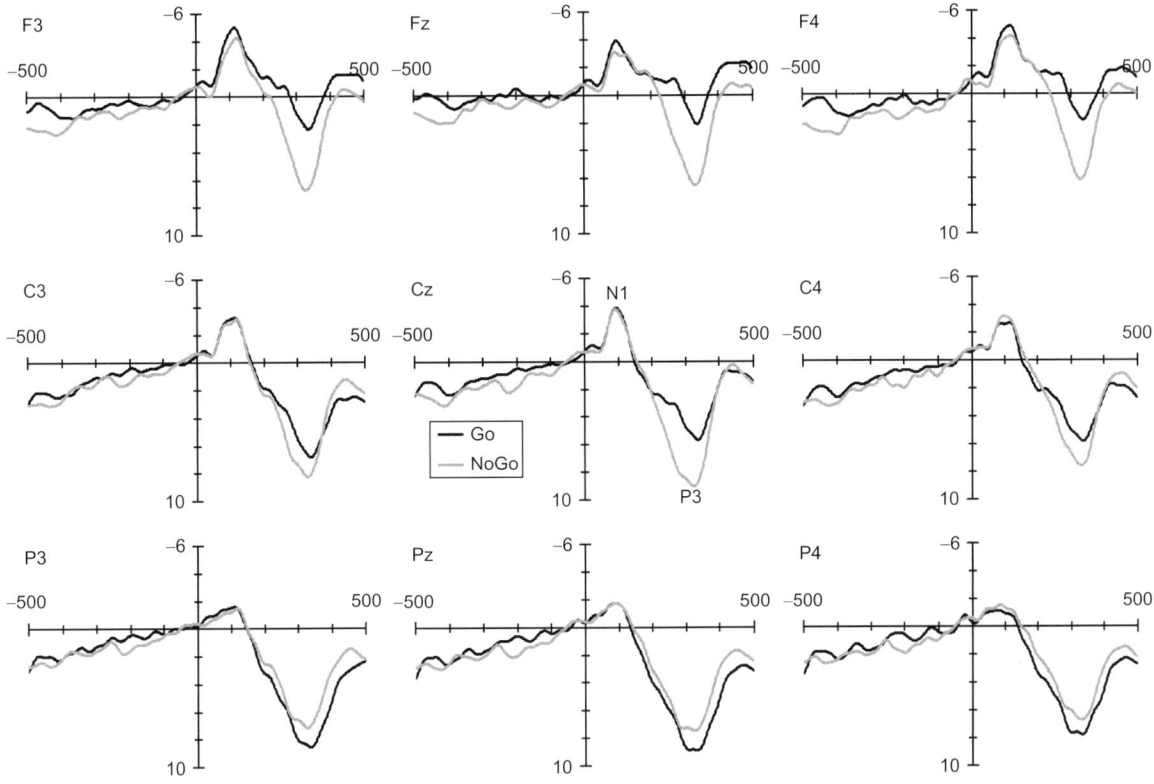

Fig. 4.　Grand mean ERPs for Go and NoGo stimuli at each analyzed site. Note the NoGo anteriorization of the P3. Vertical scale is in µV, horizontal scale is in ms relative to stimulus onset.

NoGo N1 amplitudes in *negativity* compared with positivity phases were significantly smaller at 2, 3, 4, 5, and 6 Hz, and larger at 9 Hz. Amplitudes for NoGo N1 in *negative driving* compared with positive driving phases were larger at 1, 2, 3, 4, and 5 Hz, and smaller at 8 Hz. NoGo N1 latency in *negativity* compared with positivity phases was increased at 6, 7, 8, and 9 Hz; it was decreased significantly at 11 and 12 Hz, and somewhat so at 13 Hz. In *negative driving* compared with positive driving phases, NoGo N1 latencies were significantly decreased at 4, 5, and 6 Hz and increased at 9, 10, and 11 Hz.

Go P3 amplitudes in *negativity* compared with positivity phases were significantly increased at 1 and 2 Hz, somewhat increased at 5 Hz, and significantly decreased at 3 Hz. Go P3 amplitudes in *negative driving* were decreased compared with positive driving phases at 1, 4, 5, and 7 Hz. Go

P3 latencies in *negativity* compared with positivity phases were significantly decreased at 2 and 5 Hz, increased at 4 and 7 Hz, and somewhat decreased at 8 Hz. In *negative driving* compared with positive driving phases, Go P3 latencies were increased at 1, 2, 4, 5, and 8 Hz and decreased at 3, 6, and 13 Hz. In *waxing* phases, there was some decrease in Go P3 latencies at 8 Hz.

NoGo P3 amplitudes in *negativity* compared with positivity phases were significantly increased at 1, 2, and 5 Hz, somewhat increased at 4 Hz, and significantly decreased at 3 Hz. NoGo P3 amplitudes in *negative driving* were decreased compared with positive driving phases at 1, 3, and 4 Hz and increased at 2 Hz. NoGo P3 latencies in *negativity* compared with positivity phases were significantly decreased at 2 and 5 Hz and increased at 4, 7, and 10 Hz. In *negative driving* compared with positive driving phases, NoGo P3 latencies were somewhat

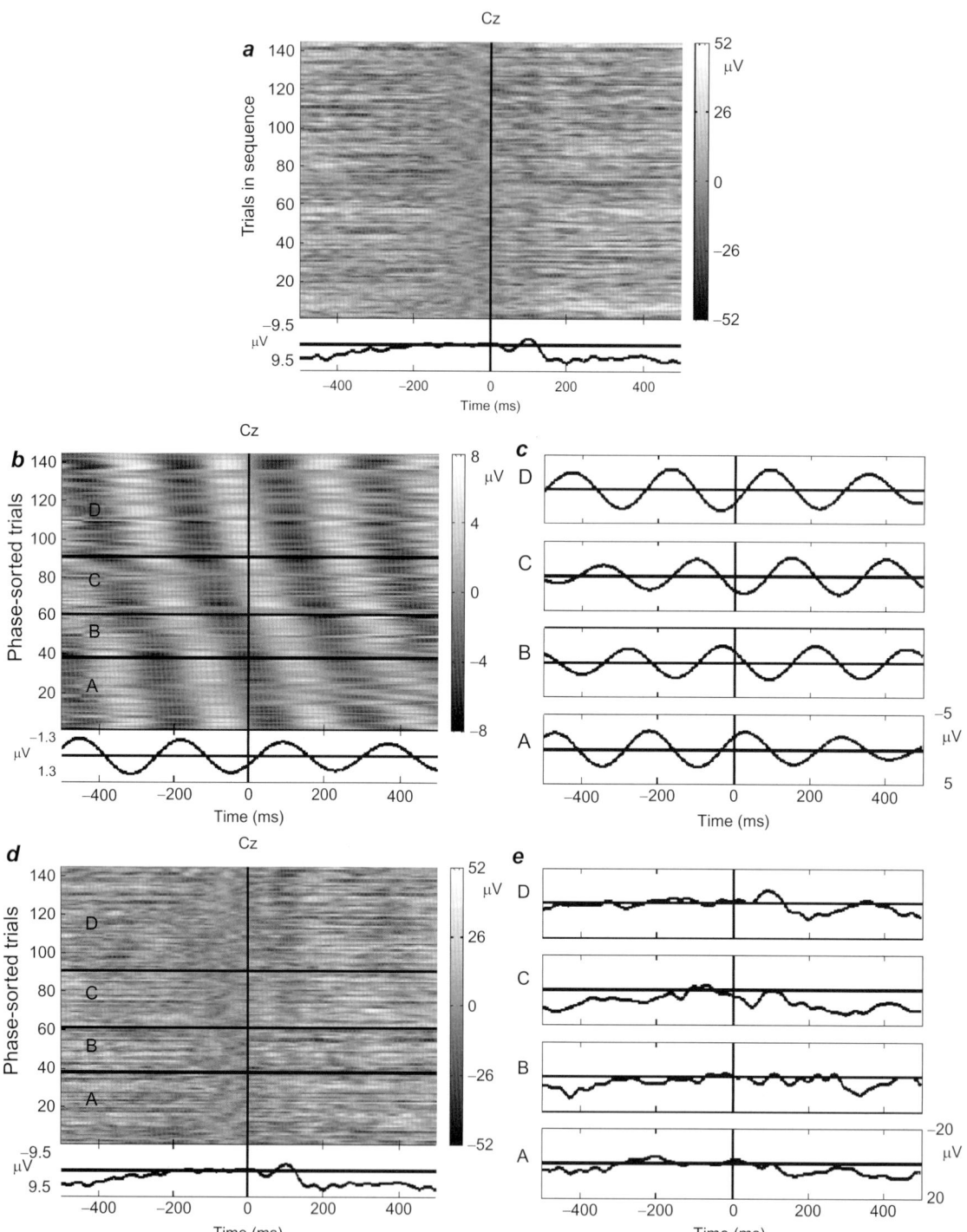

Fig. 5.   An example from a single subject of the occurrence of preferred brain states at Go stimulus onset. *a*: EEG at Cz for all accepted Go trials in order of stimulus presentation. One horizontal line per trial shows the amplitude at each time point. The mean across trials is shown below as the traditional ERP. *b*: the corresponding 4-Hz data stream sorted by the phase at stimulus onset, with the four phases as defined in Fig. 1 marked. *c*: the mean narrow-band ERP from each phase. *d*: the raw trials from panel *a* rearranged in the phase order of panel *b*, and the corresponding mean ERPs from each phase division are shown in *e*.

TABLE 1

SIGNIFICANT PHASE EFFECTS OBTAINED IN THE DEPENDENT VARIABLES AS A FUNCTION OF THE INDEPENDENT PHASE VARIABLES

Independent variable	Dependent variable	Effect	Frequency (Hz)												
			1	2	3	4	5	6	7	8	9	10	11	12	13
Negativity vs. positivity	Number	Phase	↑***	↑***	↑***	↑***	↓***				↑0.053	↑*	↑*		
	N1 amplitude	Go responses	↓0.056	↓***	↓***	↓***	↓0.080	↓***	↑***	↑***	↑***	↑**			
		NoGo responses		↑*	↑***	↑***	↑***	↑***	↑***		↑***				
	N1 latency	Go responses			↓***	↓0.081		↑***	↑***	↑***	↑***		↓***	↓***	↓***
		NoGo responses		↓0.083	↓***	↓***	↓***	↑*	↑***	↑***	↑*		↑***	↓***	↓0.078
	P3 amplitude	Go responses	↑***	↑***	↑***	↓***	↑0.055		↑***	↑***					
		NoGo responses	↑***	↑***	↓***	↑0.091	↓***		↑***	↑***					
	P3 latency	Go responses		↓***	↓***	↑***	↓***	↑*	↑***	↑***					
		NoGo responses		↓*	↓***	↑***	↓***	↓***	↑***	↓0.056		↑***			
Negative driving vs. positive driving	Number	Phase	↓***	↑*	↑***	↑***	↑***	↑***	↑***		↑*				↑**
	N1 amplitude	Go responses	↓***	↓***	↓***	↓***	↑***	↓***	↑*		↑*				
		NoGo responses	↓***	↓***	↑***	↓***	↑*	↓***			↑**				
	N1 latency	Go responses				↓***	↓***	↑***		↓*	↑***	↑***	↑***		
		NoGo responses				↓***	↓***	↓***	↓*	↑*	↑***	↑**	↑**		
	P3 amplitude	Go responses	↓***		↓*	↓***	↓*		↑***	↑***					
		NoGo responses	↓***	↑*	↓***	↓***			↓*						
	P3 latency	Go responses	↑*	↑*	↓***	↑*	↑***	↑***	↑***	↑***					↑*
		NoGo responses	↑0.099		↓***	↑***	↑***	↓***	↓***	↑***			↑***		↓0.096
Waxing vs. waning	Number	Phase	↓***	↑*											
	N1 amplitude	Go responses													
		NoGo responses													
	N1 latency	Go responses										↓***			
		NoGo responses													
	P3 amplitude	Go responses													
		NoGo responses													
	P3 latency	Go responses				↑0.069				↓0.081					
		NoGo responses													

↑: Larger for target phases; ↓: smaller for target phases; *significant at $p < 0.05$; **significant at $p < 0.01$; ***significant at $p < 0.005$; probability is indicated for effects approaching significance.

increased at 1 Hz, and significantly so at 4, 5, 8, and 11 Hz, and significantly decreased at 3 and 6 Hz, and to some extent at 13 Hz. In *waxing* phases, there was some increase in NoGo P3 latencies at 4 Hz.

In addition to the main effects in N1 and P3 amplitude and latency listed above, there were many phase-determined topographic effects obtained in these peaks, as well as main effects and topographic interactions involving pre-stimulus RMS amplitudes, post-stimulus changes in RMS amplitudes, and amplitudes of the pre-stimulus contingent negative variation (see Barry et al., 2010 for details).

3.4. Discussion

The most important results of Barry et al. (2010) relate to the existence of preferred brain states at stimulus onset. The results shown in the first line of each panel of Table 1 indicate the widespread occurrence of these phases across the frequencies investigated here. Since the Bonferroni-corrected probability of a false alarm in regard to phase occurrence was 0.05, the chance of 15 significant cases of preferential phase randomly occurring ($p = 0.05^{15}$) is vanishingly small. This strongly confirms the existence of these preferred brain states at stimulus onset in this paradigm. As predicted, these preferred phases did not differ between Go and NoGo stimuli. That is, the existence of preferred brain states was confirmed in a different paradigm and with very different EEG decomposition techniques, involving the use of FFT rather than digital filtering. This confirmation suggests the widespread existence of this aspect of brain dynamics and encourages further research into its mechanisms.

As can be seen from Table 1, some of these preferred phase states were associated with amplitude and latency effects in both the N1 and P3. Both *negativity* and *negative driving* effects, on balance, produced enhancement of both Go and NoGo N1 amplitudes, and preferred *negativity* phases produced shorter Go and NoGo N1 latencies. In relation to the P3, preferred *negativity* and *negative*

driving states were associated largely with Go and NoGo amplitude increases and latency reductions. Some effects differed between Go and NoGo stimuli, suggesting that at least some of the processing differences associated with the different stimuli were impacted by the preferred brain states. Preferred *negativity* states in alpha, and preferred *negative driving* states in theta, enhanced the amplitude of the Go N1. With the P3, preferred *negativity* states in alpha contributed to Go/NoGo latency differences. Preferred *negative driving* states in theta increased Go P3 amplitudes and, in the alpha range, decreased Go P3 latency. The results described here were limited to main effects and excluded other important topographic effects that were apparent in both ERP components (see Barry et al., 2010 for details).

These findings suggest that the preferential occurrence of particular brain states, as indicated by the non-random patterning of EEG phase in the narrow EEG bands at stimulus onset, is functionally associated with efficient stimulus processing in this paradigm. In general, N1 and P3 amplitudes were increased, and their latencies were decreased. The preferred states also appear to be involved in the differential processing of Go and NoGo stimuli, leading to some of the associated topographic differences in ERP components.

It is currently unknown whether the narrow-band phase effects are specifically related to their frequency, or if these are only examples of broader effects. Perhaps the preferred states at different frequencies are only important to the extent that they produce negativity/positivity over the cortex at particular times. That could serve to activate or deactivate cortical regions associated with aspects of stimulus processing in these tasks. Whatever the cortical mechanisms involved, the three phase dimensions used here present a simple and intuitive analysis of phase occurrence, linked to easily conceptualized EEG changes. They have served to confirm that the phase of ongoing EEG activity at a range of frequencies is reflexively adjusted to optimize performance in tasks involving repetitive stimulus presentations. These have been found to occur in different paradigms, with different EEG decomposition techniques used to obtain the narrow-band EEG streams.

To date our published work in brain dynamics has been derived from young adult samples. Our current work is extending this research with normal children, and results indicate that they show reliable preferred phase occurrence in the Go/NoGo task. The relationships between these phase states and ERP parameters have not been fully analyzed as yet. The wider aim of this child research is to provide a comparative context for research in children with AD/HD. We consider it likely that some of the functional processing differences reported in children with this disorder (such as reduced posterior P3; see Barry et al., 2003) reflect fundamental anomalies in reflexive brain dynamics, possibly those involving preferred phase states. We also have data in hand from a well-functioning elderly group, which will allow us to explore the preferred phase phenomenon across the age-span, and will later provide a context for future work in relation to Alzheimer's disease. Overall, this program is aimed at increasing our understanding of normal brain dynamics, and also determining whether disruptions in that normal functioning are relevant to specific clinical impairments.

Acknowledgments

This research was funded by a grant from the Australian Research Council Discovery funding scheme (Project Number DP0772251). My thanks are due to Frances M. De Blasio for assistance with implementing the change to FFT decomposition.

References

Barry, R.J. (2009) Evoked activity and EEG phase resetting in the genesis of auditory Go/NoGo ERPs. *Biol. Psychol.*, 80: 292–299.

Barry, R.J. and Rushby, J.A. (2006) An orienting reflex perspective on anteriorisation of the P3 of the event-related potential. *Exp. Brain Res.*, 173: 539–545.

Barry, R.J., De Pascalis, V., Hodder, D., Clarke, A.R. and Johnstone, S.J. (2003) Preferred EEG brain states at stimulus onset in a fixed interstimulus interval auditory oddball task, and their effects on ERP components. *Int. J. Psychophysiol.*, 47: 187–198.

Barry, R.J., Rushby, J.A., Johnstone, S.J., Clarke, A.R., Croft, R.J. and Lawrence, C.A. (2004) Event-related potentials in the auditory oddball as a function of EEG alpha phase at stimulus onset. *Clin. Neurophysiol.*, 115: 2593–2601.

Barry, R.J., Rushby, J.A., Smith, J.L., Clarke, A.R. and Croft, R.J. (2006) Dynamics of narrow-band EEG phase effects in the passive auditory oddball task. *Eur. J. Neurosci.*, 24: 291–304.

Barry, R.J., Rushby, J.A., Smith, J.L., Clarke, A.R., Croft, R.J. and Wallace, M.J. (2007) Brain dynamics in the active vs. passive auditory oddball task: exploration of narrow-band EEG phase effects. *Clin. Neurophysiol.*, 118: 2234–2247.

Barry, R.J., Rushby, J.A., Smith, J.L., Clarke, A.R. and Croft, R.J. (2009) Brain dynamics in the auditory oddball task as a function of stimulus intensity and task requirements. *Int. J. Psychophysiol.*, 73: 313–325.

Barry, R.J., De Blasio, F., Rushby, J.A. and Clarke, A.R. (2010) Brain dynamics in the auditory Go/NoGo task as a function of EEG frequency. *Int. J. Psychophysiol.*, 78: 115–128.

Başar, E. (1980) *EEG Brain Dynamics: Relation between EEG and Brain Evoked Potentials.* Elsevier/North-Holland Biomedical Press, Amsterdam.

Başar, E. and Stampfer, H.G. (1985) Important associations among EEG-dynamics, event-related potentials, short-term memory and learning. *Int. J. Neurosci.*, 26: 161–180.

Başar, E., Başar-Eroğlu, C., Rosen, B. and Schütt, A. (1984) A new approach to endogenous event-related potentials in man: relation between EEG and P300-wave. *Int. J. Neurosci.*, 24: 1–21.

Callaway, E. and Yeager, C.L. (1960) Relationship between reaction time and electroencephalographic alpha phase. *Science*, 132: 1765–1766.

Delorme, A. and Makeig, S. (2004) EEGLAB: an open source toolbox for analysis of single-trial EEG dynamics including independent component analysis. *J. Neurosci. Meth.*, 134: 9–21.

Jansen, B.H. and Brandt, M.E. (1991) The effect of the phase of prestimulus alpha activity on the averaged visual evoked response. *Electroenceph. Clin. Neurophysiol.*, 80: 241–250.

Makeig, S., Delorme, A., Westerfield, M., Jung, T.P., Townsend, J., Courchesne, E. and Sejnowski, T.J. (2004) Electroencephalographic brain dynamics following manually responded visual targets. *PLoS Biol.*, 2: 747–762.

Pleydell-Pearce, C.W. (1994) DC potential correlates of attention and cognitive load. *Cogn. Neuropsychol.*, 11: 149–166.

Rémond, A. and Lesèvre, N. (1967) Variations in average visual evoked potentials as a function of the alpha rhythm phase ("autostimulation"). *Electroenceph. Clin. Neurophysiol.*, Suppl. 26: 42–52.

Rockstroh, B., Elbert, T., Canavan, A., Lutzenberger, W. and Birbaumer, N. (1989) *Slow Cortical Potentials and Behaviour*, 2nd Edn. Urban and Schwarzenberg, Munich.

Trimble, J.L. and Potts, A.M. (1975) Ongoing occipital rhythms and the VER. I. Stimulation at peaks of the alpha-rhythm. *Invest. Ophthalmol. Vis. Sci.*, 14: 537–546.

Application of Brain Oscillations in Neuropsychiatric Diseases
(Supplements to Clinical Neurophysiology, Vol. 62)
Editors: E. Başar, C. Başar-Eroğlu, A. Özerdem, P.M. Rossini, G.G. Yener

Chapter 4

The in vivo topography of cortical changes in healthy aging and prodromal Alzheimer's disease

Annapaola Prestia[a], Annalisa Baglieri[b], Michela Pievani[a], Matteo Bonetti[c], Paul E. Rasser[d], Paul M. Thompson[e], Silvia Marino[b], Placido Bramanti[b] and Giovanni B. Frisoni[a,*]

[a]*Laboratory of Epidemiology, Neuroimaging and Telemedicine, IRCCS Centro San Giovanni di Dio Fatebenefratelli, The National Center for Research and Care of Alzheimer's and Mental Diseases, 25125 Brescia, Italy*
[b]*IRCCS Centro Neurolesi Bonino-Pulejo, 98124 Messina, Italy*
[c]*Service of Neuroradiology, Istituto Clinico Città di Brescia, 25125 Brescia, Italy*
[d]*Schizophrenia Research Institute, Darlinghurst, Sydney, NSW 2010, Australia and Priority Centre for Brain and Mental Health Research, University of Newcastle, Newcastle, NSW 2300, Australia*
[e]*Laboratory of Neuro Imaging, UCLA School of Medicine, Los Angeles, CA 90095-7334, USA*

ABSTRACT

Background: Gray matter atrophy is regarded as a valid marker of neurodegeneration in Alzheimer's disease (AD), but few studies have investigated in detail the topographic changes associated with normal aging. In addition, few studies have compared the changes in the earliest clinical stage of AD (prodromal AD (pAD)) with those of healthy aging. Here we aimed to investigate the topographical distribution of age-related cortical atrophy and to compare it with that associated with prodromal and estabilished AD.

Methods: Structural T1-weighted high-resolution brain magnetic resonance imaging scans were acquired from 60 healthy volunteers (20 young adults, YA: age 32.7 ± 4.5 years; 40 elderly subjects, HE: age 71.3 ± 6.2 years), 16 mild cognitive impairment subjects who converted to AD within 2 years (prodromal AD, pAD: age 72.8 ± 5.4), and 20 mild to moderate AD patients (mAD, age 72.5 ± 10.3). Cortical gray matter differences were investigated using a surface-based anatomical mesh modeling technique (cortical pattern matching) and region-of-interest (ROI) analyses based on hypothesized brain networks taught to have a functional and a structural link to each other. Differences in cortical atrophy were assessed between groups, as well as the effect of age within groups.

Results: HE compared to YA showed a 10–30% deficit in cortical gray matter in widespread frontal, temporal, and parietal regions ($p = 0.0001$ by permutation testing), 6–13% loss in the visual and sensorimotor cortices ($p < 0.01$) and up to 13% loss in the direct hippocampal pathway ROIs ($p < 0.001$). pAD patients showed on average 8–9% cortical loss compared to HE ($p < 0.0001$), mainly in the left (up to 6% loss, $p = 0.06$) and right polysynaptic hippocampal pathway ROIs (up to 8% loss, $p = 0.01$), and in the left and right olfactory/orbitofrontal cortex (up to 12–15% loss, $p < 0.001$). The pattern of cortical atrophy in mAD versus HE was similar to that in pAD, but was more severe in the direct hippocampal pathway ROIs and sensorimotor, visual and temporal cortices (13–15% loss compared with HE, $p < 0.0001$).

Correspondence to: Dr. Giovanni B. Frisoni, IRCCS Fatebenefratelli, Via Pilastroni 1, 25125 Brescia, Italy.
Tel.: +39 030 3501361;
E-mail: gfrisoni@fatebenefratelli.it

Conclusion: Gray matter loss occurs during aging with rates of atrophy even more severe than that observed during the course of AD. These changes may be caused by normal mechanisms. In pAD, cortical atrophy due to disease is milder than that due to aging, maybe resulting from a slowed down velocity of cell loss, but affects specific brain areas. These findings are consistent with the view that AD is not merely accelerated aging.

KEYWORDS

Atrophy; Aging; Alzheimer's disease; Cortical pattern matching; Gray matter loss

4.1. Introduction

Considerable advances in magnetic resonance imaging (MRI) and computer technology over the past decades have allowed the study of brain morphometry in vivo. MRI provides accurate and reproducible measures of brain changes in several physiological or pathological conditions (Thompson et al., 2004). Indeed, the quantitative assessment of structural brain changes has entered into clinic as a marker to monitor clinical outcomes and treatment effects in many diseases, such as Alzheimer disease (AD), multiple sclerosis, schizophrenia, and many others (Ge et al., 2002).

Cerebral volume loss with increasing age has been observed by many studies, but the processes/mechanisms underlying such changes (neuronal loss, incipient or asymptomatic neurodegenerative diseases) are not clear (Freeman et al., 2008). Volume loss in non-demented older individuals has been examined in both longitudinal and cross-sectional imaging studies (Resnick et al., 2003; Fotenos et al., 2005). The overall brain atrophy rate is around –0.45% per year in adulthood (Fotenos et al., 2005). Both gray and white matter volumes decreased with age, albeit with a different linear and non-linear pattern, respectively (Ge et al., 2002). Some studies used manual drawing of regions of interest (ROIs) or automated/semi-automated techniques to assess atrophy in specific brain regions. These studies show that certain cortical regions, such as the frontal cortices, seem to be more vulnerable to volume loss with aging (Allen et al., 2005; Raz and Rodrigue, 2006). Other regions are affected to a lesser extent and include the temporal, parietal, and occipital association areas (Allen et al., 2005), followed by the perirolandic cortex (Salat et al., 2004), and possibly the anterior and posterior cingulate cortices (Abe et al., 2008; Kalpouzos et al., 2009).

AD is the most prevalent neurodegenerative disease in the elderly population, generally characterized by atrophy in most of the cerebral regions mentioned above. It results from the accumulation of abnormal amyloid and tau proteins in extracellular space and neurons. This eventually leads to cell death and progressive cognitive decline. Pathologic features of AD are often observed, even if with a narrower and milder anatomical distribution, in patients affected by mild cognitive impairment (MCI), the prodromal stage of AD which includes individuals with memory problems who do not meet criteria for dementia but who annually progress to AD with a percentage of up to 15 (Petersen et al., 2001). Gray matter atrophy of temporal lobes and especially of medial-temporal regions, which are involved in memory processing, is considered one of the most accurate markers of neurodegeneration (Frisoni et al., 2010) and is regarded as a supportive feature of AD according to the new research criteria (Dubois et al., 2007). The medial temporal lobes (MTLs), together with the enthorinal and perirhinal cortices, are among the first regions affected by neurofibrillary pathology and cell loss very early in AD (Braak and Braak, 1991; Kordower et al., 2001). Extensive gray matter loss in the temporal pole, temporo-parietal association cortex, dorsal prefrontal cortex, and visual cortex follows later, while atrophy in the primary sensorimotor cortex seems to occur not earlier than the moderate stage of the disease (Frisoni et al., 2009).

The normal aging process seems to affect all those cortical regions too, but there appears to be no age-related neuronal loss (Pakkenberg et al., 2003), even though normal adults physiologically show neurofibrillary pathology in many of these areas (Price et al., 2001; Von Gunten et al., 2005).

In this study we sought to investigate the topographical distribution of age-related cortical atrophy, and to distinguish it from that associated with prodromal AD (pAD), in order to gain a better insight into the cortical areas vulnerable to age from those specifically vulnerable to AD. To this aim, a technique able to map volumetric differences over the whole cortical mantle with a spatial accuracy of a few millimeters was used.

4.2. Materials and methods

4.2.1. Study subjects and assessment

Cognitively healthy controls were selected from subjects enrolled in a previous study on the Italian brain normative archive on structural MR scans (Galluzzi et al., 2009). All participants underwent a multidimensional assessment including clinical, neurological, and neuropsychological evaluations, as described in detail elsewhere (Galluzi et al., 2009). Subjects were separated into two groups according to their age: young healthy adults (YA, age range between 20 and 40 years; $n = 20$) and elderly subjects (HE, age range between 60 and 80 years; $n = 40$).

Patients (mild to moderate AD mAD and prodromal pAD) were recruited from the Outpatient Memory Clinic of the IRCCS Centro San Giovanni di Dio Fatebenefratelli (National Center for Alzheimer's Disease), Brescia, Italy. From this group, we selected patients with a clinical diagnosis of AD (McKhann et al., 1984) (mAD, age range between 60 and 90 years, $n = 20$) and 45 MCI (Petersen et al., 2001), based on the results of a standardized protocol including physical and neurological examination, neuropsychological assessment, and an MRI scan. History was taken with a structured interview from patients' relatives (typically spouses).

MCI patients were clinically followed for at least 2 years, and 16 of them converted to AD during follow-up and were included in the study (pAD, age range between 62 and 83 years; $n = 16$).

Written informed consent was obtained from patients and controls prior to their inclusion in the study. No compensation was provided for study participation. The study was approved by the local ethics committee and performed in accordance with the ethical standards in the 1964 Declaration of Helsinki.

4.2.2. Neuropsychological assessment

Neuropsychological assessment was performed by a psychologist and included the following tests: (i) global cognitive functioning with the MMSE (Crum et al., 1993); (ii) phonological and semantic verbal fluency as well as language comprehension with the Token test; (iii) visuospatial and constructional abilities with the Rey–Osterreith figure's copy test; (iv) frontal-executive functions with the clock drawing test; and (v) learning and memory with Rey's figure and immediate and delayed recall tests of Rey's list (Lezak et al., 2004).

4.2.3. MR acquisition

MR scans were acquired for YA, HE, mAD, and pAD patients (when they were at MCI level) with a Philips Gyroscan 1.0 T scanner at the Neuroradiology Unit of the Città di Brescia Hospital. High-resolution gradient echo sagittal three-dimensional (3D) sequences (TR = 20 ms, TE = 5 ms, flip angle 30°, field of view = 220 mm, acquisition matrix = 256 × 256, and slice thickness = 1.3 mm) and fast fluid attenuated inversion recovery axial sequences were acquired. Gray matter was studied with the cortical pattern matching algorithm developed at the Laboratory of Neuroimaging (LONI) of the University of California, Los Angeles (Thompson et al., 2004). White matter damage was ascertained by computing global scores on the age-related white matter changes visual rating scale (Wahlund et al., 2001) for each participant.

The 3D images were reoriented along the anterior commissure–posterior commissure (AC-PC) line and voxels below the cerebellum were removed using the MRIcro software (http://www. cabiatl.com/mricro/mricron/index.html). The AC was manually set as the origin of the spatial coordinates for an anatomical normalization algorithm implemented in the Statistical Parametric Mapping (SPM99) software package (http://www.fil.ion.ucl. ac.uk/spm/software/spm99/). A 12-parameter affine transformation was used to normalize each image to a customized template in stereotaxic space, created from the MRI scans of 40 control subjects.

4.2.4. Cortical pattern matching

Individual brain masks for each hemisphere were extracted from normalized images with the automatic software Brainsuite (http://www.loni.ucla. edu/Software/BrainSuite), visually inspected and manually corrected with *Display*, a 3D visualization program (http://www.bic.mni.mcgill.ca/ ServicesSoftwareVisualization/HomePage) that allows the manual correction of errors in ROIs (or "masks") differentiating brain and non-brain tissues. The resulting masks were then applied to the normalized images to obtain "skull-stripped" images of each hemisphere. After automated 3D hemispheric reconstruction using an intensity threshold that best differentiated gray matter from extracerebral cerebrospinal fluid (Thompson et al., 2001a), a total of 39 sulcal lines for each hemisphere were manually traced (17 sulci on the lateral surface, 12 sulci on the medial surface, and 11 lines drawn to outline interhemispheric gyral limits of each hemisphere) by two tracers (A.P. and A.B.) blind to diagnoses on the cortical surfaces, following a detailed and extensively validated protocol (http://www. loni.ucla.edu/~khayashi/Public/medial_surface/ www.loni.ucla.edu/~esowell/new_sulcvar.html)

for each subject. The reliability of manual outlining was assessed prior to experimental subject tracing with a standard protocol requiring the same rater to trace all lateral and medial sulci of six test brains (Sowell et al., 2001). At the end of the reliability phase, the mean 3D difference of both tracers from the gold standard (Sowell et al., 2001) was <3.5 mm everywhere for medial and lateral sulci. Individual sulcal maps were averaged to create a common average sulcal map for all subjects in the study (Thompson et al., 2000). The individual cortical surfaces were parameterized, flattened, and warped. Image voxels were classified using a partial volume classifier algorithm (Thompson et al., 2000).

Gray matter density (GMD), a commonly used measure of regional gray matter volume (Frisoni et al., 2009), was computed at each cortical point as the proportion of tissue classified as gray matter in a sphere centered at that point, with a radius of 15 mm. The maps of mean GMD were then computed by averaging cortical GMD values within each group. Maps of the percentage difference in GMD were computed based on the ratio, at each cortical point, between the mean GMD value at that point in the HE group and in the YA group, and between the patient group (pAD or AD) and HE. This ratio allowed visualization of the relative deficit in gray matter at each cortical point as a proportion, or percentage, of the normal values seen in respective healthy controls.

A deformable Brodmann area (BA) atlas (Rasser et al., 2004) was applied to the left and right hemisphere average models and values of mean gray matter volume were computed from all vertices comprising a given BA. For the ROI analysis, five brain networks were hypothesized (the polysynaptic hippocampal, the olfactory, the direct hippocampal, the sensorimotor, and the visual pathway) comprising all the BAs having a functional and a structural link to each other, as previously described (Fig. 1) (Duvernoy, 1998; Frisoni et al., 2009). The mean GMD values were computed for each of these networks.

Hypothesized network	Cortical region	Comprised BAs
Polysynaptic hippocampal pathway	Posterior cingulate Retrosplenial cortex	23 + 31 + 26 + 29 + 30
Olfactory pathway	Prefrontal orbital cortex Subgenual cortex	11 + 25
Direct hippocampal pathway	Temporal pole Medial and inferior temporal cortex Prefrontal cortex	20 + 38 + 27 + 28 + 35 + 36 + 37 8+9+10+44+45+46+47
Sensorimotor pathway	Primary motor and somatosensory cortices	1+4+43
Visual pathway	Primary and associative visual cortices	17+18+19

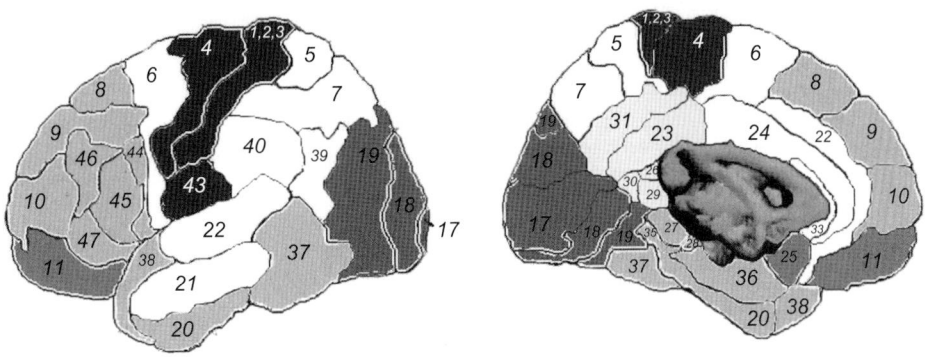

Fig. 1.   Composition of neural networks. (For color figures, please refer to the color figures in last section of the book.)

4.2.5. Statistical analysis

Cortical gray matter differences between groups were computed based on the ratio, at each cortical point, between the mean GMD value at that point in each patient group and the mean GMD in each pertinent control group (HE vs. YA, pAD vs. HE, and mAD vs. HE). This ratio allows maps of the relative deficit in gray matter to be visualized as a proportion, or percentage, of the normal values seen in pertinent control subjects (YA for HE and HE for pAD and mAD). The p values representing the significance of the differences between groups were mapped to the whole cortex, after setting a significance threshold of $p = 0.05$. Set-level correction for multiple comparisons was carried out by permutation testing at a threshold of $p = 0.05$. This analysis assesses the fraction of the cortical surface area with statistics exceeding the given threshold and compares it with a null distribution constructed empirically by randomly assigning subjects to groups. To explore the relationships between GMD and age,

Pearson's r correlations were assessed within each group (HE, pAD, and mAD) and corrected for multiple comparisons with permutation testing at a threshold of $p = 0.05$. In order to rule out the possible effect of gender on cortical GMD, we investigated GMD differences between males and females within controls (HE and YA) and patients (pAD and mAD).

Significant differences in sociodemographic, cognitive, genetic, neuropsychological, and morphostructural features (network volumes) between groups were computed using Kruskal–Wallis (with Mann–Whitney U test for post-hoc comparisons) test for non-parametrical data and chi-square test for dichotomous variables. Wilson's method was used to calculate confidence intervals for proportions.

4.3. Results

Table 1 shows that patients and elderly controls were generally in their 70s, with their mean

TABLE 1

SOCIODEMOGRAPHIC, COGNITIVE, AND GENETIC FEATURES OF THE STUDY GROUPS

	Young adults (n = 20)	Healthy elders (n = 40)	pAD (n = 16)	mAD (n = 20)	p
Age (years)	32.7±4.5*	71.3±6.2	72.8±5.4	72.5±10.3	0.0001
Gender, female (%)	11 (55%)	22 (55%)	6 (37%)	15 (75%)	0.16
Mini Mental State Exam (range)	29.4±0.6 (27–30)	28.7±0.9 (27–30)	26.0±2.5** (24–29)	20.0±4.1* (13–27)	0.0001
ARWMC global score	0.2±0.5*	3.2±3.9	4.5±3.7	4.7±4.9	0.001

Values indicate mean±S.D.
ARWMC = age-related white matter changes visual rating scale (Wahlund et al., 2001).
*, ** No or same markers denote no differences and different markers denote significant differences on Kruskal–Wallis (with Mann–Whitney post-hoc U test between groups for continuous and chi-square for dichotomous variables).

TABLE 2

NEUROPSYCHOLOGICAL FEATURES OF THE STUDY GROUPS

		YA (n = 20)	HE (n = 40)	p vs. YA	pAD (n = 16)	p vs. HE	mAD (n = 20)	p vs. HE
Learning	Rey's list immed. recall	52.1±15.4	29.1±7.1	0.0001	39.7±9.5	0.001	16.8±6.1	0.0001
	Rey's list delayed recall	13.1±2.1	4.8±5.5	0.0001	7.7±2.8	0.0001	0.6±1.3	0.0001
	Rey's figure recall	22.3±6.5	7.2±4.4	0.0001	13.3±7.4	0.005	0.7±1.3	0.0001
Language	Token	34.7±0.6	31.7±2.5	0.10	30.7±6.3	0.65	26.0±6.4	0.002
	Letter fluency	37.2±10.1	29.4±17.4	0.16	29.1±9.7	0.20	15.7±9.0	0.0001
	Category fluency	39.8±6.9	25.5±5.4	0.04	34.6±9.6	0.001	15.5±8.7	0.0001
Frontal-exec.	Clock drawing	1.0±0.3	1.9±1.3	0.01	2.3±2.1	0.62	4.6±1.4	0.0001
Visuospatial	Rey's figure copy	35.0±1.4	29.2±5.1	0.09	31.3±7.6	0.08	8.9±9.6	0.0001

Values indicate mean±S.D.
YA = young adults; HE = healthy elders; pAD = prodromal AD; mAD = mild to moderate AD.
Statistical analysis performed: Kruskal–Wallis with Mann–Whitney post-hoc U test for difference between groups.

educational level being between primary and middle school. Their global cognitive performance was as expected, based on the diagnostic categories. Gender was balanced, but with a slightly lower prevalence of women in the pAD group ($p = 0.093$). White matter damage was equally present among HE, pAD, and mAD. Young adults, as expected, had higher educational levels and lower levels of white matter damage relative to both the patients and healthy elderly groups.

Neuropsychological performance revealed increasing cognitive impairment from young to healthy elderly (Table 2) for all functions listed in Table 2 ($p < 0.04$) except for language comprehension ($p = 0.10$), verbal production ($p = 0.16$), and visuospatial abilities ($p = 0.09$). As expected, pAD when compared to HE had lower scores on tests of under score immediate ($p = 0.001$) and delayed ($p = 0.00001$) verbal memory and visuospatial memory ($p = 0.005$), as well as in semantic

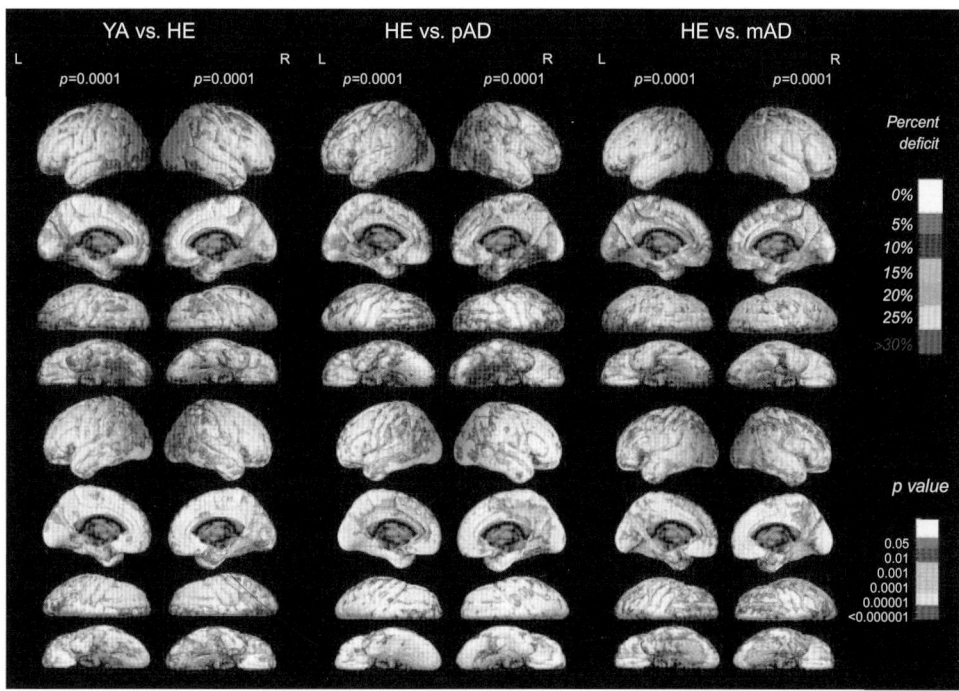

Fig. 2. Map of the differences of gray matter between study groups. Corrected set level significance on permutation test is reported on top of each hemisphere. (For color figures, please refer to the color figures in last section of the book.)

language production ($p = 0.0001$). mAD compared to HE featured severe cognitive impairments on all tests (p for all comparisons < 0.0002).

Fig. 2 shows that compared to YA, HE subjects featured cortical gray matter deficits of up to 20–35% in the superior parietal cortices and less widespread loss of up to 15–20% in the frontal, temporal, and occipital regions ($p = 0.0001$ from permutation testing for both left and right hemispheres). Compared to HE, pAD featured on average 15–20% posterior cingulate/retrosplenial and subgenual/orbitofrontal cortex gray matter loss, with less marked loss in the medial temporal (between 10% and 15%) regions ($p = 0.0001$ for both left and right hemispheres). mAD patients gray matter pattern of atrophy with respect to HE otherwise, overlapped with that of pAD, with more severe gray matter loss localized in medial temporal, parietal, and occipital cortices (these values being, on average, around 13–15% for gray matter loss, $p < 0.0001$), in direct hippocampal

neural network (15% of gray matter loss, $p < 0.0001$ for both left and right hemispheres) and also involving the temporal poles (15–25% of gray matter).

Fig. 3 shows the correlation between GMD and age for the three groups (HE, pAD, and mAD patients); while there was generally a strong linear association (Pearson's $r > -0.60$, $p < 0.0001$ for both hemispheres from permutation testing) between gray matter decline and age for HE, encompassing all parietal, frontal, and temporal areas, for pAD, the effect of age was totally obscured by the incoming pathology in the left hemisphere ($p = 0.10$ from permutation testing), while in the right hemisphere there was a strong association (Pearson's $r > -0.60$, $p = 0.002$ from permutation testing) only for specific frontal and temporal pole regions, without mapping on these particular areas of GMD found atrophic in pAD vs. HE contrast. A similar pattern of association, though milder for the right hemisphere, was found

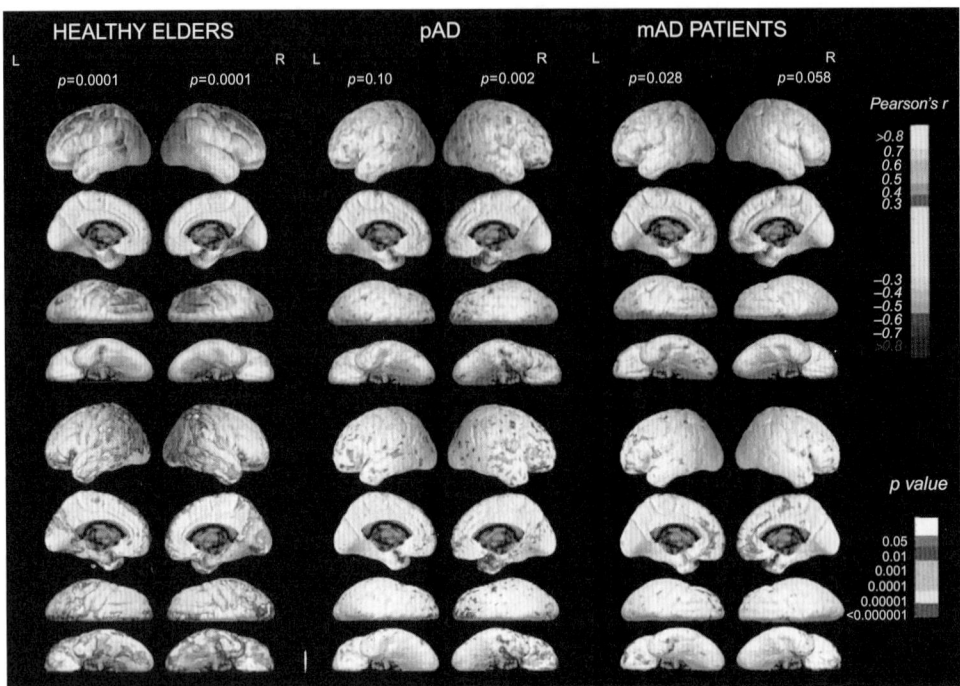

Fig. 3.   Map of correlations between age and gray matter density. Corrected set level significance on permutation test is reported on top of each hemisphere. (For color figures, please refer to the color figures in last section of the book.)

also for the mAD group (Pearson's $r > -0.060$, $p < 0.058$ from permutation testing for both hemispheres). Table 3 shows the average volume percent differences between each group of interest (HE, pAD, or mAD) and its corresponding control group (YA for HE or HE for pAD and mAD). ROIs were defined in terms of networks of functional and structural linked BAs. As expected, the atrophy pattern is similar to that in Fig. 2 but the values, being areal averages, are lower. In general, healthy elderly group featured less gray matter compared to the younger control group in all left and right brain lobes (7–13% of gray matter loss). In particular, the most affected areas were the direct hippocampal pathway ($p < 0.001$ for both hemispheres) and the sensorimotor ($p < 0.001$ for both hemispheres) and visual networks ($p < 0.007$ for both hemispheres). Other networks, such as the polysynaptic hippocampal and olfactory network, were involved in only the

pAD and mAD groups (6–15% of gray matter loss, $p < 0.06$) with respect to HE. For pAD patients a loss of gray matter was also detected in the direct hippocampal pathway, sensorimotor cortices, and in all brain lobes ($p < 0.05$), but at a level -5 to 10% with respect to the HE group. While for the mAD group the amount of gray matter loss of polysynaptic hippocampal and olfactory networks was similar to that of pAD with respect to HE (6–13% of gray matter loss, $p < 0.031$), it was greater for each other analyzed brain area (11–15% of gray matter loss, $p < 0.0001$).

The effect of gender was controlled by running an ANCOVA to compare gray matter volumes in the networks listed in Table 3 among the four groups by entering group (YA, HE, pAD, mAD) as the fixed factor, gender as the random factor, and age as a covariate. As p for each comparison was non-significant ($p > 0.22$), this indicated that gender was not a confounder of the findings of this study.

TABLE 3

REGION OF INTEREST-BASED ANALYSIS OF GRAY MATTER VOLUMES

Values reported below are mean values of gray matter volumes computed throughout all voxels comprising given network of BAs.

		Young adults (YA)	Healthy elders (HE)			Prodromal AD patients (pAD)			Mild to moderate AD patients (mAD)		
			p vs. YA		Δ HE vs. YA (±95% CI)	p vs. HE		Δ pAD vs. HE (±95% CI)	p vs. HE		Δ mAD vs. HE (±95% CI)
Network volumes											
Polysynaptic hippocampal pathway	L	10,719±887	0.67	10,632±1098	−1% (−6 to 4)	0.06	10028±1172	−6% (−12 to 0.05)	0.031	10,056±966	−6% (−11 to 0.1)
	R	10,877±1055	0.34	10,617±1228	−2% (−8 to 3)	0.04	9727±1069	−8% (−15 to −2)	0.005	9696±875	−9% (−14 to −2)
Olfactory	L	5259±388	0.06	5009±458	−5% (−9 to −0.02)	0.001	4412±478	−12% (−17 to −6)	0.0001	4487±342	−10% (−15 to −6)
	R	5471±455	0.11	5092±443	−7% (−11 to −2)	0.001	4311±501	−15% (−20 to −10)	0.0001	4447±416	−13% (−17 to −8)
Direct hippocampal pathway	L	39,667±1686	0.001	34,515±2552	−13% (−16 to −10)	0.005	31,904±3381	−7% (−12 to −3)	0.0001	29,357±2215	−15% (−19 to −11)
	R	40,219±2121	0.001	34,618±2700	−14% (−17 to −10)	0.001	31,593±3259	−9% (−13 to −4)	0.0001	29,375±2921	−15% (−20 to −11)
Sensorimotor	L	6486±517	0.001	5668±555	−13% (−17 to −8)	0.02	5314±572	−6% (−12 to −0.03)	0.0001	4891±365	−14% (−19 to −9)
	R	6664±512	0.001	5697±573	−14% (−19 to −10)	0.05	5351±464	−6% (−12 to −0.04)	0.0001	4873±374	−14% (−19 to −9)
Visual	L	12,136±946	0.007	11,351±1018	−6% (−11 to −2)	0.13	10,769±1023	−5% (−10 to 0.01)	0.0001	9779±708	−14% (−18 to −9)
	R	12,684±965	0.001	10,994±897	−13% (−7 to −9)	0.07	10,147±680	−7% (−12 to −3)	0.0001	9559±923	−13% (−18 to −8)
Lobar volumes											
Frontal lobe	L	55,803±3280	0.001	49,438±3759	−11% (−5 to −8)	0.001	44,340±4704	−10% (−15 to −5)	0.0001	43,107±3371	−13% (−17 to −9)
	R	55,614±3431	0.001	49,533±4146	−11% (−5 to −7)	0.001	44,742±3408	−10% (−14 to −5)	0.0001	43,804±3424	−12% (−16 to −7)
Parietal lobe	L	39,822±2091	0.001	37,139±2947	−7% (−10 to −3)	0.003	34,090±3131	−8% (−13 to −3)	0.0001	33,035±2575	−11% (−15 to −7)
	R	40,038±2564	0.003	37,308±3440	−7% (−11 to −2)	0.001	33,569±2644	−10% (−15 to −5)	0.0001	32,539±2496	−13% (−17 to −8)
Temporal lobe	L	34,208±1669	0.001	30,483±2266	−11% (−14 to −7)	0.011	28,734±2872	−6% (−10 to −1)	0.0001	26,462±1983	−13% (−17 to −9)
	R	34,713±1935	0.001	30,353±2589	−13% (−16 to −9)	0.008	28,012±2845	−8% (−13 to −3)	0.0001	26,165±2904	−14% (−19 to −9)
Global volumes											
Total gray matter volume	L	91,056±4202	0.0001	82,125±5639	−10% (−13 to −7)	0.001	75,216±6456	−8% (−13 to −4)	0.0001	71,505±4561	−13% (−16 to −9)
	R	91,749±4635	0.0001	81,955±5967	−11% (−14 to −7)	0.0001	74,439±5069	−9% (−13 to −5)	0.0001	71,282±5406	−13% (−17 to −9)

Volumes are mm³ mean ±S.D. Δ denotes the percent difference between gray matter concentrations for each group; L = left, R = right; CI = 95% confidence intervals around Δ % difference.
Statistical analysis performed: Kruskal–Wallis with Mann–Whitney post-hoc U test for difference between groups.

4.4. Discussion

Using an advanced, accurate, and reliable computational technique for investigating the cerebral cortex, we were able to investigate the topographical distribution of age-related cortical atrophy in healthy elderly and to distinguish normal age-related cortical changes with those pathological associated with prodromal and established AD. From this, several key conclusions may be drawn.

First, the overall pattern of observed structural MRI differences in the healthy elderly was global. This agrees with prior studies (Raji et al., 2009) of normal aging that have found that the brains of elderly adults without dementia have lower weight, reduced tissue volume, and expansion of both the cerebral ventricles and sulci, loss of neuronal cells in neocortical, hippocampal, and cerebellar areas, shrinkage of neurons, and a reduction in synaptic density (Morrison and Hof, 2007). Compared to healthy young adults, HE featured cortical gray matter loss up to 35% in the superior parietal cortices and less widespread loss of up to 15–20% in the frontal, temporal, and occipital regions. These data agree with the well-documented pattern of atrophy with age and are localized in prefrontal, frontal, temporal, occipital, and parietal cortices, cerebellum, and caudate nuclei (Good et al., 2001; Smith et al., 2007). Hippocampal and mesial temporal lobe volume losses have been reported too in normal aging (Raz et al., 1998) consistent with neuropathologic studies that find neurofibrillary tangles and neuronal loss in cognitively normal individuals (Guillozet et al., 2003). These massive volumetric brain reductions, seen in healthy aging, are thought to be related to neuronal loss to only a minor extent. Rather, reductions of synaptic spines and lower numbers of synapses probably account for the gray matter atrophy; in addition, the length of myelinated axons is greatly reduced, up to almost 50% during the aging process (Fjell and Walhovd, 2010). Moreover, despite a significant loss of total neuronal numbers, age-related decrements in brain weight and cortical thickness are strongly related to the shrinkage of large neurons resulting in increase in the number of small neurons and the neuron–glia ratio (Terry et al., 1987). Constant neuronal density coupled with diminished cortical volume (decreased brain weight and cortical thinning) and increasing number of gliar cells indicate that there is some neuronal loss with age, but it is of much lesser extent than that due to the neurodegenerative process seen in AD, where total number of neurons declines without any "compensatory" rise of small neurons: large cells do not shrink, but die in AD (Terry, 2006).

The pAD patients displayed a pattern of significant atrophy compared to healthy controls. This pattern partially overlapped the HE in temporal areas, but to a lesser degree. This finding agrees with voxel-based morphometry (Raji et al., 2009) studies. The confluence of age and AD atrophy in the MTL suggests this region to be a common target for both processes. Aging is a key risk factor for AD because it is strongly linked to many critical brain areas affected by AD. The pattern of gray matter atrophy in full blown mAD was similar to that of pAD but of greater prominence, as cortical loss was seen in virtually all areas, growing from 6% to 15% of gray matter deficit and, in line with results from previous studies (see Frisoni et al., 2010 for a review).

In both HE and pAD groups, a global pattern of atrophy was detected for all brain regions, when compared to YA and HE, respectively. For the HE group, these findings should reflect normal aging processes more than pathological processes related to a future progression to AD (Guillozet et al., 2003). In fact, correlation maps of age and GMD completely overlapped in their pattern with atrophy maps of HE in respect to YA group. The areas of gray matter showing loss were strongly associated with the aging effect and this was not the case for the pAD and mAD groups.

The gray matter loss in the polysynaptic hippocampal pathway and in the orbitofrontal cortex (the network that we defined as "olfactory" and comprising BA 11 — prefrontal orbital cortex — and BA 25 — subgenual cortex) seemed to be more specifically associated with the pAD status; in fact, there were no differences between HE and YA in those areas, thus reflecting probable pathological neuronal death processes present in pAD patients only. Moreover, those areas featured the same amount of gray matter loss in the mAD vs. HE conditions too. Losses in these critical cortical networks may occur near the beginning of the pathology and then remain stable, as atrophy progresses and encompasses other cortical areas. In support of this, neuropathological (Delacourte et al., 1999) and longitudinal MRI studies indicate early and marked alterations in the surrounding hippocampal zones of subjects at risk of developing AD, including MCI (Yamada et al., 1996), very old subjects (Kaye et al., 1997), ApoE4 carriers (Pievani et al., 2009), and asymptomatic subjects with familial AD (Schott et al., 2003). Atrophy of the subgenual/orbitofrontal cortex, involved in the perception of smell (Yousem et al., 1997), has been found repeatedly in patients with MCI and overt AD (Chételat et al., 2005), while smell discrimination seems to be reduced from the early phase of the disease (Djordjevic et al., 2008). Pathologic data indicate that this area is heavily affected by tangle and amyloid pathology (Resnick et al., 2007). Interestingly, atrophy in the orbitofrontal cortex of AD patients has been found to be more severe in men than in women (Callen et al., 2004). This is consistent with the greater, although not significant, prevalence of men in pAD compared to both young adult and healthy elderly controls in our study.

Our results fit well with our previous study (Prestia et al., 2010) that indicated those two neural networks are among the most sensitive and important areas for predicting the transition from MCI to AD. Recent studies analyzing brain areas predictive of conversion to AD reported accelerating atrophy in these networks in patients with MCI (Misra et al., 2009), identifying the cingulate gyrus and the orbitofrontal cortex as the most predictive brain areas of conversion. Considering correlation maps of atrophy and age in pAD group, we can infer two things: first, as documented by many studies (Thompson et al., 2001b), the left hemisphere seems to be more and earlier affected by AD pathology than the right. In our study, the effect of age on the left hemisphere is completely obscured by the presence of the disease (the correlation between age and GMD was not significant).

Second, for the right hemisphere, age-related differences map mainly to frontal and parietal areas, with almost total sparing of the posterior cingulate/retrosplenial and orbitofrontal cortices.

The posterior cingulate/retrosplenial cortex is the target of efferent fibers coming directly from the polysynaptic hippocampal pathway (Frisoni et al., 2009), but the orbitofrontal cortex undergoes widespread damage in AD due to the neurofibrillary tangle pathology (Van Hoesen et al., 2000). This may relate to some of the non-memory-related behavioral changes in the disorder (Shibata et al., 2008). In the mAD group, the pattern of age-related change is similar, with only the right and left frontal and parietal areas (Pearson's $r > -0.5, p = 0.03$) associated with gray matter loss.

The only apparently contrasting finding is that the difference between pAD and HE in the left hippocampal pathway shows just a trend ($p = 0.06$) toward significance: this may be explained by the presence, in HE group, of at least two subjects severely atrophic in this and many other areas who, even if considered as normal during the inclusion phase of this study, performed also more poorly on neuropsychological tests. Those two individuals may progress toward pAD and/or AD overt pathology during the coming months, so their presence in the HE group diminishes the gray matter difference between HE and pAD in areas crucial for the developing of AD.

The neuropsychological tests for which scores in the pAD group were significantly worse than in the HE group were highly related to executive functions such as the verbal fluency test, while some others were more related to memory performances highly dependent on the hippocampus.

Visuospatial memory is one of the first domains to be impaired in individuals affected by pAD (Iachini et al., 2009) and is highly related to MTL function, as well as anterior cingulate and prefrontal cortex. These findings are in accordance with our results that show a loss of gray matter in the posterior cingulated cortex and MTLs of patients affected by pAD in healthy elders but not in the same cortical areas of HE in young adults. Difference in memory and executive functions between HE and YA should depend more on aging than on a pathological loss of cortical gray matter.

This study has some limitations. Our sample size is small and as some previous reports found differences in brain atrophy between men and women (Coffey et al., 1998; Xu et al., 2000), future studies should include well-balanced groups to rule out the possible contribution of sex to the patterns of cortical atrophy. Even so, this effect should not have greatly influenced our results as indicated by our control analyses. Moreover, the YA group education level is higher than that of all patients groups. Finally, the image acquisition protocol and post-processing methods used are not directly comparable to other similar reports, although their reproducibility and stability over time seem to be good (Sowell et al., 2004).

With several promising disease-modifying candidate treatments under development, the ability to discern physiological structural changes in healthy elderly brains from changes specific to AD pathology raises hopes for the identification of more specific surrogate markers of the disease.

Acknowledgments

This work was supported by Grants Ex Art 56 533 F/B 1 and PS-Neuro Ex 56/05/11 (Italian Ministry of Health), and supported in part by a grant from the Italian Ministry of Health, Analisi dei Fattori di Rischio e di Potenziali Elementi Predittivi di Danno Neurodegenerativo Nelle Sindromi Parkinsoniane number 502/92.

P.T. is supported, in part, by NIH Grants R01 EB008281, EB008432, EB007813, AG036535, and AG020098, and by the NIBIB, NCRR, NIA, and NICHD, agencies of the U.S. National Institutes of Health.

The authors have no conflicts of interest to declare.

References

Abe, O., Yamasue, H., Aoki, S., Suga, M., Yamada, H., Kasai, K., Masutani, Y., Kato, N., Kato, N. and Ohtomo, K. (2008) Aging in the CNS: comparison of gray/white matter volume and diffusion tensor data. *Neurobiol. Aging*, 29: 102–116.

Allen, J.S., Bruss, J., Brown, C.K. and Damasio, H. (2005) Normal neuroanatomical variation due to age: the major lobes and a parcellation of the temporal region. *Neurobiol. Aging*, 26: 1245–1260.

Braak, H. and Braak, E. (1991) Neuropathological staging of Alzheimer-related changes. *Acta Neuropathol.*, 82: 239–259.

Callen, D.J., Black, S.E., Caldwell, C.B. and Grady, C.L. (2004) The influence of sex on limbic volume and perfusion in AD. *Neurobiol. Aging*, 25: 761–770.

Chételat, G., Landeau, B., Eustache, F., Mézenge, F., Viader, F., De la Sayette, V., Desgranges, B. and Baron, J.C. (2005) Using voxel-based morphometry to map the structural changes associated with rapid conversion in MCI: a longitudinal MRI study. *Neuroimage*, 27: 934–946.

Coffey, C.E., Lucke, J.F., Saxton, J.A., Ratcliff, G., Unitas, L.J., Billig, B. and Bryan, R.N. (1998) Sex differences in brain aging: a quantitative magnetic resonance imaging study. *Arch. Neurol. (Chic.)*, 55: 169–179.

Crum, R.M., Anthony, J.C., Bassett, S.S. and Folstein, M.F. (1993) Population-based norms for the Mini-Mental State Examination by age and educational level. *J. Am. Med. Ass.*, 269: 2386–2391.

Delacourte, A., David, J.P., Sergeant, N., Buée, L., Wattez, A., Vermersch, P., Ghozali, F., Fallet-Bianco, C., Pasquier, F., Lebert, F., Petit, H. and Di Menza, C. (1999) The biochemical pathway of neurofibrillary degeneration in aging and Alzheimer's disease. *Neurology*, 52: 1158–1165.

Djordjevic, J., Jones-Gotman, M., De Sousa, K. and Chertkow, H. (2008) Olfaction in patients with mild cognitive impairment and Alzheimer's disease. *Neurobiol. Aging*, 29: 693–706.

Dubois, B., Feldman, H.H., Jacova, C., Dekosky, S.T., Barberger-Gateau, P., Cummings, J., Delacourte, A., Galasko, D., Gauthier, S., Jicha, G., Meguro, K., O'Brien, J., Pasquier, F., Robert, P., Rossor, M., Salloway, S., Stern, Y., Visser, P.J. and Scheltens, P. (2007) Research criteria for the diagnosis of Alzheimer's disease: revising the NINCDS-ADRDA criteria. *Lancet Neurol.*, 6: 734–746.

Duvernoy, H.M. (1998) *The Human Hippocampus: Functional Anatomy, Vascularization and Serial Sections with MRI*. Springer, New York.

Fjell, A.M. and Walhovd, K.B. (2010) Structural brain changes in aging: courses, causes and cognitive consequences. *Rev. Neurosci.*, 21: 187–221.

Fotenos, A.F., Snyder, A.Z., Girton, L.E., Morris, J.C. and Buckner, R.L. (2005) Normative estimates of cross-sectional and longitudinal brain volume decline in aging and AD. *Neurology*, 64: 1032–1039.

Freeman, S.H., Kandel, R., Cruz, L., Rozkalne, A., Newell, K., Frosch, M.P., Hedley-Whyte, E.T., Locascio, J.J., Lipsitz, L.A. and Hyman, B.T. (2008) Preservation of neuronal number despite age-related cortical brain atrophy in elderly subjects without Alzheimer disease. *J. Neuropathol. Exp. Neurol.*, 67: 1205–1212.

Frisoni, G.B., Prestia, A., Rasser, P.E., Bonetti, M. and Thompson, P.M. (2009) In vivo mapping of incremental cortical atrophy from incipient to overt Alzheimer's disease. *J. Neurol.*, 256: 916–924.

Frisoni, G.B., Fox, N.C., Jack, C.R., Scheltens, P. and Thompson, P.M. (2010) The clinical use of structural MRI in Alzheimer disease. *Nat. Rev. Neurol.*, 6: 67–77.

Galluzzi, S., Testa, C., Boccardi, M., Bresciani, L., Benussi, L., Ghidoni, R., Beltramello, A., Bonetti, M., Bono, G., Falini, A., Magnani, G., Minonzio, G., Piovan, E., Binetti, G. and Frisoni, G.B. (2009) The Italian brain normative archive of structural MR scans: norms for medial temporal atrophy and white matter lesions. *Aging Clin. Exp. Res.*, 21: 266–276.

Ge, Y., Grossman, R.I., Babb, J.S., Rabin, M.L., Mannon, L.J. and Kolson, D.L. (2002) Age-related total gray matter and white matter changes in normal adult brain. Part I. Volumetric MR imaging analysis. *Am. J. Neuroradiol.*, 23: 1327–1333.

Good, C.D., Johnsrude, I.S., Ashburner, J., Henson, R.N.A., Friston, K.J. and Frackowiak, R.S.J. (2001) A voxel-based morphometric study of aging in 465 normal adult human beings. *Neuroimage*, 14: 21–36.

Guillozet, A.L., Weintraub, S., Mash, D.C. and Mesulam, M.M. (2003) Neurofibrillary tangles, amyloid, and memory in aging and mild cognitive impairment. *Arch. Neurol. (Chic.)*, 60: 729–736.

Iachini, I., Iavarone, A., Senese, V.P., Ruotolo, F. and Ruggiero, G. (2009) Visuospatial memory in healthy elderly, AD and MCI: a review. *Curr. Aging Sci.*, 2: 43–59.

Kalpouzos, G., Chételat, G., Baron, J.C., Landeau, B., Mevel, K., Godeau, C., Barré, L., Constans, J.M., Viader, F., Eustache, F. and Desgranges, B. (2009) Voxel-based mapping of brain gray matter volume and glucose metabolism profiles in normal aging. *Neurobiol. Aging*, 30: 112–124.

Kaye, J.A., Swihart, T., Howieson, D., Dame, A., Moore, M.M., Karnos, T., Camicioli, R., Ball, M., Oken, B. and Sexton, G. (1997) Volume loss of the hippocampus and temporal lobe in healthy elderly persons destined to develop dementia. *Neurology*, 48: 1297–1304.

Kordower, J.H., Chu, Y., Stebbins, G.T., DeKosky, S.T., Cochran, E.J., Bennett, D. and Mufson, E.J. (2001) Loss and atrophy of layer II entorhinal cortex neurons in elderly people with mild cognitive impairment. *Ann. Neurol.*, 49: 202–213.

Lezak, M., Howieson, D. and Loring, D.W. (2004) *Neuropsychological Assessment*, 4th Edn. Oxford University Press, London.

McKhann, G., Drachman, D., Folstein, M., Katzman, R., Price, D. and Stadlan, E.M. (1984) Clinical diagnosis of Alzheimer's disease: report of the NINCDS-ADRDA Work Group under the auspices of Department of Health and Human Services Task Force on Alzheimer's Disease. *Neurology*, 34: 939–944.

Misra, C., Fan, Y. and Davatzikos, C. (2009) Baseline and longitudinal patterns of brain atrophy in MCI patients, and their use in prediction of short-term conversion to AD: results from ADNI. *Neuroimage*, 44: 1415–1422.

Morrison, J.H. and Hof, P.R. (2007) Life and death of neurons in the aging cerebral cortex. *Int. Rev. Neurobiol.*, 81: 41–57.

Pakkenberg, B., Pelvig, D., Marner, L., Bundgaard, M.J., Gundersen, H.J., Nyengaard, J.R. and Regeur, L. (2003) Aging and the human neocortex. *Exp. Gerontol.*, 38: 95–99.

Petersen, R.C., Doody, R., Kurz, A., Mohs, R.C., Morris, J.C., Rabins, P.V., Ritchie, K., Rossor, M., Thal, L. and Winblad, B. (2001) Current concepts in mild cognitive impairment. *Arch. Neurol. (Chic.)*, 58: 1985–1992.

Pievani, M., Rasser, P.E., Galluzzi, S., Benussi, L., Ghidoni, R., Sabattoli, F., Bonetti, M., Binetti, G., Thompson, P.M. and Frisoni, G.B. (2009) Mapping the effect of ApoE epsilon4 on gray matter loss in Alzheimer's disease in vivo. *Neuroimage*, 45: 1090–1098.

Prestia, A., Drago, V., Rasser, P.E., Bonetti, M., Thompson, P.M. and Frisoni, G.B. (2010) Cortical changes in incipient Alzheimer's disease. *J. Alzheimers Dis.*, 22: 1339–1349.

Price, J.L., Ko, A.I., Wade, M.J., Tsou, S.K., McKeel, D.W. and Morris, J.C. (2001) Neuron number in the entorhinal cortex and CA1 in preclinical Alzheimer disease. *Arch. Neurol. (Chic.)*, 58: 1395–1402.

Raji, C.A., Lopez, O.L., Kuller, L.H., Carmichael, O.T. and Becker, J.T. (2009) Age, Alzheimer disease, and brain structure. *Neurology*, 73: 1899–1905.

Rasser, P.E., Johnston, P., Ward, P. and Thompson, P.M. (2004) A deformable Brodmann area atlas. In: R. Leahy and C. Roux (Eds.), *Proceedings of the IEEE International Symposium on Biomedical Imaging: From Macro to Nano*. IEEE, Arlington, pp. 400–403.

Raz, N. and Rodrigue, K.M. (2006) Differential aging of the brain: patterns, cognitive correlates and modifiers. *Neurosci. Biobehav. Rev.*, 30: 730–748.

Raz, N., Gunning-Dixon, F.M., Head, D., Dupuis, J.H. and Acker, J.D. (1998) Neuroanatomical correlates of cognitive aging: evidence from structural magnetic resonance imaging. *Neuropsychology*, 12: 95–114.

Resnick, S.M., Pham, D.L., Kraut, M.A., Zonderman, A.B. and Davatzikos, C. (2003) Longitudinal magnetic resonance imaging studies of older adults: a shrinking brain. *J. Neurosci.*, 23: 3295–3301.

Resnick, S.M., Lamar, M. and Driscoll, I. (2007) Vulnerability of the orbitofrontal cortex to age-associated structural and functional brain changes. *Ann. N. Y. Acad. Sci.*, 1121: 562–575.

Salat, D.H., Buckner, R.L., Snyder, A.Z., Greve, D.N., Desikan, R.S., Busa, E., Morris, J.C., Dale, A.M. and

Fischl, B. (2004) Thinning of the cerebral cortex in aging. *Cereb. Cortex*, 14: 721–730.

Schott, J.M., Fox, N.C., Frost, C., Scahill, R.I., Janssen, J.C., Chan, D., Jenkins, R. and Rossor, M.N. (2003) Assessing the onset of structural change in familial Alzheimer's disease. *Ann. Neurol.*, 53: 181–188.

Shibata, K., Narumoto, J., Kitabayashi, Y., Ushijima, Y. and Fukui, K. (2008) Correlation between anosognosia and regional cerebral blood flow in Alzheimer's disease. *Neurosci. Lett.*, 435: 7–10.

Smith, C.D., Chebrolu, H., Wekstein, D.R., Schmitt, F.A. and Markesbery, W.R. (2007) Age and gender effects on human brain anatomy: a voxel-based morphometry study in healthy elderly. *Neurobiol. Aging*, 28: 1075–1087.

Sowell, E.R., Thompson, P.M., Tessner, K.D. and Toga, A.W. (2001) Mapping continued brain growth and gray matter density reduction in dorsal frontal cortex: inverse relationships during postadolescent brain maturation. *J. Neurosci.*, 21: 8819–8829.

Sowell, E.R., Thompson, P.M., Leonard, C.M., Welcome, S.E., Kan, E. and Toga, A.W. (2004) Longitudinal mapping of cortical thickness and brain growth in normal children. *J. Neurosci.*, 24: 8223–8231.

Terry, R.D. (2006) Alzheimer's disease and the aging brain. *J. Geriatr. Psychiatry Neurol.*, 19: 125–128.

Terry, R.D., De Teresa, R. and Hansen, L.A. (1987) Neocortical cell counts in normal human adult aging. *Ann. Neurol.*, 21: 530–539.

Thompson, P.M., Woods, R.P., Mega, M.S. and Toga, A.W. (2000) Mathematical/computational challenges in creating deformable and probabilistic atlases of the human brain. *Hum. Brain Mapp.*, 9: 81–92.

Thompson, P.M., Mega, M.S., Vidal, C., Rapoport, J.L. and Toga, A.W. (2001a) Detecting disease-specific patterns of brain structure using cortical pattern matching and a population-based probabilistic brain atlas. In: M. Insana and R. Leahy (Eds.), *Lecture Notes in Computer Science 2082*. Springer, New York, pp. 488–501.

Thompson, P.M., Mega, M.S., Woods, R.P., Zoumalan, C.I., Lindshield, C.J., Blanton, R.E., Moussai, J., Holmes, C.J., Cummings, J.L. and Toga, A.W. (2001b) Cortical change in Alzheimer's disease detected with a disease-specific population-based brain atlas. *Cereb. Cortex*, 11: 1–16.

Thompson, P.M., Hayashi, K.M., Sowell, E.R., Gogtay, N., Giedd, J.N., Rapoport, J.L., De Zubicaray, G.I., Janke, A.L., Rose, S.E., Semple, J., Doddrell, D.M., Wang, Y., Van Erp, T.G., Cannon, T.D. and Toga, A.W. (2004) Mapping cortical change in Alzheimer's disease, brain development, and schizophrenia. *Neuroimage*, 23: S2–S18.

Van Hoesen, G.W., Parvizi, J. and Chu, C.C. (2000) Orbitofrontal cortex pathology in Alzheimer's disease. *Cereb. Cortex*, 10: 243–251.

Von Gunten, A., Kövari, E., Rivara, C.B., Bouras, C., Hof, P.R. and Giannakopoulos, P. (2005) Stereologic analysis of hippocampal Alzheimer's disease pathology in the oldest-old: evidence for sparing of the entorhinal cortex and CA1 field. *Exp. Neurol.*, 193: 198–206.

Wahlund, L.O., Barkhof, F., Fazekas, F., Bronge, L., Augustin, M., Sjögren, M., Wallin, A., Ader, H., Leys, D., Pantoni, L., Pasquier, F., Erkinjuntti, T. and Scheltens, P. (2001) European Task Force on Age-Related White Matter Changes. A new rating scale for age-related white matter changes applicable to MRI and CT. *Stroke*, 32: 1318–1322.

Xu, J., Kobayashi, S., Yamaguchi, S., Iijima, K., Okada, K. and Yamashita, K. (2000) Gender effects on age-related changes in brain structure. *Am. J. Neuroradiol.*, 21: 112–118.

Yamada, N., Tanabe, H., Kazui, H., Ikeda, M., Hashimoto, M., Nakagawa, Y., Wada, Y. and Eguchi, Y. (1996) Longitudinal MRI-based quantitative and neuropsychological assessments in early Alzheimer's disease. *Alzheimer's Res.*, 2: 29–36.

Yousem, D.M., Williams, S.C., Howard, R.O., Andrew, C., Simmons, A., Allin, M., Geckle, R.J., Suskind, D., Bullmore, E.T., Brammer, M.J. and Doty, R.L. (1997) Functional MR imaging during odor stimulation: preliminary data. *Radiology*, 204: 833–838.

Application of Brain Oscillations in Neuropsychiatric Diseases
(Supplements to Clinical Neurophysiology, Vol. 62)
Editors: E. Başar, C. Başar-Eroğlu, A. Özerdem, P.M. Rossini, G.G. Yener

Chapter 5

The value of spontaneous EEG oscillations in distinguishing patients in vegetative and minimally conscious states

Alexander A. Fingelkurts[a,*], Andrew A. Fingelkurts[a], Sergio Bagnato[b,c], Cristina Boccagni[b,c] and Giuseppe Galardi[b,c]

[a]*BM-Science — Brain and Mind Technologies Research Center, FI-02601 Espoo, Finland*
[b]*Neurorehabilitation Unit, Rehabilitation Department, Fondazione Istituto "San Raffaele — G. Giglio", 90015 Cefalù (PA), Italy*
[c]*Neurophysiology Unit, Rehabilitation Department, Fondazione Istituto "San Raffaele — G. Giglio", 90015 Cefalù (PA), Italy*

ABSTRACT

Objective: The value of spontaneous electroencephalography (EEG) oscillations in distinguishing patients in vegetative state (VS) and minimally conscious states (MCS) was studied.

Methods: We quantified dynamic repertoire of EEG oscillations in resting condition with closed eyes in patients in VS and MCS. The exact composition of EEG oscillations was assessed by the probability-classification analysis of short-term EEG spectral patterns.

Results: The probability of delta, theta, and slow-alpha oscillations occurrence was smaller for patients in MCS than for VS. Additionally, only patients in MCS demonstrated fast-alpha oscillation occurrence. Depending on the type and composition of EEG oscillations, the probability of their occurrence was either etiology dependent or independent. The probability of EEG oscillations occurrence differentiated brain injuries with different etiologies.

Conclusions: Spontaneous EEG oscillations have a potential value in distinguishing patients in VS and MCS.

Significance: This work may have implications for clinical care, rehabilitative programs, and medical–legal decisions in patients with impaired consciousness states following coma due to acute brain injuries.

Highlights:
- The probability of delta, theta, and slow-alpha oscillations occurrence was smaller and the probability of fast-alpha oscillations occurrence was higher for patients in MCS than for patients in VS.
- The probability of EEG oscillations occurrence differentiated brain injuries with different etiologies.
- Spontaneous EEG has a potential value in distinguishing patients in VS and MCS.

KEYWORDS

Electroencephalogram; Disorder of consciousness; EEG oscillations; Patients in vegetative and minimally conscious states

Correspondence to: Dr. Alexander A. Fingelkurts, Ph.D., Co-head of Research, BM-Science — Brain and Mind Technologies Research Center, P.O. Box 77, FI-02601 Espoo, Finland.
Tel.: +358 9 5414506; Fax: +358 9 5414507;
E-mail: alexander.fingelkurts@bm-science.com

5.1. Introduction

Severe brain injuries constitute an epidemic public health problem affecting, for example, more than 100,000 Americans annually (Winslade, 1998;

NIH Consensus Development Panel, 1999). Severe brain injuries are caused mainly either by trauma, or by vascular or anoxic events and lead to disorders of consciousness such as vegetative state (VS) or minimally conscious state (MCS) following coma. VS is "a clinical condition of unawareness of self and environment in which the patient breathes spontaneously, has a stable circulation, and shows cycles of eye closure and opening which may simulate sleep and waking" (Monti et al., 2010). The MCS is "a condition of severely altered consciousness in which minimal but definite behavioral evidence of self or environmental awareness is demonstrated. In MCS, cognitively mediated behavior occurs inconsistently, but is reproducible or sustained long enough to be differentiated from reflexive behavior" (Giacino et al., 2002).

Studies indicated that 10–17 years ago the MCS caseload in the USA was estimated at 112,000–280,000 (Strauss et al., 2000) and a VS caseload was estimated at 10,000–25,000 adults and 4000–10,000 children (The Multi-Society Task Force on PVS, 1994). Thanks to advances in critical care, VS and MCS incidence and prevalence are progressively increasing (Beaumont and Kenealy, 2005).

In spite of significant progress in neuroimaging and the introduction of clear-cut diagnostic criteria, patients with disorders of consciousness still represent an important clinical problem in terms of diagnosis, prognosis, treatment, everyday management, and end-of-life decision making. Indeed, the rate of misdiagnosis of VS/MCS has not substantially changed in the past 15 years (Schnakers et al., 2009).

Misdiagnoses of VS and MCS are common and have been shown to be as high as 37–43% (Tresch et al., 1991; Childs et al., 1993; Andrews et al., 1996; Schnakers et al., 2006). Such misdiagnoses may have a profound effect on end-of-life decision making (Andrews et al., 1996; Andrews, 2004; Gill-Thwaites, 2006). Today, almost half of all deaths in critical care units follow a decision to withhold or withdraw therapy (Smedira et al., 1990).

Misdiagnoses of VS and MCS are due to the fact that the diagnosis of VS and MCS patients is based on clinical observation of subjectively interpreted behavioral responses mostly, while conscious experience often occurs without behavioral signs. Therefore, determining whether or not noncommunicative or minimally communicative patients are phenomenally conscious is still a major clinical and ethical challenge. For this reason, additional objective measurement tools are needed for achieving more accurate diagnoses.

Electrophysiological electroencephalography (EEG) measures which permit bedside assessment could be particularly useful since EEG directly and objectively records spontaneous brain activity without requiring any behavioral response by the patient. It has been proposed that EEG oscillations act as communication networks with functional relationships to the integrative brain functions (Başar et al., 2001a). It is assumed that EEG oscillations are of fundamental importance for mediating and distributing "higher-level" processes in the human brain (Klimesch 1999; Başar et al., 2001b). Moreover, it was repeatedly demonstrated that changes in EEG oscillations are associated with cognitive deficits, and brain and mind pathologies (for the review and discussion see Başar and Güntekin, 2008; Başar, 2010). Although EEG is a routine examination in patients with disorders of consciousness, there is a considerable lack of studies which investigate explicitly the value of EEG oscillations in distinguishing MCS and VS patients. To our best knowledge there is only one such study which used EEG bispectral index (BIS; see Schnakers et al., 2008). Even though BIS seems to correlate empirically with consciousness (Myles et al., 2004), it has no clear theoretical foundation (Massimini et al., 2009).

Earlier Fingelkurts et al. (2012) using automatic advanced analysis of EEG demonstrated that particular types of EEG oscillatory phenomena were associated with awareness (the probability of the occurrence of some EEG oscillations was in the order of NORM > MCS > VS) or unawareness (the probability of the occurrence of other EEG oscillations was in the order of NORM < MCS < VS). This study was theoretically motivated and it provided an empirical support that spontaneous EEG oscillatory states have a potential value in revealing neural constitutes of consciousness. Hence, it is reasonable to assume that spontaneous EEG oscillations can be useful in distinguishing patients with disorders of consciousness with different degrees of expression of consciousness.

Therefore, the aim of the present study was to investigate the capacity of spontaneous EEG oscillations to distinguish VS and MCS patients considering different etiologies of brain damage. In this study we will consider only those differences in EEG oscillations between VS and MCS patients which demonstrated association with awareness/unawareness in earlier study (Fingelkurts et al., 2012).

5.2. Methods

5.2.1. Subjects

The study was performed on 21 non- or minimally communicative patients with severe brain injuries suffering from different consciousness disorders (Table 1), admitted to the Neurorehabilitation Unit of Fondazione Istituto "San Raffaele — G. Giglio" to carry out an intensive neurorehabilitation program.

On admission all patients underwent a thorough and comprehensive clinical neurological examination. The diagnosis of VS and MCS was made according to currently accepted diagnostic criteria (ANA Committee on Ethical Affairs, 1993; The Multi-Society Task Force on PVS, 1994; Royal College of Physicians, 2003). Additionally, the levels of cognitive functioning (LCF) score (Gouvier et al., 1987) was assessed on the day of admission and 3 days later when the EEG was recorded. We chose to use the LCF scale instead of the Glasgow Outcome Scale (Jennett and Bond, 1975), the Glasgow Coma Scale (Jennett et al., 1981), or the JFK Coma Recovery Scale (Giacino et al., 2004) because LCF evaluates not only behavioral patterns but also cognitive functions (which are closely related to consciousness rather than to behavioral patterns), and LCF has been found better related with the presence of EEG abnormalities in patients with disorders of consciousness in previous studies (Bagnato et al., 2010; Boccagni et al., 2011). The LCF scale has different grades ranging from 1 to 8 (1 = patient does not respond to external stimuli and/or command; 8 = patient is self-oriented and responds to the environment but abstract reasoning abilities decrease relative to pre-morbid levels).

Based on the strict adherence to the aforesaid diagnostic criteria, 14 of the patients (mean age 42.9 ± 20 years) were classified as being in a VS and the remaining seven patients (mean age 48.7 ± 19.8 years) were classified as being in a minimally conscious state (MCS). Patients in VS had an LCF score of 1 or 2 while patients in MCS had an LCF score of 3. In order to reduce the variability of clinical evaluation, LCF scores were assigned to all patients only if they were unchanged between the day of admission and the day of the EEG registration; otherwise, patients were excluded from the study. Other exclusion criteria were (a) a history of neurological disease before admission and (b) severe spasticity (causing constant EMG artifacts). Inclusion criteria included (a) less than 3 months after the acute brain event onset and (b) first-ever acute brain event. None of the chosen patients were excluded because the scores for all the patients in the study remained unchanged from the day of admission to the day that the EEG was recorded.

The study was approved by the local institutional ethics committee and complies with Good Medical Practice. Overt consent of subjects' legal representatives, in line with the Code of Ethics of the World Medical Association (Declaration of Helsinki) and standards established by the

TABLE 1

BASIC DEMOGRAPHIC AND CLINICAL CHARACTERISTICS OF THE PATIENTS

EEG ID	Age	Gender	Type of consciousness disorder	Etiology	CT/MRI findings (in the acute phase)	Time (in days) between acute event and EEG recording	Drugs	LCF at the EEG recording day
1	38	M	MCS	Trauma	Subdural and epidural hematoma in the right hemisphere; right fronto-temporal intraparenchymal hemorrhage; right fronto-temporal cortical contusions	36	None	3
5	19	F	MCS	Trauma	Subdural hematoma in the right hemisphere; bilateral frontal cortical contusions	74	None	3
9	64	F	MCS	Trauma	Cortical contusions in the temporal lobes and in the right parietal lobe	56	VPA 1500	3
11	61	F	MCS	Vascular	Intraparenchymal hemorrhage in the right parietal lobe	77	None	3
13	29	F	MCS	Vascular	Fronto-temporo-parietal intraparenchymal hemorrhage in the right hemisphere	45	VPA 600	3
14	60	F	MCS	Vascular	Subdural hematoma in the left hemisphere	67	CBZ 800, PB 100	3
16	70	M	MCS	Vascular	Left temporo-parietal ischemia	44	None	3
Mean±S.D. summary	48.7±19.8			TBI: 43%, NTBI: 57%	Left: 29%, right: 71%	57±16	N: 57%, D: 43%	3±0.0
2	36	M	VS	Trauma	Left parieto-temporal intraparenchymal hemorrhage; several intraparenchymal micro-hemorrhages	36	PB 100	2
3	35	M	VS	Trauma	Diffuse axonal injury; right temporal cortical contusion	42	None	1

No.	Age	Sex	Diagnosis	Etiology	Lesion		Drug	LCF
4	28	M	VS	Trauma	Subdural and epidural hematoma in the right hemisphere	46	None	2
6	55	M	VS	Trauma	Cortical contusions in the frontal lobes and in the right temporal lobe; subdural hematoma; diffuse axonal injury	37	None	2
7	14	M	VS	Trauma	Subdural hematoma in the left hemisphere; widespread intraparenchymal microhemorrhages	89	PB 100	2
8	19	M	VS	Trauma	Intraparenchymal microhemorrhages in the right frontal, temporal, and parietal lobes; diffuse axonal injury	14	None	2
10	35	M	VS	Vascular	Left subarachnoid hemorrhage and left temporo-parieto-occipital ischemia (due to vasospasm)	32	None	2
12	41	M	VS	Vascular	Fronto-temporo-parietal intraparenchymal hemorrhage in the left hemisphere	44	None	1
15	79	F	VS	Vascular	Intraparenchymal hemorrhage in left parieto-occipital region	77	LTG 200, PB 100	2
17	50	M	VS	Vascular	Hemorrhage in the right putamen	79	None	2
18	66	M	VS	Vascular	Right fronto-temporo-parietal intraparenchymal and subarachnoid hemorrhage	72	PB 100	1
19	57	M	VS	Vascular	Brainstem hemorrhage	87	PB 100	2
20	16	M	VS	Anoxia		92	None	2
21	68	M	VS	Anoxia		63	None	1
Mean±S.D. summary	42.9±20			TBI: 43%, NTBI: 57%	Left: 42%, right: 50%	57.8±25	N: 64%, D: 36%	1.7±0.5

M = male, F = female, MCS = minimally conscious state, VS = vegetative state, TBI = traumatic brain injury etiology, NTBI = nontraumatic brain injury etiology, N = no drug, D = drugs, LCF = level of cognitive functioning scale, VPA = valproic acid, CBZ = carbamazepine, PB = phenobarbital, LTG = lamotrigine.

Fondazione Istituto "San Raffaele — G. Giglio" Review Board were acquired. The use of the data was authorized by means of written informed consent of the caregivers for VS and MCS patients.

5.2.2. EEG recording

Spontaneous electrical brain activity was recorded with a 21-channel EEG data acquisition system (Neuropack electroencephalograph, Nihon Kohden, Tokyo, Japan). EEG data were collected (cephalic reference — mean of the signals from C3 and C4 electrodes; 0.5–70 Hz bandpass; 200 Hz sampling rate; around 30 min) in patients during a waking resting state (eyes closed) from 19 electrodes positioned in accordance with the International 10–20 system (i.e., O_1, O_2, P_3, P_4, P_z, T_5, T_6, C_3, C_4, C_z, T_3, T_4, F_3, F_4, F_z, F_7, F_8, Fp_1, Fp_2). Recording the full, physiologically relevant range of frequencies does not have trade-offs that would favor any frequency band at the expense of another. The impedance of recording electrodes was monitored for each subject and was always below 5 kΩ. To monitor eye movements, an electrooculogram (0.5–70 Hz bandpass) was also recorded.

The EEG recordings for all patients were performed during the late morning. EEG recordings in patients were started in all cases only if patients spontaneously had their eyes open, the eyelids were then closed by hand. At the end of the recordings all patients opened their eyes spontaneously. In order to keep a constant level of vigilance, an experimenter monitored patients EEG traces in real time, looking for signs of drowsiness and the onset of sleep (increase in "tonic" theta rhythms, K complexes, and sleep spindles). The presence of an adequate EEG signal was determined by visual inspection of the raw signal on the computer screen. Even though it may be difficult to assess precisely the level of vigilance in patients in VS, preserved sleep patterns may be observed in the majority of patients in VS (for review see Cologan et al., 2010).

5.2.3. EEG signal data processing

The presence of an adequate EEG signal was determined by visually checking each raw signal. Epochs containing artifacts due to eye movements, eyes opening, significant muscle activity, and movements on EEG channels were marked and then automatically removed from any further analysis.

Artifact-free EEG signals were filtered in the 1–30-Hz frequency range. This frequency range was chosen because approximately 98% of spectral power lies within these limits (Thatcher, 2001). Although it has recently been proposed that frequencies above 30 Hz (gamma band) may be functionally informative, there are a number of methodological issues which lead us to exclude frequencies above 30 Hz from the present analysis: (a) it was shown that volume conduction has little influence on the shape of the spectrum below about 25 Hz; however, spatial filtering is significant for frequencies around 25 Hz (Robinson et al., 2001); (b) high-frequency spindles have a very low signal-to-noise ratio, which results in considerable noise contamination of the gamma band; (c) the dynamics of high-frequency effects may be a trivial by-product of power changes in lower frequencies (Pulvermüller et al., 1995); (d) increased power in the gamma range may be due to the harmonics of activity in lower frequency ranges, and/or due to the ringing of filters by EEG spikes recurring at theta rates (Freeman, 2003); (e) the gamma band may be an artifact of (un)conscious micro-constrictions of muscles of the organism and/or face muscles (Whitham et al., 2007; Ball et al., 2008; Yuval-Greenberg et al., 2008); (f) comprising just 2% of the spectral power (Thatcher, 2001), the contribution of high-frequency band to the spectrum cannot be significant; (g) Bullock et al. (2003) demonstrated many "good" rhythms in the 2–25 Hz range which were mainly sinusoidal but did not find them in the 30–50 Hz band. In light of the above, there may be difficulties in carrying out a meaningful interpretation of effects at the high-frequency band regardless of how powerful or statistically significant they are.

DC drifts were removed using high-pass filters (1-Hz cutoff).

For each patient, a full EEG stream, free from any artifacts, was fragmented into consecutive 1-min epochs. Therefore the "VS" group (patients in VS) has 137 1-min EEGs and the "MCS" group (patients in minimally conscious state) has 87 1-min EEGs. Within each group further data processing was performed for each separate 1-min portion of the signal. Due to the technical requirements of the tools used to process the data, EEGs were re-sampled to 128 Hz. This procedure should not have affected the results since 128 Hz sampling rate meets the Nyquist criterion (Faulkner, 1969) of a sample rate greater than twice the maximum input frequency and is sufficient to avoid aliasing and pre-serves all the information about the input signal. This method was considered sufficient since the sampling rate of the source signals was significantly higher than required.

After re-sampling, EEG oscillations were iden-tified. This procedure was undertaken in three stages (Fig. 1). During the *first stage* of EEG anal-ysis, the data series from each EEG channel were separately divided into overlapping windows in order to capture EEG changing dynamics. EEG oscillations were quantified by calculation of indi-vidual short-term EEG spectral patterns (SPs). Individual power spectra were calculated in the range of 1–30 Hz with 0.5-Hz resolution, using a Fast Fourier Transform with a 2-s Hanning win-dow shifted by 50 samples (0.39 s) for each channel of 1-min EEG (Fig. 1). According to previous studies, these values have proved to be the most effective for revealing oscillatory patterns from the signal (Levy, 1987; Kaplan, 1998). A sliding spectral analysis with overlapping segments, previ-ously applied to EEG signals (Keidel et al., 1987; Tirsch et al., 1988), (a) takes the non-stationarity of the time series into account, (b) compensates for the effects of windowing, and (c) prevents loss of information due to residual activity. Addition-ally, using overlapping intervals (which just means a different aggregation scheme) cannot add any artifactual information (Muller, 1993).

After calculation of EEG short-term SPs, the total number of individual SPs for each 1-min EEG channel was 149 (Fig. 1).

During the *second stage*, with the help of a probability-classification analysis of the short-term EEG SPs (see Fingelkurts et al., 2003; Appendix in Fingelkurts and Fingelkurts, 2010a), each SP was labeled according to the class index it belonged to. Sequential single EEG SPs were adaptively clas-sified in each 1-min EEG channel using a set of standard SPs which were generated automatically from the EEG data itself (*first step*). The selection was not arbitrary: a pool of SPs ($n = 634,144$) was collated from all the SPs for all the EEG signals (all locations) for all patients. From this pool, all iden-tical SPs with dominant power peaks (peaks that rise significantly above the general average) were counted automatically. The peak detection was based on normalizing the SP to within-SP relative percentages of magnitude, where acceptance is achieved when the peak exceeds a given (60%) per-cent magnitude (100% corresponds to the magni-tude of the highest peak within the SP).

According to the preliminary study, this value has proved to be the most effective for peak detec-tion. The set of SPs with the highest count were the most probable candidates to form the "set of stan-dard SPs." Only those SPs with a minimum mutual correlation were selected. As a result, in this study the standard set included 32 SPs.

During the *second step*, the initial matrix of cross-correlations (Pearson's correlation coefficients (CC)) between standard and current individual SPs of ana-lyzed EEG was calculated for each channel sepa-rately. The current SPs that their CC passed the acceptance criteria of $r \geq 0.71$ were attributed to their respective standard classes. Therefore, the same cur-rent SPs maybe included simultaneously into differ-ent standard classes. The CC acceptance criterion r was determined such as for $r \geq 0.71$ more than 50% of the SP variances were coupled/associated.

During the *third step*, the current SPs included in a particular class were averaged within this class. The same procedure was performed for all classes separately for each EEG channel. On the back of

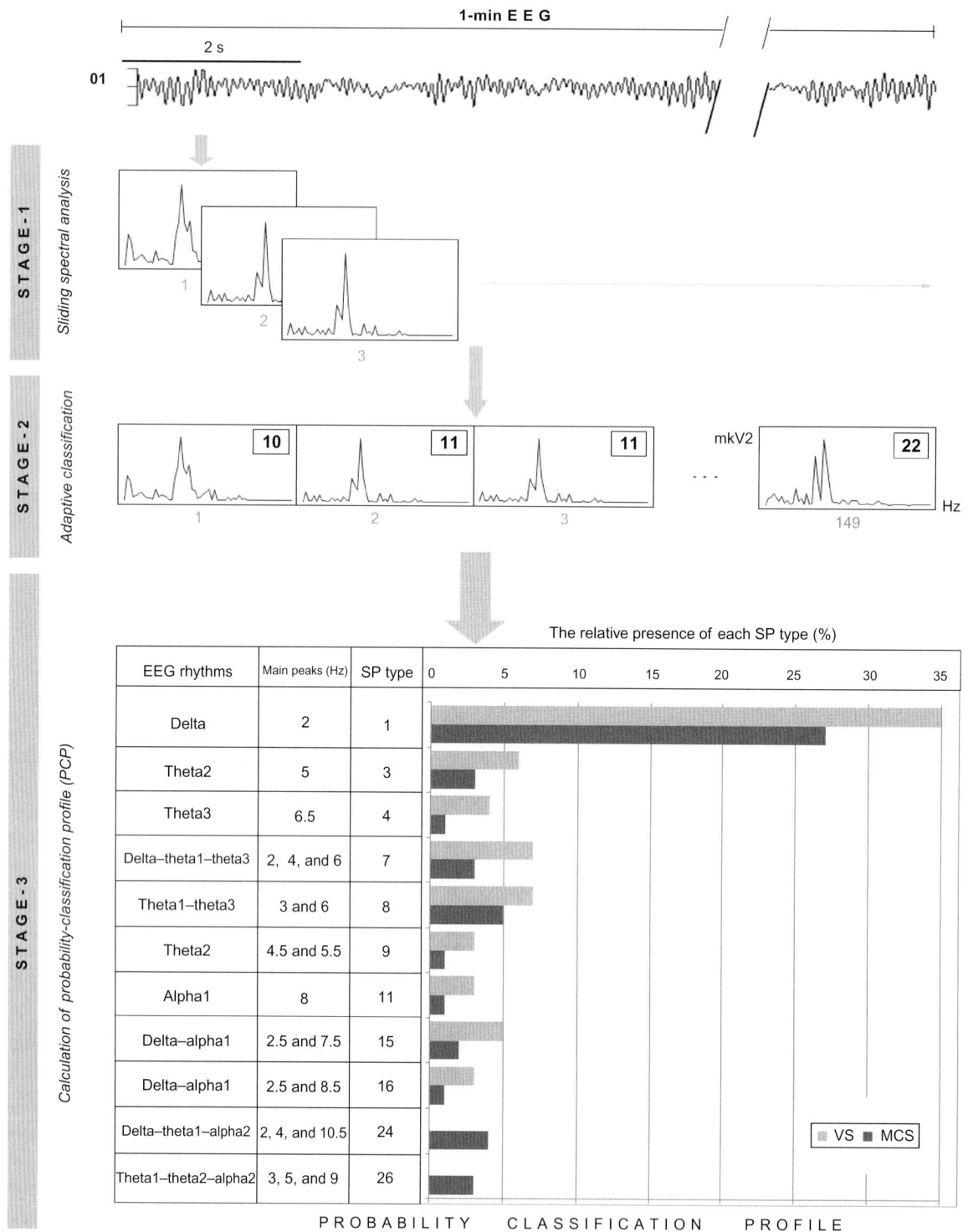

Fig. 1. The scheme of data processing. First stage: sliding spectral analysis was conducted separately for each patient and each 1-min EEG channel. O_1 = left occipital EEG channel. Second stage: adaptive classification of short-term spectral patterns (SP) was performed separately for each patient and each 1-min EEG channel. The small gray numbers under each SP represent the running numbers from 1 to 149 for a 1-min EEG. The number in the square represents the class to which a given SP was assigned during classification procedure. Third stage: probability-classification profile (PCP) separately for each patient and each 1-min EEG channel was calculated. Presented PCP illustrates an example of the composition and percent ratio of EEG oscillations in O_1 EEG channel for patients in minimally conscious state (MCS) and vegetative state (VS). "EEG rhythm(s)" = the brain oscillations which contribute the most into a particular SP. Column "Hz" represents the main dominant peak(s) in particular SP. "SP type" represents the labels of spectral pattern types. Delta: 1–2.5 Hz; theta$_1$: 3–4 Hz; theta$_2$: 4.5–5.5 Hz; theta$_3$: 6–7 Hz; alpha$_1$: 7.5–8.5 Hz; alpha$_2$: 9–13 Hz.

this, the standard spectra were reconstructed but this time taking into account the peculiarities of the spectral description of concrete channel of the particular EEG. In this way an "actualization" of the initial standard SP set was performed. In other words, standard SPs were converted into the so-called actual SP. Notice that the main frequency peaks in the *actual* SP of every class stay the same as in the corresponding *standard* SP's classes. However, overall shape of the power spectrum was automatically modulated in the direction to better represent the multitude of all SPs within each class in each given EEG channel.

An actual SP set was in turn used for the *fourth step* — the final classification of the current SPs: each of current SPs was attributed to only one actual SP class for which the CC was the *maximum* of the set of $r \geq 0.71$.

Thus, using a probability-classification procedure (Fingelkurts et al., 2003; Appendix in Fingelkurts and Fingelkurts, 2010a), each current SP was labeled according to the index of the class to which it belonged (Fig. 1). Hence, each 1-min EEG signal was reduced to a sequence of individually classified SPs. Notice that during the same time observation (2 s) different EEG channels were characterized usually by different SP types.

During the *third stage*, probability-classification profiles (PCPs) of SPs for each 1-min EEG channel in each patient were calculated. These PCPs were calculated by taking the relative number of cases of an SP type as a percentage of the total amount of all SPs within each EEG channel, presented as the histogram of relative presence of each SP type. PCPs were averaged across 87 (for MCS patients) and 137 (for VS patients) 1-min EEG signals separately for each EEG channel. It was expected that these PCPs would make it possible to illustrate in detail (in SP description) the composition of EEG oscillations and their percent ratio for MCS and VS patients.

5.2.4. Statistics

The Wilcoxon *t* test was used to reveal any statistically significant differences in the presence of each SP type in EEG between MCS and VS. Wilcoxon *t* test was chosen because in contrast to parametric statistics such as a repeated measures ANOVA, Wilcoxon *t* test is (a) distribution free, (b) suitable for statistics of small sample sizes, and (c) not influenced by outliers (extremely high or low values). As the SPs represent frequencies of events (the occurrence of a specific pattern during a time interval), they are likely not to follow normal distribution. Event frequencies may not be analyzed by parametric statistics. To control for repeated observations of the same measures, a Bonferroni correction was made. $p_{corrected}$ is the value required to keep the number of false positives at $p = 5\%$. Differences in the demographic data were assessed either by Wilcoxon *t* test or by χ^2 test.

5.3. Results

5.3.1. Demographical data

There were no significant differences between the MCS and VS groups in terms of age ($p = 0.41$) and time post brain injury ($p = 1$), as well as distribution of traumatic brain injury (TBI) and non-TBI (NTBI) etiologies (43% of TBI and 57% of non-TBI in both groups), left- and right-side lesions ($p = 0.62$), and medicated versus non-medicated patients ($p = 0.82$).

5.3.2. General description of EEG for MCS and VS patients

To estimate which of EEG oscillations within a broad frequency range (1–30 Hz) are occurred more or less frequent for MCS and VS, we examined the probability of the occurrence of SP types (which characterize EEG oscillations and/or their mixture).

Analysis revealed that (a) EEGs in both MCS and VS were characterized by the same five EEG oscillations: delta (around 2 Hz), theta$_1$ (around 3 or 4 Hz), theta$_2$ (around 5 Hz), theta$_3$ (around 6 Hz), and alpha$_1$ (around 7.5 or 8 or 8.5 Hz) and (b) only EEGs in MCS had in addition sixth EEG oscillations — alpha$_2$ (around 9 or

10.5 Hz). Each of these oscillations was present in EEG either alone or in combination with others in different EEG segments, thus exhibiting "mosaic" dynamics.

In general, MCS and VS patients differed from each other in all EEG channels: there was not a single EEG channel without statistically significant differences in the relative presence of at least 7% of SP types in PCPs between MCS and VS patients. At the same time, different cortical areas were characterized by a different number of SP types which demonstrated statistically significant difference in their relative presence in PCPs, thus indicating the magnitude of that difference (Table 2). Thus, maximal magnitude of the difference between MCS and VS patients was observed in the posterior-central part of the cortex (O_1, O_2, P_3, P_4, P_z, C_3, C_z EEG channels) ($p_{corrected} < 0.002$) — the number of SP types which demonstrated statistically significant difference in their relative presence in PCPs between MCS and VS patients reached in these areas up to 41% from all observed SP types. Medium magnitude of the difference between MCS and VS patients was in the temporal lobes of the cortex (T_4, T_5, T_6, C_4, F_7, F_8 EEG channels) (up to 26%, $p_{corrected} < 0.002$). Minimum ($p_{corrected} < 0.002$) number of SP types (up to 11%), which demonstrated statistically significant difference in their relative presence in PCPs between MCS and VS patients, was observed in the anterior part of the cortex (T_3, F_3, F_4, F_z, Fp_1, Fp_2 EEG channels; Table 2). At the same time, each from all observed SP types ($n = 14$) revealed statistically significant differences in its relative presence in PCPs between MCS and VS patients in at least 11% of EEG channels.

5.3.3. The probability of the occurrence of EEG oscillations (in terms of SP types) for MCS and VS patients

MCS and VS patients differed from each other according to the probability estimation of the occurrence of SP types in PCPs.

In the case of common EEG oscillations for both groups of patients, comparative analysis of the PCPs demonstrated that EEG during MCS was characterized by a smaller percentage of delta (SP1 (main peak at 2 Hz)), delta–alpha$_1$ (SP15 (main peaks at 2.5 and 7.5 Hz), SP16 (2.5 and 8.5 Hz)), delta–theta$_1$–theta$_3$ (SP7 (2, 4 and 6 Hz)), theta$_2$ (SP3 (5 Hz), SP9 (4.5 and 5.5 Hz)), theta$_3$ (SP4 (6.5 Hz)), theta$_1$–theta$_3$ (SP8 (3 and 6 Hz)), and alpha$_1$ (SP11 (8 Hz)) rhythmic EEG segments when compared to VS ($p_{corrected} < 0.05$–$p_{corrected} < 0.000001$ for different EEG channels and SPs) (Table 3).

TABLE 2

EEG CHANNEL GROUPS AND THE NUMBER (IN %) OF SPECTRAL PATTERN TYPES WHICH DEMONSTRATED STATISTICALLY SIGNIFICANT ($P_{CORRECTED} < 0.05$–$P_{CORRECTED} < 0.000001$) DIFFERENCE IN RELATIVE PRESENCE IN PROBABILITY-CLASSIFICATION PROFILES BETWEEN MINIMALLY CONSCIOUS STATE (MCS) AND VEGETATIVE STATE (VS)

Data averaged across 87 EEGs for MCS and 137 EEGs for VS patients.

Brain regions	EEG channels	Range (%)	Mean (%)	S.D.	Stat. significance
Posterior-central	O_1, O_2, P_3, P_4, P_z, C_3, C_z	36–50	41	1	$p_{corrected} < 0.002$
Temporal	T_4, T_5, T_6, C_4, F_7, F_8	21–29	26	0.5	$p_{corrected} < 0.002$
Anterior	T_3, F_3, F_4, F_z, Fp_1, Fp_2	7–14	11	0.5	$p_{corrected} < 0.002$

TABLE 3

SPECTRAL PATTERN TYPES WHICH DEMONSTRATED STATISTICALLY SIGNIFICANT ($p_{CORRECTED}$< 0.05–$p_{CORRECTED}$< 0.000001) DIFFERENCE IN RELATIVE PRESENCE IN PROBABILITY-CLASSIFICATION PROFILE BETWEEN MINIMALLY CONSCIOUS STATE (MCS) AND VEGETATIVE STATE (VS), SATISFYING MCS<VS AND/OR MCS>VS

Data averaged across 87 EEGs for MCS and 137 EEGs for VS only SP types which demonstrated statistically significant differences in their presence between MCS and VS in more than 1 EEG channel from 19 are considered*.

EEG rhythm(s)	SP type	Frequencies of the main peaks (Hz)	Number of EEG channels	EEG channels affected	Effect globality**
MCS < VS					
Theta$_3$	SP4	6.5	16 [79%]	All except Cz, T3, Fz, Fp1	Generalized
Theta$_1$–theta$_3$	SP8	3 and 6	13 [68.4%]	All except F3, F4, Fz, F7, Fp1, Fp2	Generalized
Delta	SP1	2	6 [31.6%]	T6, T4, F3, F7, Fp1, Fp2	Regional
Delta–alpha$_1$	SP15	2.5 and 7.5	8 [37%]	O1, O2, P4, Pz, C4, T3, F7	Regional
Alpha$_1$	SP11	8	7 [21%]	P4, T6, Cz, T4	Regional
Theta$_2$	SP3	5	3 [15.8%]	P4, Pz, F8	Local
Delta–theta$_1$–theta$_3$	SP7	2, 4, and 6	2 [10.5%]	C3, Cz	Local
Delta–alpha$_1$	SP16	2.5 and 8.5	6 [10.5%]	O2, P4,	Local
MCS > VS					
Theta$_1$–theta$_2$–alpha$_2$	SP26	3, 5, and 9	2 [10.5%]	Pz, Cz	Local
Delta–theta$_1$–alpha$_2$	SP24	2, 4, and 10.5	2 [10.5%]	P3, P4	Local

SP = spectral pattern; "EEG rhythm(s)" colomn represents the brain oscillations which contribute the most into a particular SP. "SP type" column represents the labels of spectral pattern types; [%] = percent of EEG channels which demonstrated observed effect. Delta: 1–2.5 Hz; theta$_1$: 3–4 Hz; theta$_2$: 4.5–5.5 Hz; theta$_3$: 6–7 Hz; alpha$_1$: 7.5–8.5 Hz; alpha$_2$: 9–13 Hz.
*This permits to arrive at a direct estimation of a 5% level of statistical significance ($p < 0.05$) of the observed effects: one can expect $19 \times 0.05 = 0.95$ false positives for 19 EEG channels analyzed under the null hypothesis (where 0.05 is the significance level). Based on these calculations, it is rather improbable that, a false-positive functional connection will emerge by chance simaltaneously in two EEG channels. For the existence of statistical heterogeneity of the electromagnetic field in regard to neurodynamics within quasi-stable periods in regional EEGs (see Fingelkurts and Fingelkurts, 2010b; see also Kaplan et al., 2005; Fingelkurts and Fingelkurts, 2008).
**Generalized – observed effect is found in more than 68% of EEG channels; Regional – observed effect is found in 17–67% of EEG channels; Local = observed effect is found in less than 16% of EEG channels.

Additionally, the comparative analysis of PCPs for MCS and VS patients demonstrated that there were unique SP types associated only with MCS: SP24 (main peaks at 2, 4, and 10.5 Hz) and SP26 (3, 5, and 9 Hz) (Table 3). These SPs contain alpha$_2$ components.

It can be seen that differences in the probability of the occurrence of theta$_1$ and theta$_3$ oscillations between MCS and VS were generalized, meaning that they were observed mostly in the majority of EEG channels (up to 82%, Table 3). The differences in the probability of the occurrence of delta and alpha$_1$ oscillations between MCS and VS were mostly regional — they were observed mainly in 32–42% of EEG channels. The probability of the occurrence of theta$_2$ and alpha$_2$ oscillations differed between MCS and VS mainly locally — they were observed mainly in 10.5–16% of EEG channels (Table 3).

Both groups of patients were composed of patients with disorders of consciousness as a result of different etiologies: traumatic or vascular etiology for MCS and traumatic, vascular, or anoxic etiologies for VS. Therefore, it was interesting to check whether different etiologies affect the probability of the occurrence of EEG oscillations differently. This will be examined in the next section.

5.3.4. The probability of the occurrence of EEG oscillations (in terms of SP types) and etiology of MCS and VS

Comparative analysis of the PCPs *between* MCS and VS of different etiologies demonstrated that the probability of the occurrence of SP4, SP8, SP15, SP24, and SP26 showed the same behavior as for the combined groups (Table 4A), thus being etiology independent. Simultaneously, the probability of the occurrence of SP3 was trauma dependent, whereas the probability of the occurrence of SP1, SP11, and SP16 was vascular dependent (Table 4A).

Analysis of the PCPs *within* MCS and VS of different etiologies demonstrated that EEG in MCS of traumatic etiology was characterized by less probability of the occurrence of SPs with mostly delta and/or $theta_1$ components and more probability of the occurrence of SPs with mostly $theta_2$ and/or $theta_3$ and/or $alpha_{1/2}$ components when compared to MCS of vascular etiology ($p_{corrected}$ < 0.05–$p_{corrected}$ < 0.000001 for different EEG channels and SPs; Table 4B). For EEG in VS, the probability of the occurrence of SPs with mostly delta and/or $theta_{1/2/3}$ components was the greatest for VS of anoxic etiology, lower for VS of vascular etiology, and the lowest for VS of traumatic etiology ($p_{corrected}$ < 0.05–$p_{corrected}$ $<$ 0.000001 for different EEG channels and SPs; Table 4B). Whereas the probability of the occurrence of SPs with $theta_3$ and/or $alpha_1$ components was the greatest for VS of traumatic etiology, lower for VS of vascular etiology, and the lowest

for VS of anoxic etiology ($p_{corrected}$ < 0.05–$p_{corrected}$ < 0.000001 for different EEG channels and SPs; Table 4B).

5.4. Discussion

5.4.1. Demographic factors

Since there were no significant differences between the MCS and VS groups in terms of age and time post brain injury, distribution of TBI and non-TBI etiologies, left- and right-side lesions, and distribution of medicated versus nonmedicated patients, all these factors could not be responsible for the differences in EEG parameters found between the MCS and VS groups.

It could be argued that the effects of phenobarbital and valproic acid on the EEGs could give rise to the differences between MCS and VS groups. However, these drugs induce changes in the high frequency range mostly (Sannità et al., 1980, 1990–1991; Drake et al., 1990), while our results were consistent with a differential value for delta, theta, and alpha oscillations.

Patients with epidural or subdural hematomas may potentially affect EEG results due to the lower conductivities from brain to scalp. However, the time between brain injury and EEG recording was >1 month for patients with epidural or subdural hematomas. We assume that sufficient time had lapsed for the hematoma to be reabsorbed.

5.4.2. Composition of multiple EEG oscillations for MCS and VS patients

The PCPs obtained for both MCS and VS patients revealed that all EEG channels were predominantly characterized by the same five EEG oscillations (indexed by nine SP types) in multiple frequency bands, several of which were superimposed: delta, $theta_1$, $theta_2$, $theta_3$, $alpha_1$. In addition to these EEG oscillations, MCS was characterized by unique EEG oscillation: $alpha_2$

TABLE 4

COMPARISON OF THE RELATIVE PRESENCE OF SPECTRAL PATTERN TYPES FOR MINIMALLY CONSCIOUS STATE (MCS) AND VEGETATIVE STATE (VS) OF DIFFERENT ETIOLOGIES (T-TRAUMA; V-VASCULAR; A-ANOXIA)

Data averaged across 38 EEGs (traumatic etiology) and 49 EEGs (vascular etiology) for MCS and 70 EEGs (traumatic etiology), 56 EEGs (vascular etiology) and 11 EEGs (anoxia etiology) for VS. Only SP types which demonstrated statistically significant differences in their presence between MCS and VS in more than 1 EEG channel from 19 are considered*.

A. Spectral pattern types which demonstrated statistically significant ($p_{corrected} < 0.05$–$p_{corrected} < 0.000001$) difference in relative presence in probability-classification profile between MCS and VS of different eticlogies.

EEG rhythm(s)	Delta	Theta$_2$	Theta$_3$	Theta$_1$–theta$_3$	Alpha$_1$	Delta–alpha$_1$	Delta–alpha$_1$	Delta–theta$_1$–alpha$_2$	Theta$_1$–theta$_2$–alpha$_1$
Frequencies of the main peaks (Hz)	2	5	6.5	3 and 6	8	2.5 and 7.5	2.5 and 8.5	2, 4, and 10.5	3, 5, and 9
SP type	**SP1**	**SP3**	**SP4**	**SP8**	**SP11**	**SP15**	**SP16**	**SP24**	**SP26**
(MCS-T) < (VS-T)	X		X	X		X			
(MCS-V) < (VS-V)		X	X	X		X			
(MCS-T) > (VS-T)					X		X	X	X
(MCS-V) > (VS-V)								X	X

B. Spectral pattern types which demonstrated statistically significant ($p_{corrected} < 0.05$–$p_{corrected} < 0.000001$) difference in relative presence in probability classification profile within MCS and VS of different etiologies

	(MCS-T) < (MCS-V)
SPs with mostly delta and/or theta$_1$ components	
SPs with mostly theta$_2$ and/or theta$_3$ and/or alpha$_{1/2}$ components	(MCS-T) > (MCS-V)
SPs with mostly delta and/or theta$_{1/2/3}$ components	(VS-T) < (VS-V) < (VS-A)
SPs with mostly theta$_3$ and/or alpha$_1$ components	(VS-T) > (VS-V) > (VS-A)

SP = spectral pattern; "EEG rhythm(s)" = the brain oscillations which contribute the most into a particular SP. "SP type" = represents the labels of spectral pattern types; Delta: 1–2.5 Hz; theta$_1$: 3–4 Hz; theta$_2$: 4.5–5.5 Hz; theta$_3$: 6–7 Hz; alpha$_1$: 7.5–8.5 Hz; alpha$_2$: 9–13 Hz.

*This permits to arrive at a direct estimation of a 5% level of statistical significance ($p < 0.05$) of the observed effects: one can expect $19 \times 0.05 = 0.95$ false positives for 19 EEG channels analyzed under the null hypothesis (where 0.05 is the significance level). Based on these calculations, it is rather improbable that a false-positive functional connection will emerge by chance simultaneously in two EEG channels.

(indexed by two SP types). Additionally, MCS patients differed from VS patients according to the probability estimation of the occurrence of particular EEG oscillations and/or their compositions (indexed by the relative presence of SP types in PCPs). Thus, delta, theta, and $alpha_1$ oscillations were less probable, whereas $alpha_2$ oscillations were more probable for MCS than for VS patients. Differences in the brain activity between MCS and VS patients were observed in the whole cortex (various areas to different degrees). These findings combined suggest that different degrees of consciousness expression (from its full absence in VS to its minimal expression in MCS) are reflected in the reorganization of the probability of the occurrence of several EEG oscillations and/or their composition.

Our results are in line with the observations that increase in the amount of slow EEG oscillations (mostly delta and theta) and decrease in the amount of fast-alpha oscillations are associated with stupor and alterations of consciousness (Brenner, 2005; Rusalova, 2006), decrease in mentation recall (Pivik and Foulkes, 1968), and loss of consciousness during general anesthesia (Clark and Rosner, 1973; Engelhardt et al., 1994; Sleigh and Galletly, 1997; Gugino et al., 2001; Kuizenga et al., 2001). Additionally, it was demonstrated that the amount of alpha oscillations correlated with conscious awareness (Babiloni et al., 2006) and is associated with transition of VS patients to a minimally conscious state (Kondrat'eva, 2004). Summary of functional significance of these EEG oscillations in relation to the degree of consciousness expression can be found in Fingelkurts et al. (2012).

5.4.3. Composition of multiple EEG oscillations and etiology of MCS and VS

$Theta_3$ (around 6.5 Hz) oscillation and compositions of such EEG oscillations as $theta_1$–$theta_3$ (around 3 and 6 Hz), delta–$alpha_1$ (around 2.5 and 7.5 Hz), delta–$theta_1$–$alpha_2$ (around 2, 4, and 10.5 Hz), and $theta_1$–$theta_2$–$alpha_2$ (around 3, 5, and 9 Hz) demonstrated independency from brain injury etiology. This means that the probability of the occurrence of these multiple EEG oscillations differentiates MCS and VS independently on brain injury etiology.

At the same time, several EEG oscillations were etiology dependent. Thus, the probability of the occurrence of $theta_2$ (around 5 Hz) oscillation was trauma dependent, whereas the probability of the occurrence of delta (around 2 Hz) oscillation, $alpha_1$ (around 8 Hz) oscillation, and composition of such EEG oscillations as delta–$alpha_1$ (around 2.5 and 8.5 Hz) was vascular dependent. These results may be due to the different brain damage neuropathology in TBI and NTBI (Bagnato et al., 2010).

This supposition is supported by the results of the comparative analysis of the probability of the occurrence of SP types within MCS and VS of different etiologies. Thus, for MCS it was demonstrated that the probability of the occurrence of SPs with mostly delta and/or $theta_1$ components followed the order: traumatic < vascular etiology, whereas the probability of the occurrence of SPs with mostly $theta_2$ and/or $theta_3$ and/or $alpha_{1/2}$ components followed the reverse order: traumatic > vascular etiology. Similarly, for VS the probability of the occurrence of SPs with mostly delta and/or $theta_{1/2/3}$ components followed the order: traumatic < vascular < anoxic etiology, whereas the probability of the occurrence of SPs with mostly $theta_3$ and/or $alpha_1$ components followed the reverse order: traumatic > vascular > anoxic etiology. Considering clinical significance of different types of EEG oscillations (for the review see Fingelkurts and Fingelkurts, 2010b), we may suggest that for both MCS and VS patients, the brain after the injury with traumatic etiology is characterized by better functional state than with vascular etiology: fast-theta and slow-alpha oscillations versus delta and slow-theta oscillations correspondingly. At the same time for VS patients, brain after the injury with anoxic etiology is characterized by worst functional state of the brain when compared to vascular and traumatic etiologies. Indeed, it is well known that increase in the amount of delta and slow-theta activity in resting awake EEG is usually proportional to the degree of pathological processes and reflects encephalopathy and/or structural lesions (Donnelly and Blum, 2007), whereas the increase in alpha activity reflects normalization in brain functional state (Niedermeyer, 1999).

Perhaps such differences in oscillatory descriptors of brain functional states for brain injuries of different etiologies contribute to known differences in their outcome. According to The Multi-Society Task Force on PVS (1994), patients with non-traumatic (primarily anoxic) brain injury have higher mortality figures and lower chances to recover consciousness and other functions than patients with TBI. Note that convincing signs of consciousness have so far never been reported in the post-anoxic VS (Noirhomme et al., 2008).

Summarizing, our supposition is in line with previous studies which demonstrated that a pattern of unvarying activity with the major frequency component in the delta–slow-theta (1–3 Hz) band predicts poor prognosis (Bricolo et al., 1978), whereas a peak in the alpha or fast-theta frequency band indicates a good outcome from traumatic coma (Steudel and Kruger, 1979; Cant and Shaw, 1984; Kane et al., 1998). Additionally, examination of the clinical outcome (mortality after 6 months and recovery of function (indexed by the LCF score increase) after 3 months) for the patients participated in the present study confirmed our supposition: the outcome after 3–6 months was worse for the patients with NTBI (being the worst for anoxic etiology) than for the patients with TBI (Table 5).

5.4.4. Differences in the composition of multiple EEG oscillations between MCS and VS patients and topography

Observed findings in this study demonstrated that the number of EEG oscillations which demonstrated that statistically significant difference in their relative presence in EEG between MCS and VS patients was the largest in the posterior cortex of the brain. This may suggest the importance of the posterior cortex for at least partial consciousness.

TABLE 5

THE OUTCOME FOR PATIENTS IN MCS AND VS OF DIFFERENT ETIOLOGIES

Data presented as the number (in %) of patients who died after 6 months or demonstrated some improvement (measured by LCF core) after 3 months*.

Condition	Mortality (in %) after 6 months	Recovery of function (in %) after 3 months
MCS-T	0	67
MCS-V	50	50
VS-T	17	50
VS-V	33	17
VS-A	50	0

MCS = patients in minimally conscious state, T = traumatic etiology, V = vascular etiology, A = anoxic etiology.
*To give the "Recovery rate" for all patients, we used 3 months — the time when all patients were alive.

Indeed, posterior cortex is one of the most active cerebral regions in conscious waking (Andreasen et al., 1995; Maquet et al., 1997; Gusnard and Raichle, 2001). Vogeley and Fink (2003) suggested that the parietal cortex is involved in the first-person perspective, the viewpoint of the observing self (see also Vogt and Laureys, 2005). Additionally, parts of posterior cortex such as PCC and precuneus are (a) believed to be involved in self-processing events with a visuospatial (attentional) connotation (Cavanna and Trimble, 2006), (b) considered to be involved in self integration — that is linkage of self-referential stimuli to the personal context (Northoff and Bermpohl, 2004), and (c) considered relevant for neural conscious processes, since their activity is reduced in low or absent consciousness states, such as in physiological sleep, drug-induced anesthesia or neuropsychiatric conditions (epilepsy, schizophrenia, coma, VS, and MCS) (Cavanna, 2007; Boly et al., 2008; Buckner et al., 2008).

5.5. Conclusions

Summarizing, the present study demonstrated that the resting brain activity between VS and MCS patients deferred in nearly the whole cortex, rather than in only the frontal and/or parietal areas. This was reflected in the considerable reorganization of the composition of EEG oscillations in multiple frequencies in a broad frequency range (1–30 Hz) in the majority of EEG channels. At the same time, the magnitude of the difference between VS and MCS patients was maximal in the posterior cortex of the brain.

In particular, for MCS patients, delta, theta, and slow-alpha oscillations were less probable, whereas fast-alpha oscillations were more probable in EEG when compared to VS patients. Some of the compositions of these EEG oscillations were etiology independent, whereas others were etiology dependent. Types of EEG oscillations which were etiology dependent differentiated traumatic, vascular, and anoxic etiologies of brain injury in terms of the probability of EEG oscillation occurrence.

Finally, the probability of occurrence of EEG oscillations perhaps contributes to known and observed differences in the outcome of patients with brain injuries of different etiologies after 3–6 months. However, to establish any clinical relationship between the outcome and the probability of EEG oscillation occurrence, a relevant statistical analysis in larger groups of patients should be performed.

Taken together, results in the present study suggest that automatic advanced EEG analysis may be useful in distinguishing VS and MCS patients. Such an advanced automatic analysis of EEG (the procedure, which is easy, simple, and available in most neurorehabilitation departments) may improve clinical characterization of VS and MCS patients, what may lead to a redefining of their diagnosis. This will contribute to better clinical care, resource allocation, and treatment and to more objective diagnostic criteria for consciousness and end-of-life decision making in patients with disorders of consciousness following coma caused by severe brain damages.

Future studies, including larger groups of patients with brain injuries for each etiology, are warranted to confirm these results.

Acknowledgments

The authors thank Caterina Prestandrea (neurophysiology technician), who made all the EEG recordings and Carlos Neves (computer science specialist) for programming, technical, and IT support.

This work was supported partially by BM-Science Center, Finland. The author declares that the research was conducted in the absence of any commercial or financial relationships that could be construed as a potential conflict of interest.

References

ANA Committee on Ethical Affairs (1993) Persistent vegetative state: report of the American Neurological Association Committee on Ethical Affairs. *Ann. Neurol.*, 33: 386–390.

Andreasen, N.C., O'Leary, D.S., Cizadlo, T., Arndt, S., Rezai, K., Watkins, G.L., Ponto, L.L. and Hichwa, R.D. (1995) Remembering the past: two facets of episodic memory explored with positron emission tomography. *Am. J. Psychiatry*, 152: 1576–1585.

Andrews, K. (2004) Medical decision making in the vegetative state: withdrawal of nutrition and hydration. *NeuroRehabilitation*, 19(4): 299–304.

Andrews, K., Murphy, L., Munday, R. and Littlewood, C. (1996) Misdiagnosis of the vegetative state: retrospective study in a rehabilitation unit. *Br. Med. J.*, 313: 13–16.

Babiloni, C., Vecchio, F., Miriello, M., Romani, G.L. and Rossini, P.M. (2006) Visuo-spatial consciousness and parieto-occipital areas: a high-resolution EEG study. *Cereb. Cortex*, 16: 37–46.

Bagnato, S., Boccagni, C., Prestandrea, C., Sant'Angelo, A., Castiglione, A. and Galardi, G. (2010) Prognostic value of standard EEG in traumatic and non-traumatic disorders of consciousness following coma. *Clin. Neurophysiol.*, 121: 274–280.

Ball, T., Demandt, E., Mutschler, I., Neitzel, E., Mehring, C., Vogt, K., Aertsen, A. and Schulze-Bonhage, A. (2008) Movement related activity in the high gamma range of the human EEG. *Neuroimage*, 41: 302–310.

Başar, E. (2010) *Brain–Body–Mind in the Nebulous Cartesian System: A Holistic Approach by Oscillations*. Springer, Berlin, 523 pp.

Başar, E. and Güntekin, B. (2008) A review of brain oscillations in cognitive disorders and the role of neurotransmitters. *Brain Res.*, 1235: 172–193.

Başar, E., Başar-Eroğlu, C., Karakas, S. and Schurmann, M. (2001a) Gamma, alpha, delta, and theta oscillations govern cognitive processes. *Int. J. Psychophysiol.*, 39: 241–248.

Başar, E., Schurmann, M., Demiralp, T., Başar-Eroğlu, C. and Ademoğlu, A. (2001b) Event-related oscillations are 'real brain responses' — wavelet analysis and new strategies. *Int. J. Psychophysiol.*, 39: 91–127.

Beaumont, J.G. and Kenealy, P.M. (2005) Incidence and prevalence of the vegetative and minimally conscious states. *Neuropsychol. Rehab.*, 15: 184–189.

Boccagni, C., Bagnato, S., Sant' Angelo, A., Prestandrea, C. and Galardi, G. (2011) Usefulness of standard EEG in predicting the outcome of patients with disorders of consciousness after anoxic coma. *Clin. Neurophysiol.*, 28(5): 489–492.

Boly, M., Phillips, C., Tshibanda, L., Vanhaudenhuyse, A., Schabus, M., Dang-Vu, T.T., Moonen, G., Hustinx, R., Maquet, P. and Laureys, S. (2008) Intrinsic brain activity in altered states of consciousness: how conscious is the default mode of brain function? *Ann. NY Acad. Sci.*, 1129: 119–129.

Brenner, R.P. (2005) The interpretation of the EEG of stupor and coma. *Neurologist*, 11: 271–284.

Bricolo, A., Turazzi, S., Faccioli, F., Odorizzia, F., Sciarretta, G. and Erculiania, P. (1978) Clinical application of compressed spectral array in long-term EEG monitoring of comatose patients. *Electroencephalogr. Clin. Neurophysiol.*, 45: 211–225.

Buckner, R.L., Andrews-Hanna, J.R. and Schacter, D.L. (2008) The brain's default network: anatomy, function, and relevance to disease. *Ann. NY Acad. Sci.*, 1124: 1–38.

Bullock, T.H., McClune, M.C. and Enright, J.T. (2003) Are the EEGs mainly rhythmic? Assessment of periodicity in wideband time series. *Neuroscience*, 121(1): 233–252.

Cant, B.R. and Shaw, N.A. (1984) Monitoring by compressed spectral array in prolonged coma. *Neurology*, 34: 35–39.

Cavanna, A.E. (2007) The precuneus and consciousness. *CNS Spectr.*, 12: 545–552.

Cavanna, A.E. and Trimble, M.R. (2006) The precuneus: a review of its functional anatomy and behavioual correlates. *Brain*, 129: 564–583.

Childs, N.L., Mercer, W.N. and Childs, H.W. (1993) Accuracy of diagnosis of persistent vegetative state. *Neurology*, 43: 1465–1467.

Clark, D.L. and Rosner, B.S. (1973) Neurophysiologic effects of general anesthetics. I. The electroencephalogram and sensory evoked responses in man. *Anesthesiology*, 38: 564–582.

Cologan, V., Schabus, M., Ledoux, D., Moonen, G., Maquet, P. and Laureys, S. (2010) Sleep in disorders of consciousness. *Sleep Med. Rev.*, 14(2): 97–105.

Donnelly, E.M. and Blum, A.S. (2007) Focal and generalized slowing, coma, and brain death. In: A.S. Blum and S.B. Rutkove (Eds.), *The Clinical Neurophysiology Primer*. Humana Press, Totowa, NJ, pp. 127–140.

Drake, M.E., Huber, S.J., Pakalnis, A. and Denio, L. (1990) Electroencephalographic effects of antiepileptic drug therapy. *J. Epilepsy*, 3(2): 75–79.

Engelhardt, W., Stahl, K., Marouche, A., Hartung, E. and Dierks, T. (1994) Ketamine racemate versus S(C)-ketamine with or without antagonism with physostigmine. A quantitative EEG study on volunteers. *Anaesthesist*, 43: S76–S82.

Faulkner, E.A. (1969) *Introduction to the Theory of Linear Systems*. Chapman and Hall, London.

Fingelkurts, A.A. and Fingelkurts, A.A. (2008) Brain–mind operational architectonics imaging: technical and methodological aspects. *Open Neuroimag. J.*, 2: 73–93.

Fingelkurts, A.A. and Fingelkurts, A.A. (2010a) Topographic mapping of rapid transitions in EEG multiple frequencies: EEG frequency domain of operational synchrony. *Neurosci. Res.*, 68: 207–224.

Fingelkurts, A.A. and Fingelkurts, A.A. (2010b) Short-term EEG spectral pattern as a single event in EEG phenomenology. *Open Neuroimag. J.*, 4: 130–156.

Fingelkurts, A.A., Fingelkurts, A.A. and Kaplan, A.Y. (2003) The regularities of the discrete nature of multi-variability of EEG spectral patterns. *Int. J. Psychophysiol.*, 47(1): 23–41.

Fingelkurts, AlA., Fingelkurts, AnA., Bagnato, S., Boccagni, C. and Galardi, G. (2012) EEG oscillatory states as neurophenomenology of consciousness as revealed from patients in vegetative and minimally conscious states. *Conscious Cogn.*, 21: 149–169.

Freeman, W.J. (2003) The wave packet: an action potential for the 21st century. *J. Integr. Neurosci.*, 2: 3–30.

Giacino, J.T., Ashwal, S., Childs, N., Cranford, R., Jennett, B., Katz, D.I., Kelly, J.P., Rosenberg, J.H., Whyte, J., Zafonte, R.D. and Zasler, N.D. (2002) The minimally conscious state. Definition and diagnostic criteria. *Neurology*, 58: 349–353.

Giacino, J.T., Kalmar, K. and Whyte, J. (2004) The JFK coma recovery scale-revised: measurement characteristics and diagnostic utility. *Arch. Phys. Med. Rehab.*, 85: 2020–2029.

Gill-Thwaites, H. (2006) Lotteries, loopholes and luck: misdiagnosis in the vegetative state patient. *Brain Inj.*, 20: 1321–1328.

Gouvier, W.D., Blanton, P.D., La Porte, K.K. and Nepomuceno, C. (1987) Reliability and validity of the Disability Rating Scale and the Levels of Cognitive Functioning Scale in monitoring recovery from severe head injury. *Arch. Phys. Med. Rehab.*, 68: 94–97.

Gugino, L.D., Chabot, R I, Prichep, L.S., John, E.R., Formanck, V. and Aglio, L.S. (2001) Quantitative EEG changes associated with loss and return of consciousness in healthy adult volunteers anesthetized with propofol or sevoflurane. *Br. J. Anaesth.*, 87: 421–428.

Gusnard, D.A. and Raichle, M.E. (2001) Searching for a baseline: functional imaging and the resting human brain. *Nat. Rev. Neurosci.*, 2: 685–694.

Jennett, B. and Bond, M. (1975) Assessment of outcome after severe brain damage. *Lancet*, 1: 480–484.

Jennett, B., Snoek, J., Bond, M.R. and Brooks, N. (1981) Disability after severe brain injury: observations on the use of the Glasgow Outcome Scale. *J. Neurol. Neurosurg. Psychiatry*, 44: 285–293.

Kane, N.M., Moss, T.H., Curry, S.H. and Butler, S.R. (1998) Quantitative electroencephalographic evaluation of nonfatal and fatal traumatic coma. *Electroencephalogr. Clin. Neurophysiol.*, 106(3): 244–250.

Kaplan, A.Y. (1998) Nonstationary EEG: methodological and experimental analysis. *Usp. Physiol. Nayk* (Success in Physiol. Sci.), 29: 35–55. (In Russian.)

Kaplan, A.Y., Fingelkurts, A.A., Fingelkurts, A.A., Borisov, S.V. and Darkhovsky, B.S. (2005) Nonstationary nature of the brain activity as revealed by EEG/MEG: methodological, practical and conceptual challenges. *Signal Proces.*, 85: 2190–2212.

Keidel, M., Keidel, W.D., Tirsch, W.S. and Poppl, S.J. (1987) Studying temporal order in human CNS by means of 'running' frequency and coherence analysis. In: L. Rensing, U. Van der Heiden and M.C. Mackey (Eds.), *Temporal Disorder in Human Oscillatory Systems. Springer Series in Synergetics.* Springer, Berlin, pp. 57–68.

Klimesch, W. (1999) Event-related band power changes and memory performance. Event-related desynchronization and related oscillatory phenomena of the brain. In: G. Pfurtscheller and F.H. Lopez da Silva (Eds.), *Handbook of Electroencephalography and Clinical Neurophysiology,* Revised Edn. Elsevier, Amsterdam, pp. 151–178.

Kondrat'eva, E.A. (2004) *Vegetative State: Diagnostics, Intensive Therapy, Outcome Prognosis.* M.D. Dissertation, St. Petersburg Medical Academy of Postdiploma Education, St. Petersburg. (In Russian.)

Kuizenga, K., Wierda, J.M.K.H. and Kalkman, C.J. (2001) Biphasic EEG changes in relation to loss of consciousness during induction with thiopental, propofol, etomidate, midozalam, or sevoflurane. *Br. J. Anaesth.*, 86: 354–360.

Levy, W.J. (1987) Effect of epoch length on power spectrum analysis of the EEG. *Anesthesiology*, 66(4): 489–495.

Maquet, P., Degueldre, C., Delfiore, G., Aerts, J., Peters, J.M., Luxen, A. and Franck, G. (1997) Functional neuroanatomy of human slow wave sleep. *J. Neurosci.*, 17: 2807–2812.

Massimini, M., Boly, M., Casali, A., Rosanova, M. and Tononi, G. (2009) A perturbational approach for evaluating the brain's capacity for consciousness. In: *Progress in Brain Research,* Vol. 177. Elsevier, Amsterdam, pp. 201–214.

Monti, M.M., Laureys, S. and Owen, A.M. (2010) The vegetative state. *Br. Med. Ass.*, 341: c3765.

Muller, U.A. (1993) Statistics of variables observed over overlapping intervals. Working Paper from Olsen and Associates No. 1993-06-18. File URL:http://www.olsen.ch/fileadmin/Publications/Working_Papers/931130-intervalOverlap.pdf Accessed 2011 May 2.

Myles, P.S., Leslie, K., McNeil, J., Forbes, A. and Chan, M.T. (2004) Bispectral index monitoring to prevent awareness during anaesthesia: the B-Aware randomised controlled trial. *Lancet*, 363: 1757–1763.

Niedermeyer, E. (1999) The normal EEG of the waking adult. In: E. Niedermeyer and F.H. Lopes da Silva (Eds.), *Electroencephalography: Basic Principles, Clinical Applications and Related Fields*, 4th Edn. Williams and Wilkins, Philadelphia, PA, pp. 149–173.

NIH Consensus Development Panel (1999) Rehabilitation of persons with traumatic brain injury. *J. Am. Med. Ass.*, 282: 974–983.

Noirhomme, Q., Schnakers, C. and Laureys, S. (2008) A twitch of consciousness: defining the boundaries of vegetative and minimally conscious states. *J. Neurol. Neurosurg. Psychiatry*, 79(7): 741–742.

Northoff, G. and Bermpohl, F. (2004) Cortical midline structures and the self. *Trends Cogn. Sci.*, 8(3): 102–107.

Pivik, T. and Foulkes, D. (1968) NREM mentation: relation to personality, orientation time, and time of night. *J. Consult. Clin. Psychol.*, 32: 144–151.

Pulvermüller, F., Preissl, H., Lutzenberger, W. and Birbaumer, N. (1995) Spectral responses in the gamma-band: physiological signs of higher cognitive processes? *NeuroReport*, 6: 2057–2064.

Robinson, P.A., Rennie, C.J., Wright, J.J., Bahramali, H., Gordon, E. and Rowe, D.L. (2001) Prediction of electroencephalographic spectra from neurophysiology. *Phys. Rev. E*, 63: 021903-1–021903-18.

Royal College of Physicians (2003) The vegetative state: guidance on diagnosis and management. A report of a working party of the Royal College of Physicians. *Clin. Med.*, 2: 249–254.

Rusalova, M.N. (2006) Frequency–amplitude characteristics of the EEG at different levels of consciousness. *Neurosci. Behav. Physiol.*, 36(4). (Translated from *Rossiiskii Fiziologicheskii Zhurnal imeni I. M. Sechenova*, 2005, 91 (4): 353–363.)

Sannità, W.G., Rapallino, M.V., Rodriguez, G. and Rosadini, G. (1980) EEG effects and plasma concentrations of phenobarbital in volunteers. *Neuropharmacology*, 19(9): 927–930.

Sannità, W.G., Balbi, A., Giacchino, F. and Rosadini, G. (1990–1991) Quantitative EEG effects and drug plasma concentration of phenobarbital, 50 and 100 mg single-dose oral administration to healthy volunteers: evidence of early CNS bioavailability. *Neuropsychobiology*, 23(4): 205–212.

Schnakers, C., Giacino, J., Kalmar, K., Piret, S., Lopez, E., Boly, M., Malone, R. and Laureys, S. (2006) Does the FOUR score correctly diagnose the vegetative and minimally conscious states? *Ann. Neurol.*, 60(6): 744–745.

Schnakers, C., Ledoux, D., Majerus, S., Damas, P., Damas, F., Lambermont, B., Lamy, M., Boly, M., Vanhaudenhuyse, A., Moonen, G. and Laureys, S. (2008) Diagnostic and prognostic use of bispectral index in coma, vegetative state and related disorders. *Brain Inj.*, 22(12): 926–931.

Schnakers, C., Vanhaudenhuyse, A., Giacino, J., Ventura, M., Boly, M., Majerus, S., Moonen, G. and Laureys, S. (2009) Diagnostic accuracy of the vegetative and minimally conscious state: clinical consensus versus standardized neurobehavioral assessment. *BMC Neurol.*, 9: 35 (doi:10.1186/1471-2377-9-35).

Sleigh, J.W. and Galletly, D.C. (1997) A model of the electrocortical effects of general anesthesia. *Br. J. Anaesth.*, 78: 260–263.

Smedira, N.G., Evans, B.H., Grais, L.S., Cohen, N.H., Lo, B., Cooke, M., Schecter, W.P., Fink, C., Epstein-Jaffe, E., May, C., et al. (1990) Withholding and withdrawal of life support from the critically ill. *N. Engl. J. Med.*, 322: 309–315.

Steudel, W.I. and Kruger, J. (1979) Using the spectral analysis of the EEG for prognosis of severe brain injuries in the first post-traumatic week. *Acta Neurochir. Suppl.*, 28: 40–42.

Strauss, D.J., Ashwal, S., Day, S.M. and Shavelle, R.M. (2000) Life expectancy of children in vegetative and minimally conscious states. *Pediatr. Neurol.*, 23: 312–319.

Thatcher, R.W. (2001) Normative EEG databases and EEG biofeedback. *J. Neurother.*, 3: 1–29.

The Multi-Society Task Force on PVS (1994) Medical aspects of the persistent vegetative state. *N. Engl. J. Med.*, 330: 1499–1508.

Tirsch, W.S., Keidel, M. and Poppl, S.J. (1988) Computer-aided detection of temporal patterns in human CNS dynamics. In: J.L. Willems, J.H. Van Bemmel and J. Michel (Eds.), *Progress in Computer-Assisted Function Analysis*. Elsevier/North-Holland, Amsterdam, pp. 109–118.

Tresch, D.D., Sims, F.H., Duthie, E.H., Goldstein, M.D. and Lane, P.S. (1991) Clinical characteristics of patients in the persistent vegetative state. *Arch. Intern. Med.*, 151: 912–930.

Vogeley, K. and Fink, G.R. (2003) Neural correlates of the first-person perspective. *Trends Cogn. Sci.*, 7: 38–42.

Vogt, B.A. and Laureys, S. (2005) Posterior cingulate, precuneal and retrosplenial cortices: cytology and components of the neural network correlates of consciousness. In: *Progress in Brain Research*, Vol. 150. Elsevier, Amsterdam, pp. 205–217.

Whitham, E.M., Pope, K.J., Fitzgibbon, S.P., Lewis, T., Clark, C.R., Loveless, S., Broberg, M., Wallace, A., De los Angeles, D., Lillie, P., Hardy, A., Fronsko, R., Pulbrook, A. and Willoughby, J.O. (2007) Scalp electrical recording during paralysis: quantitative evidence that EEG frequencies above 20 Hz are contaminated by EMG. *Clin. Neurophysiol.*, 118: 1877–1888.

Winslade, W.J. (1998) *Confronting Traumatic Brain Injury*. Yale University Press, New Haven, CT.

Yuval-Greenberg, S., Tomer, O., Keren, A.S., Nelken, I. and Deouell, L.Y. (2008) Transient induced gamma-band response in EEG as a manifestation of miniature saccades. *Neuron*, 58: 429–441.

Application of Brain Oscillations in Neuropsychiatric Diseases
(Supplements to Clinical Neurophysiology, Vol. 62)
Editors: E. Başar, C. Başar-Eroğlu, A. Özerdem, P.M. Rossini, G.G. Yener

Chapter 6

The auditory steady-state response (ASSR): a translational biomarker for schizophrenia

Brian F. O'Donnell[a,b,c,*], Jenifer L. Vohs[b,c], Giri P. Krishnan[d], Olga Rass[a], William P. Hetrick[a,b,c] and Sandra L. Morzorati[c]

[a]*Department of Psychological and Brain Sciences, Indiana University, Bloomington, IN 47405, USA*
[b]*Department of Psychiatry, Indiana University School of Medicine, Indianapolis, IN 46222, USA*
[c]*Larue D. Carter Memorial Hospital, Indianapolis, IN 46222, USA*
[d]*Department of Cell Biology and Neuroscience, University of California Riverside, Riverside, CA 92521, USA*

ABSTRACT

Electrophysiological methods have demonstrated disturbances of neural synchrony and oscillations in schizophrenia which affect a broad range of sensory and cognitive processes. These disturbances may account for a loss of neural integration and effective connectivity in the disorder. The mechanisms responsible for alterations in synchrony are not well delineated, but may reflect disturbed interactions within GABAergic and glutamatergic circuits, particularly in the gamma range. Auditory steady-state responses (ASSRs) provide a non-invasive technique used to assess neural synchrony in schizophrenia and in animal models at specific response frequencies. ASSRs are electrophysiological responses entrained to the frequency and phase of a periodic auditory stimulus generated by auditory pathway and auditory cortex activity. Patients with schizophrenia show reduced ASSR power and phase locking to gamma range stimulation. We review alterations of ASSRs in schizophrenia, schizotypal personality disorder, and first-degree relatives of patients with schizophrenia. In vitro and in vivo approaches have been used to test cellular mechanisms for this pattern of findings. This translational, cross-species approach provides support for the role of N-methyl-D-aspartate and GABAergic dysregulation in the genesis of perturbed ASSRs in schizophrenia and persons at risk.

KEYWORDS

Auditory steady-state response; Translational biomarker; Schizophrenia; Schizotypal personality disorder

6.1. Introduction

Schizophrenia (SZ) is a debilitating mental disorder associated with psychotic symptoms, such as

---

Correspondence to: Dr. Brian F. O'Donnell, Department of Psychological and Brain Sciences, Indiana University, 1101 East 10th Street, Bloomington, IN 47405, USA.
Tel.: +1 812 856 4164;
E-mail: bodonnel@indiana.edu

hallucinations and delusions, which affects nearly 0.8% of the population (Saha et al., 2005). Disturbances of auditory perception are among the most characteristic features of SZ. Interview measures of perceptual abnormalities, as distinct from hallucinations, indicate that auditory distortions are more frequent than distortions in any other sensory modality, occurring in 42% of patients with SZ compared to 17% of healthy adults (Bunney et al., 1999). Consistent with these subjective reports, behavioral measures of auditory processing have demonstrated deficits in time estimation (Carroll et al., 2009), spatial localization (Perrin et al., 2010), sound intensity discrimination (Bach et al., 2011), pitch discrimination (Leitman et al., 2008), and echoic memory (Strous et al., 1995). Event-related potential (ERP) findings suggest that auditory processing is affected within 50–200 ms of stimulus onset, including reduction of the P50 response to the first click of a paired click paradigm, impaired P50 gating, reduction of the auditory N100 component, and reduced mismatch negativity (see Hirayasu et al., 1998; Turetsky et al., 2007). Auditory hallucinations are a diagnostic criterion for SZ, and patients with auditory hallucinations show altered brain activation in left superior temporal gyrus and middle temporal gyrus compared to non-hallucinating individuals (Kuhn and Gallinat, 2010). Consequently, the auditory system can provide a window into one of the key neurobehavioral symptoms.

The neural mechanisms which produce symptoms of SZ remain poorly understood, but accumulating evidence suggests that disturbances in neural synchrony and oscillatory activity may contribute to failures of effective connectivity and neural integration in the illness (Whittington, 2008; Uhlhaas and Singer, 2010; Başar, 2011). While non-invasive measures currently cannot detect cellular signaling at the level of individual neurons and circuits in humans, the electroencephalogram (EEG) and magnetoencephalogram (MEG) can detect the synchronous activity of ensembles of neurons. Moreover, since both EEG and MEG are primarily generated by postsynaptic potentials, they are often highly sensitive to alterations in neurotransmission secondary to brain dysfunction or pharmacological manipulations (Luck et al., 2011). Thus, these measures have the potential to serve as biomarkers for disturbance of synchrony and oscillations in SZ.

6.1.1. Auditory steady-state responses

The auditory steady-state responses (ASSRs) is a type of ERP which can test the integrity of auditory pathways and the capacity of these pathways to generate synchronous activity at specific frequencies (Brenner et al., 2009). ASSRs are elicited by temporally modulated auditory stimulation, such as a train of clicks with a fixed inter-click interval, or an amplitude-modulated (AM) tone. After the onset of the stimulus, the EEG or MEG rapidly entrains to the frequency and phase of the stimulus. Testing the capacity of auditory circuits to support entrainment provides a non-invasive method to determine the relationship of the power or phase of the output (EEG) to the characteristics of the periodic input. If the auditory system is unable to support neural synchronization, particularly at higher gamma frequencies (>30 Hz), this would be evident in the amplitude or phase variability of the ASSR.

The ASSR is generated by activity within the auditory pathway. The ASSR for modulation frequencies up to 50 Hz is generated from the auditory cortex based on EEG (Pantev et al., 1996; Herdman et al., 2002), MEG (Ross et al., 2002), and animal studies (Dolphin and Mountain, 1992; Conti et al., 1999). Higher frequencies of modulation (>80 Hz) are thought to originate from brainstem areas (Herdman et al., 2002). The type of stimulus may also affect the region of activation within the auditory cortex. AM tones and click train stimuli are commonly used stimuli to evoke the ASSR (Picton et al., 2003). AM tones are generated by temporally modulating a tone (or sine wave) using another sine wave modulation resulting in variation of the amplitude of the tone over time. The frequency of the tone is referred to as the carrier frequency and the frequency of the modulation envelope is called the modulation frequency. The click train stimuli, on the other hand, consist of clicks which are brief but broad spectrum sound stimuli. Thus, the click stimulus has several harmonics, while the modulation frequency of AM tones has only one peak at the stimulus frequency. Due to tonotopic mapping of the auditory cortex, the carrier frequency or the frequency content in individual stimuli determines the region of the auditory cortex that is activated. In the case of the AM tones, only a small region that responds to the carrier frequency responds, while click stimuli activate a larger area. This is reflected in the amplitude of the ASSR responses, as clicks generate higher amplitude ASSR than AM tones. The mechanisms of generation of ASSRs differ as a function of frequency, but likely represent both the superposition of individual evoked potentials to each click or cycle of modulation, as well as intrinsic oscillatory processes in the auditory pathways. For further discussion of this issue, see Krishnan et al. (2009).

6.1.2. Time–frequency analysis of ASSRs

Entrainment is apparent in the ASSR averaged in the time domain (Fig. 1A and B), but the frequency response can be more accurately quantified using time–frequency analysis. One approach is to apply a Fast Fourier Transform (FFT) to the period of stimulation, or to the ASSR averaged across stimulus periods to improve signal to noise by isolating phase-locked activity (Fig. 1C). The FFT decomposes the time domain ASSR into a sum of sinusoidal waveforms varying in power and phase. A power spectrum displays the coefficients for each frequency measured by the FFT as a graph of power values (usually in μV^2), as shown in Fig. 1C. In Fig. 1, the ASSR was elicited by a 40-Hz AM tone (1-s duration) with a 1000-Hz carrier frequency. The power spectrum in Fig. 1C shows a prominent peak in power at 40 Hz, which has a larger value in the control group compared to the group of patients with SZ. The ASSR in humans shows a peak response at about 40–45 Hz (Fig. 2).

More recently, signal analysis procedures have allowed trial-to-trial differentiation of phase consistency of the ASSR, and change in power from baseline. The phase-locking factor (PLF), or inter-trial phase coherence, is a measure of phase synchronization of EEG activity across trials at particular temporal intervals and frequencies (Delorme and Makeig, 2004). In order to compute PLF, a baseline normalized spectrogram is first obtained by applying FFT using a time sliding window on single trial data. This results in a

time–frequency transform consisting of a complex number for every time point, frequency, and trial. This complex output is divided by its complex norm (absolute value), which is then averaged across trials. The complex norm of this averaged value results in PLF for different time and frequency points. PLF values can range from 0 (absence of synchronization) to 1 (perfect synchronization, or phase reproducibility across trials at a given latency). In contrast, mean power (MP) difference from baseline (also called event-related spectral perturbation (ERSP)) measures the power in a frequency band relative to baseline. MP is obtained by first subtracting the power from the prestimulus baseline period and then averaging across trials. This measure represents the average change in power at a given frequency from the mean baseline power and so can detect changes in power that are induced by, but are not necessarily phase-locked to, stimulus onset. Fig. 1D and E shows time–frequency plots comparing MP (or ERSP) and PLF (inter-trial coherence) for subjects with and without SZ to the 40-Hz AM tone.

6.1.3. ASSRs in schizophrenia

ASSRs are usually reduced in power or phase locking in patients with schizophrenia to 40 Hz stimulation (Table 1). Kwon et al. (1999) first reported that SZ patients showed a reduction in the ASSR. Short, 500-ms click trains were used to elicit the ASSR at three frequencies: 20, 30, and 40 Hz. Patients with schizophrenia showed a reduction in power at 40 Hz, but not at 20 or 30 Hz. Moreover, patients showed delayed onset of phase synchronization and delayed desynchronization to the 40-Hz click trains. Subsequently, a reduction in 40-Hz power or PLF in SZ has been observed in most (Light et al., 2006; Vierling-Classen et al., 2008; Wilson et al., 2008; Spencer et al., 2009; Mulert et al., 2011) but not all (Hong et al., 2004) studies. The 30- and 40-Hz PLF ASSR reductions have been observed in first episode SZ (Spencer et al., 2008) and in adolescents with a diagnosis of a psychotic disorder (Wilson et al.,

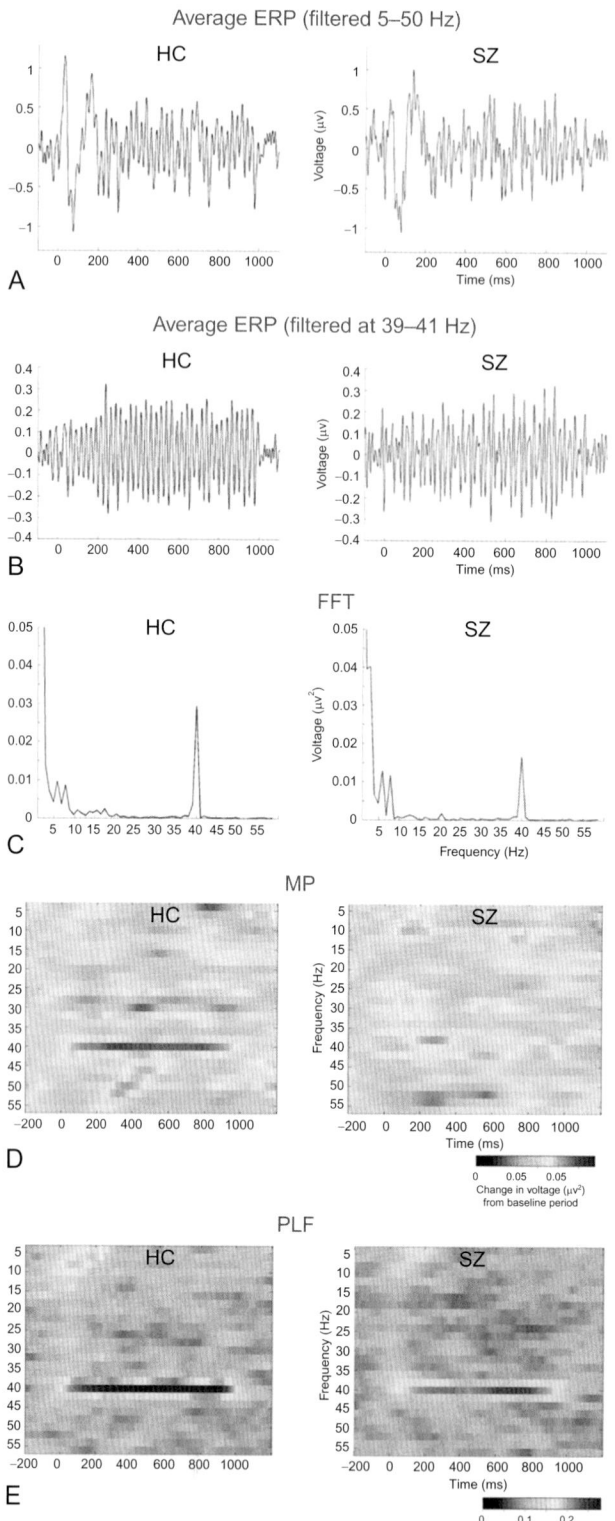

Fig. 1. Auditory steady-state responses (ASSRs) to a 1-s, 40-Hz amplitude-modulated tone recorded at Cz in a healthy control group (HC; $N = 21$) and in patients with schizophrenia (SZ; $N = 21$). (A) The ERP in the time domain averaged across subjects, showing both a large onset response as well as the 40-Hz oscillation. In (B), the averaged wave form has been filtered between 39 and 41 Hz. (C) A power spectrum obtained by applying a Fast Fourier Transform on the ERPs in the two groups, showing the 40-Hz response in the HC group which is reduced in magnitude in the SZ group. (D) Mean power (MP) across the epoch which indicates the average change in power at a given frequency from the mean baseline power. The x-axis represents time in milliseconds, the y-axis represents frequency in Hertz, and the colors represent the magnitude of power. (E) The phase-locking factor (PLF) across trials. The x-axis indicates time in milliseconds, the y-axis indicates frequency, and the colors represent phase reproducibility across trials ranging from 0 (absence of synchronization) to 1 (perfect synchronization). (For color figures, please refer to the color figures in last section of the book.)

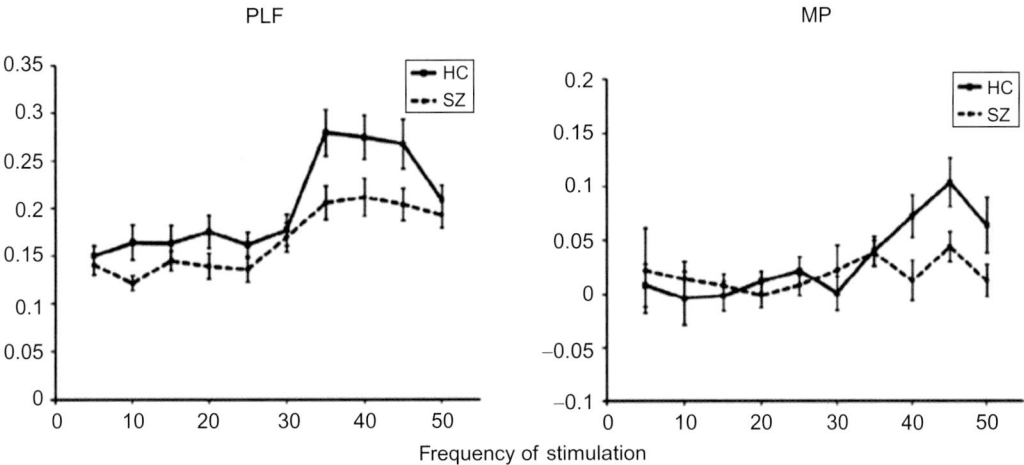

Fig. 2. The modulation transfer function (MTF) for the ASSR recorded at Cz from healthy control (HC; $N = 21$) and schizophrenia (SZ; $N = 21$) groups. The MTFs for the each stimulus frequency are displayed. Each data point is the mean value across the entire stimulus period averaged across subjects within the group. The error bars indicate standard errors. Note the large decrement in schizophrenia for both PLF and MP between 35 and 50 Hz.

2008) indicating that the deficit is probably not due to chronic illness or long-term medication effects. Type of stimulus may affect the specificity of the deficit to gamma range (>30 Hz) frequencies. Studies which used AM tones rather than clicks to elicit the ASSR have found that power was reduced from 11 to 82 Hz (Brenner et al., 2003), and both power and PLF were reduced from 5 to 50 Hz (Krishnan et al., 2009). Hamm et al. (2011) used broad-band noise bursts and found that 5-, 40-, and 80-Hz ASSRs were attenuated in SZ, while 20-Hz was unaffected. Similar to findings by Hamm et al. (2011), unpublished data from the Krishnan et al. (2009) study also revealed an 80-Hz ASSR deficit in SZ. There is also evidence that the ASSR 40-Hz deficit is associated with genetic risk, although not with schizotypal personality characteristics. In the only study to examine first-degree relatives of SZ patients, Hong et al. (2004) reported that relatives showed a reduction in the 40-Hz power. In contrast, individuals with schizotypal personality disorder, a phenotype which shares symptoms with schizophrenia, did not show a deficit in power at 42 Hz or at any other frequency between 11 and 82 Hz (Brenner et al., 2003).

ASSR deficits in 30–40 Hz range are suggestive of auditory cortex disturbances. Auditory cortex involvement in SZ has also been indicated by both imaging and neuropathological findings. Reduction of the gray matter volume of the posterior superior temporal gyrus, including auditory cortex, is a consistent neuroanatomical finding in SZ (Shenton et al., 2001). At the cellular level, Sweet et al. (2003) have reported reduction of the volume of pyramidal neurons in the deep layer of primary and secondary auditory cortex in post-mortem tissue from patients with SZ.

6.1.4. Summary

Patients with SZ have typically demonstrated a deficit in ASSR power or PLF, which is most consistent at 40 Hz. This deficit is apparent for both EEG and MEG ASSR measures and is present at the first psychotic episode. The disturbance in synchrony affects a broader range of frequencies when AM tones, rather than clicks, are used as stimuli. Since the auditory cortex is the primary generator for scalp recorded ASSRs in the 40–50 Hz frequency range, these electrophysiological findings are convergent

TABLE 1

STUDIES OF AUDITORY STEADY-STATE RESPONSES (ASSRs) IN SCHIZOPHRENIA AND RELATED DISORDERS

Author	Stimulus frequency (Hz)	Stimulus type	Group	Results (power, MP or PLF)
Kwon et al., 1999	20, 30, 40	Clicks	SZ	Reduced 40 Hz
Brenner et al., 2003	11, 22, 31, 42, 51, 62, 82	AM tones	SZ	Reduced across multiple frequencies
Brenner et al., 2003	11, 22, 31, 42, 51, 62, 82	AM tones	SPD	No reduction at any frequency
Hong et al., 2004	20, 30, 40	Clicks	SZ	No reduction at 40 Hz
Hong et al., 2004	20, 30, 40	Clicks	First-degree relatives	Reduced 40 Hz
Light et al., 2006	20, 30, 40	Clicks	SZ	Reduced 40 Hz
Spencer et al., 2008	20, 30, 40	Clicks	First-episode psychosis: SZ	Reduced 30, 40 Hz, reduced PLF of 40 Hz harmonic of 20 Hz ASSR
Teale et al., 2008	40	AM tones	SZ	Reduced 40 Hz
Vierling-Classen et al., 2008	20, 30, 40	Clicks	SZ	Reduced 40 Hz, but increased 20 Hz
Wilson et al., 2008	40	Clicks	Adolescent psychosis: SZ, BP	Reduced 40 Hz
Krishnan et al., 2009	5–50	AM tones	SZ	Broad-band reduction
Spencer et al., 2009	40	Clicks	SZ	Reduced 40 Hz
Mulert et al, 2011	40	Clicks	SZ	Reduced 40 Hz
Hamm et al., 2011	5, 20, 40, 80, 160	Broad-band noise bursts	SZ	Reduced 5 Hz and 80 Hz, reduced 40 Hz in right hemisphere

Abbreviations: SZ = schizophrenia; SPD = schizotypal personality disorder; MP = mean power; PLF = phase-locking factor.

with other imaging data, demonstrating abnormalities in auditory cortex anatomy and function. The 40-Hz deficit also appears in first-degree relatives, suggesting that it may reflect genetic risk or shared environmental factors, but not in individuals with schizotypal personality disorder.

6.2. Cellular mechanisms, pharmacology, and animal models

ASSRs demonstrate alterations in a key system affected by SZ, the auditory pathways and auditory cortex. The interpretation of this deficit and its value as a biomarker depend in part on understanding the cellular mechanisms responsible for synchrony and oscillatory activity within neural networks, and how these are disturbed by putative pathophysiological processes. Consequently, in vitro and in vivo studies of neurobiological mechanisms in animal models will likely play a critical role in further understanding cellular mechanism and evaluating novel treatments in both preclinical and clinical stages of development. Gamma range oscillatory activity (30–80 Hz) has been widely studied across a range of mammalian species (Ehrlichman et al., 2009; Lazarewicz et al., 2010).

6.2.1. Generation of gamma oscillations

Neural oscillations are a putative mechanism for sensory, attentional, mnemonic, and motoric processes (Singer, 1999; Başar, 2011). A number of models have been developed to identify important components and network properties associated with neural synchronization. Data from both in vitro and in vivo investigations support the role of synaptic inhibition in the generation of neuronal oscillations, either in an interneuronal network or in a reciprocal excitatory–inhibitory loop (Wang, 2010).

In vitro studies suggest that two major cell types, excitatory principal neurons and inhibitory interneurons, and two specific receptor types, gamma-aminobutyric acid (GABA$_A$) and N-methyl-D-aspartate (NMDA), are critical for neural synchronization (Roopun et al., 2008) in the gamma frequency range. It was originally postulated that among interneuron networks, precise, in-phase firing modulates excitatory glutamatergic pyramidal neuron activity (Whittington et al., 1995; Gray and McCormick, 1996; Traub et al., 1996; Whittington, 2008).Once activated by glutamatergic (NMDA) receptors, GABAergic interneurons generate post-synaptic interneuronal potentials (Traub et al., 1996) and engage in ongoing mutual inhibition and a recurrent feedback loop (Whittington et al., 1995). It has since been demonstrated that trains of fast, somatic inhibitory post-synaptic potentials mediated by the GABA$_A$ receptor are present in all forms of gamma oscillations (Roopun et al., 2008).

High-frequency synchronization is likely propagated through networks in a cycle of GABA$_A$-mediated inhibition followed by rebound excitation and then inhibition (Lewis and Gonzalez-Burgos, 2008). The NMDA receptor is thought to contribute to the generation of network oscillations via modulation of both interneuron to interneuron and interneuron to pyramidal neuron, cell connections. A recent in vitro study demonstrated that the effects of altering NMDA function via ketamine administration may be region specific. Roopun et al. (2008) used horizontal cortical slices to examine the effects of NMDA antagonism of beta$_2$ (20–29 Hz) and gamma (30–80 Hz) range oscillations. This study showed that, following the administration of ketamine, beta$_2$ power increased in association with prelimbic cortices,

while gamma range power was decreased in slice recordings of several regions (medial entorhinal, perirhinal, insular, and medial orbital cortices). Of the areas studied, NMDA-induced increase in gamma power was only detected in auditory cortex. In an in vivo study involving rodents, Pinault (2008) showed that acute blockade of NMDA receptors (with ketamine and MK-801) increased gamma activity in a dose-dependent manner. It could, therefore, be speculated that blocking excitation of inhibitory interneurons decreased phasic inhibitory post-synaptic potentials onto pyramidal cells, resulting in a net excitatory effect on the neuronal network.

In summary, while NMDA antagonists cause an increase in in vitro gamma activity in several brain regions, the auditory cortex appears to show the opposite effect for acute blockade. In vivo studies have shown an increase in gamma activity after acute NMDA blockade. These variations in synchronization patterns may result from intrinsic differences in NMDA signaling in different regions, or interactions among regions that are evident in in vivo studies (Kuwada et al., 2002; Roopun et al., 2008).

6.2.2. Pharmacological effects on ASSRs

The anatomical and functional organization of auditory pathways in humans and other mammalian species is comparable, allowing for the use of animals such as rodents to study ASSR in cross-species studies of schizophrenia-related phenotypes. However, an important issue is whether a specific animal model demonstrates the same frequency response function as that observed in humans. For example, while the healthy human brain has an ASSR resonant frequency at 40 Hz (Kwon et al., 1999), rat ASSRs appear to be maximal at about 50 Hz (Fig. 3; Vohs et al., 2010). It has been argued that this difference should not preclude the use of rodents in ASSR studies because the observed frequency shift is likely secondary to brain volume differences (see Leiser et al., 2011 for further information).

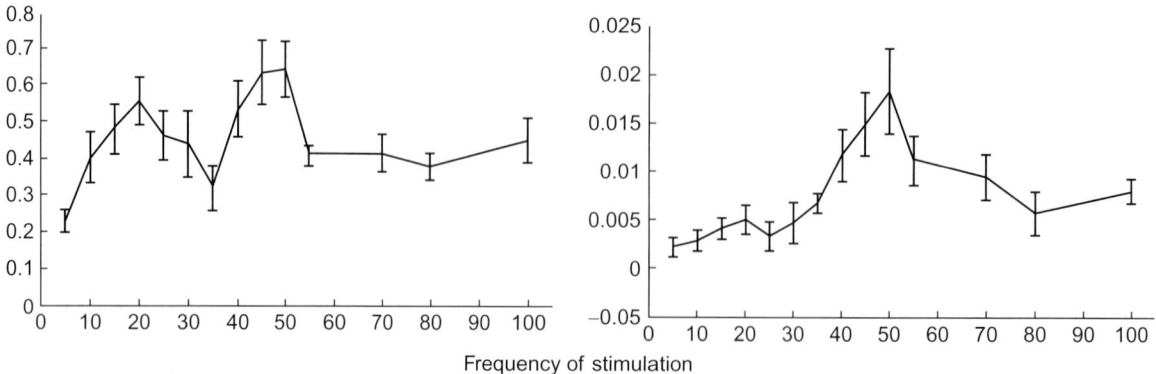

Fig. 3. Modulation transfer function of phase-locking factor (PLF, left panel) and mean power (MP, right panel) to 10-s click trains in eight male rats, with frequency of stimulation on the *x*-axis. The peak frequency of response for both phase locking and mean power is at a slightly higher frequency in rats than in humans (between 45 and 50 Hz).

Because NMDA and GABAergic interneurons are thought to be the most likely candidate mechanisms for ASSR generation, studies examining pharmacological effects on this response have focused on these transmitter systems. However, few studies have utilized pharmacological manipulation on ASSRs. NMDA receptor antagonism via phencyclidine (PCP), MK-801, or ketamine administration induces schizophrenic-like symptoms in healthy individuals (Javitt and Zukin, 1991; Krystal et al., 1994) and exacerbates psychoses in patients with schizophrenia (Lahti et al., 1995; Malhotra et al., 1997). These effects likely reflect dysregulation of the glutamatergic system, and more specifically the NMDA receptor, in the disorder (Tsai et al., 1998). NMDA receptor antagonism not only induces positive (similar to amphetamine psychosis), but also mimics negative and cognitive symptoms associated with schizophrenia. As in patients with schizophrenia and healthy subjects (Plourde et al., 1997), NMDA antagonism (ketamine MK-801 PCP) produces an increase in baseline (unevoked) gamma power in vivo local field potentials and EEG in awake rodents (Pinault, 2008; Ehrlichman et al., 2009; Hakami et al., 2009; Lazarewicz et al., 2010). While these studies mostly examined baseline gamma magnitude and suggested that NMDA antagonism increased gamma, none specifically tested ASSRs. In humans, it has been demonstrated that ketamine increased

the 40-Hz ASSR in healthy individuals (Plourde et al., 1997). Ehrlichman et al. (2009), however, examined both baseline and evoked gamma band responses. These investigators found that subanesthetic (20 mg/kg) doses of ketamine produced increased baseline, but not evoked gamma response. Interestingly, dopamine agonism (D-amphetamine) did not alter gamma band response, suggesting that dopamine may not play a direct role in the gamma deficits observed in patients with schizophrenia.

6.2.3. ASSRs in rodent models of schizophrenia phenotypes

EEG synchronization has recently been studied in rodent models of schizophrenia (Pinault, 2008; Ehrlichman et al., 2009; Lazarewicz et al., 2010). However, limited data have been obtained using the ASSR protocol commonly employed in patients with schizophrenia in animal models. One such study (Vohs et al., 2010) elicited 40-Hz ASSRs from neonatal ventral hippocampal lesion (NVHL) model rats, an established rat model of schizophrenia. In addition, a pharmacological manipulation targeting the $GABA_A$ receptor was also performed to further elucidate this receptor's role in ASSR generation and its status in the NVHL model. The authors found that agonism of the $GABA_A$ receptor yielded a strong lesion by drug interaction, with ASSR magnitude and synchronization decreased in NVHL and increased in sham rats (Vohs et al., 2010). These data suggested an alteration in GABA$_A$ receptor function in NVHL rats and altered inhibitory transmission in the neuronal networks responsible for ASSR generation in NVHL rats.

6.2.4. Summary

A key question in the application of a translational biomarker is whether a comparable neural response can be obtained in human and in an animal model. The ASSR can be elicited from a wide range of species, although initial studies suggest the need for better characterization of the frequency response function to both click and AM tone stimuli in rodent models. In vitro studies suggest that gamma range oscillations in cortical circuits are entrained by GABA$_A$ neurons and are reduced by NMDA receptor antagonists. Importantly, the effect of NMDA antagonists on gamma activity may vary across cortical regions, and between in vitro and in vivo preparations. Thus, while the sensitivity of gamma range activity has been demonstrated by both types of preparation, study of local circuit activity and neural populations in vivo will be required to better characterize the basis of specific pharmacological effects. Several studies have examined ASSRs in rodent models of schizophrenia-related phenotypes and suggest that this approach may offer a flexible vehicle for cross-species studies of pathophysiological mechanisms and medication effects.

6.3. Discussion

ASSRs, particularly in the gamma frequency range (>30 Hz), are reduced in power and phase synchronization in schizophrenia. Because synchronized neural activity appears to be critical for a wide range of perceptual, cognitive, and motoric processes, oscillatory deficits may index a key mechanism for functional disconnection or integration in SZ

(Başar et al., 2001; Whittington, 2008; Uhlhaas and Singer, 2010). ASSRs therefore appear to have the potential to serve as a translational, cross-species biomarker for schizophrenia and related disorders. However, the functional significance of the ASSR deficit and its implications regarding the pathophysiology of SZ must be better characterized for this response to be effectively utilized as an informative biomarker in studying etiological factors, mechanisms, and intervention effects.

The ASSR represents only one of a variety of EEG and MEG paradigms which can capture disturbances of neural synchrony or oscillations in schizophrenia (Başar et al., 2001; Uhlhaas and Singer, 2010; Başar, 2011). Gamma activity, for example, may also be evoked by the onset of an auditory stimulus, or induced by working memory demands in patients with schizophrenia. Moreover, gamma activity deficits have been observed in other disorders as well, including attention-deficit hyperactivity disorder and bipolar disorder (see Başar and Güntekin, 2008, for review), and therefore are not specific to schizophrenia. Given the dependence on gamma oscillations on interactions among GABAergic and glutamatergic neurons within cortical circuits, it is not surprising that oscillatory deficits would be sensitive to a range of neuropsychiatric disorders.

From a clinical perspective, the relationship of ASSRs to the development and course of the illness, treatment, and outcomes is incompletely characterized. While it has been established, the motoric, cognitive, and social behavior deficits are often present in children who develop schizophrenia later in life (O'Donnell, 2007), there are no studies of ASSRs in high-risk or prodromal individuals who later develop the illness. A single study (Hong et al., 2004) has reported that the 40-Hz ASSR deficit occurs in non-psychotic relatives of patients with schizophrenia, consistent with an effect of familial or genetic risk factors. No longitudinal studies have been conducted, and long-term test–retest reliability of the measure in SZ has not been evaluated. The relationship of ASSR deficits to long-term outcomes or treatment response has not been studied. Hong et al. (2004) reported that patients receiving novel antipsychotic medication may show an enhanced 40-Hz activity, but no studies have examined ASSRs in patients before and after receiving antipsychotic medications.

The ease of recording ASSRs in animal models of SZ phenotypes suggests that these measures could also be highly informative in testing neurophysiological models of the disorder, particularly with respect to glutamate and GABAergic interactions. ASSRs can test cellular mechanisms that are not accessible through non-invasive measures in humans and could provide a preclinical measure to test novel antipsychotic treatments. The potential of a combined human and animal model approach to treatment development is especially intriguing and merits exploration in future research.

Acknowledgments

This work was supported by the National Institutes of Mental Health (R01 MH62150, 1 R21 MH091774-01, and CTSA UL1RR025761-01 to B.F.O., and R01 MH074983 to W.P.H.).

References

Bach, D.R., Buxtorf, K., Strik, W.K., Neuhoff, J.G. and Seifritz, E. (2011) Evidence for impaired sound intensity processing in schizophrenia. *Schizophr. Bull.*, 37: 426–431.

Başar, E. (2011) *Brain–Body–Mind in the Nebulous Cartesian System: A Holistic Approach by Oscillations.* Springer, New York, p. 523.

Başar, E. and Güntekin, B. (2008) A review of brain oscillations in cognitive disorders and the role of neurotransmitters. *Brain Res.*, 1235: 172–193.

Başar, E., Başar-Eroğlu, C., Karakas, S. and Schurmann, M. (2001) Gamma, alpha, delta, and theta oscillations govern cognitive processes. *Int. J. Psychophysiol.*, 39: 241–248.

Brenner, C.A., Sporns, O., Lysaker, P.H. and O'Donnell, B.F. (2003) EEG synchronization to modulated auditory tones in schizophrenia, schizoaffective disorder, and schizotypal personality disorder. *Am. J. Psychiatry*, 160: 2238–2240.

Brenner, C.A., Krishnan, G.P., Vohs, J.L., Ahn, W.Y., Hetrick, W.P., Morzorati, S.L. and O'Donnell, B.F. (2009) Steady state responses: electrophysiological assessment of sensory function in schizophrenia. *Schizophr. Bull.*, 35: 1065–1077.

Bunney, W.E., Hetrick, W.P., Bunney, B.G., Patterson, J.V., Patterson, J.V., Jin, Y., Potkin, S.G. and Sandman, C.A. (1999) Structured interview for assessing perceptual anomalies. *Schizophr. Bull.*, 25: 577–592.

Carroll, C.A., O'Donnell, B.F., Shekhar, A. and Hetrick, W.P. (2009) Timing dysfunctions in schizophrenia span from millisecond to several-second durations. *Brain Cogn.*, 70: 181–190.

Conti, G., Santarelli, R., Grassi, S., Ottaviani, F. and Azzena, B. (1999) Auditory steady-state responses to click trains from the rat temporal cortex. *Clin. Neurophysiol.*, 110: 62–70.

Delorme, A. and Makeig, S. (2004) EEGLAB: an open source toolbox for analysis of single-trial EEG dynamics including independent component analysis. *J. Neurosci. Meth.*, 134: 9–21.

Dolphin, W.F. and Mountain, D.C. (1992) The envelope following response: scalp potentials elicited in the Mongolian gerbil using sinusoidally AM acoustic signals. *Hearing Res.*, 58: 70–78.

Ehrlichman, R.S., Gandal, M.J., Maxwell, C.R., Lazarewicz, M.T., Finkel, L.H., Contreras, D., Turetsky, B.I. and Siegel, S.J. (2009) N-Methyl-D-aspartic acid receptor antagonist-induced frequency oscillations in mice recreate pattern of electrophysiological deficits in schizophrenia. *Neuroscience*, 158: 705–712.

Gray, C.M. and McCormick, D.A. (1996) Chattering cells: superficial pyramidal neurons contributing to the generation of synchronous oscillations in the visual cortex. *Science*, 274: 109–113.

Hakami, T., Jones, N.C., Tolmacheva, E.A., Gaudias, J., Chaumont, J., Salzberg, M., O'Brien, T.J. and Pinault, D. (2009) NMDA receptor hypofunction leads to generalized and persistent aberrant gamma oscillations independent of hyperlocomotion and the state of consciousness. *PLoS One*, 4: e6755.

Hamm, J.P., Gilmore, C.S., Picchetti, N.A., Sponheim, S.R. and Clementz, B.A. (2011) Abnormalities of neuronal oscillations and temporal integration to low- and high-frequency auditory stimulation in schizophrenia. *Biol. Psychiatry*, 69: 989–996.

Herdman, A.T., Lins, O., Van Roon, P., Stapells, D.R., Scherg, M. and Picton, T.W. (2002) Intracerebral sources of human auditory steady-state responses. *Brain Topogr.*, 15: 69–86.

Hirayasu, Y., Potts, G.F., O'Donnell, B.F., Kwon, J.S., Arakaki, H., Akdag, S.J., Levitt, J.J., Shenton, M.E. and McCarley, R.W. (1998) Auditory mismatch negativity in schizophrenia: topographic evaluation with a high-density recording montage. *Am. J. Psychiatry*, 155: 1281–1284.

Hong, L.E., Summerfelt, A., McMahon, R., Adami, H., Francis, G., Elliott, A., Buchanan, R.W. and Thaker, G.K. (2004) Evoked gamma band synchronization and the liability for schizophrenia. *Schizophr. Res.*, 70: 293–302.

Javitt, D.C. and Zukin, S.R. (1991) Recent advances in the phencyclidine model of schizophrenia. *Am. J. Psychiatry*, 148: 1301–1308.

Krishnan, G.P., Hetrick, W.P., Brenner, C.A., Shekhar, A., Steffen, A.N. and O'Donnell, B.F. (2009) Steady state and induced auditory gamma deficits in schizophrenia. *Neuroimage*, 47: 1711–1719.

Krystal, J.H., Karper, L.P., Seibyl, J.P., Freeman, G.K., Delaney, R., Bremner, J.D., Heninger, G.R., Bowers, M.B., Jr. and Charney, D.S. (1994) Subanesthetic effects of the noncompetitive NMDA antagonist, ketamine, in humans. Psychotomimetic, perceptual, cognitive, and neuroendocrine responses. *Arch. Gen. Psychiatry*, 51: 199–214.

Kuhn, S. and Gallinat, J. (2010) Quantitative meta-analysis on state and trait aspects of auditory verbal hallucinations in schizophrenia. *Schizophr. Bull.*, 22 December: published online.

Kuwada, S., Anderson, J.S., Batra, R., Fitzpatrick, D.C., Teissier, N. and D'Angelo, W.R. (2002) Sources of the scalp-recorded amplitude-modulation following response. *J. Am. Acad. Audiol.*, 13: 188–204.

Kwon, J.S., O'Donnell, B.F., Wallenstein, G.V., Greene, R.W., Hirayasu, Y., Nestor, P.G., Hasselmo, M.E., Potts, G.F., Shenton, M.E. and McCarley, R.W. (1999) Gamma frequency range abnormalities to auditory stimulation in schizophrenia. *Arch. Gen. Psychiatry*, 56: 1001–1005.

Lahti, A.C., Koffel, B., Laporte, D. and Tamminga, C.A. (1995) Subanesthetic doses of ketamine stimulate psychosis in schizophrenia. *Neuropsychopharmacology*, 13: 9–19.

Lazarewicz, M.T., Ehrlichman, R.S., Maxwell, C.R., Gandal, M.J., Finkel, L.H. and Siegel, S.J. (2010) Ketamine modulates theta and gamma oscillations. *J. Cogn. Neurosci.*, 22: 1452–1464.

Leiser, S.C., Dunlop, J., Bowlby, M.R. and Devilbiss, D.M. (2011) Aligning strategies for using EEG as a surrogate biomarker: a review of preclinical and clinical research. *Biochem. Pharmacol.*, 81: 1408–1421.

Leitman, D.I., Laukka, P., Juslin, P.N., Saccente, E., Butler, P. and Javitt, D.C. (2008) Getting the cue: sensory contributions to auditory emotion recognition impairments in schizophrenia. *Schizophr. Bull.*, 36: 545–556.

Lewis, D.A. and Gonzalez-Burgos, G. (2008) Neuroplasticity of neocortical circuits in schizophrenia. *Neuropsychopharmacology*, 33: 141–165.

Light, G.A., Hsu, J.L., Hsieh, M.H., Meyer-Gomes, K., Sprock, J., Swerdlow, N.R. and Braff, D.L. (2006) Gamma band oscillations reveal neural network cortical coherence dysfunction in schizophrenia patients. *Biol. Psychiatry*, 60: 1231–1240.

Luck, S.J., Mathalon, D.H., O'Donnell, B.F., Hämäläinen, M.S., Spencer, K.M., Javitt, D.C. and Uhlhaas, P.J. (2011) A roadmap for the development and validation of event-related potential biomarkers in schizophrenia research. *Biol. Psychiatry*, 70: 28–34.

Malhotra, A.K., Pinals, D.A., Adler, C.M., Elman, I., Clifton, A., Pickar, D. and Breier, A. (1997) Ketamine-induced exacerbation of psychotic symptoms and cognitive impairment in neuroleptic-free schizophrenics. *Neuropsychopharmacology*, 17: 141–150.

Mulert, C., Kirsch, V., Pascual-Marqui, R., McCarley, R.W. and Spencer, K.M. (2011) Long-range synchrony of gamma oscillations and auditory hallucination symptoms in schizophrenia. *Int. J. Psychophysiol.*, 79: 55–63.

O'Donnell, B.F. (2007) Cognitive impairment in schizophrenia: a life span perspective. *Am. J. Alzheimer's Dis. Other Demen.*, 22: 398–405.

Pantev, C., Roberts, L.E., Elbert, T., Ross, B. and Wienbruch, C. (1996) Tonotopic organization of the sources of human auditory steady-state responses. *Hearing Res.*, 101: 62–74.

Perrin, M.A., Butler, P.D., Di Constanzo, J., Forchelli, G., Silipo, G. and Javitt, D.C. (2010) Spatial localization deficits and auditory cortical dysfunction in schizophrenia. *Schizophr. Res.*, 124: 161–168.

Picton, T.W., John, M.S., Dimitrijević, A. and Purcell, D. (2003) Human auditory steady-state responses. *Int. J. Audiol.*, 42: 177–219.

Pinault, D. (2008) *N*-Methyl-D-aspartate receptor antagonists ketamine and MK-801 induce wake-related aberrant gamma oscillations in the rat neocortex. *Biol. Psychiatry*, 63: 730–735.

Plourde, G., Baribeau, J. and Bonhomme, V. (1997) Ketamine increases the amplitude of the 40-Hz auditory steady-state response in humans. *Br. J. Anaesth.*, 78: 524–529.

Roopun, A.K., Cunningham, M.O., Racca, C., Alter, K., Traub, R.D. and Whittington, M.A. (2008) Region-specific changes in gamma and beta$_2$ rhythms in NMDA receptor dysfunction models of schizophrenia. *Schizophr. Bull.*, 34: 962–973.

Ross, B., Picton, T.W. and Pantev, C. (2002) Temporal integration in the human auditory cortex as represented by the development of the steady-state magnetic field. *Hearing Res.*, 165: 68–84.

Saha, S., Chant, D., Welham, J. and McGrath, J. (2005) A systematic review of the prevalence of schizophrenia. *PLoS Med.*, 2: e141.

Shenton, M.E., Dickey, C.C., Frumin, M. and McCarley, R.W. (2001) A review of MRI findings in schizophrenia. *Schizophr. Res.*, 49: 1–52.

Singer, W. (1999) Neuronal synchrony: a versatile code for the definition of relations? *Neuron*, 24(49–65): 111–125.

Spencer, K.M., Salisbury, D.F., Shenton, M.E. and McCarley, R.W. (2008) Gamma-band auditory steady-state responses are impaired in first episode psychosis. *Biol. Psychiatry*, 64: 369–375.

Spencer, K.M., Niznikiewicz, M.A., Nestor, P.G., Shenton, M.E. and McCarley, R.W. (2009) Left auditory cortex gamma synchronization and auditory hallucination symptoms in schizophrenia. *BMC Neurosci.*, 10: 85.

Strous, R.D., Cowan, N., Ritter, W. and Javitt, D.C. (1995) Auditory sensory ("echoic") memory dysfunction in schizophrenia. *Am. J. Psychiatry*, 152: 1517–1519.

Sweet, R.A., Pierri, J.N., Auh, S., Sampson, A.R. and Lewis, D.A. (2003) Reduced pyramidal cell somal volume in auditory association cortex of subjects with schizophrenia. *Neuropsychopharmacology*, 28: 599–609.

Teale, P., Collins, D., Maharajh, K., Rojas, D.C., Kronberg, E. and Reite, M. (2008) Cortical source estimates of gamma band amplitude and phase are different in schizophrenia. *Neuroimage*, 42: 1481–1489.

Traub, R., Whittington, M.A., Stanford, I.M. and Jefferys, J.G.R. (1996) A mechanism for generation of long-range synchronous fast oscillations in the cortex. *Nature (London)*, 383: 621–624.

Tsai, G., Van Kammen, D.P., Chen, S., Kelley, M.E., Grier, A. and Coyle, J.T. (1998) Glutamatergic neurotransmission involves structural and clinical deficits of schizotrenia. *Biol. Psychiatry*, 44: 667–674.

Turetsky, B.I., Calkins, M.E., Light, G.A., Olincy, A., Radant, A.D. and Swerdlow, N.R. (2007) Neurophysiological endophenotypes of schizophrenia: the viability of selected candidate measures. *Schizophr. Bull.*, 33: 69–94.

Uhlhaas, P.J. and Singer, W. (2010) Abnormal neural oscillations and synchrony in schizophrenia. *Nat. Rev. Neurosci.*, 11: 100–113.

Vierling-Classen, D., Siekmeier, P., Stufflebeam, S. and Kopell, N. (2008) Modeling GABA alterations in schizophrenia: a link between impaired inhibition and altered gamma and beta range auditory entrainment. *J. Neurophysiol.*, 99: 2656–2671.

Vohs, J.L., Chambers, R.A., Krishnan, G.P., O'Donnell, B.F., Berg, S. and Morzorati, S.L. (2010) GABAergic modulation of the 40 Hz auditory steady-state response in a rat model of schizophrenia. *Int. J. Neuropsychopharmacol.*, 13: 487–497.

Wang, X.J. (2010) Neurophysiological and computational principles of cortical rhythms in cognition. *Physiol. Rev.*, 90: 1195–1268.

Whittington, M.A. (2008) Can brain rhythms inform on underlying pathology in schizophrenia? Biol. *Psychiatry*, 63: 728–729.

Whittington, M.A., Traub, R. and Jefferys, J.G.R. (1995) Synchronized oscillations in interneuron networks driven by metabotropic glutamate receptor activation. *Nature (Lond.)*, 373: 612–615.

Wilson, T.W., Hernandez, O.O., Asherin, R.M., Teale, P.D., Reite, M.L. and Rojas, D.C. (2008) Cortical gamma generators suggest abnormal auditory circuitry in early-onset psychosis. *Cereb. Cortex*, 18: 371–378.

Application of Brain Oscillations in Neuropsychiatric Diseases
(Supplements to Clinical Neurophysiology, Vol. 62)
Editors: E. Başar, C. Başar-Eroğlu, A. Özerdem, P.M. Rossini, G.G. Yener

Chapter 7

Clinical relevance of animal models of schizophrenia

Michael Koch*

*Department of Neuropharmacology, Brain Research Institute, University of Bremen, PO Box 330440,
D-28334 Bremen, Germany*

ABSTRACT

Animal models and endophenotypes of mental disorders are regarded as preclinical heuristic approaches aiming at understanding the etiopathogenesis of these diseases, and at developing drug treatment strategies. A frequently used translational model of sensorimotor gating and its deficits in some neuropsychiatric disorders is prepulse inhibition (PPI) of startle. PPI is reduced in schizophrenia patients, but the exact relationship between symptoms and reduced PPI is still unclear. Recent findings suggest that the levels of PPI in humans and animals may be predictive of certain cognitive functions. Hence, this simple measure of reflex suppression may be of use for clinical research.

PPI is the reduction of the acoustic startle response that occurs when a weak prestimulus is presented shortly prior to a startling noise pulse. It is considered a measure of sensorimotor gating and is regulated by a cortico-limbic striato-pallidal circuit. However, PPI does not only occur in the domain of startle. PPI of alpha, gamma, and theta oscillations at frontal and central locations has been found, suggesting a relationship between PPI and cognitive processes. In fact, levels of PPI in healthy subjects and in animals predict their performance in cognitive tasks mainly mediated by the frontal cortex. Taken together, PPI might reflect a more general filtering performance leading to gating of intrusive sensory, motor, and cognitive input, thereby improving cognitive function. Hence, PPI might be used in clinical settings to predict the impact of drugs or psychotherapy on cognitive performance in neuropsychiatric patients.

KEYWORDS

EEG; Oscillation; Sensorimotor gating; Working memory

7.1. Introduction

Animal models of neuropsychiatric diseases are an indispensable part of biological psychiatry and experimental neurology (Koch, 2006). They have traditionally been regarded as preclinical heuristic

models aiming at: first, understanding the etiopathogenesis of these diseases and, second, developing drug treatment strategies with high therapeutic potential and little side effects. However, it might be possible that they have direct relevance as biomarkers for clinical research.

Generally, it is understood that an animal model never corresponds to a disorder in toto, but always strives to model distinct aspects of the disease, e.g., etiopathogenic factors, certain symptoms or neuropathology. Animal models are validated on the basis of their face, predictive and construct validity (Koch, 2006). A very influential

---

Correspondence to: Prof. M. Koch, Department of Neuropharmacology, Brain Research Institute, University of Bremen — FB 2, PO Box 330440, D-28334 Bremen, Germany.
Tel.: +49-421-21862970; Fax: +49-421-21862984;
E-mail: michael.koch@uni-bremen.de

conceptual approach to establishing an animal model for a certain disease was put forward by Gottesman and Gould (2003): the concept of endophenotypes (or intermediate phenotypes) postulates that relatively simple quantifiable phenotypes that are intermediate between the genotype and a complex phenotype of an organism can be used to experimentally address genetic or physiological underpinnings of the disease. These endophenotypes appear to be ideal candidates for translational animal models. Among the endophenotypes for schizophrenia research are working memory, oculomotor function and sensory, as well as sensorimotor gating (Gottesman and Gould, 2003). The question arises though whether or not these endophenotypes are related to each other, and/or whether or not they are related to clinical symptoms.

A frequently used operational model of sensorimotor gating and its deficits in some neuropsychiatric disorders is prepulse inhibition (PPI) of startle. PPI is reduced in schizophrenia patients and in a number of other neuropsychiatric disorders, but the exact relationship between neuropathology, symptoms, and reduced PPI is still unclear and empirical data dealing with this issue are still scarce (Weike et al., 2000; Braff et al., 2001; Swerdlow et al., 2006a). More than 10 years ago, it has been suggested that early gating processes leading to PPI — albeit probably mediated by different neuronal circuits — may also be relevant for the attentional blink, backward masking, negative priming, as well as for complex neuropsychological tasks (Filion et al., 1999). Interestingly, recent findings suggest that the levels of PPI in humans and animals may be predictive of certain cognitive functions. Hence, this simple measure of reflex suppression may be of use for clinical research. The aim of the present contribution is to discuss the neurophysiological basis of PPI, to review recent findings of human and animal PPI research and to take soundings on the possible relevance of PPI as a predictor of cognitive performance.

7.2. Results

PPI is the reduction of the acoustic startle response (ASR) magnitude that occurs when a weak prestimulus (sometimes termed "lead stimulus") is presented some 25–1020 ms prior to the startling noise pulse (Fig. 1). The inhibition of the ASR is normally around 70%, depending upon the exact stimulus settings and interstimulus interval (ISI). PPI is considered a cross-species measure of sensorimotor gating and is regulated by a cortico-limbic striato-pallidal circuit (Koch, 1999; Fendt et al., 2001; Geyer et al., 2001). However, it should be noted that PPI is not restricted to the modulation of the ASR, but also occurs in other domains of information processing in the central nervous system (vide infra). One influential theory for the explanation of the function of PPI is that the automatic response to the prepulse protects its processing from disruption by the ensuing startle stimulus and/or response (Graham et al., 1975). Similar forms of gating of a second stimulus by a preceding stimulus is the P50 event-related potential (ERP) suppression paradigm where, normally, the ERP to the second of a paired set of stimuli is reduced (Adler et al., 1999). It is noteworthy that the neuronal events induced by the prepulse, which can occur in different sensory domains (Ison and Hammond, 1971), are still not exactly characterized although they might be relevant for the understanding of PPI (Csomor et al., 2005; Yee and Feldon, 2009). Recently, we have shown that one early component of the acoustic prepulse-elicited reaction is a motor response following 40 ms after prepulse onset (Brosda et al., 2011). However, it is very likely that early sensory (bottom up) and late perceptual components of this stimulus are also relevant for the inhibition of the ASR and other effects of the prepulse.

Deficits in PPI of the ASR experimentally induced in animals aim at modeling PPI deficits in humans under pathological conditions and perhaps help to understand the mechanisms underlying different aspects of the disease

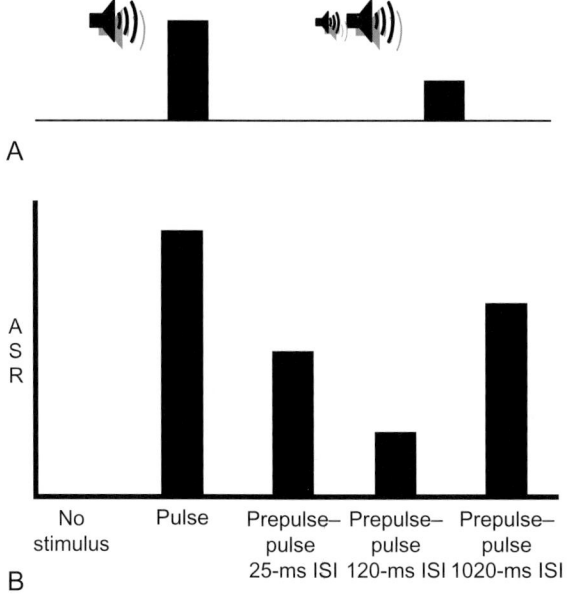

A

B

Fig. 1. Schematic depiction of the basic principle of PPI of the acoustic startle response (ASR). (A) A shortly preceding prepulse markedly reduces the magnitude of the ASR. PPI strongly depends on the interstimulus interval (ISI) between prepulse and startling pulse (B). However, PPI is found in a relatively wide range of ISIs (data are extracted from Brosda et al. (2011) and depict arbitrary stabilimeter readings for the ASR of rats).

(etiopathogenesis, symptomatology, and neuropathology). There are numerous reports on reduced PPI induced by dopamine, serotonin or cannabinoid receptor agonists, as well as glutamate N-methyl-D-aspartate receptor antagonists, and the influence of antipsychotic drugs thereupon (Geyer et al., 2001; Brosda et al., 2011) that provide models supporting the classical pharmacological theories of schizophrenia. Furthermore, several models capitalized on the neurodevelopmental theory of the etiology of schizophrenia, suggesting that the disease may result from sequential noxious events early (e.g., pre- or perinatally) and late (e.g., puberty and adolescence) during development (Weinberger, 1995; Beckmann, 2001). Especially the neonatal lesion as well as the maternal or social deprivation

models were successfully showing PPI deficits (Geyer et al., 2001; Van den Buuse et al., 2003; Lipska, 2004; Koch, 2006).

However, not very many studies in animals have tried to systematically relate reduced PPI with other behavioral measures. We have used a genetic top-down approach to study the relationship between low or high PPI and cognitive performance in rats. Based on their individual levels of PPI, male and female rats were selectively bred for high or low PPI. Already after two generations, the "low" group showed stable PPI levels of around 10% that were mitigated by both typical and atypical neuroleptic drugs (Hadamitzky et al., 2007). In a systematic study on animals of the fourth and sixth filial generation of low PPI breeding, we found reduced PPI at all prepulse intensities, ISIs and at all developmental stages tested, as well as deficits in short-term habituation of the ASR (Schwabe et al., 2007). Interestingly, the rats of the low PPI breeding line showed normal behavior in spatial learning and memory, but showed enhanced perseverative behavior in response switching between different navigation rules on the maze, as well as in an operant task in a Skinner box, suggesting reduced response flexibility in low PPI rats (Freudenberg et al., 2007). In addition, rats of the low PPI group showed impaired social behavior and reduced reward-related behavior (Dieckmann et al., 2007). Taken together, these findings suggest that reduced PPI of the ASR is related to other behavioral markers in rats that might be relevant for schizophrenia.

Although PPI is usually measured as inhibition of the ASR in humans and in animals, it probably does not only occur in the domain of startle. Conceptually, PPI is thought to reflect a filter mechanism that gates intrusive sensory or cognitive information out of an already activated neuronal program, in order to protect the processing routine of the sensory prepulse (Koch, 1998). Hence, it is very likely that PPI is not confined to startle but also to other neuronal processes. Given the fact that PPI of the ASR is found at ISIs of circa

20–1000 ms, it is conceivable that both short-latency bottom-up sensory or motor events and top-down cognitive events of longer latency, are involved in PPI.

ERPs, defined as the measured EEG signal time-locked to an event, allow disentangling different modulatory factors of a behavioral response in the time domain. Concurrent PPI and EEG studies have shown that prominent evoked potentials such as the P50, P1, N1, P2, and P300 are reduced for acoustic stimuli when preceded by a prepulse, although the extent to which these potentials are influenced by the prepulse is not correlated with the PPI of the ASR, indicating that PPI of startle and that of evoked potentials are mediated by different, but perhaps overlapping, neuronal mechanisms (Schall et al., 1997; Ford and Roth, 1999; Campbell et al., 2007). The P50 reflects bottom-up processing ("sensory gating"), while the P1 and N1 are already modulated by focused attention and perceptual binding. The P3 reflects top-down cognitive events related to decision making, memory, and allocation of attentional resources (Başar-Eroğlu et al., 1992; Polich, 2007). Furthermore, ERPs are determined by superimposed event-related oscillations (EROs) in different frequency bands (Başar, 2006). Within the first 500-ms post-stimulus onset, PPI is observed for the oscillatory theta (4–7 Hz), alpha (8–13 Hz), and gamma (28–48 Hz) response. Interestingly, delta band EROs (0.5–4 Hz) were broader in the prepulse–pulse conditions at ISIs of 60 and 120 ms, but not 240 ms, compared to pulse-alone conditions (Kedzior et al., 2006, 2007). The topographic pattern of the PPI modulation indicated involvement of brain areas related to auditory sensory processing and cognition. Thus, studies on ERPs indicate that prepulses may impact on both bottom-up as well as top-down processing. In accordance, modulations of the ERPs and EROs do not fully explain but seem to contribute to the observed motor response, i.e., PPI of the blink (Ford and Roth, 1999; Kedzior et al., 2007).

PPI deficits in patients with schizophrenia are also reflected in ERPs. Reduction of the P1 elicited by a tone, which was preceded by a prepulse, was observed in healthy controls but not in patients with schizophrenia. Furthermore, at temporal sites, patients with schizophrenia showed a dominant N1 and P1 at the right hemisphere, which was not observed in healthy subjects (Schall et al., 1997). Similar results were described for the P2. Enhancement of the N1, expected for the pulse after long prepulse–pulse intervals, which allow focusing attention on the pulse after sufficient processing of the prepulse, is also lacking in patients with schizophrenia (Ford et al., 1999). These results suggest disturbed balancing between inhibition and facilitation to select and process relevant information in patients with schizophrenia.

Although not explicitly investigated, it might also be assumed that the oscillatory brain response might be altered during PPI paradigms for similar reasons. For example, higher levels of PPI have been associated with better recovery in a backward masking task in healthy volunteers (Wynn et al., 2004), while schizophrenia patients showed reduced gamma band activity and poorer performance in backward masking (Wynn et al., 2005). Furthermore, auditory processing has been often associated with a reduction of the oscillatory gamma band response (Haig et al., 2000; Lee et al., 2003; Spencer et al., 2004; Herrmann and Demiralp, 2005). However, it seems that the consistency of the response over trials, i.e., presumably the effectively utilized brain activity, is especially affected. When looking at single events the oscillatory response might be enhanced and even encompass to brain areas not related to auditory processing (Başar-Eroğlu et al., 2011). Furthermore, not only gamma but all frequency bands are disturbed in patients with schizophrenia (for review see Başar-Eroğlu et al., Ch. 8, this volume). Thus, auditory stimuli might be processed less selectively in timing but also with regard to the information transfer between brain areas and frequency bands.

Levels of PPI in healthy subjects and in animals predict their performance in cognitive tasks mainly mediated by the frontal cortex, for example, response flexibility, selective attention, planning, and Stroop tasks (Bitsios and Giakoumaki, 2005; Bitsios et al., 2006; Giakoumaki et al., 2006; Freudenberg et al., 2007). Interestingly, PPI performance correlated with working memory performance in a recent study on the influence of single nucleotide polymorphisms in genes associated with schizophrenia risk (Roussos et al., 2011). Since impaired working memory in schizophrenia patients appears to be partly due to sensory encoding deficits (Mathes et al., 2005; Dias et al., 2011), it is conceivable that PPI can be used as a feasible test for possible treatment effects on cognitive performance.

Studies in healthy humans have shown that the atypical antipsychotic drugs sertindole, quetiapine, or clozapine increased PPI in subjects with low PPI performance (Swerdlow et al., 2006b; Vollenweider et al., 2006; Holstein et al., 2011). Clozapine also slightly improved attention and working memory. However, no direct correlation between PPI and cognitive performance was found (Vollenweider et al., 2006). In another study by the Swerdlow group, the relationship in schizophrenia patients between PPI and various parametric, demographic, clinical, and cognitive parameters (e.g., sex, symptom severity, medication, and cognitive performance) was assessed. The results of that study suggest that levels of PPI strongly depend on the prepulse–pulse interval (impaired PPI in patients only at the 60-ms interval), on the smoking and medication status (nicotine and atypical neuroleptic drugs increase PPI), and on sex (PPI higher in male patients). There was a significant correlation between PPI and global assessment of function scores in male patients. However, cognitive performance and symptom severity were not related to PPI levels (Swerdlow et al., 2006a).

With respect to neuropathology, there is also a link between reduced PPI in animal models and some measures of cognitive performance. Among the diverse neuropathological findings in schizophrenia (Harrison, 1999), a reduced amount of the calcium-binding protein, parvalbumine, has been found in GABAergic interneurons in the prefrontal cortex (Lewis et al., 2005). Reduced prefrontal parvalbumine has also been shown in neonatal lesion models of schizophrenia that are characterized by reduced PPI (Lipska et al., 2003; Schneider and Koch, 2005; Klein et al., 2008). Interestingly, a recent study has shown that these interneurons play an essential role in prefrontal cognitive function and gamma oscillations (Sohal et al., 2009). Disrupted GABA functioning in the prefrontal cortex has been implicated in abnormal oscillatory activity and cognitive deficits in schizophrenia (Uhlhaas and Singer, 2010). However, very recent experiments in rats showed no correlation between the levels of PPI and T-maze learning or delayed alternation performance (Fig. 2). Since these results in animals point toward differences between healthy subjects and rats with respect to the relationship between working memory and PPI, further experiments are planned to scrutinize this issue.

7.3. Conclusions

Taken together, PPI might reflect a more general filtering process leading to gating of intrusive sensory, motor, and cognitive input, thereby improving cognitive function. Hence, PPI might be used in clinical settings to predict the impact of drugs or psychotherapy on cognitive performance in neuropsychiatric patients. Since PPI has both sensory and cognitive aspects, correlates with oscillations and other endophenotypes for schizophrenia, it would be interesting to measure PPI of oscillations in neuropsychiatric patients.

Acknowledgments

I thank Dr. Birgit Mathes (University of Bremen) for helpful comments on the manuscript and Ellen Irrsack for running the behavioral tests.

118

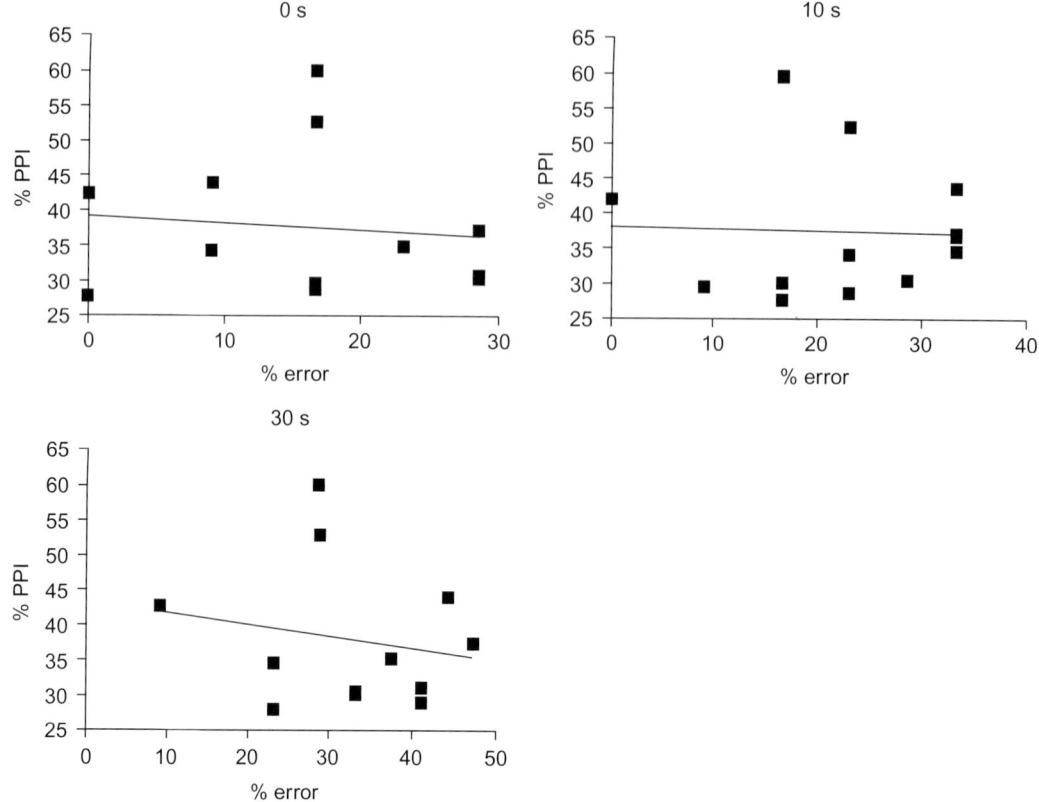

Fig. 2. No significant correlation between PPI of the ASR and working memory in a T-maze (correlation coefficients = −0.09 for 0 s; −0.03 for 10 s; −0.19 for 30 s, $p >0.05$; $n = 12$ rats). Percent PPI data are pooled across 68, 72, and 76 dB prepulse intensities presented 120 ms prior to 105 dB broadband noise startle pulses. T-maze data present percent number of errors during acquisition (0 s) of the task and during delayed (10 and 30 s) alternation.

References

Adler, L.E., Freedman, R., Ross, R.G., Olincy, A. and Waldo, M.C. (1999) Elementary phenotypes in the neurobiological and genetic study of schizophrenia. *Biol. Psychiatry*, 46: 8–18.

Başar, E. (2006) The theory of the whole-brain work. *Int. J. Psychophysiol.*, 60: 133–138.

Başar-Eroğlu, C., Başar, E., Demiralp, T. and Schurmann, M. (1992) P300-response: possible psychophysiological correlates in delta and theta frequency channels. A review. *Int. J. Psychophysiol.*, 13: 161–179.

Başar-Eroğlu, C., Mathes, B., Brand, A. and Schmiedt-Fehr, C. (2011) Occipital gamma response to auditory stimulation in patients with schizophrenia. *Int. J. Psychophysiol.*, 79: 3–8.

Beckmann, H. (2001) Neuropathology of the endogenous psychoses. In: F. Henn, N. Sartorius, H. Helmchen and H. Lauer

(Eds.), *Contemporary Psychiatry*. Springer, Berlin, pp. 81–100.

Bitsios, P. and Giakoumaki, S.G. (2005) Relationship of prepulse inhibition of the startle reflex to attentional and executive mechanisms in man. *Int. J. Psychophysiol.*, 55: 229–241.

Bitsios, P., Giakoumaki, S.G., Theou, K. and Frangou, S. (2006) Increased prepulse inhibition of the acoustic startle response is associated with better strategy formation and execution times in healthy males. *Neuropsychologia*, 44: 2494–2499.

Braff, D.L., Geyer, M.A. and Swerdlow, N.R. (2001) Human studies of prepulse inhibition of startle: normal subjects, patient groups, and pharmacological studies. *Psychopharmacology*, 156: 234–258.

Brosda, J., Hayn, L., Klein, C., Koch, M., Meyer, C., Schallhorn, R. and Wegener, N. (2011) Pharmacological and parametrical investigation of prepulse inhibition of startle and prepulse elicited reactions in Wistar rats. *Pharmacol. Biochem. Behav.*, 99: 22–28.

Campbell, L.E., Hughes, M., Budd, T.W., Cooper, G., Fulham, W.R., Karayanidis, F., Hanlon, M.C., Stojanov, W., Johnston, P., Case, V. and Schall, U. (2007) Primary and secondary neural networks of auditory prepulse inhibition: a functional magnetic resonance imaging study of sensorimotor gating of human acoustic startle response. *Eur. J. Neurosci.*, 26: 2327–2333.

Csomor, P.A., Vollenweider, F.X., Feldon, J. and Yee, B.K. (2005) On the feasibility to detect and to quantify prepulse-elicited reaction in prepulse inhibition of the acoustic startle reflex in humans. *Behav. Brain Res.*, 162: 256–263.

Dias, E.C., Butler, P.D., Hoptman, M.J. and Javitt, D.C. (2011) Early sensory contributions to contextual encoding deficits in schizophrenia. *Arch. Gen. Psychiatry*, 68: 654–664.

Dieckmann, M., Freudenberg, F., Klein, S., Koch, M. and Schwabe, K. (2007) Disturbed social behavior and motivation in rats selectively bred for deficient sensorimotor gating. *Schizophr. Res.*, 97: 250–253.

Fendt, M., Li, L. and Yeomans, J.S. (2001) Brain stem circuits mediating prepulse inhibition of the startle reflex. *Psychopharmacology*, 156: 216–224.

Filion, D.L., Kelly, K.A. and Hazlett, E.A. (1999) Behavioral analogies of short lead interval startle inhibition. In: M.E. Dawson, A.M. Schell and A.H. Böhmelt (Eds.), *Startle Modification: Implications for Neuroscience, Cognitive Science, and Clinical Science*. Cambridge University Press, Cambridge, MA, pp. 269–283.

Ford, J. and Roth, W. (1999) Event-related potential components and startle. In: M.E. Dawson, A.M. Schell and A.H. Böhmelt (Eds.), *Startle Modification: Implications for Neuroscience, Cognitive Science and Clinical Science*. Cambridge University Press, Cambridge, MA, pp. 284–299.

Ford, J.M., Roth, W.T., Menon, V. and Pfefferbaum, A. (1999) Failures of automatic and strategic processing in schizophrenia: comparisons of event-related brain potential and startle blink modification. *Schizophr. Res.*, 37: 149–163.

Freudenberg, F., Dieckmann, M., Winter, S., Koch, M. and Schwabe, K. (2007) Selective breeding for deficient sensorimotor gating is accompanied by increased perseveration in rats. *Neuroscience*, 148: 612–622.

Geyer, M.A., Krebs-Thomson, K., Braff, D.L. and Swerdlow, N.R. (2001) Pharmacological studies of prepulse inhibition models of sensorimotor gating deficits in schizophrenia: a decade in review. *Psychopharmacology*, 156: 117–154.

Giakoumaki, S.G., Bitsios, P. and Frangou, S. (2006) The level of prepulse inhibition in healthy individuals may index cortical modulation of early information processing. *Brain Res.*, 1078: 168–170.

Gottesman, I.I. and Gould, T.D. (2003) The endophenotype concept in psychiatry: etymology and strategic intentions. *Am. J. Psychiatry*, 160: 636–645.

Graham, F.K., Putnam, L.E. and Leavitt, L.A. (1975) Lead-stimulation effects on human cardiac orienting and blink reflexes. *J. Exp. Psychol. Hum. Percept. Perform.*, 104: 161–169.

Hadamitzky, M., Harich, S., Koch, M. and Schwabe, K. (2007) Deficient prepulse inhibition induced by selective breeding of rats can be restored by the dopamine D2 antagonist haloperidol. *Behav. Brain Res.*, 177: 364–367.

Haig, A.R., Gordon, E., De Pascalis, V., Meares, R.A., Bahramali, H. and Harris, A. (2000) Gamma activity in schizophrenia: evidence of impaired network binding. *Clin. Neurophysiol.*, 111: 1461–1468.

Harrison, P.J. (1999) The neuropathology of schizophrenia. A critical review of the data and their interpretation. *Brain*, 122: 593–624.

Herrmann, C.S. and Demiralp, T. (2005) Human EEG gamma oscillations in neuropsychiatric disorders. *Clin. Neurophysiol.*, 116: 2719–2733.

Holstein, D.H., Csomor, P.A., Geyer, M.A., Huber, T., Brugger, N., Studerus, E. and Vollenweider, F.X. (2011) The effects of sertindole on sensory gating, sensorimotor gating, and cognition in healthy volunteers. *J. Psychopharmacol.*, 25: 1600–1613.

Ison, J.R. and Hammond, G.R. (1971) Modification of the startle reflex in the rat by changes in the auditory and visual environments. *J. Comp. Psychol.*, 75: 435–452.

Kedzior, K.K., Koch, M. and Başar-Eroğlu, C. (2006) Prepulse inhibition (PPI) of auditory startle reflex is associated with PPI of auditory-evoked theta oscillations in healthy humans. *Neurosci. Lett.*, 400: 246–251.

Kedzior, K.K., Koch, M. and Başar-Eroğlu, C. (2007) Auditory-evoked EEG oscillations associated with prepulse inhibition (PPI) of auditory startle reflex in healthy humans. *Brain Res.*, 1163: 111–118.

Klein, S., Koch, M. and Schwabe, K. (2008) Neuroanatomical changes in the adult rat brain after neonatal lesion of the medial prefrontal cortex. *Exp. Neurol.*, 209: 199–212.

Koch, M. (1998) How can adaptive behavioural plasticity be implemented in the mammalian brain? *Z. Naturforsch.*, 53c: 593–598.

Koch, M. (1999) The neurobiology of startle. *Prog. Neurobiol.*, 59: 107–128.

Koch, M. (2006) Animal models of schizophrenia. In: M. Koch (Ed.), *Animal Models of Neuropsychiatric Diseases*, Imperial College Press, London, pp. 227–402.

Lee, K.H., Williams, L.M., Breakspear, M. and Gordon, E. (2003) Synchronous gamma activity: a review and contribution to an integrative neuroscience model of schizophrenia. *Brain Res. Rev.*, 41: 57–78.

Lewis, D.A., Hashimoto, T. and Volk, D.W. (2005) Cortical inhibitory neurons and schizophrenia. *Nat. Rev. Neurosci.*, 6: 312–324.

Lipska, B.K. (2004) Using animal models to test a neurodevelopmental hypothesis of schizophrenia. *J. Psychiatry Neurosci.*, 29: 282–286.

Lipska, B.K., Lerman, D.N., Khaing, Z.Z. and Weinberger, D.R. (2003) The neonatal ventral hippocampal lesion model of schizophrenia: effects on dopamine and GABA mRNA markers in the rat midbrain. *Eur. J. Neurosci.*, 18: 3097–3104.

Mathes, B., Wood, S.J., Proffitt, T.M., Stuart, G.W., Buchanan, J.M., Velakoulis, D., Brewer, W.J., McGorry, P.D. and Pantelis, C. (2005) Early processing deficits in object working memory in first-episode schizophreniform psychosis and established schizophrenia. *Psychol. Med.*, 35: 1053–1062.

Polich, J. (2007) Updating P300: an integrative theory of P3a and P3b. *Clin. Neurophysiol.*, 118: 2128–2148.

Roussos, P., Giakoumaki, S.G., Adamaki, E., Anastasios, G., Nikos, R.K. and Bitsios, P. (2011) The association of schizophrenia risk D-amino acid oxydase polymorphisms with sensorimotor gating, working memory and personality in healthy males. *Neuropsychopharmacology*, 36: 1677–1688.

Schall, U., Schön, A., Zerbin, D., Bender, S., Eggers, C. and Oades, R.D. (1997) A left temporal lobe impairment of auditory information processing in schizophrenia: an event-related potential study. *Neurosci. Lett.*, 229: 25–28.

Schneider, M. and Koch, M. (2005) Behavioral and morphological alterations following neonatal excitotoxic lesions of the medial prefrontal cortex in rats. *Exp. Neurol.*, 195: 185–198.

Schwabe, K., Freudenberg, F. and Koch, M. (2007) Selective breeding of reduced sensorimotor gating in Wistar rats. *Behav. Genet.*, 37: 706–712.

Sohal, V.S., Zhang, F., Yizhar, O. and Deisseroth, K. (2009) Parvalbumin neurons and gamma rhythms enhance cortical circuit performance. *Nature (London)*, 459: 698–702.

Spencer, K.M., Nestor, P.G., Perlmutter, R., Niznikiewicz, M.A., Klump, M.C., Frumin, M., Shenton, M.E. and McCarley, R.W. (2004) Neural synchrony indexes disordered perception and cognition in schizophrenia. *Proc. Natl. Acad. Sci. USA*, 101: 17288–17293.

Swerdlow, N.R., Light, G.A., Cadenhead, K.S., Sprock, J., Hsieh, M.H. and Braff, D.L. (2006a) Startle gating deficits in a large cohort of patients with schizophrenia. *Arch. Gen. Psychiatry*, 63: 1325–1335.

Swerdlow, N.R., Talledo, J., Sutherland, A.N., Nagy, G. and Shoemaker, J.M. (2006b) Antipschotic effects on prepulse inhibition in normal 'low gating' humans and rats. *Neuropsychopharmacology*, 31: 2011–2021.

Uhlhaas, P.J. and Singer, W. (2010) Abnormal neural oscillations and synchrony in schizophrenia. *Nat. Rev. Neurosci.*, 11: 100–113.

Van den Buuse, M., Garner, B. and Koch, M. (2003) Neurodevelopmental animal models of schizophrenia: effects on prepulse inhibition. *Curr. Mol. Med.*, 3: 459–471.

Vollenweider, F.X., Barro, M., Csomor, P.A. and Feldon, J. (2006) Clozapine enhances prepulse inhibition in healthy humans with low but not with high prepulse inhibition levels. *Biol. Psychiatry*, 60: 597–603.

Weike, A.I., Bauer, U. and Hamm, A.O. (2000) Effective neuroleptic medication removes prepulse inhibition deficits in schizophrenia patients. *Biol. Psychiatry*, 47: 61–70.

Weinberger, D.R. (1995) Schizophrenia as a neurodevelopmental disorder. In: S.R. Hirsch and D.R. Weinberger (Eds.), *Schizophrenia*. Blackwell Science, Oxford, pp. 293–323.

Wynn, J.K., Dawson, M.E. and Schell, A.M. (2004) The functional relationship between visual backward masking and prepulse inhibition. *Psychophysiology*, 41: 306–312.

Wynn, J.K., Light, G.A., Breitmeyer, B., Nuechterlein, K.H. and Green, M.F. (2005) Event-related gamma activity in schizophrenia patients during a visual backward-masking task. *Am. J. Psychiatry*, 162: 2330–2336.

Yee, B.K. and Feldon, J. (2009) Distinct forms of prepulse inhibition disruption distinguishable by the associated changes in prepulse-elicited reaction. *Behav. Brain Res.*, 204: 387–395.

Chapter 8

Auditory-evoked alpha oscillations imply reduced anterior and increased posterior amplitudes in schizophrenia

Canan Başar-Eroğlu*, Christina Schmiedt-Fehr and Birgit Mathes

Institute of Psychology and Cognition Research, University of Bremen, D-28359 Bremen, Germany

ABSTRACT

Objective: Most of the work on disturbed oscillatory activity during auditory tasks in schizophrenia has focused on reduced gamma oscillations at fronto-central sites. Recent studies of our group, however, indicate a more general disturbance affecting the spatial distribution of oscillatory brain activity of gamma as well as slow frequencies, such as alpha oscillations.
Methods: During a passive auditory listening task, electroencephalography was recorded from healthy controls and patients with schizophrenia. Stimulus-locked alpha activity within the first 250 ms after stimulus onset was analyzed from midline electrodes.
Results: Healthy controls showed the common fronto-central maximum of the early alpha response, while patients with schizophrenia showed lower fronto-central and larger parieto-occipital alpha activity than controls, leading to a more similar amplitude distribution across the midline electrode sites.
Conclusions: The present results indicate malfunctioning long-range inhibition of task-irrelevant cortical areas in schizophrenia, which may disturb functional integration of perception and attention. We emphasize the importance of the whole-brain network theory for the understanding of schizophrenia since it proposes that integrative brain function is based on the coexistence and cooperative action of many interwoven and interacting sub-mechanisms.
Significance: Neuropsychiatric illnesses such as schizophrenia are marked by communication and coordination failures between different brain regions and different frequency bands.

KEYWORDS

Schizophrenia; EEG; Alpha oscillation; Auditory evoked potential

8.1. Introduction

8.1.1. Abnormal neural synchronization in schizophrenia

Brain oscillatory activity in schizophrenia, as measured by electroencephalography (EEG), indicates

---
Correspondence to: Dr. Canan Başar-Eroğlu, Ph.D., Institute of Psychology and Cognition Research, University of Bremen, Grazer Str. 4, D-28359 Bremen, Germany.
Tel.: +49 (0)421-218 68700; Fax: +49 (0)421-218 68719; E-mail: cbasar@uni-bremen.de

abnormal temporal integration and interregional connectivity of brain networks as a core disturbance (for reviews see Lee et al., 2003; Ford et al., 2007; Başar and Güntekin, 2008; Uhlhaas and Singer, 2010). It is suggested that such integrative brain functions are obtained through multiple oscillatory processes in different frequency bands and are a necessity for temporal coherence of perceptions and actions (Başar et al., 2001; Başar, 2006, 2011).

Most of the work on disturbed oscillatory activity in schizophrenia has focused on gamma oscillations. Mainly reduced synchrony or magnitude of gamma responses in schizophrenia is reported (e.g., Haig et al., 2000; Lee et al., 2003; Spencer et al., 2003, 2004, 2008; Herrmann and Demiralp, 2005). This finding is suggested to reflect a disturbance in coordinated activity within local neuronal circuits in sensory cortex, which is, however, essential for both perception and subsequent higher order cognition (see also Leavitt et al., 2007; Javitt, 2009). However, not all studies find reduced early gamma responses related to sensory processing (Blumenfeld and Clementz, 2001; Brockhaus-Dumke et al., 2008; Brenner et al., 2009; Başar-Eroğlu et al., 2011).

8.1.2. Abnormal neural synchrony related to auditory sensory processing

Studies on auditory processing remain somewhat inconsistent due to differences in methodological approaches and disease characteristics between studies. Some studies indicate that auditory gamma oscillations during continuous performance or target detection may be more thoroughly affected while processing targets when compared to non-targets (Gallinat et al., 2004; Spencer et al., 2008), whereas others find disturbances in gamma oscillations for non-targets (Haig et al., 2000; Leicht et al., 2010) or even for both when looking at single trial instead of averaged gamma responses (Başar-Eroğlu et al., 2009). Our recent study on auditory gamma responses indicates abnormal topographical distribution of gamma oscillations in schizophrenia, i.e., an increased occipital gamma response after auditory stimuli in patients with schizophrenia (Başar-Eroğlu et al., 2011). This could be related to changes in spatial integration mechanisms.

However, changes in oscillatory brain activity in patients with schizophrenia are multifold and can be reflected in multiple frequency bands (e.g., Herrmann and Demiralp, 2005; Schmiedt et al., 2005; Başar-Eroğlu et al., 2007, 2009, 2011; Uhlhaas et al., 2008; Ramos-Loyo et al., 2009; Haenschel et al., 2010), including delta ($\sim$0.5–4 Hz), theta ($\sim$4–7 Hz), alpha ($\sim$8–15 Hz),

beta ($\sim$15–30 Hz), and gamma ($\sim$30–80 Hz) oscillations. Our previous studies on visual and auditory modalities specifically indicate a disturbance in the temporal integration and spatial distribution of all frequency components (Schmiedt et al., 2005; Başar-Eroğlu et al., 2007, 2008, 2009; Ergen et al., 2008).

Increases of the alpha response in the time range up to 250-ms poststimulus have been implicated to reflect integrity of sensory and preparatory phases of cognitive processing (Başar et al., 1997; Dinse et al., 1997; Schürmann et al., 1997, 2000; Schürmann and Başar, 2001; Klimesch et al., 2004). Hence, investigations of alpha activity are especially important to understand disturbed sensory processing in schizophrenia (e.g., Başar-Eroğlu et al., 2008; Haenschel et al., 2010). Supporting this assumption, we found that during an auditory oddball task early stimulus-locked alpha activity in patients was reduced at fronto-central leads for non-targets but not for targets (Başar-Eroğlu et al., 2009).

However, given that in oddball tasks non-targets are randomly intermixed with targets, auditory stimuli in these tasks are processed with more attentional load than auditory stimuli in a passive listening context. Thus, investigation of low cognitive demand context could help to understand the occurrence and meaning of altered auditory alpha oscillations.

8.1.3. Present study

Given that schizophrenia is characterized by multiple impairments, it is surprising that studies on lower frequency bands have been little acknowledged and main attention is presently paid to gamma oscillations. The present study complements our previous work and focuses on topographical changes in stimulus-locked auditory alpha oscillations related to early auditory stimulus processing during low cognitive demand. The auditory stimuli and stimulus presentation sequence were matched to our previous auditory oddball study to allow a more direct comparison of the results and estimation of cognitive demand effects (Başar-Eroğlu et al., 2009). Averaged responses in the time window 0–250-ms post-stimulus were evaluated to analyze general group differences in amplitude and midline amplitude distribution.

8.2. Methods

8.2.1. Participants

A total of 9 in-patients (two females, mean age: 35.6 ± 9.8 years) and 10 healthy controls (5 females, mean age: 31.8 ± 4.1 years) gave informed consent and participated in the study. All patients were interviewed using a structured diagnostic interview and were required to meet DSM-IV criteria for schizophrenia (American Psychiatric Association, 1994). Mean illness duration was 8 years. All patients were recruited as in-patients after clinical stabilization of an acute psychotic episode. Four patients received atypical medication at the time of assessment (clozapine, olanzapine, risperidone, and aripiprazol); four patients received typical medication (mainly fluxpentixol). Medication for one patient is unknown. Exclusion criteria for patients and controls were a history of substance abuse in the past 6 months, known history of learning difficulties, evidence of head trauma with loss of consciousness, or disease of the central nervous system other than schizophrenia. All participants, except one patient, were right-handed and all had normal or corrected-to-normal vision.

8.2.2. Procedure

Passive auditory processing was investigated using sinusoidal tone stimuli with different durations and frequencies. Subjects were instructed to passively listen to a tone series presented one at a time over loudspeakers. All tones were presented at an intensity of 80 dB SPL. To ensure comparability with our previous auditory oddball study, the same tones and tone sequence were used in this study (Başar-Eroğlu et al., 2009): two tones — 1400 and 1480 Hz, respectively — were presented in pseudo-randomized sequence with a stimulus duration of either 100 or 300 ms. Each of the four stimulus types occurred with equal probability. The interstimulus interval was 1000 ms, with a total of 100 trials.

8.2.3. EEG recording, processing, and data analysis

EEG activity was recorded during the task in a dimly lit, soundproof, and electromagnetically shielded room using Ag–AgCl electrodes at Fz, Cz, Pz, Oz locations, with linked earlobes as reference. EEG was recorded at 1000 Hz, with band limits of 0.5–70 Hz by means of a Nihon Kohden electroencephalograph (Model EEG-4421 G), and a 50-Hz notch filter (36 dB/octave) was applied. EOG was recorded from electrodes placed above and to the right of the right eye and epochs contaminated by eye or other artifacts were manually rejected offline. The EEG data were processed in 1-s long epochs (250-ms prestimulus/750-ms post-stimulus). The number of artifact-free epochs included in the analysis was kept comparable between groups (mean for patients: 62.7 ± 19.3; mean for healthy controls: 65.6 ± 13.7).

The data were digitally filtered in the alpha range (8–13 Hz) using Fast Fourier Transformation (FFT). Digital filtering produces visual displays of time courses of oscillatory components within the frequency limits of the utilized filters. The digital filters are advantageous because they do not produce phase shifts characteristic for electronic filters. The filtered and averaged data were used to estimate maximum peak-to-peak poststimulus amplitudes for each electrode position and subject within the first 250 ms after stimulus onset. The time windows were selected after inspection of the filtered single subject and group grand averages (see Fig. 1).

124

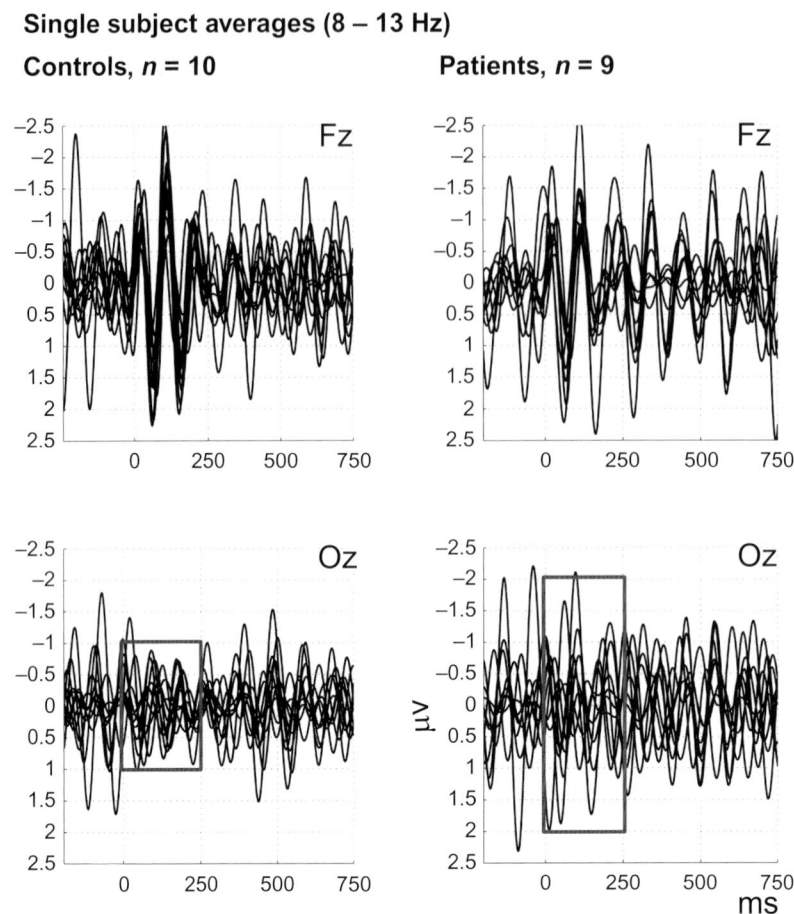

Single subject averages (8 – 13 Hz)

Controls, *n* = 10 **Patients, *n* = 9**

Fig. 1.   Superimposed single subject averages of event-related alpha oscillations in controls (left) and patients with schizophrenia (right) at frontal (top) and occipital (bottom) electrode positions elicited during passive auditory processing. Zero indicates stimulus onset. Note that alpha oscillations for controls have a frontal maximum. Note that for healthy controls the alpha activity at occipital locations tended to decrease after stimulus onset (similar to alpha blocking). This stimulus-induced alteration cannot be observed in patients.

8.2.4. Statistical analysis

The averaged poststimulus alpha response was analyzed using a mixed design repeated measures analysis of variance using two groups (patients vs. controls) × four electrode locations (Fz, Cz, Pz, Oz). Huynh–Feldt corrections were applied to the degrees of freedom where needed, with the corrected probabilities reported. For post hoc comparisons by *t* tests, *p* values are corrected using the Sidak procedure.

8.3. Results

Fig. 1 presents superimposed single subject averages of event-related alpha oscillations in controls (left) and patients with schizophrenia (right) at frontal (top) and occipital (bottom) electrode positions elicited during passive auditory processing. It can be seen that alpha oscillations have a frontal maximum for controls only. In patients, the alpha response appears to be more similar between Fz and Oz. Phase locking between participants is restricted to anterior electrode positions for both groups. For healthy controls, the alpha activity at occipital locations tended to decrease after stimulus onset (similar to alpha blocking). This stimulus-induced alteration was not observed in patients.

Fig. 2 presents the maximum peak-to-peak alpha amplitude for all midline electrodes between 0 and 250 ms following stimulus onset. The amplitudes in patients were more similar across all measured midline sites than in healthy controls.

The statistical analysis of the maximum peak-to-peak alpha amplitude revealed a fronto-central maximum (F (3, 51) $= 27.1, p < 0.001$). Post hoc comparisons confirmed larger amplitudes at fronto-central than parieto-occipital and at parietal than occipital locations (Fz $=$ Cz $>$ Pz $>$ Oz, $p < 0.05$ for all post hoc comparisons). In accordance with the observations described above for Figs. 1 and 2, the significant interaction between electrode $\times$ group (F (3, 51) $= 3.3$, $p < 0.05$) indicated that this topographic pattern occurred only for the healthy controls (Fz $=$ Cz $>$ Pz $>$ Oz, $p < 0.05$ for all post hoc comparisons for controls only).

8.4. Discussion

This study examined the amplitude distribution of early stimulus-locked auditory alpha oscillations evoked by frequently occurring tones in a passive listening task. The early auditory alpha band response is suggested to reflect mechanisms of sensory processing of auditory stimuli (e.g., Başar and Schürmann, 1994) and in general alpha oscillations are thought to indicate integrity of inter-areal interactions (e.g., Von Stein and Sarnthein, 2000). In our previous studies, we found that altered topographical distribution of oscillatory activity in schizophrenia was present for visual alpha responses (Başar-Eroğlu et al., 2008) and for auditory gamma responses (Başar-Eroğlu et al., 2011) in both passive sensory tasks and oddball tasks. The current study on auditory alpha is consistent with these findings: While healthy controls showed a clear fronto-central distribution of alpha responses, the amplitudes in patients were less distinctly distributed with similar amplitudes across the midline sites.

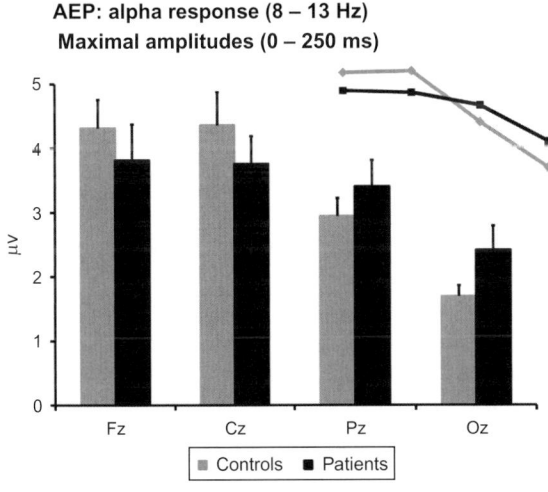

AEP: alpha response (8 – 13 Hz)
Maximal amplitudes (0 – 250 ms)

Fig. 2. Maximum amplitudes of alpha oscillations within the first 250 ms after stimulus onset averaged over single subjects. Error bars represent the standard error. Note that the maximum alpha amplitude in controls drops between anterior (Fz, Cz) and posterior electrode positions (Pz, Oz) while the maximum amplitudes in patients with schizophrenia were more similar across the entire scalp (as schematically illustrated in the right-hand corner).

8.4.1. Alpha response to auditory stimuli in the healthy brain

Oscillatory activity is thought to control the timing of neuronal discharges and provide a mechanism for precise temporal resolution for the encoding of information (for review see e.g., Uhlhaas and Singer, 2010). Synchronous oscillatory activity is thought to be a mechanism to increase the salience of signals, to facilitate their transmission across different networks, and to ensure selective routing. There is a growing consensus that in the healthy brain stimulus-locked alpha oscillations in the first 250-ms poststimulus are related to the early ERP components in visual, auditory, and somatosensory modalities (e.g., Jansen and Brandt, 1991; Başar, 1997; Başar et al., 1997; Makeig et al., 2002; Klimesch et al., 2004; Palva et al., 2005; Haenschel et al., 2010). Early ERP components in healthy participants in the auditory domain are, thereby, maximal at fronto-central electrode sites (e.g., Freedman et al., 1987). Functionally, the early stimulus-locked alpha response is suggested to index integrity of sensory processing and the degree of conscious attention paid to the stimuli (for review see Başar et al., 1997). The amplitude of alpha activity has been shown to be larger when participants devote greater attention to a visual stimulus (e.g., Herrmann et al., 2004) or consciously perceive somatosensory stimulation (e.g., Palva et al., 2005). Thus, the stimulus-locked alpha response in the present study, which is largest at fronto-central sites in controls, is most probably functionally linked to efficient neuronal mechanisms underlying behavioral phenomena, such as attention and sensory awareness (Başar and Schürmann, 1994; Başar et al., 1997; Schürmann and Başar, 2001; Palva and Palva, 2007).

8.4.2. Alpha response to auditory stimuli in patients with schizophrenia

The less distinct alpha response distribution in patients with schizophrenia has two main implications: First, compared to the healthy controls, the patients in this study showed a less prominent anterior alpha response, which most probably indicates less efficient processing of the external auditory input as suggested by the alpha studies presented above (see Section 8.4.1). This finding is in line with our previous auditory oddball study showing reduced alpha responses for non-targets (Başar-Eroğlu et al., 2009), as well as with a wide range of other studies suggesting deficits throughout the auditory cortex (e.g., Rojas et al., 2002; Whitford et al., 2005) and at both early and late

levels of auditory processing in schizophrenia (Freedman et al., 1987; Ford et al., 2001; Lee et al., 2003; Bramon et al., 2004; O'Donnell et al., 2004; Spencer et al., 2004; Whitford et al., 2005; Javitt, 2009; Leicht et al., 2010; Salisbury et al., 2010).

Second, patients with schizophrenia showed a less distinct distribution of alpha oscillations with larger alpha amplitudes at occipital sites. Slow oscillations, including alpha, have been suggested to play an important role for long-range information transfer in brain (Von Stein and Sarnthein, 2000). Given that communication and coordination failures between different brain regions have been suggested to account for a wide range of problems in schizophrenia (Ford et al., 2007; Uhlhaas et al., 2008), it can be speculated that the present alpha results can be linked to malfunctioning long-range inhibition of task-irrelevant cortical areas. The determinants of increased alpha activity in a passive listening task at posterior regions in patients with schizophrenia need further evaluation. For instance, such a finding was not given during active detection of acoustic targets, which implies a possible modification of this finding by cognitive demand or task context (Bernstein et al., 1985; Başar-Eroğlu et al., 2009). Furthermore, in a recent study on auditory gamma oscillations, we found that schizophrenia was related to larger occipital gamma oscillations (Başar-Eroğlu et al., 2011), which is similar to the alpha findings presented in this study.

In our earlier study, we found no alterations of the alpha response during auditory target detection and, therefore, assumed that the alterations for non-targets might be related to sensory processes (Başar-Eroğlu et al., 2009). The results of the current study, which uses a simple passive listening task with comparable stimuli and stimuli sequences, support this assumption. Attention toward the target might lead at least to a partial compensation of the early alpha response, possibly underlying similar mechanisms as described by Herrmann et al. (2004). Attentional compensation might not occur for the concurrent and subsequent delta, theta and gamma responses, indicating that the transmission of sensory stimuli in cognitive processing remains disturbed (Schürmann et al., 1995; Başar-Eroğlu et al., 2009). The wealth of studies on altered gamma and the fewer studies on slow oscillations in schizophrenia mentioned in Section 8.1 may reflect interrelated mechanisms. For example, long-distance coordination of gamma oscillations is currently proposed to be influenced by alpha oscillations. In a recent study by White et al. (2010) altered correlation of alpha and evoked gamma oscillations in schizophrenia during perception of sensory stimuli was reported. Using a joint independent component analysis on EEG and functional magnetic resonance imaging data, they found that in healthy individuals the strongest component was dominated by alpha oscillations and was associated not only with activity in somatosensory regions but also in the insula and anterior cingulate cortex. Whereas, in patients with schizophrenia, the strongest component had low alpha power and activity was limited mainly to somatosensory regions. Moreover, in the healthy participants, but not the patients, significant correlation was given between the strongest component and stimulus-locked gamma power. The authors hypothesize that gamma localized to sensory cortex elicits stimulus locking of spatially distinct, large-scale ongoing alpha oscillations. White et al. (2010) link their results to a salience network, including insula and anterior cingulate cortex, which is believed to play a role in directing brain processing resources from internally generated mental activity to the processing of sensory input to alpha oscillations (e.g., Sridharan et al., 2008), and which appears to be dysfunctional in schizophrenia.

Taken together, the present results are in line with accumulating evidence of dysfunctional synchronization of slow frequencies that are assumed to reflect disturbances of functional integration of perception and attention in schizophrenia (Jansen and Brandt, 1991; Röschke et al., 1996; Schmiedt et al., 2005; Başar-Eroğlu et al., 2008; Ergen et al., 2008; Haenschel et al., 2010). Our study shows that sensory processing in schizophrenia is not only related to reductions of amplitude and abnormalities in higher frequencies.

8.4.3. Limitations of the study

The study has some limitations common to studies of schizophrenia. Patients were taking various antipsychotic medications in different dosages. Therefore, we cannot rule out the effects of medication. However, many studies reported that the cognitive deficits are attributable to schizophrenia itself rather than medication (e.g., Goldberg et al., 1993; Gallinat et al., 2004). We should also emphasize here that our results are based on patients with dominant negative symptoms. Furthermore, it should be noted that the presented results must be considered preliminary as the number of patients is very limited.

8.5. Conclusion

The present alpha results in schizophrenia indicate a combination of both a deficient mechanism related to sensory processing (i.e., reduced anterior response) and a deficient mechanism engaging long-range inhibition of task-irrelevant cortical areas (i.e., larger alpha amplitudes at occipital sites). Future understanding of neuropsychiatric illnesses might profit when not restricting the analysis to single frequency bands or isolated brain regions. Based on our results, we emphasize the importance of the whole-brain network theory (Başar, 2006, 2011), which proposes that integrative brain function is based on the coexistence and cooperative action of many interwoven and interacting sub-mechanisms. We tentatively conclude that all of our recent studies on schizophrenia indicate a malfunction of such a coexistence and cooperative action with deficits being reflected in alterations in multiple frequency bands.

128

Acknowledgments

We thank Dr. Andreas Brand, M.D., and Prof. Dr. Jörg Zimmermann, M.D., for clinical assessment of the patients as well as Edwin Hoff and Claudia Schieber for data recording.

The authors report no biomedical financial interests or potential conflicts of interest.

References

American Psychiatric Association (1994) *Diagnostic and Statistical Manual of Mental Disorders IV from the American Psychiatric Association.* American Psychiatric Press, New York.

Başar, E. (1997) Functional correlates of alpha's panel discussion of the conference 'Alpha Processes in the Brain'. *Int. J. Psychophysiol.*, 26: 455–474.

Başar, E. (2006) The theory of the whole-brain work. *Int. J. Psychophysiol.*, 60: 133–138.

Başar, E. (2011) *Brain–Body–Mind in the Nebulous Cartesian System: A Holistic Approach by Oscillations.* Springer, New York.

Başar, E. and Güntekin, B. (2008) A review of brain oscillations in cognitive disorders and the role of neurotransmitters. *Brain Res.*, 1235: 172–193.

Başar, E. and Schürmann, M. (1994) Functional aspects of evoked alpha and theta responses in humans and cats. Occipital recordings in "cross modality" experiments. *Biol. Cybern.*, 72: 175–183.

Başar, E., Schürmann, M., Başar-Eroğlu, C. and Karakas, S. (1997) Alpha oscillations in brain functioning: an integrative theory. *Int. J. Psychophysiol.*, 26: 5–29.

Başar, E., Başar-Eroğlu, C., Karakas, S. and Schürmann, M. (2001) Gamma, alpha, delta, and theta oscillations govern cognitive processes. *Int. J. Psychophysiol.*, 39: 241–248.

Başar-Eroğlu, C., Brand, A., Hildebrandt, H., Karolina Kedzior, K., Mathes, B. and Schmiedt, C. (2007) Working memory related gamma oscillations in schizophrenia patients. *Int. J. Psychophysiol.*, 64: 39–45.

Başar-Eroğlu, C., Schmiedt-Fehr, C., Marbach, S., Brand, A. and Mathes, B. (2008) Altered oscillatory alpha and theta networks in schizophrenia. *Brain Res.*, 1235: 143–152.

Başar-Eroğlu, C., Schmiedt-Fehr, C., Mathes, B., Zimmermann, J. and Brand, A. (2009) Are oscillatory brain responses generally reduced in schizophrenia during long sustained attentional processing? *Int. J. Psychophysiol.*, 71: 75–83.

Başar-Eroğlu, C., Mathes, B., Brand, A. and Schmiedt-Fehr, C. (2011) Occipital gamma response to auditory stimulation in patients with schizophrenia. *Int. J. Psychophysiol.*, 79: 3–8.

Bernstein, A.S., Riedel, J.A., Pava, J., Schnur, D. and Lubowsky, J. (1985) A limiting factor in the "normalization" of schizophrenic orienting response dysfunction. *Schizophr. Bull.*, 11: 230–254.

Blumenfeld, L.D. and Clementz, B.A. (2001) Response to the first stimulus determines reduced auditory evoked response suppression in schizophrenia: single trial analysis using MEG. *Clin. Neurophysiol.*, 112: 1650–1659.

Bramon, E., Rabe-Hesketh, S., Sham, P., Murray, R.M. and Frangou, S. (2004) Meta-analysis of the P300 and P50 waveforms in schizophrenia. *Schizophr. Res.*, 70: 315–329.

Brenner, C.A., Kieffaber, P.D., Clementz, B.A., Johannesen, J.K., Shekhar, A., O'Donnell, B.F. and Hetrick, W.P. (2009) Event-related potential abnormalities in schizophrenia: a failure to "gate in" salient information? *Schizophr. Res.*, 113: 332–338.

Brockhaus-Dumke, A., Mueller, R., Faigle, U. and Klosterkoetter, J. (2008) Sensory gating revisited: relation between brain oscillations and auditory evoked potentials in schizophrenia. *Schizophr. Res.*, 99: 238–249.

Dinse, H.R., Kruger, K., Akhavan, A.C., Spengler, F., Schoner, G. and Schreiner, C.E. (1997) Low-frequency oscillations of visual, auditory and somatosensory cortical neurons evoked by sensory stimulation. *Int. J. Psychophysiol.*, 26: 205–227.

Ergen, M., Marbach, S., Brand, A., Başar-Eroğlu, C. and Demiralp, T. (2008) P3 and delta band responses in visual oddball paradigm in schizophrenia. *Neurosci. Lett.*, 440: 304–308.

Ford, J.M., Mathalon, D.H., Kalba, S., Marsh, L. and Pfefferbaum, A. (2001) N1 and P300 abnormalities in patients with schizophrenia, epilepsy, and epilepsy with schizophrenia-like features. *Biol. Psychiatry*, 49: 848–860.

Ford, J.M., Krystal, J.H. and Mathalon, D.H. (2007) Neural synchrony in schizophrenia: from networks to new treatments. *Schizophr. Bull.*, 33: 848–852.

Freedman, R., Adler, L.E., Gerhardt, G.A., Waldo, M., Baker, N., Rose, G.M., Drebing, C., Nagamoto, H., Bickford-Wimer, P. and Franks, R. (1987) Neurobiological studies of sensory gating in schizophrenia. *Schizophr. Bull.*, 13: 669–678.

Gallinat, J., Winterer, G., Herrmann, C.S. and Senkowski, D. (2004) Reduced oscillatory gamma-band responses in unmedicated schizophrenic patients indicate impaired frontal network processing. *Clin. Neurophysiol.*, 115: 1863–1874.

Goldberg, T.E., Greenberg, R.D., Griffin, S.J., Gold, J.M., Kleinman, J.E., Pickar, D., Schulz, S.C. and Weinberger, D.R. (1993) The effect of clozapine on cognition and psychiatric symptoms in patients with schizophrenia. *Br. J. Psychiatry*, 162: 43–48.

Haenschel, C., Linden, D.E., Bittner, R.A., Singer, W. and Hanslmayr, S. (2010) Alpha phase locking predicts residual working memory performance in schizophrenia. *Biol. Psychiatry*, 68: 595–598.

Haig, A.R., Gordon, E., De Pascalis, V., Meares, R.A., Bahramali, H. and Harris, A. (2000) Gamma activity in schizophrenia: evidence of impaired network binding? *Clin. Neurophysiol.*, 111: 1461–1468.

Herrmann, C.S. and Demiralp, T. (2005) Human EEG gamma oscillations in neuropsychiatric disorders. *Clin. Neurophysiol.*, 116: 2719–2733.

Herrmann, C.S., Senkowski, D. and Rottger, S. (2004) Phase-locking and amplitude modulations of EEG alpha: two measures reflect different cognitive processes in a working memory task. *Exp. Psychol.*, 51: 311–318.

Jansen, B.H. and Brandt, M.E. (1991) The effect of the phase of prestimulus alpha activity on the averaged visual evoked response. *Electroenceph. Clin. Neurophysiol.*, 80: 241–250.

Javitt, D.C. (2009) When doors of perception close: bottom-up models of disrupted cognition in schizophrenia. *Annu. Rev. Clin. Psychol.*, 5: 249–275.

Klimesch, W., Schack, B., Schabus, M., Doppelmayr, M., Gruber, W. and Sauseng, P. (2004) Phase-locked alpha and theta oscillations generate the P1–N1 complex and are related to memory performance. *Cogn. Brain Res.*, 19: 302–316.

Leavitt, V.M., Molholm, S., Ritter, W., Shpaner, M. and Foxe, J.J. (2007) Auditory processing in schizophrenia during the middle latency period (10–50 ms): high-density electrical mapping and source analysis reveal subcortical antecedents to early cortical deficits. *J. Psychiatry Neurosci.*, 32: 339–353.

Lee, K.H., Williams, L.M., Breakspear, M. and Gordon, E. (2003) Synchronous gamma activity: a review and contribution to an integrative neuroscience model of schizophrenia. *Brain Res. Rev.*, 41: 57–78.

Leicht, G., Kirsch, V., Giegling, I., Karch, S., Hantschk, I., Möller, H.J., Pogarell, O., Hegerl, U., Rujescu, D. and Mulert, C. (2010) Reduced early auditory evoked gamma-band response in patients with schizophrenia. *Biol. Psychiatry*, 67: 224–231.

Makeig, S., Westerfield, M., Jung, T.P., Enghoff, S., Townsend, J., Courchesne, E. and Sejnowski, T.J. (2002) Dynamic brain sources of visual evoked responses. *Science*, 295: 690–694.

O'Donnell, B.F., Vohs, J.L., Hetrick, W.P., Carroll, C.A. and Shekhar, A. (2004) Auditory event-related potential abnormalities in bipolar disorder and schizophrenia. *Int. J. Psychophysiol.*, 53: 45–55.

Palva, S. and Palva, J.M. (2007) New vistas for alpha-frequency band oscillations. *Trends Neurosci.*, 30: 150–158.

Palva, S., Linkenkaer-Hansen, K., Näätänen, R. and Palva, J.M. (2005) Early neural correlates of conscious somatosensory perception. *J. Neurosci.*, 25: 5248–5258.

Ramos-Loyo, J., Gonzalez-Garrido, A.A., Sanchez-Loyo, L.M., Medina, V. and Başar-Eroğlu, C. (2009) Event-related potentials and event-related oscillations during identity and facial emotional processing in schizophrenia. *Int. J. Psychophysiol.*, 71: 84–90.

Rojas, D.C., Bawn, S.D., Carlson, J.P., Arciniegas, D.B., Teale, P.D. and Reite, M.L. (2002) Alterations in tonotopy and auditory cerebral asymmetry in schizophrenia. *Biol. Psychiatry*, 52: 32–39.

Röschke, J., Wagner, P., Mann, K., Fell, J., Grozinger, M. and Frank, C. (1996) Single trial analysis of event related potentials: a comparison between schizophrenics and depressives. *Biol. Psychiatry*, 40: 844–852.

Salisbury, D.F., Collins, K.C. and McCarley, R.W. (2010) Reductions in the N1 and P2 auditory event-related potentials in first-hospitalized and chronic schizophrenia. *Schizophr. Bull.*, 36: 991–1000.

Schmiedt, C., Brand, A., Hildebrandt, H. and Başar-Eroğlu, C. (2005) Event-related theta oscillations during working memory tasks in patients with schizophrenia and healthy controls. *Cogn. Brain Res.*, 25: 936–947.

Schürmann, M. and Başar, E. (2001) Functional aspects of alpha oscillations in the EEG. *Int. J. Psychophysiol.*, 39: 151–158.

Schürmann, M., Başar-Eroğlu, C., Kolev, V. and Başar, E. (1995) A new metric for analyzing single-trial event-related potentials (ERPs): application to human visual P300 delta response. *Neurosci. Lett.*, 197: 167–170.

Schürmann, M., Başar-Eroğlu, C. and Başar, E. (1997) A possible role of evoked alpha in primary sensory processing: common properties of cat intracranial recordings and human EEG and MEG. *Int. J. Psychophysiol.*, 26: 149–170.

Schürmann, M., Demiralp, T., Başar, E. and Başar-Eroğlu, C. (2000) Electroencephalogram alpha (8–15 Hz) responses to visual stimuli in cat cortex, thalamus, and hippocampus: a distributed alpha network? *Neurosci. Lett.*, 292: 175–178.

Spencer, K.M., Nestor, P.G., Niznikiewicz, M.A., Salisbury, D.F., Shenton, M.E. and McCarley, R.W. (2003) Abnormal neural synchrony in schizophrenia. *J. Neurosci.*, 23: 7407–7411.

Spencer, K.M., Nestor, P.G., Perlmutter, R., Niznikiewicz, M.A., Klump, M.C., Frumin, M., Shenton, M.E. and McCarley, R.W. (2004) Neural synchrony indexes disordered perception and cognition in schizophrenia. *Proc. Natl. Acad. Sci. USA*, 101: 17288–17293.

Spencer, K.M., Niznikiewicz, M.A., Shenton, M.E. and McCarley, R.W. (2008) Sensory-evoked gamma oscillations in chronic schizophrenia. *Biol. Psychiatry*, 63: 744–747.

Sridharan, D., Levitin, D.J. and Menon, V. (2008) A critical role for the right fronto-insular cortex in switching between central-executive and default-mode networks. *Proc. Natl. Acad. Sci. USA*, 105: 12569–12574.

Uhlhaas, P.J. and Singer, W. (2010) Abnormal neural oscillations and synchrony in schizophrenia. *Nat. Rev. Neurosci.*, 11: 100–113.

Uhlhaas, P.J., Haenschel, C., Nikolic, D. and Singer, W. (2008) The role of oscillations and synchrony in cortical networks and their putative relevance for the pathophysiology of schizophrenia. *Schizophr. Bull.*, 34: 927–943.

Von Stein, A. and Sarnthein, J. (2000) Different frequencies for different scales of cortical integration: from local gamma to long range alpha/theta synchronization. *Int. J. Psychophysiol.*, 38: 301–313.

White, T.P., Joseph, V., O'Regan, E., Head, K.E., Francis, S.T. and Liddle, P.F. (2010) Alpha-gamma interactions are disturbed in schizophrenia: a fusion of electroencephalography and functional magnetic resonance imaging. *Clin. Neurophysiol.*, 121: 1427–1437.

Whitford, T.J., Farrow, T.F., Gomes, L., Brennan, J., Harris, A.W. and Williams, L.M. (2005) Grey matter deficits and symptom profile in first episode schizophrenia. *Psychiatry Res.*, 139: 229–238.

Application of Brain Oscillations in Neuropsychiatric Diseases
(Supplements to Clinical Neurophysiology, Vol. 62)
Editors: E. Başar, C. Başar-Eroğlu, A. Özerdem, P.M. Rossini, G.G. Yener
© 2013 Elsevier B.V. All rights reserved

Chapter 9

Early auditory gamma band response abnormalities in first hospitalized schizophrenia

Grantley W. Taylor[a,b], Robert W. McCarley[a,c] and Dean F. Salisbury[a,b,d,*]

[a]*Department of Psychiatry, Harvard Medical School, Boston, MA 02115, USA*
[b]*Cognitive Neuroscience Laboratory, McLean Hospital, Belmont, MA 02478, USA*
[c]*Boston Veterans Affairs Healthcare System, Brockton Division, Brockton, MA 02301, USA*
[d]*Current address: Department of Psychiatry, Western Psychiatric Institute and Clinic, University of Pittsburgh School of Medicine, Pittsburgh, PA 15213, USA*

ABSTRACT

Background: Abnormalities in coherent cortical circuit functioning, reflected in gamma band activity ($\sim$40 Hz), may be a core deficit in schizophrenia. The early auditory gamma band response (EAGBR) is a neurophysiologically simple probe of circuit functioning in primary auditory cortex. We examined the EAGBR in first hospitalized schizophrenia to assess whether it was reduced at first hospitalization.
Method: Wavelet evoked power and intertrial phase locking of the EAGBR at Fz to standard tones during an oddball target detection task were examined in 28 first hospitalized schizophrenia patients (10 female) and 44 control subjects (17 female).
Results: At first hospitalization EAGBR trial-to-trial phase locking and evoked power were significantly reduced in patients. Although reduced overall in patients, greater total symptoms were significantly associated with greater gamma phase locking and power. Additionally, greater EAGBR power was marginally associated with greater positive factor scores, hallucinations, and thinking disturbance.
Conclusions: Abnormalities of gamma band functioning in local auditory sensory circuits are present in schizophrenia at first hospitalization further evidence that basic sensory processes are impaired in schizophrenia. It remains to be determined whether the EAGBR becomes permanently impaired with disease progression, and if its reduction is specific to schizophrenia.

KEYWORDS

Schizophrenia; Gamma band response; Oscillation; EEG; Evoked potential; Auditory oddball

9.1. Introduction

9.1.1. Integration and connectivity in schizophrenia

Schizophrenia reflects a disintegration of many facets of distributed and parallel brain functioning, characterized by failure of integration between domains, e.g., poor coordination of mental and emotional processes, and disorder within domains, e.g., cognitive disorganization. Abnormalities of functional and structural connectivity within and between brain regions are apparent (Andreasen et al., 1998; Uhlhaas et al., 2006; Ford et al., 2007; Zhou et al., 2007; Roopun et al., 2008; Stephan et al., 2009), suggesting an underlying pathophysiological and anatomical disconnection. The formation of flexible, dynamic neural assemblies, both local and long-range, is thought to underlie distributed cerebral processing and is

Correspondence to: Dean F. Salisbury, PhD, Clinical Neurophysiology Research Laboratory, Western Psychiatric Institute and Clinic, Oxford Building, 3501 Forbes Ave, Pittsburgh, PA 15213, USA.
Tel.: +1 (412) 246-5123
E-mail: salisburyd@upmc.edu

likely due to temporal synchrony of neural firing within and between brain regions. There has been particular interest in gamma frequency (30–80 Hz) because of its relation to perceptual binding in animals (Freeman and Van Dijk 1987; Singer 1993; Engel and Singer, 2001) and higher-order cognition in humans (Başar et al., 1999; Rodriguez et al., 1999; Tallon-Baudry and Bertrand, 1999; Herrmann et al., 2004; Kaiser and Lutzenberger, 2005; Jensen et al., 2007).

9.1.2. Wavelet analysis of oscillations

Interest in frequency analysis of the EEG has undergone resurgence in tandem with development of methods that provide amplitude and phase measures superior to windowed Fourier transforms or restricted bandpass techniques. The wavelet method uses windowed or edge-modulated sinusoidals for frequency-in-time analyses, such as the Morlet wavelet which uses a Gaussian-modulated sinusoid. Measures of primary interest within the gamma range are power and the intertrial phase-locking factor (PLF). Power measures the energy within specific frequency bands and is the square of amplitude. PLF is a measure of the variance in phase across trials and thus reflects the temporal stability of oscillatory activity from trial to trial at specific sites. Though phase and amplitude are independent — clearly a low amplitude signal can be in phase from trial to trial — evoked power and PLF interact substantially as a high amplitude signal when averaged can appear smaller if out of phase between trials.

9.1.3. Gamma band responses

Gamma responses have been categorized into evoked and induced forms. Evoked responses are time locked to stimulus onset and generally occur earlier in the processing stream. These types of event-related oscillations (EROs) are thought to reflect basic perceptual mechanisms such as sensory registration. Evoked power is typically extracted from the averaged response across trials (i.e., the wavelet of the averaged response) and is analogous to the stimulus-locked event-related potential (ERP), where temporal variability between trials reduces the signal. Induced power represents the averaged wavelets of trials and thus does not "average out" non-stimulus-locked activity. Induced responses generally occur later and show varying onset times relative to stimulus onset. Like long-latency ERPs, these EROs are thought to reflect greater endogenous cognitive activity related to more complex internal operations and transforms of perceptual information. For an excellent review of gamma and other oscillations in cognitive and psychiatric disorders, see Başar and Güntekin (2008).

9.1.4. Gamma band responses in schizophrenia

Although recent work has focused on later induced gamma activity associated with complex perceptual phenomena (e.g., illusory contours) in schizophrenia (Spencer et al., 2003; Uhlhaas et al., 2006), it is important to determine whether more basic sensory processes are also impaired in the disorder. Coordinated activity within local processing circuits in sensory cortex is not only necessary for perception, but also for subsequent complex cognition. Recent ERP work has provided evidence of abnormalities in early sensory ERPs in schizophrenia (Leavitt et al., 2007; Javitt, 2009; Salisbury et al., 2010). One type of sensory-driven or evoked gamma oscillation, the steady-state evoked potential, uses repetitive click stimuli to cause the EEG to oscillate at the driving frequency. Deficits exist in gamma driving in schizophrenia (Kwon et al., 1999a,b; Light et al., 2006) even at first hospitalization (Spencer et al., 2008b). However, this response reflects the super-position of many responses to many stimuli and a subsequent reverberation of local circuits which cannot be purely sensory in nature.

Another gamma burst occurs early within the auditory system to discrete stimuli and may serve as a simple probe of coherent cortical circuit functioning. This early auditory gamma band response (EAGBR) to simple stimuli occurs early in the information processing stream and allows for a more reductionistic probing of basic cortical architecture in primary sensory areas (Brosch et al., 2002). Like other sensory processes, the EAGBR appears to be enhanced by selective attention (Tiitinen et al., 1993; Debener et al., 2003), and possibly task difficulty, perhaps through anterior cingulate modulation (Mulert et al., 2007). EAGBR abnormalities in schizophrenia would be consistent with basic low level processing deficits in schizophrenia as suggested by some recent studies (Leavitt et al., 2007; Javitt 2009).

9.1.5. Auditory pathophysiology in schizophrenia

Gray matter deficits throughout the auditory cortex have been noted in schizophrenia, even at first hospitalization (Kwon et al., 1999a,b; Hirayasu et al., 2000; Rojas et al., 2002; Kasai et al., 2003; Whitford et al., 2005). Moving down from complex to simple auditory processes, it is apparent that auditory system dysfunction in schizophrenia spans multiple levels of processing complexity. The presence of auditory hallucinations is a hallmark of schizophrenia and has been associated with abnormal primary auditory cortex activation (Lennox et al., 2000; Wible et al., 2009) and abnormal temporo-frontal white matter connectivity (Hubl et al., 2004). Abnormalities in the P300 to auditory oddballs (Roth et al., 1980; Bramon et al., 2004; Van der Stelt et al., 2005) and in the P200 and N100 to standard and oddball stimuli (Ford et al., 2001; O'Donnell et al., 2004) in schizophrenia are well established and present even at first hospitalization for schizophrenia (Salisbury et al., 1999, 2010). The P50/P1 auditory ERP is abnormal in schizophrenia (Freedman et al., 1987). Thus, ERPs spanning late endogenous and early exogenous processes are abnormal in schizophrenia.

9.1.6. EAGBR in schizophrenia

Consequently, it seems likely that the EAGBR would be reduced in schizophrenia. Results to date have been inconsistent. Six studies have used odd-ball-type target detection paradigms to examine the EAGBR. Gallinat et al. (2004) used a modified paradigm with click pairs as standard stimuli (500 ms separation) and tones as targets. Significant differences between patients and controls for EAGBR activity were not detected, although activity at Cz to standard clicks appears to be approximately 40% smaller in patients than controls. PLF was not reported. Spencer et al. (2008a) measured EAGBR power and PLF in 23 schizophrenics versus 21 controls. They did not detect significant EAGBR reductions in schizophrenia. Roach and Mathalon (2008) suggested that wavelet parameters might play a role in detection of group differences and detected reduced EAGBR PLF in 21 patients relative to 22 controls. Power was not assessed. Hall et al. (2011) reported reduced evoked EAGBR power and PLF in schizophrenics and their ill and well twins, leading Hall et al. (2011) to propose EAGBR as a putative endophenotype for the disorder. Leicht et al. (2010) found both reduced evoked power and PLF of EAGBR using wavelets in 90 patients versus 90 healthy comparison subjects. A recent report by Başar-Eroğlu et al. (2011) compared averaged and single trial responses to ignored single tone trains and to attended oddball trains. They reported that the averaged EAGBR did not differ between 10 patients and 10 controls, but that EAGBR power was increased in patients on individual trials over occipital areas. They suggested that trial-to-trial variability might be a crucial parameter for understanding the basic underlying pathophysiology of schizophrenia. Another extant report of early gamma activity in schizophrenia did not, in fact, measure the same phenomenon. Symond et al. (2005) used a standard two-tone oddball task and reported gamma phase across a windowed Fast Fourier Transform (FFT) from 37 to 41 Hz from −150 to 150 ms post stimulus. They did not examine intertrial PLF at specific sites, but measured synchrony between sites (anterior vs. posterior, left vs. right). They detected lower synchrony in 40 first episode schizophrenia subjects versus 40 controls, but they did not measure EAGBR per se with, for example, some peaks preceding stimulus onset. Thus, six studies have assessed the EAGBR in response to attended oddball-type tasks in schizophrenia, with equivocal results: half found reductions of the averaged responses, half did not.

Several studies examined EAGBR to clicks in the P50-gating paradigm, where click pairs (∼500 ms ISI) are passively attended with a long ITI (∼10 s). The EAGBR to clicks may not be identical to the EAGBR to tones (clicks include broad spectrum energy unlike pure tones), but it is likely that these EROs are highly similar. Click-gating tasks have generally reported lower but non-significantly different EAGBR to the first click (S1) and relatively normal gamma gating to the second click (S2). Using selective bandpass methods (not frequency in time methods like wavelets), Clementz et al. (1997) reported normal MEG and EEG measurement of S1 EAGBR, and that MEG detected an S2 EAGBR-gating defect in schizophrenia, but ERP measures (recorded from Cz) did not. Clementz and Blumenfeld (2001) used multi-channel EEG to determine if more dense recordings might detect ERP differences in the EAGBR and associated gating. They found no group differences in EAGBR between groups, but rather found differences in the low frequency component (LFR; theta and beta ranges). Johannesen et al. (2005) reported reduced spectral power of the EAGBR responses in schizophrenia (PCA-extracted component of restricted bandpass data submitted to FFT). They did not find any differences in EAGBR power between paranoid versus non-paranoid schizophrenia. Like Clementz and Blumenfeld (2001), they found reductions in the LFR. Later, Johannesen et al. (2008) used the Sensory Gating Inventory (Hetrick et al., 2012),

to classify schizophrenia patients with perceptual and attentional anomalies versus those without, and found that EAGBR power was smaller to S1 in schizophrenia subjects with high SGI scores than in controls, but greater in those with normal range scores than in controls, although only the two patient subgroups were significantly different. Hong et al. (2004) used a restricted bandpass method and found no difference in S1 gamma between schizophrenics and controls. Brockhaus-Dumke et al. (2008) reported similar phase locking in patients and controls to the first of two paired clicks.

Thus, analyses using click stimuli have generally not found reductions of EAGBR. Three of the six studies examining EAGBR to tones have reported EAGBR reductions. It is not clear why EAGBR results have been discrepant. In addition to the differences in the physical characteristics of the stimuli, one notable difference is that three positive tone studies used continuous wavelet analyses, whereas most of the gating data used restricted bandpass analyses. Wavelets are thought to be more sensitive to EROs than other methods (Lee and Yamamoto, 1994), but it is likely that Roach and Mathalon's (2008) caveat about wavelet parameters influencing measures is also important. Too, oddball tasks generally demand selective attention, but gating paradigms are passive, but this cannot account for inconsistent results in oddball tasks. Other factors such as prolonged medication, illness progression, and increased auditory thresholds in chronic schizophrenic populations (Rabinowicz et al., 2000) may affect EAGBR measures. Diagnostic subtype may play a role, although Johannesen et al. (2005) did not detect an effect. We suspect the actual paradigms used play a great role, as the low signal-to-noise ratio of the EAGBR makes it difficult to detect. Tasks that use many pure tone pip stimuli should be best able to visualize the $<1\,\mu V$ response. In addition, studies with large samples have generally been better able to detect group differences in this small response, as the effect size is very small.

9.1.7. Current aims

The present study examined the EAGBR in subjects at or near first hospitalization, free from potential chronicity-related confounds. The presence of EAGBR abnormalities early in the disease is crucial if the EAGBR is truly an endophenotype. Studying subjects at first hospitalization reduces the contribution of prolonged medication and progressive cortical reduction and allows for longitudinal study early in the disease to evaluate changes reflective or predictive of deterioration.

9.2. Methods

9.2.1. Subjects

Twenty-eight first hospitalized schizophrenia subjects (FHSz) at or within 1 year of first hospitalization (mean (S.D.) 18.4 (19.9) days), diagnosed via SCID-P interview for DSM-IV criteria and chart review (15 paranoid, 1 disorganized, 2 undifferentiated, 8 schizoaffective (5 bipolar subtype, 3 depressed subtype), 1 schizophreniform, and 1 delusional disorder, paranoid subtype), participated. Forty-four healthy control subjects (HC) were recruited from the local community through newspaper and online advertisements and were free of Axis I or II disorders (structured clinical interview for DSM-IV non-patient edition (SCID-NP); structured clinical interview for DSM-IV Axis II personality disorders (SCID II)), as well as a history of Axis I disorders in first-degree relatives by report. Groups were matched for age, handedness, WAIS information and vocabulary scaled scores, gender distributions, and parental SES. Subjects met these inclusion criteria: (1) right-handed (Edinburgh Handedness Inventory); (2) no ECT; (3) no history of neurological illness; (4) no alcohol or drug dependence or "detox" within the last 5 years; and (5) estimated verbal IQ above 75. Patients had slightly lower Mini-Mental State Exam (MMSE) and WAIS working memory task scores than controls, consistent with effects of acute psychosis, but were generally bright and high functioning (Table 1). The McLean Hospital IRB approved this study. After complete description of the study to the subjects, written informed consent was obtained. Subjects were paid $15/h for their participation.

9.2.2. Procedure

Subjects detected low probability Target tones (15%, 1.2 kHz, 73 dB SPL, 50 ms pips, 5 ms rise/fall times) among Standard tones (1 kHz, 73 dB SPL, 50 ms pips, 5 msc rise/fall times) presented over insert headphones (Etymotic/Earlink) with an ISI jittered equally between 800, 900, 1000, 1100, and 1200 ms. A total of 200 tones were presented with the exception of latter subjects to whom 400 tones were presented (for increased signal-to-noise ratios). Only the first 200 trials for these subjects were used in the present study so that averages had the same inherent signal-to-noise-ratio and equal habituation and refractory effects. Stimulus delivery and digital triggers were generated with Superlab Pro v.2 (Cedrus). Subjects kept a mental count of the Target tones.

9.2.3. EEG recording and processing

EEG activity was recorded from 60 scalp sites and the nose tip using a 64-channel cap (custom designed Electro-Cap International sintered Ag-AgCl caps). Activity was recorded continuously using SynAmps and Scan Acquire (Neuroscan/Compumedics, USA). The right mastoid served as the reference, except for two bipolar electrooculogram channels. Two electrodes medial to the right eye, one above and one below, monitored vertical eye movements and blinks. Electrodes at the outer canthi of the eyes monitored horizontal eye movements. The forehead served as ground. Electrode impedances were below 5 kΩ. The EEG bandpass was 0.10 (6 dB/octave roll-off) to 100 Hz (24 dB/octave roll-off). EEG was digitized at 500 Hz.

TABLE 1

DEMOGRAPHIC AND CLINICAL INFORMATION

	Patients	HC	Statistic	p
Gender (M/F)	18/10	27/17	$\chi^2 = 0.15$	0.70
Age	24.8 (7.6)	26.3 (8.0)	$t(70) = 0.80$	0.42
Handedness	0.77 (0.21)	0.81 (0.14)	$t(65) = 0.76$	0.45
SES	3.4 (1.3)	2.2 (0.8)	$t(66) = 4.56$	<0.0012
PSES	1.70 (1.0)	1.70 (1.1)	$t(65) = 0.03$	0.97
Minimental State	28.7 (1.3)	29.4 (0.6)	$t(65) = 2.91$	0.009
WAIS info	12.8 (2.4)	13.0 (2.3)	$t(65) = 0.29$	0.77
WAIS vocab	13.4 (2.3)	14.2 (2.8)	$t(65) = 1.17$	0.25
WAIS digit span	9.9 (2.3)	12.0 (2.2)	$t(65) = 3.81$	<0.001
WAIS symbol digit D	7.8 (2.0)	13.0 (8.9)	$t(65) = 2.75$	0.008
MEDS	299.9 (252.0)			
GAS	34.0 (8.2)			
PANSS total	75.6 (14.0)			
PANSS positive	20.4 (4.3)			
PANSS negative	18.7 (6.6)			
PANSS td	11.2 (3.8)			
SAPS	10.3 (6.3)			
SANS	11.5 (5.9)			

Note: values are mean (S.D.). Less df reflects data unavailable for some subjects. SES = socio-economic status; PSES = parental SES; WAIS info = Wechsler Adult Intelligence Scale information scaled score; WAIS vocab = Wechsler Adult Intelligence Scale vocabulary scaled score; WAIS digit span = Wechsler Adult Intelligence Scale digit span scaled score; WAIS symbol digit = Wechsler Adult Intelligence Scale digit symbol scaled score; MEDS = daily antipsychotic medication dosage, chlorpromazine equivalents; GAS = global assessment scale, equivalent to global assessment of functioning scale; PANSS = positive and negative syndrome scale; PANSS positive = PANSS positive symptom factor; PANSS negative = PANSS negative symptom factor; PANSS td = PANSS thought disturbance factor; SAPS = scale for the assessment of positive symptoms; SANS = scale for the assessment of negative symptoms.

Off-line processing was performed with BrainVision Analyzer (Brain Products GMBH). EEG was rereferenced to averaged mastoids and segmented for Standard stimuli into epochs of 1100-ms duration, including a 100 ms pre-stimulus baseline.

To illustrate the major time-averaged ERP correlates of the EAGBR ERO, voltage in time averages was constructed for controls using restricted passband filtering (Clementz and Blumenfeld, 2001). The EAGBR was visualized by restricted filtering from 35 to 45 Hz. Middle and high frequency contributions to the standard ERPs were visualized by high pass filtering at 8 Hz. Low frequency contributions to the ERP were visualized by low pass filtering at 8.5 Hz, with eye movement correction using the method of Gratton et al. (1983). Epochs were baseline corrected by subtraction of the average pre-stimulus voltage at each site. Subsequently, epochs containing eye movements exceeding $\pm 50\,\mu V$ at F7, F8, FP1, or FP2 were rejected.

For wavelet-derived frequency in time measures, the EEG was digitally high pass filtered at 8 Hz (24 dB/octave roll-off) to remove eye movement artifact, drift, and low frequency components. Standard tone epochs (processed as above) underwent time frequency analysis in Matlab for intertrial phase locking and evoked power (software provided by C. Torrence and G. Compo; http://atoc.colorado.edu/research/wavelets). A complex Morlet wavelet with

Morlet's constant $f/s_f = 6$ and a fixed cycle length of 6 was used over the 20–80 Hz range with 11 frequency bins. Baseline correction for each frequency bin used the 100 ms pre-stimulus interval. Evoked power was derived from the squared amplitude coefficient of the wavelet transform of the ERP. Phase was calculated as the arc tangent of the ratio of the imaginary and real coefficients of the transform for each individual trial. PLF was calculated as 1 minus the variance of phase across trials, the circular variance, for each time-frequency point (Tallon-Baudry et al., 1996). A peak-picking method based on Mulert et al. (2007), modified to diminish the likelihood of missing a peak on either side of 40 Hz, was used. Based on the grand average maximum ± 25 ms, the peak value from 50 to 100 ms post stimulus among 3 frequency bins centered at 40, 46, and 53 Hz was selected for each individual. Analysis focused on the Fz and Cz chains, including left (F1, C1), midline (Fz, Cz), and right (F2, C2) sites for standard stimuli. Repeated measures ANOVA utilizing Huynh-Feldt epsilon for position (left, middle, right) was used to test for effects. Follow-up tests used t tests. Correlations used Pearson correlations. Significance was achieved at $p \leq 0.05$.

9.3. Results

9.3.1. Morphology

Comparison of HC grand averaged standard stimuli waveforms (Fig. 1) shows that the EAGBR overlaps with the P1/P50 response, as expected (Pantev and Elbert, 1994; Clementz et al., 1997; Clementz and Blumenfeld, 2001). Both the EAGBR and the P1 are partially overlapped by the descending slope of the N100.

9.3.2. Power

Mean central (f) of EAGBR power tended to be ~46 Hz in both groups. HC showed a well defined burst of EAGBR evoked power, by contrast with patients who showed a weaker signal (Fig. 2A presents frequency-in-time maps for Fz; mean peak values of EAGBR evoked power for each site are presented in Table 2). Patients showed an evoked power reduction ($F_{1, 70} = 3.89$, $p = 0.05$). Hemispheres differed in evoked power ($F_{2, 140} = 5.03$, $p = 0.01$, $\varepsilon = 0.88$), which interacted with chain location ($F_{2, 140} = 4.36$, $p = 0.03$, $\varepsilon = 0.74$). Power was greatest at the midline for both chains, but was relatively larger over the left hemisphere than the right for the frontal chain, and relatively larger over the left hemisphere than the right for the central chain (Table 2). There was no significant main effect for chain location and no other significant interactions.

9.3.3. Phase

HC showed greater trial-to-trial phase synchrony of the EAGBR than patients ($F_{1, 70} = 5.74$, $p = 0.02$; Fig. 2B presents frequency-in-time maps for Fz PLF; Table 3 presents PLF means for all sites). Additionally, frontal sites showed greater PLF than central sites ($F_{1, 70} = 24.49$, $p < 0.001$) in both groups. PLF was largest at midline sites ($F_{2, 140} = 7.78$, $p = 0.001$, $\varepsilon = 0.97$), but the laterality of PLF interacted with chain location ($F_{2, 140} = 4.12$, $p = 0.02$, $\varepsilon = 0.94$), with the left frontal site larger than the right, whereas left and right central sites were symmetrical (Table 3).

9.3.4. Correlations with symptoms

EAGBR evoked power and PLF measures were highly correlated at all sites in both groups. Controls showed the weakest correlation between power and PLF at C1 ($r = 0.63$, $p < 0.001$) and greatest at C2 ($r = 0.71$, $p < 0.001$). Correlations between different sites ranged from 0.35 to 0.75. Patients showed the weakest correlation between power and PLF at F2 ($r = 0.77$, $p < 0.001$) and greatest at C1 ($r = 0.85$, $p < 0.001$). Correlations between different sites ranged from 0.61 to 0.87.

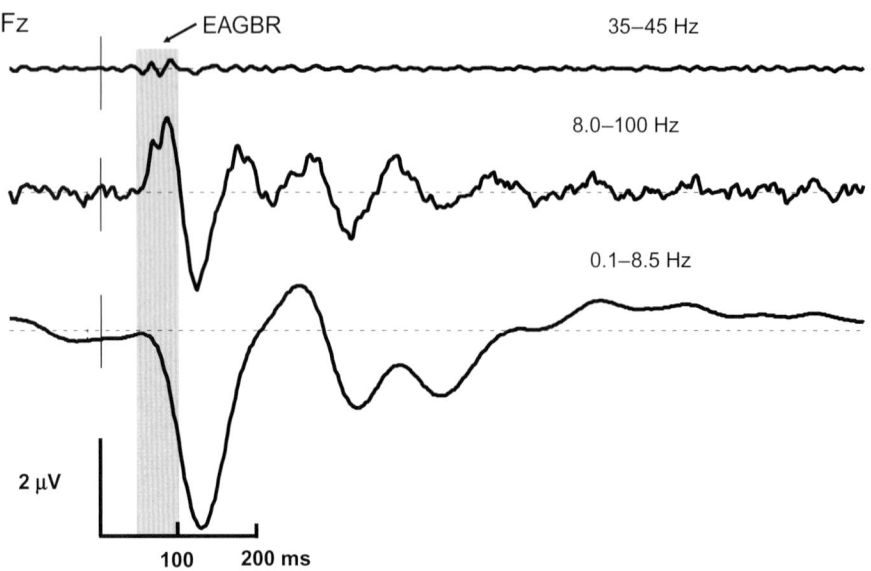

Fig. 1. Voltage in time restricted passband control subject grand averaged ERPs to standard stimuli illustrating different neurophysiological signals and their overlap. The shaded box indicates 50–100 ms post stimulus. The top trace shows the averaged EAGBR response. The middle trace highlights the P1/P50 response, which appears to overlap to a great degree with the EAGBR. The bottom trace shows N1/N100 and P2/P200. Note that the N1 response begins at approximately 75 ms and overlaps partially with the EAGBR and P1.

Evoked gamma power and PLF at Fz and Cz in control subjects were not correlated with WAIS information, vocabulary, or symbol digit scores, but EAGBR PLF at Fz correlated marginally with digit span ($r = 0.29$, $p = 0.056$). There were no significant correlations with EAGBR evoked power or PLF and semantic or working memory measures in patients. Within patients, PLF at Fz and Cz was correlated positively with PANSS total scores ($r = 0.47$, $p = 0.024$, $r = 0.43$, $p = 0.04$, respectively, Fig. 3) but not with positive, negative, or thought disturbance PANSS factors, SANS, SAPS, GAS, or medication dosages (chlorpromazine equivalents). EAGBR power at Fz and Cz was correlated positively with PANSS total scores ($r = 0.71$, $p < 0.001$, $r = 0.61$, $p = 0.002$, respectively, Fig. 3), but not with SANS, SAPS, GAS, or medication dosages. In addition, EAGBR evoked power at Fz correlated marginally with PANSS hallucinations ($r = 0.39$, $p = 0.066$), PANSS positive factor ($r = 0.39$, $p = 0.065$), and PANSS thought disturbance factor ($r = 0.41, p = 0.051$).

9.4. Discussion

9.4.1. Precis

The current study showed reduction in EAGBR evoked power and phase locking in first hospitalized schizophrenia. These findings support the presence of functional local circuit deficits in schizophrenia early in the sensory processing stream and early during disease course. Deficits at first hospitalization rather than emergence with disease course are consistent with the EAGBR's identification as a candidate endophenotype.

9.4.2. Underlying pathophysiology

It is not clear whether EAGBR deficits reflect cortical or subcortical processing abnormalities. The EAGBR is contemporaneous with the high frequency component of the P1 (Fig. 1). Some

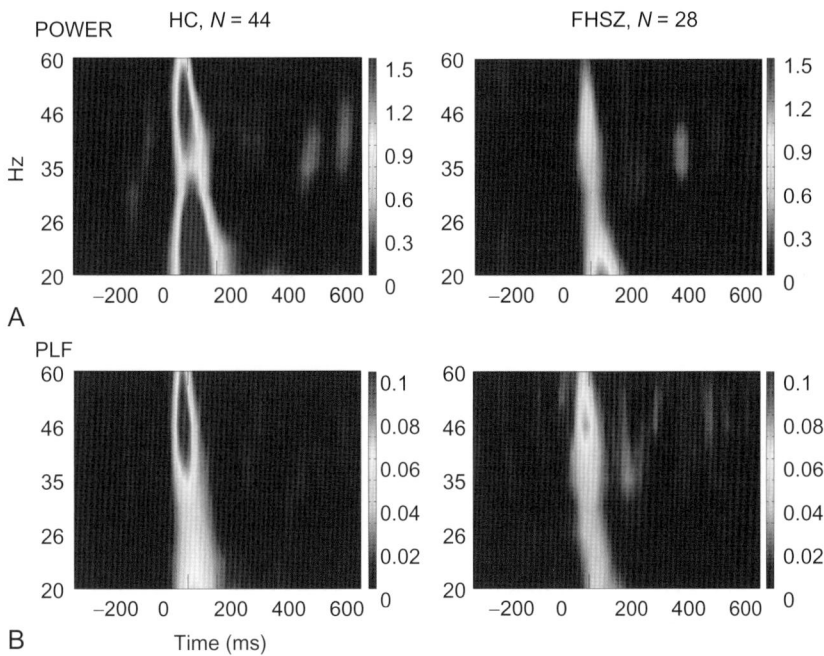

Fig. 2. (A) Frequency in time maps of evoked power at Cz for each group for standard stimuli. Note that patients show attenuated evoked power in that time interval relative to controls. The lower (f) activity reflects N1 and P2. (B) Phase-locking factor at Cz for each group for standard stimuli. Although maximum evoked power was observed at 46 Hz in controls, their maximum PLF was lower, closer to 40 Hz. Patients showed very little phase consistency across trials. (For color figures, please refer to the color figures in last section of the book.)

TABLE 2

MEAN PEAK EAGBR EVOKED POWER (70–90 ms, μV)

	F1	Fz	F2
HC	1.32 (1.77)	1.42 (1.73)	1.17 (1.46)
Patients	0.60 (1.00)	0.67 (1.11)	0.61 (1.04)
	C1	Cz	C2
HC	1.03 (1.78)	1.20 (1.84)	1.18 (2.05)
Patients	0.33 (0.65)	0.49 (1.03)	0.57 (0.97)

evidence exists suggesting subcortical, thalamic sources for the P1 (Velasco and Velasco, 1986), although most data suggest sources in Heschl's gyrus (Liégeois-Chauvel et al., 1994). EAGBR deficits may reflect local abnormalities in primary auditory cortex in schizophrenia, but may also be related to feedforward and feedback communication between thalamus (medial geniculate nucleus) and primary auditory cortex. Recent fMRI work suggests co-activation of auditory cortex and thalamus during the EAGBR (Mulert et al., 2010). In terms of pathophysiology, when coupled with other gamma band defects spanning sensory-perceptual and cognitive tasks, it is possible that wide-range gamma

TABLE 3

MEAN PEAK EAGBR PLF (70–90 ms)

	F1	Fz	F2
HC	0.10 (0.08)	0.10 (0.07)	0.07 (0.07)
Patients	0.06 (0.06)	0.06 (0.06)	0.05 (0.06)
	C1	Cz	C2
HC	0.07 (0.07)	0.08 (0.07)	0.07 (0.06)
Patients	0.03 (0.06)	0.05 (0.07)	0.04 (0.06)

band deficits reflect an ubiquitous cortical circuit deficit in schizophrenia that spans various types of cortical architecture, even sensory (Javitt, 2009). Dysfunction of coherent synchrony in cell assemblies of varying complexity may be a core deficit in schizophrenia. It is not clear if such deficits in local circuit function lead to an overall reduction of gamma power, reduced time-locking of gamma band response which leads to apparent power reduction following averaging (Başar-Eroğlu et al., 2011), or some combination of both defects.

9.4.3. Endophenotypes

Deficits in early primary sensory processes in the visual system P1 have recently been demonstrated in schizophrenia patients (Foxe et al., 2001) and their relatives (Yeap et al., 2006) and may serve as an endophenotype. Several other ERPs have been identified via family and twin studies as putative endophenotypes for schizophrenia (Hall et al., 2007). Following up the demonstration of reduced auditory N1 in family members (Force et al., 2008), we suggested that auditory N1 reduction may be endophenotypic for schizophrenia due to its presence at first hospitalization (Salisbury et al., 2010). Our recent collaborative study (Hall et al., 2011) showed reductions in EAGBR evoked power and PLF in schizophrenia, and their ill and well twins, suggesting that the EAGBR is endophenotypic. The current demonstration of

EAGBR deficits in first hospitalized schizophrenia strengthens the contention that this simple ERO is an endophenotype for schizophrenia. Neurophysiological measures of auditory sensory processing as early as the P1 and the EAGBR (and analogues in the visual system) may be valid biomarkers for genetic risk factors for schizophrenia. It is important to examine EAGBR in other major psychiatric illnesses, such as bipolar disorder, to determine whether the reduction is specific to schizophrenia or associated with psychosis or some other pathophysiological condition more generally.

9.4.4. Sensory or cognitive deficit?

Although neurophysiological deficits exist in schizophrenia early in auditory sensory processing, it is unclear whether this reduction reflects a true sensory deficit or a deficit in the ability to use top-down attention to modulate auditory signals. Most oddball tasks demonstrating EAGBR deficits in schizophrenia used an active oddball target detection task, while most P50 gating studies that have not seen EAGBR reductions have used a passive paired-click task. Force et al. (2008) indicated that family members did modulate auditory N1 with attention in contrast to schizophrenic and bipolar subjects, and Hall et al. (2011) showed reduced EAGBR in family members on an oddball task (where presumably they modulated sensory signals as a

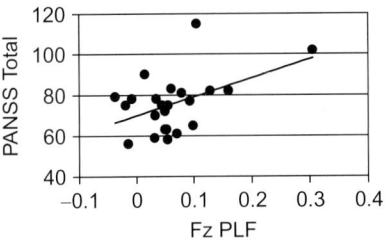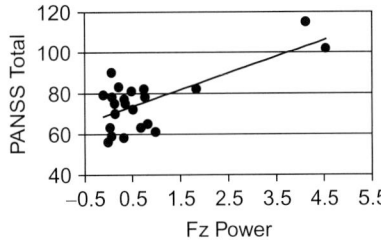

Fig. 3. Correlations between EAGBR power and PLF to standard tones and total PANSS scores in first hospitalized schizophrenia.

function of selective attention). These findings are consistent with a true sensory defect, but attention effects need to be quantified. Currently, we are recording EAGBR during attend and ignore conditions to assess selective attention effects in first hospitalized subjects and matched controls.

9.4.5. Variability in literature

Among tasks using oddball paradigms, the present study supports the findings of Roach and Mathalon (2008), Leicht et al. (2010), and Hall et al. (2011). Nevertheless, there have been two negative studies looking at the auditory EAGBR on oddball tasks. Gallinat et al. (2004) used click stimuli as standards and a restricted wavelet analysis, which may have affected results (note that their response looks attenuated in midline and left hemisphere sites in their Fig. 3). Spencer et al. (2008a) did not find reductions in a chronic population in the auditory EAGBR, though early gamma band abnormalities were present to visual stimuli. In addition to analytical difference, as discussed by Roach and Mathalon (2008), we note here that measurement methods of wavelets may affect results. For example, our use of peak picking resulted in larger values than when a static interval was used. There is a substantial amount in individual variability in the EAGBR and different measurement schemes may be differentially sensitive to this variability. Finally, the between-group EAGBR differences are quite small in magnitude, and the effect size

is not large. Both Leicht et al. (2010) and Hall et al. (2011) tested large numbers of subjects, with effect sizes around 0.3 and 0.4, respectively. The utility of the EAGBR may be somewhat lessened by this fact, which indicates substantial group distribution overlap.

9.4.6. EAGBR and symptoms

Correlations between PANSS totals and EAGBR evoked power and PLF were found, but were paradoxically positive. This indicates that the most symptomatic patients showed the greatest power and trial-to-trial temporal stability. Remember, however, that the patient means were overall lower than control means. Although somewhat counter-intuitive, this finding appears to be consistent with previous studies showing positive correlations between hallucinations and steady-state gamma parameters (Spencer et al., 2003, 2008a). The observed relationships were influenced somewhat by two outliers in the patient group, although the correlations remained (albeit weaker) using Spearman's rank order methods. Further research is needed to determine if, within overall reduced patient gamma measures, higher values are associated with greater symptoms.

9.4.7. Caveats

Several issues related to the EAGBR need to be clarified. The reliability of the EAGBR, its variability over the course of disease, and its specificity to schizophrenia need to be assessed. Further, correlations with baseline temporal lobe auditory gray matter volumes and progressive auditory cortex gray matter changes during the early course of the disease need to be determined. Wavelet-derived measures of EEG and their application to psychiatry is an emerging and developing field. Roach and Mathalon (2008) have recently reviewed neural synchrony measures and indicated several methodological issues that the field is still addressing, such as the most appropriate baseline correction method. Comparison of baseline in HC and first hospitalized schizophrenia indicated that the choice used in the current study did not influence the results, but the field has not adopted a standard method. Evoked power and intertrial phase-locking are highly correlated. Nevertheless, they are not entirely redundant measures. It remains to be determined what neurophysiological processes are manifested in these two measures.

9.4.8. Summary

Evoked power and PLF of the EAGBR were reduced in schizophrenia patients at their first hospitalization for psychosis. Cortical dysfunctions related to abnormalities of local circuit synchrony are present in schizophrenia relatively early in cortical sensory processing. This may relate to a ubiquitous defect in GABA and glutaminergic regulation of cell assemblies, although several different neurotransmitters and neuromodulators are involved in gamma oscillations (Uhlhaas et al., 2008). When coupled with our demonstration of similarly reduced EAGBR measures in the well twins of schizophrenic individuals (Hall et al., 2011), and EAGBR reductions in long-term schizophrenia subjects (Roach and Mathalon, 2008; Leicht et al., 2010), the presence of this deficit in first hospitalized subjects suggests that EAGBR may be a physiologically simple, yet potentially powerful, endophenotype for detecting genetic risk variants associated with schizophrenia,

particularly if a means of increasing group differences and hence effect size can be developed.

Acknowledgments

The Authors would like to thank our Research Assistants Rachel Berman, Akanksha Thakur, Courtney Brown, KC Collins, Katherine Tyler, Diane Ventura, and Toni Mahowald for help in collecting and analyzing the data. Drs Taylor and Salisbury had full access to all the data in the study and take responsibility for the integrity of the data and the accuracy of the data analysis.

The authors report no biomedical financial interests or potential conflicts of interest.

Supported by the National Institutes of Health R01 MH58704 (D.F.S.) and R01 MH40799 (R.W.M.), and the Department of Veterans Affairs Merit Award, Schizophrenia Center Award, and Middleton Award (R.W.M.).

References

Andreasen, N.C., Paradiso, S. and O'Leary, D.S. (1998) "Cognitive dysmetria" as an integrative theory of schizophrenia: a dysfunction in cortical–subcortical–cerebellar circuitry? *Schizophr. Bull.*, 24: 203–218.

Başar, E. and Güntekin, B. (2008) A review of brain oscillations in cognitive disorders and the role of neurotransmitters. *Brain Res.*, 1235: 172–193.

Başar, E., Başar-Eroğlu, C., Karakas, S. and Schürmann, M. (1999) Are cognitive processes manifested in event-related gamma, alpha, theta and delta oscillations in the EEG? *Neurosci. Lett.*, 259: 165–168.

Başar-Eroğlu, C., Mathesa, B., Brand, A. and Schmiedt-Fehra, C. (2011) Occipital gamma response to auditory stimulation in patients with schizophrenia. *Int. J. Psychophysiol.*, 79: 3–8.

Bramon, E., Rabe-Hesketh, S., Sham, P., Murray, R.M. and Frangou, S. (2004) Meta-analysis of the P300 and P50 waveforms in schizophrenia. *Schizophr. Res.*, 70: 315–329.

Brockhaus-Dumke, A., Schultze-Lutter, F., Mueller, R., Tendolkar, I., Bechdolf, A., Pukrop, R., Klosterkoetter, J. and Ruhrmann, S. (2008) Sensory gating in schizophrenia: P50 and N100 gating in antipsychotic-free subjects at risk, first-episode, and chronic patients. *Biol. Psychiatry*, 64: 376–384.

Brosch, M., Budinger, E. and Scheich, H. (2002) Stimulus-related gamma oscillations in primate auditory cortex. *J. Neurophysiol.*, 87: 2715–2725.

Clementz, B. and Blumenfeld, L. (2001) Multichannel electroencephalographic assessment of auditory evoked response suppression in schizophrenia. *Exp. Brain Res.*, 139: 377–390.

Clementz, B.A., Blumenfeld, L.D. and Cobb, S. (1997) The gamma band response may account for poor P50 suppression in schizophrenia. *NeuroReport*, 8: 3889–3893.

Debener, S., Herrmann, C.S., Kranczioch, C., Gembris, D. and Engel, A.K. (2003) Top-down attentional processing enhances auditory evoked gamma band activity. *NeuroReport*, 14: 683–686.

Engel, A.K. and Singer, W. (2001) Temporal binding and the neural correlates of sensory awareness. *Trends Cogn. Sci.*, 5: 16–25.

Force, R.B., Venables, N.C. and Sponheim, S.R. (2008) An auditory processing abnormality specific to liability for schizophrenia. *Schizophr. Res.*, 103: 298–310.

Ford, J.M., Mathalon, D.H., Kalba, S., Marsh, L. and Pfefferbaum, A. (2001) N1 and P300 abnormalities in patients with schizophrenia, epilepsy, and epilepsy with schizophrenia-like features. *Biol. Psychiatry*, 49: 848–860.

Ford, J.M., Krystal, J.H. and Mathalon, D.H. (2007) Neural synchrony in schizophrenia: from networks to new treatments. *Schizophr. Bull.*, 33: 848–852.

Foxe, J.J., Doniger, G.M. and Javitt, D.C. (2001) Early visual processing deficits in schizophrenia: impaired P1 generation revealed by high-density electrical mapping. *NeuroReport*, 12: 3815–3820.

Freedman, R., Adler, L.E., Gerhardt, G.A., Waldo, M., Baker, N., Rose, G.M., Drebing, C., Nagamoto, H., Bickford-Wimer, P. and Franks, R. (1987) Neurobiological studies of sensory gating in schizophrenia. *Schizophr. Bull.*, 13: 669–678.

Freeman, W.J. and Van Dijk, B.W. (1987) Spatial patterns of visual cortical fast EEG during conditioned reflex in a rhesus monkey. *Brain Res.*, 422: 267–276.

Gallinat, J., Winterer, G., Herrmann, C.S. and Senkowski, D. (2004) Reduced oscillatory gamma-band responses in unmedicated schizophrenic patients indicate impaired frontal network processing. *Clin. Neurophysiol.*, 115: 1863–1874.

Gratton, G., Coles, M.G. and Donchin, E. (1983) A new method for off-line removal of ocular artifact. *Electroencephalogr. Clin. Neurophysiol.*, 55: 468–484.

Hall, M.H., Rijsdijk, F., Picchioni, M., Schulze, K., Ettinger, U., Toulopoulou, T., Bramon, E., Murray, R.M. and Sham, P. (2007) Substantial shared genetic influences on schizophrenia and event-related potentials. *Am. J. Psychiatry*, 164: 804–812.

Hall, M.H., Taylor, G., Sham, P., Schulze, K., Rijsdijk, F., Picchioni, M., Toulopoulou, T., Ettinger, U., Bramon, E., Murray, R.M. and Salisbury, D.F. (2011) The early auditory gamma-band response is heritable and a putative endophenotype of schizophrenia. *Schizophr. Bull.*, 37: 778–787.

Herrmann, C.S., Munk, M.H.J. and Engel, A.K. (2004) Cognitive functions of gamma-band activity: memory match and utilization. *Trends Cogn. Sci.*, 8: 347–355.

Hetrick, W.P., Erickson, M.A. and Smith, D.A. (2012) Phenomenological dimensions of sensory gating. *Schizophr. Bull.*, 38(1): 178–191.

Hirayasu, Y., McCarley, R.W., Salisbury, D.F., Tanaka, S., Kwon, J.S., Frumin, M., Snyderman, D., Yurgelun-Todd, D., Kikinis, R., Jolesz, F.A. and Shenton, M.E. (2000) Planum temporale and Heschl gyrus volume reduction in schizophrenia: a magnetic resonance imaging study of first-episode patients. *Arch. Gen. Psychiatry*, 57: 692–699.

Hong, L.E., Summerfelt, A., McMahon, R., Adami, H., Francis, G., Elliott, A., Buchanan, R.W. and Thaker, G.K. (2004) Evoked gamma band synchronization and the liability for schizophrenia. *Schizophr. Res.*, 70: 293–302.

Hubl, D., Koenig, T., Strik, W., Federspiel, A., Kreis, R., Boesch, C., Maier, S.E., Schroth, G., Lovblad, K. and Dierks, T. (2004) Pathways that make voices: white matter changes in auditory hallucinations. *Arch. Gen. Psychiatry*, 61: 658–668.

Javitt, D.C. (2009) When doors of perception close: bottom-up models of disrupted cognition in schizophrenia. *Annu. Rev. Clin. Psychol.*, 5: 249–275.

Jensen, O., Kaiser, J. and Lachaux, J.P. (2007) Human gamma-frequency oscillations associated with attention and memory. *Trends Neurosci.*, 30: 317–324.

Johannesen, J.K., Kieffaber, P.D., O'Donnell, B.F., Shekhar, A., Evans, J.D. and Hetrick, W.P. (2005) Contributions of subtype and spectral frequency analyses to the study of P50 ERP amplitude and suppression in schizophrenia. *Schizophr. Res.*, 78: 269–284.

Johannesen, J., Bodkins, M., O'Donnell, B., Shekhar, A. and Hetrick, W. (2008) Perceptual anomalies in schizophrenia co-occur with selective impairments in the gamma frequency component of midlatency auditory ERPs. *J. Abnorm. Psychol.*, 117: 106–118.

Kaiser, J. and Lutzenberger, W. (2005) Human gamma-band activity: a window to cognitive processing. *NeuroReport*, 16: 207–211.

Kasai, K., Shenton, M.E., Salisbury, D.F., Hirayasu, Y., Onitsuka, T., Spencer, M.H., Yurgelun-Todd, D.A., Kikinis, R., Jolesz, F.A. and McCarley, R.W. (2003) Progressive decrease of left Heschl gyrus and planum temporale gray matter volume in first-episode schizophrenia: a longitudinal magnetic resonance imaging study. *Arch. Gen. Psychiatry*, 60: 766–775.

Kwon, J.S., McCarley, R.W., Hirayasu, Y., Anderson, J.E., Fischer, I.A., Kikinis, R., Jolesz, F.A. and Shenton, M.E. (1999a) Left planum temporale volume reduction in schizophrenia. *Arch. Gen. Psychiatry*, 56: 142–148.

Kwon, J.S., O'Donnell, B.F., Wallenstein, G.V., Greene, R.W., Hirayasu, Y., Nestor, P.G., Hasselmo, M.E., Potts, G.F., Shenton, M.E. and McCarley, R.W. (1999b) Gamma frequency-range abnormalities to auditory stimulation in schizophrenia. *Arch. Gen. Psychiatry*, 56: 1001–1005.

Leavitt, V.M., Molholm, S., Ritter, W., Shpaner, M. and Foxe, J.J. (2007) Auditory processing in schizophrenia during the middle latency period (10–50 ms): high-density electrical mapping and source analysis reveal subcortical antecedents to early cortical deficits. *J. Psychiatry Neurosci.*, 32: 339–353.

Lee, D. and Yamamoto, A. (1994) Wavelet analysis: theory and applications. *Hewlett-Packard J.*, 44–52.

Leicht, G., Kirsch, V., Giegling, I., Karch, S., Hantschk, I., Möller, H.J., Pogarell, O., Hegerl, U., Rujescu, D. and Mulert, C. (2010) Reduced early auditory evoked gamma-band response in patients with schizophrenia. *Biol. Psychiatry*, 67: 224–231.

Lennox, B.R., Park, S.B.G., Medley, I., Morris, P.G. and Jones, P.B. (2000) The functional anatomy of auditory hallucinations in schizophrenia. *Psychiatry Res*, 100: 13–20.

Liégeois-Chauvel, C., Musolino, A., Badier, J.M., Marquis, P. and Chauvel, P. (1994) Evoked potentials recorded from the auditory cortex in man: evaluation and topography of the middle latency components. *Electroenceph. Clin. Neurophysiol.*, 92: 204–214.

Light, G.A., Hsu, J.L., Hsieh, M.H., Meyer-Gomes, K., Sprock, J., Swerdlow, N.R. and Braff, D.L. (2006) Gamma band oscillations reveal neural network cortical coherence dysfunction in schizophrenia patients. *Biol. Psychiatry*, 60: 1231–1240.

Mulert, C., Leicht, G., Pogarell, O., Mergl, R., Karch, S., Juckel, G., Möller, H.-J. and Hegerl, U. (2007) Auditory cortex and anterior cingulate cortex sources of the early evoked gamma-band response: relationship to task difficulty and mental effort. *Neuropsychologia*, 45: 2294–2306.

Mulert, C., Leicht, G., Hepp, P., Kirsch, V., Karch, S., Pogarell, O., Reiser, M., Hegerl, U., Jäger, L., Möller, H.J. and McCarley, R.W. (2010) Single-trial coupling of the gamma-band response and the corresponding BOLD signal. *NeuroImage*, 49: 2238–2247.

O'Donnell, B.F., Vohs, J.L., Hetrick, W.P., Carroll, C.A. and Shekhar, A. (2004) Auditory event-related potential abnormalities in bipolar disorder and schizophrenia. *Int. J. Psychophysiol.*, 53: 45–55.

Pantev, C. and Elbert, T. (1994) The transient auditory evoked gamma-band field. In: C. Pantev (Ed.), *Proceedings of NATO Advanced Research Workshop on Oscillatory Event-Related Brain Dynamics*. Plenum Press, New York, pp. 219–230.

Rabinowicz, E.F., Silipo, G., Goldman, R. and Javitt, D.C. (2000) Auditory sensory dysfunction in schizophrenia: imprecision or distractibility? *Arch. Gen. Psychiatry*, 57: 1149–1155.

Roach, B.J. and Mathalon, D.H. (2008) Event-related EEG time-frequency analysis: an overview of measures and an analysis of early gamma band phase locking in schizophrenia. *Schizophr. Bull.*, 34: 907–926.

Rodriguez, E., George, N., Lachaux, J.P., Martinerie, J., Renault, B. and Varela, F.J. (1999) Perception's shadow: long-distance synchronization of human brain activity. *Nature (Lond.)*, 397: 430–433.

Rojas, D.C., Bawn, S.D., Carlson, J.P., Arciniegas, D.B., Teale, P.D. and Reite, M.L. (2002) Alterations in tonotopy and auditory cerebral asymmetry in schizophrenia. *Biol. Psychiatry*, 52: 32–39.

Roopun, A.K., Cunningham, M.O., Racca, C., Alter, K., Traub, R.D. and Whittington, M.A. (2008) Region-specific changes in gamma and beta$_2$ rhythms in NMDA receptor dysfunction models of schizophrenia. *Schizophr. Bull.*, 34: 962–973.

Roth, W.T., Pfefferbaum, A., Horvath, T.B. and Kopell, B.S. (1980) P300 and reaction time in schizophrenics and controls. *Prog. Brain Res.*, 54: 522–525.

Salisbury, D.F., Shenton, M.E. and McCarley, R.W. (1999) P300 topography differs in schizophrenia and manic psychosis. *Biol. Psychiatry*, 45: 98–106.

Salisbury, D.F., Collins, K.C. and McCarley, R.W. (2010) Reductions in the N1 and P2 auditory event-related potentials in first-hospitalized and chronic schizophrenia. *Schizophr. Bull.*, 36: 991–1000.

Singer, W. (1993) Synchronization of cortical activity and its putative role in information processing and learning. *Annu. Rev. Physiol.*, 55: 349–374.

Spencer, K.M., Nestor, P.G., Niznikiewicz, M.A., Salisbury, D.F., Shenton, M.E. and McCarley, R.W. (2003) Abnormal neural synchrony in schizophrenia. *J. Neurosci.*, 23: 7407–7411.

Spencer, K.M., Niznikiewicz, M.A., Shenton, M.E. and McCarley, R.W. (2008a) Sensory-evoked gamma oscillations in chronic schizophrenia. *Biol. Psychiatry*, 63: 744–747.

Spencer, K.M., Salisbury, D.F., Shenton, M.E. and McCarley, R.W. (2008b) Gamma-band auditory steady-state responses are impaired in first episode psychosis. *Biol. Psychiatry*, 64: 369–375.

Stephan, K.E., Friston, K.J. and Frith, C.D. (2009) Dysconnection in schizophrenia: from abnormal synaptic plasticity to failures of self-monitoring. *Schizophr. Bull.*, 35: 509–527.

Symond, M.P., Harris, A.W., Gordon, E. and Williams, L.M. (2005) "Gamma synchrony" in first-episode schizophrenia: a disorder of temporal connectivity? *Am. J. Psychiatry*, 162: 459–465.

Tallon-Baudry, C. and Bertrand, O. (1999) Oscillatory gamma activity in humans and its role in object representation. *Trends Cogn. Sci.*, 3: 151–162.

Tallon-Baudry, C., Bertrand, O., Delpuech, C. and Pernier, J. (1996) Stimulus specificity of phase-locked and non-phase-locked 40 Hz visual responses in human. *J. Neurosci.*, 16: 4240–4249.

Tiitinen, H.T., Sinkkonen, J., Reinikainen, K., Alho, K., Lavikainen, J. and Näätänen, R. (1993) Selective attention enhances the auditory 40-Hz transient response in humans. *Nature (Lond.)*, 364: 59–60.

Uhlhaas, P.J., Linden, D.E., Singer, W., Haenschel, C., Lindner, M., Maurer, K. and Rodriguez, E. (2006) Dysfunctional long-range coordination of neural activity during Gestalt perception in schizophrenia. *J. Neurosci.*, 26: 8168–8175.

Uhlhaas, P.J., Haenschel, C., Nikolic, D. and Singer, W. (2008) The role of oscillations and synchrony in cortical networks and their putative relevance for the pathophysiology of schizophrenia. *Schizophr. Bull.*, 34: 927–943.

Van der Stelt, O., Lieberman, J.A. and Belger, A. (2005) Auditory P300 in high-risk, recent-onset and chronic schizophrenia. *Schizophr. Res.*, 77: 309–320.

Velasco, M. and Velasco, F. (1986) Subcortical correlates of the somatic, auditory and visual vertex activities. II. Referential EEG responses. *Electroenceph. Clin. Neurophysiol.*, 63: 62–67.

Whitford, T.J., Farrow, T.F., Gomes, L., Brennan, J., Harris, A.W. and Williams, L.M. (2005) Grey matter deficits and symptom profile in first episode schizophrenia. *Psychiatry Res.*, 139: 229–238.

Wible, C.G., Lee, K., Molina, I., Hashimoto, R., Preus, A.P., Roach, B.J., Ford, J.M., Mathalon, D.H., McCarthey, G., Turner, J.A., Potkin, S.G., O'Leary, D., Belger, A.,

Diaz, M., Voyvodic, J., Brown, G.G., Notestine, R., Greve, D. and Lauriello, J. (2009) fMRI activity correlated with auditory hallucinations during performance of a working memory task: data from the FBIRN consortium study. *Schizophr. Bull.*, 35: 47–57.

Yeap, S., Kelly, S.P., Sehatpour, P., Magno, E., Javitt, D.C., Garavan, H., Thakore, J.H. and Foxe, J.J. (2006) Early visual sensory deficits as endophenotypes for schizophrenia: high-density electrical mapping in clinically unaffected first-degree relatives. *Arch. Gen. Psychiatry*, 63: 1180–1188.

Zhou, Y., Liang, M., Jiang, T., Tian, L., Liu, Y., Liu, Z., Liu, H. and Kuang, F. (2007) Functional dysconnectivity of the dorsolateral prefrontal cortex in first-episode schizophrenia using resting-state fMRI. *Neurosci. Lett.*, 417: 297–302.

Chapter 10

Early auditory gamma-band responses in patients at clinical high risk for schizophrenia

Veronica B. Perez[a,b], Brian J. Roach[a,b], Scott W. Woods[c], Vinod H. Srihari[c], Thomas H. McGlashan[c], Judith M. Ford[a,b,c] and Daniel H. Mathalon[a,b,c,*]

[a]*Department of Psychiatry, University of California, San Francisco (UCSF), San Francisco, CA 94121, USA*
[b]*San Francisco Veterans Administration Medical Center, 4150 Clement Street, San Francisco, CA 94121, USA*
[c]*Department of Psychiatry, Yale University, 300 George Street, New Haven, CT 06511, USA*

ABSTRACT

Background: Gamma-band oscillations and their synchronization have been implicated in the coordination of activity between distributed neuronal assemblies in the service of sensory registration of stimuli and perceptual binding of their features. Prior electroencephalographic (EEG) studies of chronic schizophrenia patients have documented deficits in the magnitude and/or phase synchrony of stimulus-evoked gamma oscillations, findings that have been linked to neurotransmission abnormalities involving GABA and NMDA-glutamate receptors. However, it remains unclear whether these abnormalities are present at the onset of the illness, or indeed, whether they are present during the prodromal period preceding illness onset. Accordingly, we examined the magnitude and phase synchrony of the transient gamma-band response (GBR) elicited by an auditory stimulus in young patients with schizophrenia and in patients at clinical high risk for psychosis based on their manifestation of putatively prodromal symptoms.
Methods: EEG was recorded during an auditory oddball target detection task in three groups: young schizophrenia patients early in their illness (YSZ; $n = 19$), patients at clinical high risk for psychosis (CHR; $n = 55$), and healthy controls (HC; $n = 42$). Single-trial EEG epochs and the average event-related potential time-locked to standard tones from the oddball task were subjected to time-frequency decomposition using Morlet wavelet transformations. The GBR between 50 and 100 ms following the tone onset was quantified in terms of evoked power, total power, and the phase-locking factor (PLF) reflecting cross-trial phase synchrony.
Results: GBR evoked power was significantly reduced in YSZ ($p < 0.01$) and CHR ($p < 0.05$) patients, relative to HC. Similarly, GBR PLF was significantly reduced in YSZ ($p < 0.01$) and showed a marginal reduction in CHR patients ($p = 0.057$), relative to HC. GBR total power was not reduced in CHR patients ($p = 0.68$) and showed only a trend level reduction in YSZ ($p = 0.072$). Within the CHR group, there were no significant GBR differences between the patients who converted to a psychotic disorder and those who did not convert to psychosis during a 12-month follow-up period.
Conclusion: Reductions in the transient auditory GBR, as reflected by evoked power and phase synchrony, are evident in the early stages of schizophrenia and appear to precede psychosis onset. However, the absence of total power GBR abnormalities in CHR patients, with only a trend toward reduction in YSZ patients, suggests that the magnitude of the GBR is intact early in the course

---

Correspondence to: Dr. Daniel H. Mathalon, Ph.D., M.D., San Francisco Veterans Administration Medical Center, Bldg. 8, Room 9B, 116D, 4150 Clement Street, San Francisco, CA 94121, USA.
Tel.: +1 (415) 221-4810, ext. 3860; Fax: +1 (415) 750-6622;
E-mail: daniel.mathalon@ucsf.edu

of schizophrenia, whereas the phase synchrony of this response is deficient. Given that the GBR failed to distinguish the CHR patients who converted to psychosis from those who did not convert, the role of GBR disruption in the emergence of psychosis warrants further investigation. Asynchronous gamma activity may represent an elemental neurobiological abnormality in schizophrenia that is also evident in patients at high clinical risk for psychosis regardless of their longer-term clinical outcomes.

KEYWORDS

Schizophrenia; Clinical high risk; Auditory; Gamma; Total power; Evoked power; Phase-locking factor

10.1. Introduction

Synchronization of neural activity in the gamma range (30–80 Hz) is thought to be a mechanism for integrating sensory information across different modalities and cortical areas, thereby creating a coherent cortical representation of complex external sensory stimuli (Singer, 1999; Başar et al., 2000; Engel et al., 2001). The coordination of sensory gamma oscillations has been shown to contribute to sensory registration and perceptual processes (Clementz et al., 1997; Hong et al., 2004a), as well as higher order cognitive operations such as attention and expectation (Başar-Eroğlu and Başar, 1991; Tiitinen et al., 1993; Tallon-Baudry et al., 1997; Gurtubay et al., 2001; Debener et al., 2003; Gurtubay et al., 2004). It has been hypothesized that the widespread cognitive deficits consistently observed in schizophrenia may be attributable to core abnormalities in the timing, synchronization, and efficiency of neuro-oscillatory activity, particularly in the gamma band, that subserves the binding and integration of information processed across different brain regions (see Uhlhaas and Singer, 2010).

Patients with schizophrenia have been shown to have abnormal electroencephalographic (EEG) gamma-band responses (GBRs) associated with sensory (Kwon et al., 1999; Haig et al., 2000b; Gallinat et al., 2004; Light et al., 2006; Roach and Mathalon, 2008; Spencer et al., 2008b; Leicht et al., 2010; Hall et al., 2011a,b), perceptual (Spencer et al., 2003), attentional (Haig et al., 2000a; Symond et al., 2005), and cognitive control (Cho et al., 2006) processes. We and others have recently reported decreased early gamma activity in response to auditory stimuli in patients with schizophrenia, as reflected by evoked power (Leicht et al., 2011; Hall et al., 2011a,b) and phase-locking factor (Roach and Mathalon, 2008; Leicht et al., 2010; Hall et al., 2011b; Roach et al., 2013, this volume). In auditory oddball paradigms, schizophrenia has been associated with an abnormal reduction of GBRs to target (Haig et al., 2000b; Symond et al., 2005) and non-target (Haig et al., 2000b; Roach and Mathalon, 2008; Hall et al., 2011b) auditory tones, suggesting that the early evoked GBRs to auditory stimuli are either compromised by a lack of phase consistency across trials, reduced response magnitude, or some combination of the two. While gamma oscillation abnormalities are evident in chronic schizophrenia patients (Kwon et al., 1999; Gallinat et al., 2004; Light et al., 2006; Roach and Mathalon, 2008; Hall et al., 2011a,b; Roach et al., 2013), in first-episode psychosis (Symond et al., 2005; Spencer et al., 2008a; Williams et al., 2009), and to a lesser degree, in unaffected relatives (Hong et al., 2004b; Hall et al., 2011b; Leicht et al., 2011; but see also Hall et al., 2011a), it remains unclear whether they are present in individuals at clinical high risk for the development of psychosis.

10.2. Mechanisms of gamma-band oscillations

Fast spiking inhibitory γ-aminobutyric acid (GABA) interneurons expressing the calcium-binding protein parvalbumin have been implicated in the mediation of gamma oscillatory activity (Sohal et al., 2009; Gonzalez-Burgos et al., 2010; Carlen et al., 2011; Lewis et al., 2011). The inhibition of pyramidal cell and interneuron networks by GABAergic interneurons produces gamma-band oscillations through an inhibition and rebound excitation cycle that is modulated by $GABA_A$ receptors (Whittington et al., 1995; Sohal et al., 2009). Moreover, glutamatergic neurotransmission at NMDA receptors provides excitatory regulation of parvalbumin fast-spiking interneurons, contributing to the generation of gamma oscillations in pyramidal cell networks (Doheny et al., 2000; Roopun et al., 2008; Carlen et al., 2011) Gamma oscillatory activity non-invasively measured by EEG in patients with schizophrenia is of interest because disrupted GABAergic and glutamatergic cortical activities have been implicated in the pathophysiology of the illness (Benes, 2000; Gonzalez-Burgos and Lewis, 2008; Roopun et al., 2008; Lewis et al., 2005, 2008, 2011).

10.3. Early gamma-band responses in schizophrenia

The auditory GBR has been quantified with different methods, typically involving the transformation of the time-voltage domain EEG or event-related potential (ERP) signal into the time-frequency domain. Repeated applications of Fourier, Hilbert, or wavelet transformations produce time-frequency decompositions of EEG or ERP signals. Our analysis focuses on measures of total power, evoked power, and phase-locking factor (PLF), and typically these effects are fronto-centrally distributed across EEG channels. Total power (or event-related spectral perturbation (Delorme and Makeig, 2004)) is a measure of the event-related change in power across individual trials, including both phase synchronous and asynchronous activity. Evoked power describes only phase-locked event-related changes in power because the time-frequency transformation is derived from the time-domain averaged ERP waveform. Finally, PLF (also called intertrial phase coherence (Delorme and Makeig, 2004)) is a measure of phase consistency across trials from a single electrode or source.

Several studies have investigated the early, evoked auditory GBR associated with sensory registration of auditory stimuli (Pantev et al., 1991), using evoked power or PLF measures in schizophrenia. Clementz et al. (1997) initially observed early abnormalities in auditory evoked gamma power, and multiple subsequent studies (Hirano et al., 2008; Roach and Mathalon, 2008; Teale et al., 2008; Başar-Eroğlu et al., 2009; Krishnan et al., 2009; Leicht et al., 2010, 2011; Hall et al., 2011a,b; Lenz et al., 2011), but not all (Blumenfeld and Clementz, 2001; Brockhaus-Dumke et al., 2008a,b; Brenner et al., 2009), have reported reduced evoked power or PLF in the gamma band. However, the selective examination of these two measures limits our ability to adequately describe the stimulus-driven activity of neuronal assemblies. Evoked power reflects the amplitude of the oscillations that are phase-locked to a stimulus event, since averaging across trials tends to cancel out non-phase-locked oscillatory activity.

Accordingly, because the evoked power measure initially requires some consistency of phase across single trials, and then depends on the average magnitude of the phase-locked signal, evoked power deficits could be due to decreased phase-locking or to reduced single-trial amplitude. Given that many previous studies have acknowledged the increase in phase variance (i.e., latency jitter) in measures of neural activity in patients with schizophrenia (Ford et al., 1994), it is surprising that very few studies (Krishnan et al., 2009) have assessed total power of the early auditory GBR in this population to separate magnitude from phase-locking abnormalities.

Furthermore, it is unknown whether abnormalities in transient GBRs observed in schizophrenia patients predate the onset of psychosis, or co-occur with illness onset. This question can be addressed by studying patients at clinical high risk (CHR) for developing psychosis. Being at "clinical high risk" is defined by the Criteria of Prodromal Syndromes (COPS; Miller et al., 2002) and the similar criteria for At Risk Mental States (ARMS; Yung and McGorry, 1996). The North American prodromal longitudinal study (NAPLS) consortium reported that 35% of patients meeting COPS criteria converted to a psychotic disorder within a 2.5-year follow-up period (Cannon, 2008). An increasing number of studies are finding that electrophysiological abnormalities associated with schizophrenia are evident in clinical high risk patients (Brockhaus-Dumke et al., 2008b; Shin et al., 2009; Van Tricht et al., 2010; Bodatsch et al., 2011; Perez et al., 2011a,b; Jahshan et al., 2012); however, none has assessed whether GBRs are abnormal in these patients. GBR abnormalities in CHR patients may reflect vulnerability to the disorder and/or abnormal neurodevelopment, particularly in connection with abnormal function of NMDA and $GABA_A$ receptors. A major motivation for identifying neurophysiological abnormalities in a CHR sample is to enhance the accuracy of the prediction of which at risk patients will convert to psychosis, setting the stage for development of targeted preventive interventions aimed at those patients at greatest risk.

10.4. Design of present study

In order to assess whether transient GBRs quantified with total power, evoked power, and PLF time-frequency measures are compromised early in the course of schizophrenia, we compared young schizophrenia patients, clinical high risk patients, and healthy controls on these measures. Based on previous studies reporting reduced gamma-band evoked power and PLF in schizophrenia, we predicted that young schizophrenia patients, still early in their illness course, would show diminished evoked power and PLF in the GBR. Based on the hypothesis that abnormal GBRs may be physiological risk markers for the development of psychosis, we predicted that patients at clinical high risk for psychosis would also be abnormal on these measures. However, given the heterogeneous nature of clinical high risk samples, with only a minority of patients destined to convert to schizophrenia, we predicted that, as a group, their abnormalities would be intermediate relative to early illness schizophrenia patients and healthy controls.

Finally, we predicted that clinical high risk patients who subsequently converted to psychosis would have greater GBR abnormalities.

10.5. Method

10.5.1. Participants

Study participants included 43 patients at clinical high risk (CHR) for psychosis based on the Structured Interview for Prodromal Syndromes (SIPS; Miller et al., 2002), 19 young patients with DSM-IV schizophrenia (YSZ) based on the Structured Clinical Interview for DSM-IV (SCID), and 42 healthy control (HC) subjects. CHR patients met criteria for *at least* one of the three sub-syndromes defined by the COPS (Miller et al., 2002): (1) attenuated positive symptoms (APS), (2) brief intermittent psychotic states (BIPS), and/or (3) genetic risk with deterioration in social/occupational functioning (GRD). Interviews were conducted by a trained research assistant, psychiatrist, or clinical psychologist.

HCs were recruited by advertisements and word-of-mouth. Exclusion criteria for HC included a past or current DSM-IV Axis I disorder based on an SCID interview or having a first-degree relative with a psychotic disorder. Exclusion criteria for all groups included history of substance dependence or abuse within the past year, a history of a significant medical or neurological illness, or a history of head injury resulting in loss of consciousness. The study was approved by the Yale University institutional review board, and adult participants provided written informed consent. In the case of minors, parents provided written informed consent; youths provided written informed assent. Group demographics are included in Table 1.

10.5.2. Clinical ratings

Within 1 month of EEG assessment ($\bar{M} = 9.8$, SD = 22.99 days), a clinically trained research assistant, psychiatrist, or clinical psychologist rated YSZ symptoms using the Positive and Negative

TABLE 1

GROUP DEMOGRAPHIC DATA[a]

	CHR patients (n = 43)		YSZ patients (n = 19)		HCs (n = 42)		X^2	p value	
	n	%	n	%	n	%			
Gender							2.0	0.363	
Female	17	39.5	4	21.1	15	35.7			
Male	26	60.5	15	78.9	27	64.3			
Handedness[b]							1.7	0.787	
Right	36	83.7	16	84.2	35	83.3			
Left	3	7.0	1	5.3	5	11.9			
Both	4	9.3	2	10.5	2	4.8			
Diagnostic subtype									
Paranoid			12	63.2					
Disorganized			1	5.3					
Undifferentiated			2	10.5					
Residual			1	5.3					
Schizoaffective			3	15.7					
Schizophreniform									
Clinical high risk criteria[c]									
APS	41	95.3							
BIPS	1	2.3							
GRD	1	2.3							
Antipsychotic type									
Atypical	10	23.3	14	73.7					
Typical	0	0.0	0	0.0					
Both	0	0.0	3	15.8					
None	33	76.7	2	10.5					

	M	SD	M	SD	M	SD	F	p value	Post hoc contrasts
Age (years)	16.86	3.5	23.91	6.2	19.89	5.5	13.93	<.001	YSZ>HC>CHR
Parental socioeconomic status[d]	26.9	14.8	40.44	9.1	27.61	13.0	7.89	<.001	HC<CHR = YSZ
PANSS symptom total[e]			70.14	15.50					
SOPS symptom total	37.40	15.60							

[a]Note: Values are given as number and percentage of subjects for gender, handedness, diagnostic subtype, clinical high risk criteria, and antipsychotic type. Group means with the standard deviation for age, parental socioeconomic status, PANSS, and SOPS are reported. Gender and handedness were analyzed with Pearson chi-square tests. Age and parental socioeconomic status were analyzed with one-way ANOVA and Tukey–Kramer *post hoc* tests.

Abbreviations: CHR, clinical high risk patients; YSZ, young schizophrenia patients; HCs, healthy controls; APS, attenuated positive symptoms; BIPS, brief intermittent psychotic symptoms; GRD, genetic risk and deterioration; PANSS, positive and negative syndrome scale; SOPS, scale of prodromal symptoms.

[b]The Crovitz–Zener (1962) questionnaire was used to measure handedness.

[c]Clinical high risk criteria APS, BIPS, and GRD are not mutually exclusive.

[d]The Hollingshead (1975) four-factor index of parental socioeconomic status (SES) is based on a composite of maternal education, paternal education, maternal occupational status, and paternal occupational status. Lower scores represent higher SES. SES values are missing from 2 YSZ patients (n = 2).

[e]PANSS scores are missing from 5 YSZ patients (n = 5).

Syndrome Scale (PANSS; Kay and Opler, 1987) and CHR symptoms using the Scale of Prodromal Symptoms (SOPS; Miller et al., 2002). Symptom scores are listed in Table 1.

10.5.3. Conversion to psychosis

Of the 43 CHR patients, 15 converted to a psychotic disorder within 2.5 years of study participation. Conversion to psychosis was defined by a rating of 6 on at least one of the positive symptom items from the SIPS, indicating the presence of a full-blown psychotic syndrome. A positive symptom is given a rating of 6 if it has reached a high intensity level (e.g., delusional conviction) and exceeds a frequency or duration threshold (≥ 1 h/day for ≥ 4 days/week during the past month), or if it has a seriously disorganizing or dangerous impact on the patient (Cannon, 2008). Only CHR patients who were clinically followed for a minimum of 12 months ($n = 16$) and had not yet converted to a psychotic disorder were included in the non-conversion group.

10.5.4. Gamma-band response paradigm

Subjects listened to a random series of infrequent ($n = 45, 10\%$) high tones (1000 Hz), infrequent novel sounds ($n = 45, 10\%$), and frequent ($n = 360, 80\%$) low tones (500 Hz). Subjects were asked to press a response key to each occurrence of the infrequent, high tone (i.e., target stimulus). Transient GBRs were assessed from the frequent tones exclusively. These tones were 80 dB SPL and 50 ms in duration presented with a stimulus-onset asynchrony of 1.25 s. Sounds were delivered via Etymotic ER-3A insert earphones at 80 dB SPL through a STIM audio box (Compumedics Neuroscan).

10.5.5. EEG acquisition

EEG data were acquired at 1000 Hz from 20 sites (Fp1, Fp2, F7, F3, Fz, F4, F8, T3, C3, Cz, C4, T4, T5, P3, Pz, P4, T6, O1, Oz, O2), bandpass filtered between 0.05 and 100 Hz, and referenced to linked ears. Additional electrodes were placed on the outer canthi of both eyes and above and below the left eye to record eye movements and blinks (vertical and horizontal electro-oculogram; VEOG, HEOG). All impedances were maintained at or below 10 kΩ throughout the recording session with most EEG sites below 5 kΩ.

Single-trial EEG epochs were stimulus-locked to the onset of each tone, including data from 250 ms before the tone onset and 750 ms after its onset. Individual trials were baseline corrected using the 100-ms period preceding the tone onset after correcting for eye movements and blinks using EOG data (Gratton et al., 1983). Finally, trials containing artifacts (voltages exceeding ± 100 µV) in any of the central nine electrodes (F3, Fz, F4, C3, Cz, C4, P3, Pz, or P4) were rejected.

10.5.6. EEG time-frequency analysis

Time-frequency analysis of the EEG gamma activity was based on Morlet wavelets using the freely distributed FieldTrip (http://fieldtrip.fcdonders.nl/) software in Matlab (http://www.mathworks.com/products/matlab/), as in our prior work (Roach and Mathalon, 2008). The Morlet wavelet has a Gaussian shape that is defined by a ratio ($\sigma_f = f/C$) and a wavelet duration ($6 \sigma_t$), where f is the center frequency and $\sigma_t = 1/(2\pi\sigma_f)$. In a classic wavelet analysis, C is a constant (e.g., 7), ensuring an equal number of cycles in the mother wavelet for each frequency. In this approach, as the frequency (f) increases, the spectral bandwidth ($6 \sigma_f$) increases. This method was used to decompose single-trial time-frequency values between 20 and 60 Hz for the central nine electrodes.

After applying this method, PLF was calculated as 1 minus the circular phase angle variance, as described by Tallon-Baudry et al. (1997). PLF provides a measure of the phase consistency of frequency-specific oscillations with respect to stimulus onset across trials on a millisecond basis. In addition, event-related total power was calculated by averaging the squared single-trial magnitude values in each 1 Hz frequency bin on a millisecond basis. The average total power values were $10\log_{10}$ transformed and then baseline corrected by subtracting the average of the pre-stimulus baseline (-100 to 0 ms) from each time point separately for every frequency. The resulting event-related change in total power values (relative to baseline) are in decibels (dB).

10.5.7. ERP time-frequency analysis

To quantify evoked power, single-trial EEG epochs were averaged to create event-related potentials (ERPs). ERP data were subjected to the wavelet decomposition described above, and evoked power was calculated by squaring the output. The evoked power values were $10\log_{10}$ transformed and then baseline corrected by subtracting the average of the pre-stimulus baseline (-100 to 0 ms) from each time point separately for every frequency. The resulting event-related change in evoked power values (relative to baseline) are in decibels (dB).

10.5.8. Principal component analysis of time-frequency data

To capture and quantify the GBR, a time-frequency principal component analysis (TF-PCA) approach similar to that implemented by others (Bernat et al., 2005) was adopted. In particular, total power, evoked power, and PLF measures were down-sampled to reduce the number of points (originally 1 ms × 1 Hz) in the TF matrices by sampling every 2 Hz (e.g., 20, 22, 24 Hz ...) between 20 and 60 Hz and every 5 ms (e.g., -50, -45, -40 ms...) between -50 and 150 ms. The TF-PCA was then calculated separately for total power, evoked power, and PLF by rearranging the 2-D TF data into 1-D by transposing the frequency data at the first time point (-50 ms) and concatenating it with similarly transposed vectors at all other time points. This results in 861 sample row vectors for each electrode ($n = 9$) and each subject ($n = 104$), which were submitted to a covariance matrix PCA implemented in Matlab (Kayser and Tenke, 2003). All components were

retained and subjected to a varimax rotation, yielding orthogonal factors corresponding to major TF components. To produce interpretable TF factor loadings, 1-D factor loadings were rearranged back into the original order of the 2-D TF measures, and individual subject and electrode factor scores corresponding to the transient GBR component were saved for subsequent analyses.

10.5.9. Statistical correction for normal aging effects

To control for the effects of normal aging, we derived a single age-corrected value for each subject for total power, evoked power, and PLF scores. First, total power PCA factor scores were regressed on age in the HC group (age range 12–37 years). Next, the resulting regression equation was used to derive age-specific predicted values that were subtracted from the observed values and divided by the standard error of regression, yielding age-corrected total power factor z-scores for subjects across all groups. The resulting age-corrected z-scores reflected deviations in standard units from the values expected for a normal healthy subject of a given age. This method has been used previously to correct for normal aging effects in structural MRI data (Pfefferbaum et al., 1992). The method is preferable to using age as a covariate in an ANCOVA because it removes normal aging effects while preserving any pathological aging effects present in the patient data. This procedure was repeated to acquire age-corrected evoked power factor z-scores and PLF factor z-scores for all subjects across groups.

10.5.10. Statistical analysis

Separate 3 group (HC, CHR, YSZ) × 2 site (Fz, Cz) repeated measures analysis of variance (ANOVA) models were performed on each of the age-corrected GBR-dependent variables (total power, evoked power, PLF). Significant group effects were further parsed with *a priori* planned contrasts. Converters and non-converters were compared on total power, evoked power, and PLF, using a 2 group (converters, non-converters) × 2 site (Fz, Cz) repeated measures ANOVA.

To assess the relationship between symptom severity and total power, evoked power, and PLF in the YSZ group, GBR factor scores from each measure were correlated with positive (sum of PANSS positive symptom ratings) and negative (sum of PANSS negative symptom ratings) symptom summary scores. Correlations with SOPS positive and negative symptom summary scores were performed in the CHR group. A Bonferonni correction was applied for the number of correlations performed within each patient group, maintaining the corrected alpha level at $p = 0.05$.

10.6. Results

10.6.1. GBR PCA factor loadings

Inspection of the factor loadings for total power (Fig. 1A) revealed that the first factor peaked at ~40 Hz and 50 ms, corresponding to the GBR, and accounted for 12.59% of the variance. Inspection of the factor loadings for evoked power (Fig. 1B) revealed that the first factor peaked at ~40 Hz and 50 ms, corresponding to the GBR, and accounted for 7.62% of the variance. Inspection of the factor loadings for PLF (Fig. 1C) revealed that the third factor peaked at ~40 Hz and 50 ms, corresponding to the GBR, and accounted for 14.96% of the variance.

Furthermore, scalp topographies of the extracted PCA factor scores are consistent with the expected fronto-central distribution of the auditory gamma-band response, as shown in Fig. 1A–C.

10.6.2. Group differences in GBR PCA factor scores

The factor scores corresponding to the GBR components shown in Fig. 1 were extracted for electrode sites Fz and Cz, subjected to age-correction procedures described previously, and used in the group analyses (see Table 2). Age-corrected mean

total power, evoked power, and PLF z-scores (± S.E.) are plotted for each group in Fig. 2. Note that because z-scores are normed relative to the HC group data, the HC group has mean z-score values of zero for each measure.

10.6.3. Group differences in age-corrected PCA total power GBR

The repeated measures ANOVA revealed an absence of any significant group differences (HC, CHR, YSZ) in the total power GBR (Figs. 1A and 2A). Furthermore, the site and group × site interaction effects were not significant. A priori pairwise comparisons showed that age-corrected total power GBR factor z-scores were marginally reduced in YSZ relative to HC (Cohen's $d = 0.43$; $p = 0.072$). No reduction in total power GBR was observed in the CHR group relative to the HC group (Cohen's $d = 0.09$; $p = 0.687$).

10.6.4. Group differences in age-corrected PCA evoked power GBR

The repeated measures ANOVA showed a significant main effect of group (HC, CHR, YSZ) for the evoked power GBR (Figs. 1B and 2B). The site and group × site interaction effects were not significant. As reported in Table 2, age-corrected evoked power GBR factor z-scores were reduced in the YSZ and CHR groups relative to the HC group (YSZ vs. HC: Cohen's $d = 0.69$; $p = 0.004$; CHR vs. HC: Cohen's $d = 0.50$; $p = 0.011$).

10.6.5. Group differences in age-corrected PCA phase-locking factor GBR

The repeated measures ANOVA showed a significant main effect of group (HC, CHR, YSZ) for the PLF of the GBR (Figs. 1C and 2C). Neither the site effect nor the group × site interaction was significant. Group analyses are presented in Table 2, where age-corrected PLF z-scores were reduced in the YSZ relative to

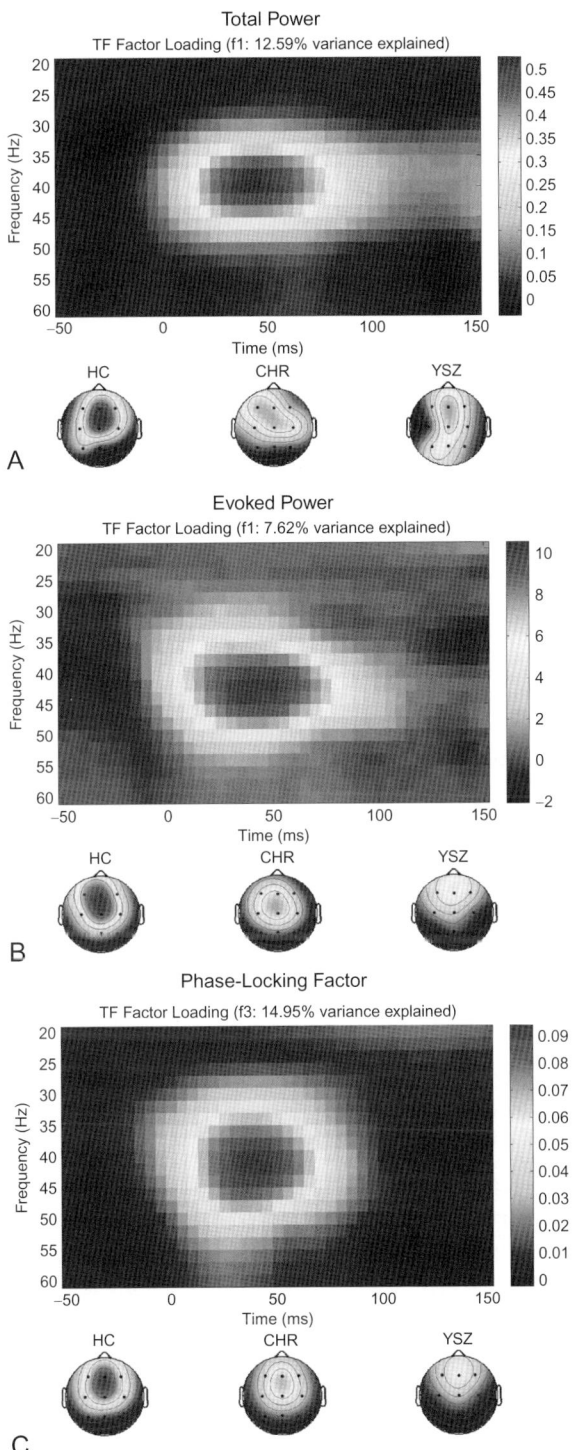

Fig. 1. GBR factor loadings. Time-frequency (TF) factor loadings are plotted from a principal component analysis (PCA) with varimax rotation for (A) total power, (B) evoked power, and (C) phase-locking factor gamma-band responses (GBR). Time (ms) is plotted on the *x*-axis; EEG frequency (Hz) is plotted on the *y*-axis. Stimulus onset occurred at 0 ms. Below each TF plot, scalp topography maps for each group (healthy control (HC), clinical high risk (CHR), and young schizophrenia (YSZ)) show a fronto-central distribution for each GBR across groups. YSZ shows reduced GBRs relative to HC. CHR is intermediate to the HC and YSZ groups. Scaling was uniform across groups. Greater total power and evoked power GBRs, and greater phase-locking consistency across trials, are shown in hot colors (red), as indicated on the color scale to the right of each TF plot. (For color figures, please refer to the color figures in last section of the book.)

156

TABLE 2

GROUP DIFFERENCES ON MEASURES OF GAMMA-BAND RESPONSE[a]

ANOVA Results (HC, CHR, YSZ)	Cohen's d	df	F	p value
Group analyses for age-corrected total power gamma-band response				
Group		2, 101	1.72	0.19
Site (Fz, Cz)		1, 101	0.00	0.98
Group × site		2, 101	1.1	0.34
Planned group comparisons				
HC vs. YSZ	0.431			0.072
HC vs. CHR	0.088			0.687
Group analyses for age-corrected evoked power gamma-band response				
Group		2, 101	5.45	**0.006**
Site (Fz, Cz)		1, 101	0.001	0.97
Group × site		2, 101	0.901	0.41
Planned group comparisons:				
HC vs. YSZ	0.688			**0.004**
HC vs. CHR	0.503			**0.011**
Group analyses for age-corrected phase-locking factor of the gamma-band response				
Group		2, 101	4.51	**0.013**
Site (Fz, Cz)		1, 101	0.00	0.99
Group × site		2, 101	1.36	0.26
Planned group comparisons				
HC vs. YSZ	0.791			**0.005**
HC vs. CHR	0.372			**0.057**

[a]One-way ANOVA comparing young schizophrenia (YSZ), clinical high risk (CHR), and healthy control (HC) groups on age-corrected total power, evoked power, and phase-locking factor principal component analysis (PCA) z-scores in gamma-band responses at Fz and Cz. Simple planned contrasts compared HC to patient groups. Significance based on alpha = 0.05, two-tailed.

the HC group (Cohen's $d = 0.79$; $p = 0.005$). Analyses also revealed marginally reduced age-corrected PLF scores in the CHR relative to the HC group (Cohen's $d = 0.37$; $p = 0.057$).

10.6.6. Converters vs. non-converters

There were no differences between converters and non-converters for total power ($p = 0.83$), evoked power ($p = 0.92$), or PLF ($p = 0.26$).

10.6.7. Demographic differences between groups

Pearson chi-square analysis showed that HC had significantly higher parental socioeconomic status (SES) than both patient groups, which did not differ from each other ($p = 0.62$). Thus, after ruling out group differences in the slopes of the relationships between parental SES and each of the GBR measures (group × parental SES interaction: total power: $p = 0.75$; evoked power: $p = 0.79$; PLF: $p = 0.76$) and dropping

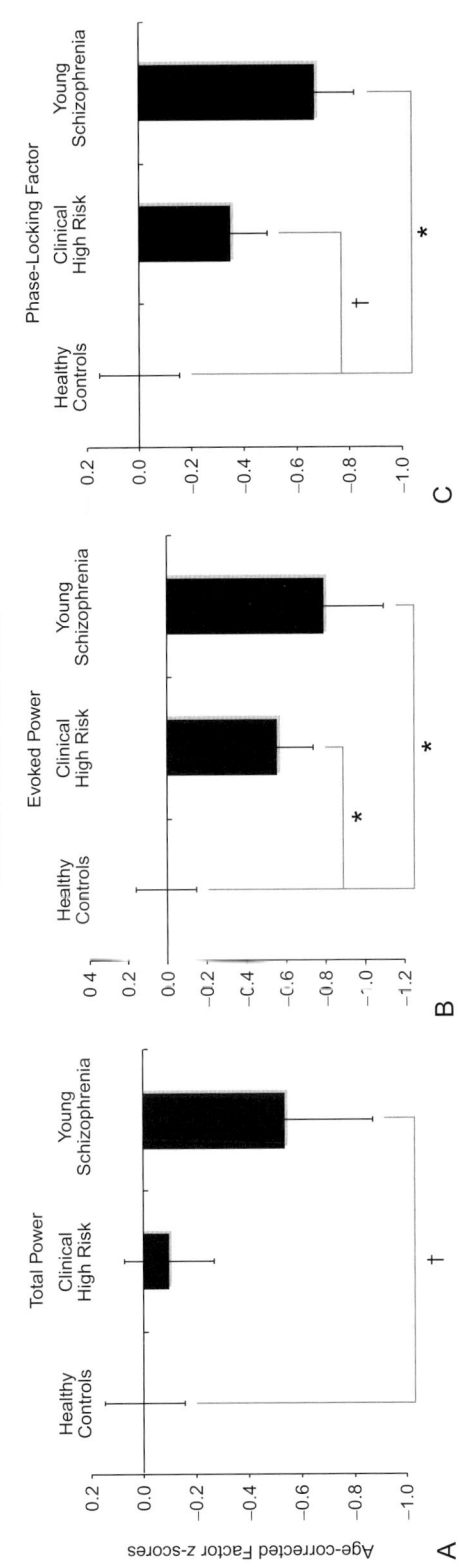

Fig. 2.   Group differences in age-corrected GBR PCA factor scores. Mean ($\pm$ S.E.) age-corrected PCA factor z-scores for the GBR in the healthy control (HC) group, clinical high risk (CHR) group, and young schizophrenia (YSZ) patients to frequent stimuli during the auditory oddball task. In (A), marginal group differences between the YSZ and HC groups for total power are plotted. CHR did not show a difference in total power from HC. In (B), significant CHR and YSZ deviations from HC evoked power are plotted. In (C), YSZ shows reductions in phase-locking factor relative to HC, with a trend for CHR to have reduced values relative to HC. * $p < 0.02$, † $p < 0.08$.

158

the interaction terms, group × site ANCOVAs were performed on each of the GBR measures using parental SES as a covariate. The parental SES effect was not significant for any of the GBR measures (total power: $p = 0.29$; evoked power: $p = 0.65$; PLF: $p = 0.92$), and the group effects were essentially the same as those resulting from the ANOVA models described above.

10.6.8. Correlational analyses with clinical ratings

PANSS positive and negative symptom subscales were not significantly correlated with total power, evoked power, or PLF scores in the YSZ sample. Similarly in the CHR patients, SOPS positive and negative symptom subscales were not significantly correlated with total power, evoked power, or PLF scores.

10.7. Discussion

We examined the early auditory gamma-band response evoked by frequently occurring standard tones from an oddball task, a signal that reflects mechanisms of sensory registration of auditory stimuli (Gurtubay et al., 2001, 2004). Previously, we showed that the early evoked gamma-band response to tones is poorly synchronized in schizophrenia (Roach and Mathalon, 2008) consistent with other reports of abnormalities in the early auditory GBR in chronic schizophrenia patients (for review, see Gandal et al., 2012), first episode patients (Symond et al., 2005; Williams et al., 2009), and unaffected relatives (Hong et al., 2004b; Hall et al., 2011b; Leicht et al., 2011). Here, we replicated earlier studies (Symond et al., 2005; Spencer et al., 2008b;) showing that young schizophrenia patients demonstrate significantly decreased evoked power in the gamma band. Furthermore, patients at clinical high risk for psychosis demonstrated significantly decreased evoked power in the gamma band relative to healthy controls, although the magnitude of the abnormality in gamma-band evoked power was less pronounced

in the CHR patients than in the young schizophrenia patients, as quantified by the effect sizes. These findings are consistent with other findings of reduced evoked power GBRs in unaffected co-twins of patients with schizophrenia (Hall et al., 2011b) and suggest that reduced auditory evoked gamma power may reflect the risk for developing schizophrenia.

Another aim of this study was to assess patients on the phase synchrony of the GBR using PLF. Consistent with other studies of older chronic patients (Slewa-Younan et al., 2004; Roach and Mathalon, 2008; Spencer et al., 2009; Mulert et al., 2011; Roach et al., 2013), the current study showed significantly diminished PLF of the GBR in young schizophrenia patients. Interestingly, marginal deficits in GBR phase consistency were present in CHR patients, where the degree of reduction in gamma synchrony was intermediate to healthy controls and young schizophrenia patients. Our findings of an intermediate effect in the at-risk group relative to healthy controls and schizophrenia patients are similar to findings in the literature (e.g., Brockhaus-Dumke et al., 2005, 2008b; van der Stelt et al., 2005; Perez et al., 2011a) reporting that CHR groups demonstrate intermediate effects that are not statistically distinguishable from either comparison group (i.e., the HC or SZ groups). In light of this, the nearly significant reduction of gamma PLF in the CHR patients suggests that deficient early auditory gamma-band phase synchrony predates the onset of schizophrenia.

Very few of the previously published GBR studies of patients with schizophrenia (Krishnan et al., 2009) examined the combination of synchronous and asynchronous neural activity by reporting total power. Accordingly, our study, which includes the total power GBR in schizophrenia patients and patients at risk for developing psychosis, represents a significant extension of prior studies. The fact that total gamma power was not reduced in CHR patients, and only showed a trend toward reduction in our young schizophrenia patients, suggests that the magnitude of early auditory gamma-band activity is relatively spared early in the course of schizophrenia. Moreover, this lack of total power deficit suggests that the significant evoked gamma power reduction in the patients mainly resulted from poor gamma phase synchrony across trials rather than from reduced magnitude of the gamma oscillations.

Unlike the results of the current study, a significant reduction of early auditory gamma total power was observed in a sample of chronic schizophrenia patients, along with significant reductions in phase synchrony (Roach et al., this volume). Many factors may contribute to this apparent discrepancy between the findings from these two studies from our laboratory, including the fact that total power measurements in the gamma range are hampered by a relatively poor signal-to-noise ratio compared to evoked power measurements. This is due to the inherently greater noise present in single trial EEG epochs relative to the ERP derived by averaging them. However, another possibility is that reduction in the magnitude of early auditory gamma oscillations is a late developing abnormality that is only evident robustly in chronic schizophrenia patients, whereas reduced gamma phase synchrony and associated reductions in evoked gamma power are present early in the illness course, possibly even before illness onset during the prodromal period. While speculative, this hypothesis is consistent with the idea that the mechanisms subserving the phase synchronization of gamma oscillations with respect to an auditory stimulus are dissociable from the mechanisms governing the magnitude of these oscillations. Moreover, to the extent that the magnitude of gamma oscillations depends on the quantity or extent of underlying neural networks in the cortex, the emergence of deficient gamma oscillation magnitudes in chronic patients is consistent with accumulating longitudinal MRI evidence of progressive gray matter volume loss over the illness course of schizophrenia (e.g., De Lisi, 1999; Mathalon et al., 2001; Hulshoff Pol and Kahn, 2008; Andreasen et al., 2011).

Attenuated GBRs were not related to positive or negative symptoms in young schizophrenia or CHR patients. This finding is consistent with some (Haig et al., 2000b), but not all (Leicht et al., 2010; Hall

et al., 2011b), prior efforts to relate abnormal oscillations in the gamma frequency range to symptoms. It is worth noting, however, that some studies have found relationships between diminished gamma response and "treatment-resistant" symptoms including disorganization (Gordon et al., 2001) and psychomotor poverty (Gordon et al., 2001; Lee et al., 2003). Additional studies have reported associations between reductions in gamma and disrupted perceptual (Johannesen et al., 2008) and cognitive ability (Uhlhaas et al., 2006), including impaired working memory (Winterer et al., 2004; Light et al., 2006). However, other studies have reported unexpected correlations between *enlarged* gamma-band response and positive symptoms (Lee et al., 2003; Spencer et al., 2004, 2008b, 2009; Uhlhaas et al., 2006; Hirano et al., 2008). Further clarification is needed about whether the same clinical and cognitive abnormalities are associated with different gamma measures (e.g., total power vs. evoked power vs. intertrial phase coherence). Thus, whether the gamma-band abnormalities are a general characteristic of schizophrenia or are more specifically associated with certain symptom domains remains unclear.

The present findings of abnormal gamma-band responses in CHR patients that are intermediate between young schizophrenia patients and healthy controls indicate that these abnormalities predate psychosis onset, at least in a subset of CHR patients. While the pathophysiological mechanisms giving rise to these gamma-band abnormalities remain to be elucidated, it is reasonable to hypothesize that these mechanisms involve dysfunction of the GABAergic and NMDA glutamatergic microcircuitry known to subserve gamma oscillations (Sohal et al., 2009; Carlen et al., 2011) that have already been implicated in the pathophysiology of schizophrenia (Benes, 2000; Doheny et al., 2000; Hashimoto et al., 2003; Lewis et al., 2005, 2008, 2011; Gonzalez-Burgos and Lewis, 2008; Roopun et al., 2008; Gonzalez-Burgos et al., 2010). In line with previous studies reporting impaired GBR measures in unaffected siblings (Leicht et al., 2011) and unaffected co-twins of schizophrenia patients (Hall et al., 2011b), the current findings suggest that abnormal early auditory gamma-band response may be a biomarker reflecting the clinical risk for the development of psychosis. However, we did not find abnormal gamma-band responses to predict conversion to psychosis among CHR patients. While the lack of a converter vs. non-converter effect may indicate that abnormal gamma-band responses reflect clinical vulnerability for psychosis, with other factors determining whether a psychotic disorder subsequently develops, larger sample sizes are needed to address this question definitively. Such large sample CHR studies are currently underway (e.g., Cannon et al., 2008).

References

Andreasen, N.C., Nopoulos, P., Magnotta, V., Pierson, R., Ziebell, S. and Ho, B.C. (2011) Progressive brain change in schizophrenia: a prospective longitudinal study of first-episode schizophrenia. *Biol. Psychiatry*, 70: 672–679.

Başar, E., Başar-Eroğlu, C., Karakas, S. and Schurmann, M. (2000) Brain oscillations in perception and memory. *Int. J. Psychophysiol.*, 35: 95–124.

Başar-Eroğlu, C. and Başar, E. (1991) A compound P300–40 Hz response of the cat hippocampus. *Int. J. Neurosci.*, 60: 227–237.

Başar-Eroğlu, C., Schmiedt-Fehr, C., Mathes, B., Zimmermann, J. and Brand, A. (2009) Are oscillatory brain responses generally reduced in schizophrenia during long sustained attentional processing? *Int. J. Psychophysiol.*, 71: 75–83.

Benes, F.M. (2000) Emerging principles of altered neural circuitry in schizophrenia. *Brain Res. Rev.*, 31: 251–269.

Bernat, E.M., Williams, W.J. and Gehring, W.J. (2005) Decomposing ERP time-frequency energy using PCA. *Clin. Neurophysiol.*, 116: 1314–1334.

Blumenfeld, L.D. and Clementz, B.A. (2001) Response to the first stimulus determines reduced auditory evoked response suppression in schizophrenia: single trials analysis using MEG. *Clin. Neurophysiol.*, 112: 1650–1659.

Bodatsch, M., Ruhrmann, S., Wagner, M., Muller, R., Schultze-Lutter, F., Frommann, I., Brinkmeyer, J., Gaebel, W., Maier, W., Klosterkotter, J. and Brockhaus-Dumke, A. (2011) Prediction of psychosis by mismatch negativity. *Biol. Psychiatry*, 69: 959–966.

Brenner, C.A., Kieffaber, P.D., Clementz, B.A., Johannesen, J.K., Shekhar, A., O'Donnell, B.F. and Hetrick, W.P. (2009) Event-related potential abnormalities in schizophrenia: a failure to "gate in" salient information? *Schizophr. Res.*, 113: 332–338.

Brockhaus-Dumke, A., Tendolkar, I., Pukrop, R., Schultze-Lutter, F., Klosterkotter, J. and Ruhrmann, S. (2005) Impaired mismatch negativity generation in prodromal subjects and patients with schizophrenia. *Schizophr. Res.*, 73: 297–310.

Brockhaus-Dumke, A., Mueller, R., Faigle, U. and Klosterkoetter, J. (2008a) Sensory gating revisited: relation between brain oscillations and auditory evoked potentials in schizophrenia. *Schizophr. Res.*, 99: 238–249.

Brockhaus-Dumke, A., Schultze-Lutter, F., Mueller, R., Tendolkar, I., Bechdolf, A., Pukrop, R., Klosterkoetter, J. and Ruhrmann, S. (2008b) Sensory gating in schizophrenia: P50 and N100 gating in antipsychotic-free subjects at risk, first-episode, and chronic patients. *Biol. Psychiatry*, 64: 376–384.

Cannon, T.D. (2008) Neurodevelopment and the transition from schizophrenia prodrome to schizophrenia: research imperatives. *Biol. Psychiatry*, 64: 737–738.

Cannon, T.D., Cadenhead, K., Cornblatt, B., Woods, S.W., Addington, J., Walker, E., Seidman, L.J., Perkins, D., Tsuang, M., McGlashan, T. and Heinssen, R. (2008) Prediction of psychosis in youth at high clinical risk: a multisite longitudinal study in North America. *Arch. Gen. Psychiatry*, 65: 28–37.

Carlen, M., Meletis, K., Siegle, J.H., Cardin, J.A., Futai, K., Vierling-Claassen, D., Ruhlmann, C., Jones, S.R., Deisseroth, K., Sheng, M., Moore, C.I. and Tsai, L.H. (2011) A critical role for NMDA receptors in parvalbumin interneurons for gamma rhythm induction and behavior. *Mol. Psychiatry*, Epub ahead of print 5 April 2011.

Cho, R.Y., Konecky, R.O. and Carter, C.S. (2006) Impairments in frontal cortical gamma synchrony and cognitive control in schizophrenia. *Proc. Natl. Acad. Sci. USA*, 103: 19878–19883.

Clementz, B.A., Blumenfeld, L.D. and Cobb, S. (1997) The gamma band response may account for poor P50 suppression in schizophrenia. *NeuroReport*, 8: 3889–3893.

Crovitz, H.F. and Zener, K. (1962) A group-test for assessing hand- and eye-dominance. *Am J Psychol.*, 75: 271–276.

Debener, S., Herrmann, C.S., Kranczioch, C., Gembris, D. and Engel, A.K. (2003) Top-down attentional processing enhances auditory evoked gamma band activity. *NeuroReport*, 14: 683–686.

De Lisi, L.E. (1999) Regional brain volume change over the lifetime course of schizophrenia. *J. Psychiat. Res.*, 33: 535–541.

Delorme, A. and Makeig, S. (2004) EEGLAB: an open source toolbox for analysis of single-trial EEG dynamics including independent component analysis. *J. Neurosci. Meth.*, 134: 9–21.

Doheny, H.C., Faulkner, H.J., Gruzelier, J.H., Baldeweg, T. and Whittington, M.A. (2000) Pathway-specific habituation of induced gamma oscillations in the hippocampal slice. *NeuroReport*, 11: 2629–2633.

Engel, A.K., Fries, P. and Singer, W. (2001) Dynamic predictions: oscillations and synchrony in top-down processing. *Nat. Rev. Neurosci.*, 2: 704–716.

Ford, J.M., White, P., Lim, K.O. and Pfefferbaum, A. (1994) Schizophrenics have fewer and smaller P300s: a single-trial analysis. *Biol. Psychiatry*, 35: 96–103.

Gallinat, J., Winterer, G., Herrmann, C.S. and Senkowski, D. (2004) Reduced oscillatory gamma-band responses in unmedicated schizophrenic patients indicate impaired frontal network processing. *Clin. Neurophysiol.*, 115: 1863–1874.

Gandal, M.J., Edgar, J.C., Klook, K. and Siegel, S.J. (2012) Gamma synchrony: towards a translational biomarker for the treatment-resistant symptoms of schizophrenia. *Neuropharmacology*, 62: 1504–1518.

Gonzalez-Burgos, G. and Lewis, D.A. (2008) GABA neurons and the mechanisms of network oscillations: implications for understanding cortical dysfunction in schizophrenia. *Schizophr. Bull.*, 34: 944–961.

Gonzalez-Burgos, G., Hashimoto, T. and Lewis, D.A. (2010) Alterations of cortical GABA neurons and network oscillations in schizophrenia. *Curr. Psychiatry Rep.*, 12: 335–344.

Gordon, E., Williams, L.M., Haig, A., Wright, J. and Meares, R.A. (2001) Symptom profile and "gamma" processing in schizophrenia. *Cogn. Neuropsychiatry*, 6: 7–19.

Gratton, G., Coles, M.G. and Donchin, E. (1983) A new method for off-line removal of ocular artifact. *Electroenceph. Clin. Neurophysiol.*, 55: 468–484.

Gurtubay, I.G., Alegre, M., Labarga, A., Malanda, A., Iriarte, J. and Artieda, J. (2001) Gamma band activity in an auditory oddball paradigm studied with the wavelet transform. *Clin. Neurophysiol.*, 112: 1219–1228.

Gurtubay, I.G., Alegre, M., Labarga, A., Malanda, A. and Artieda, J. (2004) Gamma band responses to target and non-target auditory stimuli in humans. *Neurosci. Lett.*, 367: 6–9.

Haig, A.R., Gordon, E., Wright, J.J., Meares, R.A. and Bahramali, H. (2000a) Synchronous cortical gamma-band activity in task-relevant cognition. *NeuroReport*, 11: 669–675.

Haig, A.R., Gordon, E., De Pascalis, V., Meares, R.A., Bahramali, H. and Harris, A. (2000b) Gamma activity in schizophrenia: evidence of impaired network binding? *Clin. Neurophysiol.*, 111: 1461–1468.

Hall, M.H., Taylor, G., Salisbury, D.F. and Levy, D.L. (2011a) Sensory gating event-related potentials and oscillations in schizophrenia patients and their unaffected relatives. *Schizophr. Bull.*, 37: 1187–1199.

Hall, M.H., Taylor, G., Sham, P., Schulze, K., Rijsdijk, F., Picchioni, M., Toulopoulou, T., Ettinger, U., Bramon, E., Murray, R.M. and Salisbury, D.F. (2011b) The early auditory gamma-band response is heritable and a putative endophenotype of schizophrenia. *Schizophr. Bull.*, 37: 778–787.

Hashimoto, T., Volk, D.W., Eggan, S.M., Mirnics, K., Pierri, J.N., Sun, Z., Sampson, A.R. and Lewis, D.A. (2003) Gene expression deficits in a subclass of GABA neurons in the prefrontal cortex of subjects with schizophrenia. *J. Neurosci.*, 23: 6315–6326.

Hirano, S., Hirano, Y., Maekawa, T., Obayashi, C., Oribe, N., Kuroki, T., Kanba, S. and Onitsuka, T. (2008) Abnormal neural oscillatory activity to speech sounds in schizophrenia: a magnetoencephalography study. *J. Neurosci.*, 28: 4897–4903.

Hollingshead, A.A. (1975) *Four-Factor Index of Social Status*. Yale University.

Hong, L.E., Summerfelt, A., McMahon, R.P., Thaker, G.K. and Buchanan, R.W. (2004a) Gamma/beta oscillation and sensory gating deficit in schizophrenia. *NeuroReport*, 15: 155–159.

Hong, L.E., Summerfelt, A., McMahon, R., Adami, H., Francis, G., Elliott, A., Buchanan, R.W. and Thaker, G.K. (2004b) Evoked gamma band synchronization and the liability for schizophrenia. *Schizophr. Res.*, 70: 293–302.

Hulshoff Pol, H.E. and Kahn, R.S. (2008) What happens after the first episode? A review of progressive brain changes in chronically ill patients with schizophrenia. *Schizophr. Bull.*, 34: 354–366.

Jahshan, C., Cadenhead, K.S., Rissling, A.J., Kirihara, K., Braff, D.L. and Light, G.A. (2012) Automatic sensory

information processing abnormalities across the illness course of schizophrenia. *Psychol. Med.*, 42: 85–97.

Johannesen, J.K., Bodkins, M., O'Donnell, B.F., Shekhar, A. and Hetrick, W.P. (2008) Perceptual anomalies in schizophrenia co-occur with selective impairments in the gamma frequency component of midlatency auditory ERPs. *J. Abnorm. Psychol.*, 117: 106–118.

Kay, S. and Opler, L. (1987) The positive-negative dimension in schizophrenia: its validity and significance. *Psychiatr. Dev.*, 5: 79–103.

Kayser, J. and Tenke, C.E. (2003) Optimizing PCA methodology for ERP component identification and measurement: theoretical rationale and empirical evaluation. *Clin. Neurophysiol.*, 114: 2307–2325.

Krishnan, G.P., Hetrick, W.P., Brenner, C.A., Shekhar, A., Steffen, A.N. and O'Donnell, B.F. (2009) Steady state and induced auditory gamma deficits in schizophrenia. *Neuroimage*, 47: 1711–1719.

Kwon, J.S., O'Donnell, B.F., Wallenstein, G.V., Greene, R.W., Hirayasu, Y., Nestor, P.G., Hasselmo, M.E., Potts, G.F., Shenton, M.E. and McCarley, R.W. (1999) Gamma frequency-range abnormalities to auditory stimulation in schizophrenia. *Arch. Gen. Psychiatry*, 56: 1001–1005.

Lee, K.H., Williams, L.M., Haig, A. and Gordon, E. (2003) "Gamma (40 Hz) phase synchronicity" and symptom dimensions in schizophrenia. *Cogn. Neuropsychiatry*, 8: 57–71.

Leicht, G., Kirsch, V., Giegling, I., Karch, S., Hantschk, I., Möller, H.J., Pogarell, O., Hegerl, U., Rujescu, D. and Mulert, C. (2010) Reduced early auditory evoked gamma-band response in patients with schizophrenia. *Biol. Psychiatry*, 67: 224–231.

Leicht, G., Karch, S., Karamatskos, E., Giegling, I., Möller, H.J., Hegerl, U., Pogarell, O., Rujescu, D. and Mulert, C. (2011) Alterations of the early auditory evoked gamma-band response in first-degree relatives of patients with schizophrenia: hints to a new intermediate phenotype. *J. Psychiat. Res.*, 45: 699–705.

Lenz, D., Fischer, S., Schadow, J., Bogerts, B. and Herrmann, C.S. (2011) Altered evoked gamma-band responses as a neurophysiological marker of schizophrenia? *Int. J. Psychophysiol.*, 79: 25–31.

Lewis, D.A., Hashimoto, T. and Volk, D.W. (2005) Cortical inhibitory neurons and schizophrenia. *Nat. Rev. Neurosci.*, 6: 312–324.

Lewis, D.A., Cho, R.Y., Carter, C.S., Eklund, K., Forster, S., Kelly, M.A. and Montrose, D. (2008) Subunit-selective modulation of GABA type A receptor neurotransmission and cognition in schizophrenia. *Am. J. Psychiatry*, 165: 1585–1593.

Lewis, D.A., Fish, K.N., Arion, D. and Gonzalez-Burgos, G. (2011) Perisomatic inhibition and cortical circuit dysfunction in schizophrenia. *Curr. Opin. Neurobiol.*, 21: 866–872.

Light, G.A., Hsu, J.L., Hsieh, M.H., Meyer-Gomes, K., Sprock, J., Swerdlow, N.R. and Braff, D.L. (2006) Gamma band oscillations reveal neural network cortical coherence dysfunction in schizophrenia patients. *Biol. Psychiatry*, 60: 1231–1240.

Mathalon, D.H., Sullivan, E.V., Lim, K.O. and Pfefferbaum, A. (2001) Progressive brain volume changes and the clinical course of schizophrenia in men: a longitudinal magnetic resonance imaging study. *Arch. Gen. Psychiatry*, 58: 148–157.

162

Miller, T.J., McGlashan, T.H., Rosen, J.L., Somjee, L., Markovich, P.J., Stein, K. and Woods, S.W. (2002) Prospective diagnosis of the initial prodrome for schizophrenia based on the structured interview for prodromal syndromes: preliminary evidence of interrater reliability and predictive validity. *Am. J. Psychiatry*, 159: 863–865.

Mulert, C., Kirsch, V., Pascual-Marqui, R., McCarley, R.W. and Spencer, K.M. (2011) Long-range synchrony of gamma oscillations and auditory hallucination symptoms in schizophrenia. *Int. J. Psychophysiol.*, 79: 55–63.

Pantev, C., Makeig, S., Hoke, M., Galambos, R., Hampson, S. and Gallen, C. (1991) Human auditory evoked gamma-band magnetic fields. *Proc. Natl. Acad. Sci. USA*, 88: 8996–9000.

Perez, V.B., Ford, J.M., Roach, B.J., Loewy, R.L., Stuart, B.K., Vinogradov, S. and Mathalon, D.H. (2011a) Auditory cortex responsiveness during talking and listening: early illness schizophrenia and patients at clinical high-risk for psychosis. *Schizophr. Bull.* Epub ahead of print 11 October 2011.

Perez, V.B., Ford, J.M., Woods, S.W., McGlashan, T.H., Srihari, V.H., Roach, B.J., Loewy, R.L., Vinogradov, S. and Mathalon, D.H. (2011b) Error monitoring dysfunction across the illness course of schizophrenia. *J. Abnorm. Psychol.* Epub ahead of print 7 November 2011.

Pfefferbaum, A., Lim, K.O., Zipursky, R.B., Mathalon, D.H., Rosenbloom, M.J., Lane, B., Ha, C.N. and Sullivan, E.V. (1992) Brain gray and white matter volume loss accelerates with aging in chronic alcoholics: a quantitative MRI study. *Alcohol Clin. Exp. Res.*, 16: 1078–1089.

Roach, B.J. and Mathalon, D.H. (2008) Event-related EEG time-frequency analysis: an overview of measures and an analysis of early gamma band phase locking in schizophrenia. *Schizophr. Bull.*, 34: 907–926.

Roach, B.J., Ford, J.M., Hoffman, R.E. and Mathalon, D.H. (2013) Converging evidence for gamma synchrony deficits in schizophrenia. *Suppl. Clin. Neurophysiol.*, 62: Ch. 11 (this volume).

Roopun, A.K., Cunningham, M.O., Racca, C., Alter, K., Traub, R.D. and Whittington, M.A. (2008) Region-specific changes in gamma and beta$_2$ rhythms in NMDA receptor dysfunction models of schizophrenia. *Schizophr. Bull.*, 34: 962–973.

Shin, K.S., Kim, J.S., Kang, D.H., Koh, Y., Choi, J.S., O'Donnell, B.F., Chung, C.K. and Kwon, J.S. (2009) Pre-attentive auditory processing in ultra-high-risk for schizophrenia with magnetoencephalography. *Biol. Psychiatry*, 65: 1071–1078.

Singer, W. (1999) Neuronal synchrony: a versatile code for the definition of relations? *Neuron*, 24, 49–65: 111–125.

Slewa-Younan, S., Gordon, E., Harris, A.W., Haig, A.R., Brown, K.J., Flor-Henry, P. and Williams, L.M. (2004) Sex differences in functional connectivity in first-episode and chronic schizophrenia patients. *Am. J. Psychiatry*, 161: 1595–1602.

Sohal, V.S., Zhang, F., Yizhar, O. and Deisseroth, K. (2009) Parvalbumin neurons and gamma rhythms enhance cortical circuit performance. *Nature (Lond.)*, 459: 698–702.

Spencer, K.M., Nestor, P.G., Niznikiewicz, M.A., Salisbury, D.F., Shenton, M.E. and McCarley, R.W. (2003) Abnormal neural synchrony in schizophrenia. *J. Neurosci.*, 23: 7407–7411.

Spencer, K.M., Nestor, P.G., Perlmutter, R., Niznikiewicz, M.A., Klump, M.C., Frumin, M., Shenton, M.E. and McCarley, R.W. (2004) Neural synchrony indexes disordered perception and cognition in schizophrenia. *Proc. Natl. Acad. Sci. USA*, 101: 17288–17293.

Spencer, K.M., Salisbury, D.F., Shenton, M.E. and McCarley, R.W. (2008a) Gamma-band auditory steady-state responses are impaired in first episode psychosis. *Biol. Psychiatry*, 64: 369–375.

Spencer, K.M., Niznikiewicz, M.A., Shenton, M.E. and McCarley, R.W. (2008b) Sensory-evoked gamma oscillations in chronic schizophrenia. *Biol. Psychiatry*, 63: 744–747.

Spencer, K.M., Niznikiewicz, M.A., Nestor, P.G., Shenton, M.E. and McCarley, R.W. (2009) Left auditory cortex gamma synchronization and auditory hallucination symptoms in schizophrenia. *BMC Neurosci.*, 10: 85.

Symond, M.P., Harris, A.W., Gordon, E. and Williams, L.M. (2005) "Gamma synchrony" in first-episode schizophrenia: a disorder of temporal connectivity? *Am. J. Psychiatry*, 162: 459–465.

Tallon-Baudry, C., Bertrand, O., Delpuech, C. and Permier, J. (1997) Oscillatory gamma-band (30–70 Hz) activity induced by a visual search task in humans. *J. Neurosci.*, 17: 722–734.

Teale, P., Collins, D., Maharajh, K., Rojas, D.C., Kronberg, E. and Reite, M. (2008) Cortical source estimates of gamma band amplitude and phase are different in schizophrenia. *Neuroimage*, 42: 1481–1489.

Tiitinen, H., Sinkkonen, J., Reinikainen, K., Alho, K., Lavikainen, J. and Näätänen, R. (1993) Selective attention enhances the auditory 40-Hz transient response in humans. *Nature (Lond.)*, 364: 59–60.

Uhlhaas, P.J. and Singer, W. (2010) Abnormal neural oscillations and synchrony in schizophrenia. *Nat. Rev. Neurosci.*, 11: 100–113.

Uhlhaas, P.J., Linden, D.E., Singer, W., Haenschel, C., Lindner, M., Maurer, K. and Rodriguez, E. (2006) Dysfunctional long-range coordination of neural activity during Gestalt perception in schizophrenia. *J. Neurosci.*, 26: 8168–8175.

Van der Stelt, O., Lieberman, J.A. and Belger, A. (2005) Auditory P300 in high-risk, recent-onset and chronic schizophrenia. *Schizophr. Res.*, 77: 309–320.

Van Tricht, M.J., Nieman, D.H., Koelman, J.H., Van der Meer, J.N., Bour, L.J., De Haan, L. and Linszen, D.H. (2010) Reduced parietal P300 amplitude is associated with an increased risk for a first psychotic episode. *Biol. Psychiatry*, 68: 642–648.

Whittington, M.A., Traub, R.D. and Jefferys, J.G. (1995) Synchronized oscillations in interneuron networks driven by metabotropic glutamate receptor activation. *Nature (Lond.)*, 373: 612–615.

Williams, L.M., Whitford, T.J., Gordon, E., Gomes, L., Brown, K.J. and Harris, A.W. (2009) Neural synchrony in patients with a first episode of schizophrenia: tracking relations with grey matter and symptom profile. *J. Psychiatry Neurosci.*, 34: 21–29.

Winterer, G., Coppola, R., Goldberg, T.E., Egan, M.F., Jones, D.W., Sanchez, C.E. and Weinberger, D.R. (2004) Prefrontal broadband noise, working memory, and genetic risk for schizophrenia. *Am. J. Psychiatry*, 161: 490–500.

Yung, A.R. and McGorry, P.D. (1996) The initial prodrome in psychosis: descriptive and qualitative aspects. *Aust. NZ J. Psychiatry*, 30: 587–599.

Application of Brain Oscillations in Neuropsychiatric Diseases
(Supplements to Clinical Neurophysiology, Vol. 62)
Editors: E. Başar, C. Başar-Eroğlu, A. Özerdem, P.M. Rossini, G.G. Yener

Chapter 11

Converging evidence for gamma synchrony deficits in schizophrenia

B.J. Roach[a,b], J.M. Ford[a,b,c], R.E. Hoffman[d] and D.H. Mathalon[a,b,c,*]

[a]*Northern California Institute for Research and Education, San Francisco, CA 94121, USA*
[b]*Mental Health Service, 116D, VA Medical Center, San Francisco, CA 94121, USA*
[c]*Department of Psychiatry, University of California at San Francisco, San Francisco, CA 94121, USA*
[d]*Department of Psychiatry, Yale University, 300 George Street, New Haven, CT 06511, USA*

ABSTRACT

Background: In electroencephalogram (EEG) studies of auditory steady-state responses (ASSRs), patients with schizophrenia show a deficit in power and/or phase-locking, particularly at the 40 Hz frequency where these responses resonate. In addition, studies of the transient gamma-band response (GBR) elicited by single tones have revealed deficits in gamma power and phase-locking in schizophrenia. We examined the degree to which the 40 Hz ASSR and the transient GBR to single tones are correlated and whether they assess overlapping or distinct gamma-band abnormalities in schizophrenia.
Methods: EEG was recorded during 40 Hz ASSR and auditory oddball paradigms from 28 patients with schizophrenia or schizoaffective disorder (SZ) and 25 age- and gender-matched healthy controls (HC). The ASSR was elicited by 500 ms click trains, and the transient GBR was elicited by the standard tones from the oddball paradigm. Gamma phase and magnitude values, calculated using Morlet wavelet transformations, were used to derive total power and phase-locking measures.
Results: Relative to HC, SZ patients had significant deficits in total gamma power and phase-locking for both ASSR- and GBR-based measures. Within both groups, the 40 Hz ASSR and GBR phase-locking measures were significantly correlated, with a similar trend evident for the total power measures. Moreover, co-varying for GBR substantially reduced 40 Hz ASSR power and phase-locking differences between the groups.
Conclusions: 40 Hz ASSR and transient GBR measures provide very similar information about auditory gamma abnormalities in schizophrenia, despite the overall enhancement of 40 Hz ASSR total power and phase-locking values relative to the corresponding GBR values.

KEYWORDS

Schizophrenia; Gamma; Steady-state gamma-band response; Transient gamma-band response; EEG

11.1. Introduction

Correspondence to: Dr. Daniel H. Mathalon, Ph.D., M.D., Mental Health Service, 116D, San Francisco VA Medical Center, 4150 Clement Street, San Francisco, CA 94121, USA.
Tel.: +1 (415) 221-4810, ext. 3860; Fax: +1 (415) 750-6622;
E-mail: daniel.mathalon@ucsf.edu

The auditory gamma-band response (GBR) is a 40 Hz sinusoidal component that occurs in the first 100 ms of the auditory evoked potential or field in electroencephalographic (EEG) or magneto-encephalographic (MEG) recordings (Başar et al.,

1987; Pantev et al., 1991, 1993). When an auditory stimulus is repeated at a fixed rate or frequency, it drives the auditory steady-state response (ASSR) in EEG/MEG at the same rate (Galambos et al., 1981). Although higher and lower frequencies have been tested, the ASSR reaches a maximum at a 40 Hz repetition rate (Galambos et al., 1981; Pastor et al., 2002; O'Donnell et al., 2004). This maximum could be due to the phase-synchronized overlap of individual GBRs that span 100 ms and linearly summate to produce a peak ASSR amplitude when stimuli are presented every 25 ms (i.e., at a 40 Hz frequency) (Bohorquez and Özdamar, 2008). Alternatively, the 40 Hz ASSR may reflect distinct physiological properties of the circuitry subserving gamma-band oscillations that only emerge when the circuits are externally driven at 40 Hz (Pantev et al., 1993; Ross et al., 2005; Plourde, 2006). Synthetic 40 Hz ASSRs, constructed with auditory GBRs, have been compared to the 40 Hz ASSR in order to address whether they represent physiologically distinct phenomena (Santarelli et al., 1995; Plourde and Villemure, 1996; Bohorquez and Özdamar, 2008; Presacco et al., 2010). However, we are unaware of any study that directly correlated the two measures. In addition, despite multiple reports of abnormal GBR (Hirano et al., 2008; Roach and Mathalon, 2008; Teale et al., 2008; Hall et al., 2009, 2011; Leicht et al., 2010; Lenz et al., 2011) and 40 Hz ASSR (Kwon et al., 1999; Brenner et al., 2003; Light et al., 2006; Spencer et al., 2008b, 2009; Teale et al., 2008; Vierling-Claassen et al., 2008; Wilson et al., 2008; Krishnan et al., 2009; Hamm et al., 2011) in schizophrenia, no study has examined the relationship between these measures in the same patient sample to determine if they reflect distinct pathophysiological processes. Accordingly, the present study examines the relationship between GBR and ASSR in healthy controls and patients with schizophrenia, and further compares the relative sensitivity of these measures to the pathophysiology underlying deficient gamma oscillations in schizophrenia.

The transient auditory GBR to the onset of a sound is of interest to multiple disciplines, including audiology, anesthesiology, cognitive neuroscience, and psychiatry. It was initially viewed as a reflection of sensory registration (Başar, 1972; Pantev et al., 1991), having potential applications in audiology for determining hearing thresholds (Galambos et al., 1981) and in anesthesiology for confirming consciousness (Plourde and Villemure, 1996; Dutton et al., 1999). The auditory GBR latency (20–100 ms) and frequency (40 Hz) overlap with the auditory middle latency response (MLR) (Galambos et al., 1981), but MEG studies have identified separate cortical generators of each (Pantev et al., 1993; Ross et al., 2002). Throughout this text, GBR refers to the transient gamma oscillation that occurs in the MLR temporal window of the auditory evoked potential, which is typically estimated using some form of spectral decomposition to isolate the 40 Hz contribution to the signal. Research showing GBR sensitivity to physical stimulus characteristics (Schadow et al., 2007) as well as attention (Tiitinen et al., 1993; Debener et al., 2003) indicates both bottom-up and top-down influences on this component, broadening potential research applications. As described below, GBR abnormalities have also been observed in schizophrenia.

The ASSR, particularly when the rate of stimulation is 40 Hz, is also relevant to research in various fields. In the first report of the 40 Hz ASSR, Galambos et al. (1981) theorized that the 40 Hz ASSR was nothing more than the sum of overlapping GBRs that can be recorded efficiently by taking advantage of the phase overlap of successive GBRs when stimuli are presented every 25 ms, allowing a large number of stimuli to be presented in a relatively short time period (Galambos et al., 1981). This initially made the measure appealing to audiology and anesthesiology researchers because it was a more efficient method of GBR data collection. However, Galambos' seminal theory of 40 Hz ASSR generation was challenged by converging evidence: failed attempts to build ASSRs synthetically by superimposing GBRs (Santarelli et al., 1995; Plourde and Villemure, 1996); the differential effects of anesthetics on GBRs and ASSRs (Plourde and Villemure, 1996), and MEG evidence of non-overlapping generators in auditory cortex (Pantev et al., 1993; Ross et al., 2002). Moreover, unlike the transient GBR, the ASSR takes 200–300 ms to reach a stable magnitude and is perturbed for more than one gamma cycle if a short noise burst is presented within the driving stimulus (Ross et al., 2005; Krishnan et al., 2009). However, a compelling quantitative approach using low-jitter steady-state stimulation and deconvolution to extract the transient GBR from within the ASSR has provided new support for the overlapping GBR theory of ASSR generation (Bohorquez and Özdamar, 2008; Presacco et al., 2010). Thus, whether the ASSR represents the summation of superimposed GBRs or the two components represent distinct neural phenomena is still a matter of some debate in the literature.

Despite the controversy over its relationship to GBR, the 40 Hz ASSR has continued to be of interest in many disciplines, especially because of the evidence implicating gamma oscillations in the synchronization of neural activity across distributed brain regions (Gray and Singer, 1989) and in the associated coding (Buszáki and Draguhn, 2004) and binding of information necessary for the formation of percepts (Tallon-Baudry et al., 1997). This interest has been particularly prominent in schizophrenia research because of the dependence of gamma-band oscillations on neurotransmitter receptors implicated in the illness, particularly gamma-aminobutryic acid ($GABA_A$) (Impagnatiello et al., 1998; Hashimoto et al., 2003; Lewis et al., 2005, 2008; Deng and Huang, 2006; Gonzalez-Burgos and Lewis, 2008; Sohal et al., 2009) and glutamatergic N-methyl-D-aspartate (NMDA) (Doheny et al., 2000; Krystal et al., 2002; Coyle et al., 2003; Roopun et al., 2008) receptors.

Selective deficits in 40 Hz ASSR in schizophrenia were first reported by Kwon et al. (1999). Subsequent ASSR studies have replicated this reduced 40 Hz ASSR deficit in schizophrenia (see Brenner et al., 2009, for a review) except in one case (Hong et al., 2004). Early auditory GBR abnormalities in schizophrenia were first reported by Clementz et al. (1997), a finding that has been replicated by some but not other subsequent studies (see Gandal et al., 2012, for a review). Both 40 Hz ASSR and GBR abnormalities have been found in the first-degree relatives of schizophrenia patients (Hong et al., 2004; Leicht et al., 2011), suggesting that abnormal gamma oscillations in response to auditory stimuli may be an endophenotypic marker of genetic risk for the illness. Despite this accumulating literature, a few studies have reported both single stimulus GBR and 40 Hz ASSR abnormalities in the same sample of schizophrenia patients (Teale et al., 2008; Krishnan et al., 2009), with no studies to date providing direct comparisons of the two in terms of their sensitivity to schizophrenia. Moreover, no studies have reported on the correlation between the gamma abnormalities obtained from the two methods in the same patient sample. This issue is important because of the evidence described above suggesting that 40 Hz ASSR and the transient auditory GBR may reflect distinct physiological processes.

Accordingly, we asked if the ASSRs elicited by passive, steady-state stimulation at 40 Hz and the transient GBR elicited by a single auditory stimulus converge in patients with schizophrenia and in healthy controls. Furthermore, we asked whether gamma-band oscillation abnormalities in schizophrenia are more pronounced when based on ASSR or GBR measures. Specifically, the following hypotheses were tested: (1) Schizophrenia patients show selective 40 Hz ASSR deficits in EEG power and phase synchrony, relative to 20 and 30 Hz ASSR conditions. (2) Schizophrenia patients show deficits in the power and phase synchrony of the transient GBR to single tones. (3) 40 Hz ASSR and the transient GBR measures are differentially sensitive to the pathophysiology of schizophrenia. (4) However, 40 Hz ASSR and the transient GBR show at least some correlation or convergence in schizophrenia patients and healthy controls. (5) Despite the relationship, the deficits in the 40 Hz ASSR in schizophrenia patients cannot be fully accounted for by their deficits intransient GBR, consistent with the measures being sensitive to at least some distinctive pathophysiological processes.

11.2. Methods and materials

11.2.1. Participants

EEG data were acquired from 33 patients with schizophrenia or schizoaffective disorder and 26 healthy comparison subjects. Data from one patient and one control were excluded due to outlier EEG values (> 3 S.D. above group mean for multiple measures). Four other patients were excluded because more than 30% of trials in one or more conditions were rejected by automated artifact inspection routines. There were 28 patients with schizophrenia ($n = 18$) or schizoaffective disorder ($n = 10$) (SZ) and 25 healthy comparison (HC) subjects remaining. The demographic and clinical data for these subjects are summarized in Table 1.

SZ patients were recruited from inpatient and outpatient services of the Connecticut Mental Health Center and the Veterans Affairs Healthcare System in West Haven, CT, USA. All SZ were on stable doses of antipsychotic medications for at least 2 weeks prior to testing and met DSM-IV criteria for schizophrenia or schizoaffective disorders based either on the diagnosis from a structured clinical interview for DSM-IV (First and Frances, 1995) conducted by a psychiatrist or psychologist, or by consensus of an SCID interview conducted by a trained research assistant and a clinical interview by a psychiatrist or psychologist. Patient symptom severity was assessed using the positive and negative syndrome scale (PANSS) (Kay et al., 1987). SZ were excluded if they met DSM-IV criteria for alcohol or drug abuse within 1 month prior to the recording session. In addition, SZ and HC subjects were excluded for head injuries resulting in a greater than 30 min loss of consciousness, neurological disorders, significant hearing loss in either ear, or other medical illnesses compromising the central nervous system.

HC were recruited by posted advertisements and word-of-mouth, screened by telephone using SCID screening questions (First and Frances, 1995) and excluded for any history of a major Axis I psychiatric disorder based on the SCID. All subjects provided written informed consent to participate in this study approved by the Yale Human Investigation Committee.

11.2.2. Experimental paradigms

11.2.2.1. Auditory steady-state response paradigm
The ASSR paradigm was similar to the one used by Kwon et al. (1999). Subjects were seated comfortably in a sound-attenuated booth and listened to sounds while maintaining visual fixation on a white cross centered on a black screen. The sounds consisted of trains of 1 ms rarefaction clicks presented at a frequency of 20 Hz (9 clicks, 1 every 50 ms), 30 Hz (14 clicks, 1 every 33.33 ms), or 40 Hz (19 clicks, 1 every 25 ms). Each frequency was presented in a separate block of 150 click trains with a 700 ms inter-stimulus interval, using a uniform block order (20, 30, 40 Hz) across subjects. Sounds were delivered via headphones at 80 dB SPL through a STIM audio box (Compumedics Neuroscan).

11.2.2.2. Gamma-band response paradigm
We assessed the transient GBR elicited by the standard tones presented as part of a 3-stimulus auditory oddball task, described in more detail elsewhere (Ford et al., 2008; Mathalon et al., 2010). The high probability ($p = 0.7$) standard stimuli were 500 Hz, 50 ms tones presented with a stimulus-onset asynchrony of 1.25 s 210 times over the course of the task. Sounds were delivered at 80 dB SPL in the manner described above for the ASSR paradigm. In terms of paradigm

TABLE 1

DEMOGRAPHIC AND CLINICAL DATA FOR SCHIZOPHRENIA PATIENTS AND HEALTHY CONTROLS

	Schizophrenia patients ($n = 28$)				Healthy controls ($n = 25$)			
	Mean	S.D.	Min	Max	Mean	S.D.	Min	Max
Age (years)	39.3	10.7	22.1	56.1	36.1	12.5	21.8	59.3
Average parental SES[‡]	33.82	17.4	11	69	33.78	14.7	11	62
Education (years)*	13.7	1.7	10	16	16	2.3	12	20
PANSS[a] positive[†]	15.4	5	7	25				
PANSS negative	14.3	5.2	7	22				
PANSS general	30.4	9.1	17	54				
Race	22 Caucasian, 5 African American, 1 Asian				16 Caucasian, 4 African American, 3 Hispanic, 2 Asian			
Handedness	27 right, 1 left				22 right, 2 left, 1 ambidextrous			
Gender	21 males, 7 females				14 males, 11 females			
Diagnosis	Paranoid schizophrenia (16) Undifferentiated schizophrenia (2) Schizoaffective depressed type (6) Schizoaffective bipolar type (4)							
Antipsychotic medication	2 typical, 20 atypical, 6 both							

[‡]Socioeconomic status (SES) based on Hollingshead scale; higher scores indicate lower socioeconomic status.
*$p < 0.05$ with independent samples t test.
[a]Positive and negative syndrome scale.
[†]Ratings not available for two patients.

order, the auditory oddball task was always presented first, and the ASSR paradigm was always last.

11.2.2.3. EEG acquisition

EEG data were acquired at 1000 Hz from 26 sites (F7, F3, Fz, F4, F8, FT7, FC3, FC4, FT8, T3, C3, Cz, C4, T4, TP7, CP3, CP4, TP8, T5, P3, Pz, P4, T6, O1, Oz, O2), bandpass filtered between 0.05 and 100 Hz, and referenced to linked ears. Additional electrodes were placed on the outer canthi of both eyes and above and below the left eye to record eye movements and blinks (vertical and horizontal electro-oculogram; VEOG, HEOG). All impedances were maintained at or below 10 kΩ throughout the recording session with most EEG sites below 5 kΩ.

Single-trial EEG epochs were stimulus locked to the onset of each click train or standard tone, including data from 300 ms before the start of the sound and 900 ms after it. Individual trials were baseline corrected using the 100 ms period preceding sound onset after correcting for eye movements and blinks using EOG data (Gratton et al., 1983). Finally, trials containing artifacts (voltages exceeding ±75 μV) in any of the central 9 electrodes examined in the present study (F3, Fz, F4, C3, Cz, C4, P3, Pz, or P4) were rejected.

11.2.2.4. EEG time-frequency analysis: phase-locking factor and total power

Time-frequency analysis of EEG single-trial data was done with a Morlet wavelet decomposition using freely distributed FieldTrip (http://fieldtrip.fcdonders.nl/) software in Matlab (http://www.mathworks.com/products/matlab/). This method has been described previously (Tallon-Baudry et al., 1997), but it is important to note the specific parameters used here. The Morlet wavelet has a Gaussian shape that is defined by a ratio ($\sigma_f = f/C$) and a wavelet duration (6 σ_t), where f is the center frequency and $\sigma_t = 1/(2\pi\sigma_f)$. In a classic wavelet analysis, C is a constant, ensuring an equal number of cycles in the mother wavelet for each frequency. Such an approach was used to create wavelets for the GBR analysis, as was done in our prior study (Roach and Mathalon, 2008). In this approach, as the frequency (f) increases, the spectral bandwidth (6 σ_f) increases. In the ASSR analysis, the constant (C) was varied (20 Hz $C = 7$; 30 Hz $C = 10.5$; 40 Hz $C = 14$) such that the spectral bandwidth was equal (6 $\sigma_f = 17.1429$ Hz) at 20, 30, and 40 Hz, minimizing frequency overlap without excessive loss of temporal resolution. For the remaining 1 Hz bins calculated, C was 7 for frequencies less than 20, 14 for frequencies greater than 40, and linearly spaced between 7 and 14 for frequencies between 20 and 40 Hz. This method was used to decompose single-trial time-frequency values between 10 and 100 Hz for the central nine electrodes.

After applying this method, phase-locking factor (PLF) was calculated as 1 minus the circular phase angle variance, as described by Tallon-Baudry et al. (1997). PLF provides a measure of the phase consistency of frequency specific oscillations with respect to stimulus onset across trials on a millisecond basis. In addition, event-related total power was calculated by averaging the squared single-trial magnitude values in each 1 Hz frequency bin on a millisecond basis. The average total power values were $10\log_{10}$ transformed and then baseline corrected by subtracting the average of the pre-stimulus baseline (-100 to 0 ms) from each time point separately for every frequency (Fig. 1). The resulting event-related change in total power values (relative to baseline) is in decibels (dB), as this calculation is equivalent to

$$
\begin{aligned}
\text{Total power}(t,f) &= 10 * \log_{10} \\
&\quad \left(\text{power}_{t,f} / \text{baseline power}_f \right) \\
&= \left(10 * \log_{10} \text{power}_{t,f} \right) \\
&\quad - \left(\log_{10} \sum_{i=-100 \text{ ms}}^{0 \text{ ms}} \text{power}_{i,f} / 100 \right)
\end{aligned}
$$

11.2.3. Statistical analysis

ASSR PLF and total power values were extracted by averaging the data across a 200–400 ms time window in 5 Hz bins centered on 20, 30, and 40 Hz, representing the response at each driving frequency. The time window was selected to capture a stable SSR period between onset and offset of the response. Each of these time-frequency measures was subjected to a 3-way repeated measures analysis of variance (ANOVA) with group (SZ, HC) as a between-subjects factor, and frequency (20, 30, 40 Hz) and lead (Fz, Cz) as within-subjects factors.

Transient GBR PLF and total power values from the time-frequency analysis of oddball task standard tones were extracted by averaging across 35–50 Hz frequencies within the 20–60 ms post-stimulus time window, as done previously (Roach and Mathalon, 2008). Each of these time-frequency measures was subjected to a 2-way repeated measures ANOVA with group (SZ, HC) as the between-subjects factor and lead (Fz, Cz) as the within-subjects factor.

To test the sensitivity of these paradigms to the presence of schizophrenia, 40 Hz ASSR and standard tone GBR time-frequency measures (PLF and total power) were analyzed using a 3-way ANOVA with group (SZ, HC) as the between-subjects factor, and paradigm (ASSR, GBR) and lead (Fz, Cz) as within-subjects factors.

Analysis of covariance (ANCOVA) models were applied to the 40 Hz ASSR measures with

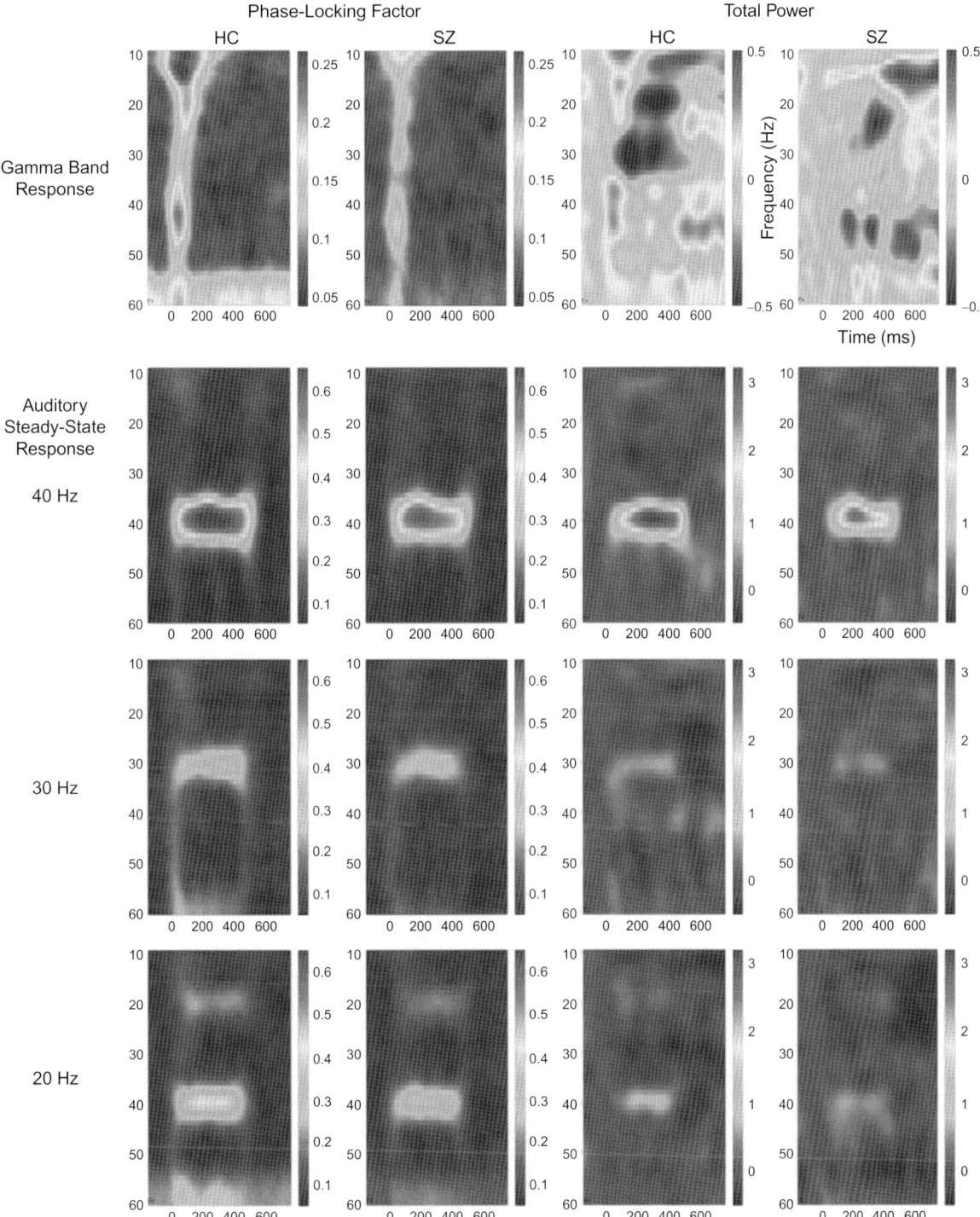

Fig. 1. Grand-average time-frequency maps from 25 healthy controls (HC) and 28 schizophrenia patients (SZ) are plotted with frequencies on the *y*-axis and time on the *x*-axis. Gamma-band responses are plotted on the top row while auditory steady-state responses for 40, 30, and 20 Hz driving conditions are shown on the second, third, and fourth rows, respectively. Dark red colors indicate little phase variance across trials in the first two columns, whereas dark blue colors indicate equally distributed phase variance across trials. In the third and fourth columns, total power data are plotted in decibel (dB) units, with dark red and blue showing magnitude increases or decreases relative to a 100 ms baseline. (For color figures, please refer to the color figures in last section of the book.)

group (SZ, HC) as the between-subjects factor and GBR as the covariate. This was done separately for PLF and total power measures averaged over the two electrodes. After first ruling out significant slope differences between the two groups, the ANCOVA model allowed us to assess (a) whether there was a significant relationship between the 40 Hz ASSR and standard tone GBR and (b) whether the group difference in 40 Hz ASSR persisted after controlling for GBR.

In addition, based on a prior study showing intact or enhanced 40 Hz ASSR power and PLF in patients with schizoaffective disorder (Reite et al., 2010), ANOVA was used to compare the subgroup of schizoaffective disorder (SAD) patients with the remaining SZ patients and the HC subjects on both the 40 Hz ASSR and GBR total power and PLF measures.

To examine relationships between clinical symptoms and gamma-band measures in the SZ group, we conducted Pearson correlations between PANSS positive and negative symptom sub-scale scores and the PLF and total power measures assessed in the 40 Hz ASSR and GBR paradigms.

All p values are Greenhouse–Geisser corrected when appropriate and higher order interactions were parsed with lower order ANOVAs.

11.3. Results

11.3.1. ASSR

Results of the 3-way repeated measures ANOVAs for the PLF and total power measures from the ASSR paradigm are presented in Table 2. Because our focus was on examining group differences in these measures, we primarily describe the highest order significant interaction effects involving

TABLE 2

ANOVA RESULTS FOR AUDITORY STEADY-STATE RESPONSE (ASSR) AND GAMMA-BAND RESPONSE (GBR) PHASE-LOCKING FACTOR (PLF) AND TOTAL POWER

Source	PLF			Total power		
	df	F	p	df	F	p
ASSR						
Group	1, 51	**4.139**	**0.047**	1, 51	3.477	0.068
Frequency	2, 102	**135.541**	**0.000**	2, 102	**82.824**	**0.000**
Group × frequency	2, 102	2.720	0.072	2, 102	**4.225**	**0.033**
20 Hz frequency: group	1, 51	0.131	0.719	1, 51	0.050	0.824
30 Hz frequency: group	1, 51	1.909	0.173	1, 51	0.058	0.810
40 Hz frequency: group	1, 51	**5.298**	**0.025**	1, 51	**4.459**	**0.040**
Lead	1, 51	**75.028**	**0.000**	1, 51	**46.270**	**0.000**
Group × lead	1, 51	2.152	0.148	1, 51	1.438	0.236
Frequency × lead	2, 102	**12.419**	**0.000**	2, 102	**23.394**	**0.000**
Group × frequency × lead	2, 102	0.570	0.558	2, 102	1.145	0.317
GBR						
Group	1, 51	**5.829**	**0.019**	1, 51	**5.773**	**0.020**
Lead	1, 51	**56.823**	**0.000**	1, 51	**17.702**	**0.000**
Group × lead	1, 51	2.978	0.090	1, 51	1.491	0.228

* Significant effects are in bold font.

group or, in the absence of interactions, the main effects of group.

PLF. As can be seen in Table 2, the 3-way frequency × lead × group interaction was not significant. However, there was a trend ($p = 0.072$) toward a significant frequency × group interaction. To parse this interaction, separate ANOVAs were conducted for each frequency. The models examining 20 and 30 Hz driving frequencies revealed no significant group effects, but a significant effect did emerge for the 40 Hz model ($p = 0.025$). This effect was driven by greater 40 Hz ASSR in HC compared to SZ (Fig. 2, left).

There were some additional significant effects worth noting. A significant main effect of frequency indicated, as expected, that 40 Hz driving produces a significantly greater PLF than 30 and 20 Hz driving frequencies ($p < 0.001$), and further, that 30 Hz PLF was significantly greater than 20 Hz PLF ($p < 0.001$). There was a significant lead effect due to greater responses at Fz than Cz ($p < 0.001$). A significant frequency × lead interaction indicated that the stronger Fz PLF relative to Cz PLF was most pronounced for the 40 Hz driving condition.

Total power. Table 2 shows that, like PLF, the 3-way interaction was not significant. However, there was a significant frequency × group interaction. To parse this interaction, separate ANOVAs were conducted for each frequency. The models examining 20 and 30 Hz driving frequencies revealed no significant group effects, but a significant

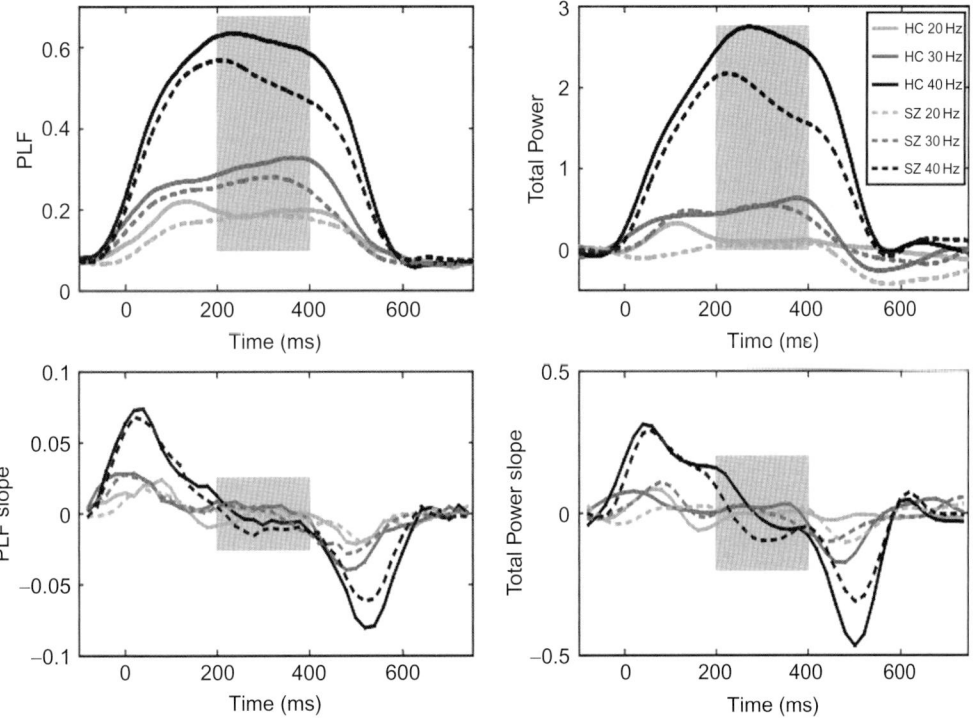

Fig. 2. Healthy control (HC, solid lines) and schizophrenia (SZ, dashed lines) group mean time-frequency data for 40 Hz (black), 30 Hz (green), and 20 Hz (orange) driving conditions are plotted for phase-locking factor (PLF) (left) and total power (right) measures on the top row. The rate of change (i.e., slope) in 20 ms increments from each measure in all conditions are plotted on the bottom row. All values are based on the group average taken in bands ±2 Hz around the stimulated frequency. Gray shading between 200 and 400 ms highlights the period of the auditory steady-state response with greatest stability across all conditions, groups, and measures. (For color figures, please refer to the color figures in last section of the book.)

effect did emerge for the 40 Hz model ($p = 0.04$) due to reduced 40 Hz total power in SZ (Fig. 2, right).

A significant main effect of frequency matched the PLF pattern with significantly greater 40 Hz driving power compared to 30 and 20 Hz driving frequencies ($p < 0.001$), while 30 Hz power was significantly greater than 20 Hz power ($p < 0.001$). Similar to PLF, a significant frequency × lead effect was due to enhanced Fz power relative to Cz, which was most pronounced for the 40 Hz driving condition.

11.3.2. GBR

Results of the 2-way repeated measures ANOVAs for the PLF and total power measures from the GBR paradigm are presented in Table 2.

PLF. There were main effects of group and lead. As previously reported (Roach and Mathalon, 2008), HC showed greater PLF GBRs than SZ, and Fz was greater than Cz ($p < 0.001$), but lead did not interact with group.

Total power. Much like PLF, there was a group difference in total power (HC > SZ). A main effect of lead was driven by greater power at Fz compared to Cz ($p < 0.001$), but lead did not significantly interact with group.

11.3.3. Comparing GBR and ASSR data

Results of the 3-way repeated measures ANOVAs for the PLF and total power from the paradigm comparison are presented in Table 3. We focus on the main effect of paradigm and its interactions below because other effects are redundant with the individual paradigm models.

PLF. There was a main effect of paradigm driven by greater PLF in 40 Hz ASSR compared to GBR. While the group × paradigm interaction failed to reach significance, there was a significant group × paradigm × lead interaction. This interaction was parsed by conducting 2-way ANOVAs for each level of the third factor (Table 3). The main

source of the 3-way interaction was the presence of a significant paradigm × lead interaction in SZ ($p < 0.001$) but not in HC ($p = 0.289$). Inspection of Fig. 3 (bottom left) indicates that in SZ there was a greater drop off in PLF from Fz to Cz for the 40 Hz ASSR paradigm than for the GBR paradigm, resulting in a greater paradigm difference at Fz than at Cz. In contrast, HC showed comparable declines in PLF from Fz to Cz across the two paradigms, resulting in equivalent paradigm effects at each lead. Interestingly, when 2-way group × paradigm ANOVAs were run at each lead, there was only an interaction trend ($p = 0.082$) at Cz and a non-significant interaction at Fz. Thus, while there was a tendency for the group effect at Cz to be larger for the ASSR paradigm ($p = 0.021$) than for the GBR paradigm ($p = 0.045$), the difference was quite modest and failed to reach statistical significance.

Total power. The total power model produced the same paradigm effect as PLF (ASSR > GBR; Fig. 3, right panel). The group × paradigm and group × paradigm × lead interactions both failed to reach significance.

11.3.4. Relationship between GBR and ASSR

PLF. The group difference in the 40 Hz ASSR PLF, controlling for GBR PLF, was assessed using an ANCOVA after ruling out a group difference in the slopes of the ASSR vs. GBR regression lines (group × GBR interaction: $F (1, 49) = 0.644$, $p = 0.426$) and dropping the interaction term from the model. In the resulting model (see Table 4), GBR PLF was directly related to 40 Hz ASSR PLF ($p = 0.018$; Fig. 4, left). Controlling for the GBR, the group effect (i.e., group difference in regression line intercepts shown in Fig. 4, left) did not reach significance ($p = 0.139$).

Total power. After establishing that the ASSR vs. GBR regression line slopes were equivalent between the groups (group × GBR interaction: $F (1, 49) = 0.313$, $p = 0.578$) and dropping the interaction term, an ANCOVA model (see Table 4) examined group differences in 40 Hz ASSR total power while covarying for GBR.

TABLE 3

GROUP × PARADIGM × LEAD ANOVA RESULTS FOR PHASE-LOCKING FACTOR (PLF) AND TOTAL POWER

Source	PLF			Total power		
	df	F	p	df	F	p
Group	1, 51	**7.438**	**0.009**	1, 51	**6.072**	**0.017**
Paradigm	1, 51	**288.057**	**0.000**	1, 51	**123.446**	**0.000**
Group × paradigm	1, 51	2.147	0.149	1, 51	2.592	0.114
Lead	1, 51	**87.630**	**0.000**	1, 51	**56.469**	**0.000**
Group × lead	1, 51	0.287	0.595	1, 51	0.001	0.978
Paradigm × lead	1, 51	**13.708**	**0.001**	1, 51	**38.607**	**0.000**
Group × paradigm × lead	1, 51	**4.696**	**0.035**	1, 51	0.562	0.457
Paradigm × lead in each group						
HC: paradigm × lead	1, 24	1.174	0.289			
SZ: paradigm × lead	1, 27	**17.480**	**0.000**			
SZ Fz: paradigm	1, 27	**163.682**	**0.000**			
SZ Cz: paradigm	1, 27	**73.188**	**0.000**			
Group × paradigm at each lead						
Fz: group × paradigm	1, 51	1.000	0.322			
Cz: group × paradigm	1, 51	3.152	0.082			
Cz GBR: group	1, 51	4.212	**0.045**			
Cz ASSR: group	1, 51	5.681	**0.021**			
Group × lead in each paradigm						
GBR: group × lead	1, 51	2.978	0.090			
ASSR: group × lead	1, 51	2.152	0.148			

* Significant effects are in bold tont.

GBR total power showed a trend toward a significant positive relationship ($p = 0.069$) with ASSR total power (Fig. 4, right). Controlling for this relationship, the group effect (i.e., group difference in regression line intercepts shown in Fig. 4, right) on 40 Hz ASSR total power was not significant ($p = 0.152$).

11.3.5. Schizoaffective disorder subgroup analysis

The ANOVA planned contrasts comparing the subgroup of SAD patients with HC subjects showed significant or trend level reductions in the SAD patients across gamma measures and paradigms (40 Hz ASSR: PLF ($p = 0.032$), total power ($p = 0.073$); GBR: PLF ($p = 0.009$), total power ($p = 0.032$)). The SAD and SZ patient subgroups did not significantly differ from each other on any of the gamma measures (40 Hz ASSR: PLF ($p = 0.444$), total power ($p = 0.531$); GBR: PLF ($p = 0.176$), total power ($p = .394$)).

11.3.6. Symptom correlations

In the SZ patients, PANSS positive and negative symptom sub-scale scores were not significantly correlated with PLF or total power for the 40 Hz ASSR and GBR measures at Fz and Cz (all p values > 0.29).

11.4. Discussion

In this study, we assessed 40 Hz ASSRs and GBRs in patients with schizophrenia (including

174

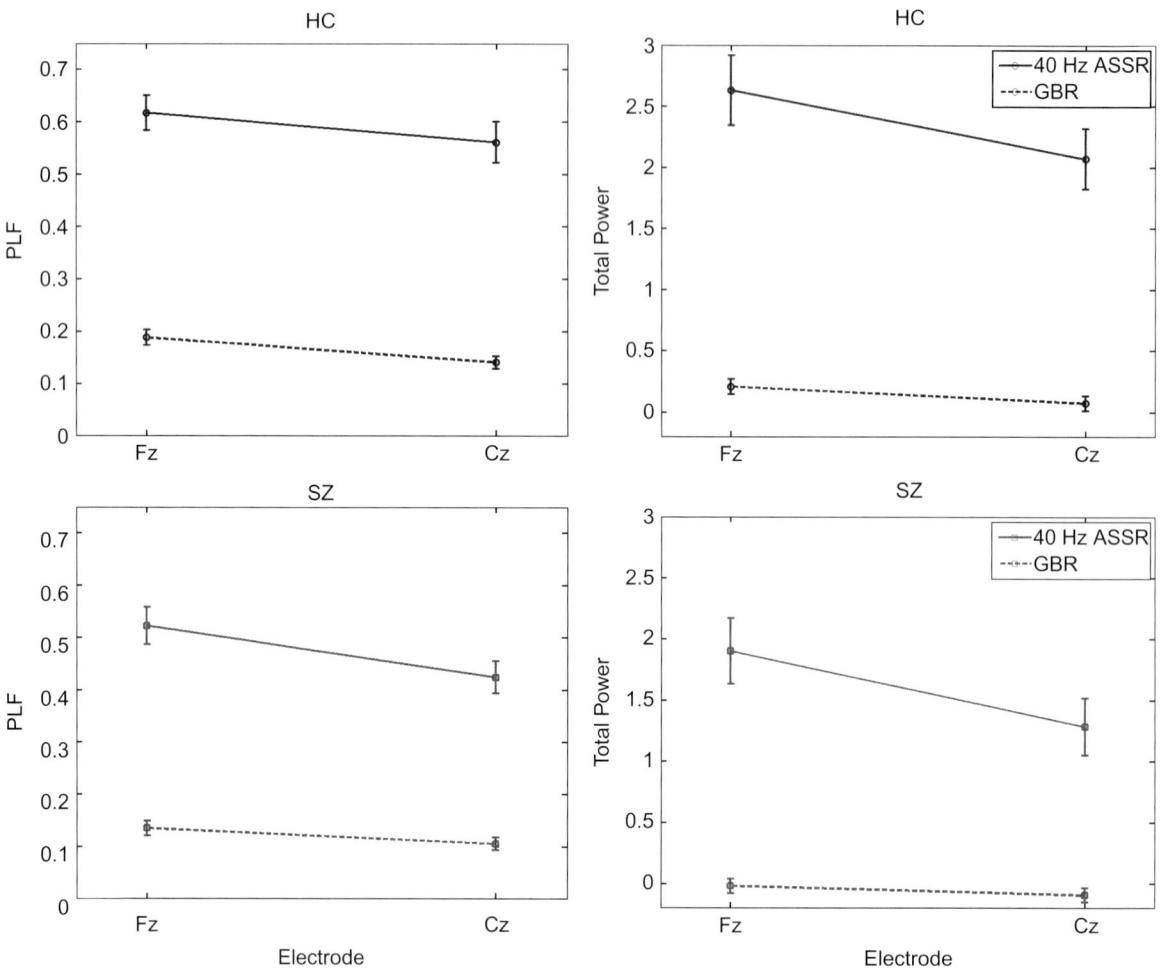

Fig. 3.   Healthy control (HC, blue lines) and schizophrenia (SZ, red lines) group means and standard error bars from gamma-band response (GBR) and 40 Hz auditory steady-state response (ASSR) conditions at electrodes Fz and Cz are plotted for phase-locking factor (PLF) (left) and total power (right). (For color figures, please refer to the color figures in last section of the book.)

schizoaffective patients) and healthy control subjects, comparing the groups on each paradigm and examining the relative sensitivity of each paradigm to schizophrenic pathophysiology. Patients showed abnormal reductions in auditory gamma-band phase synchrony and total power when assessed as an ASSR to 40 Hz click trains or as a GBR to standard tones from an oddball task. These results indicate that schizophrenia is associated with both deficient phase resetting and diminished magnitude of gamma oscillations in response to auditory stimuli. In addition, the

40 Hz ASSR and auditory GBR were only modestly correlated, sharing only about 5–10% of their variance. Despite the limited overlap between the ASSR and GBR measures, they converged in their sensitivity to the pathophysiology of schizophrenia. The equivalent sensitivity to schizophrenia was demonstrated by the lack of a significant group × paradigm interaction as well as the elimination of the 40 Hz ASSR group effect after controlling for auditory GBR differences. Thus, while the 40 Hz ASSR and GBR measures are largely independent,

TABLE 4

GROUP ANCOVA RESULTS FOR 40 HZ AUDITORY STEADY-STATE RESPONSE (ASSR), COVARYING FOR AUDITORY GAMMA-BAND RESPONSE, FOR PHASE-LOCKING FACTOR (PLF) AND TOTAL POWER MEASURES AVERAGED OVER ELECTRODES FZ AND CZ

Source	PLF			Total power		
	df	F	p	df	F	p
GBR	1, 50	**5.952**	**0.018**	1, 50	3.453	0.069
Group	1, 50	2.258	0.139	1, 50	2.121	0.152

* Significant effects are in bold font.

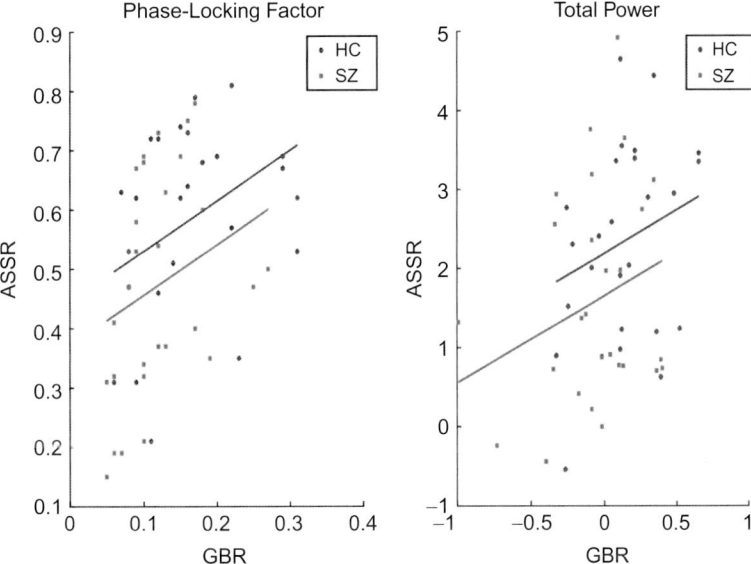

Fig. 4. The relationship between standard tone gamma-band response (GBR: x-axis) and 40 Hz auditory steady-state response (ASSR: y-axis) is illustrated with separate scatter plots for phase-locking factor (PLF, left) and total power (right). Each point represents single subject (schizophrenia (SZ): red square; healthy control (HC): blue circle) data, averaged across 35–50 Hz and 20–60 ms for the GBR or across 38–42 Hz and 200–400 ms for the ASSR. Regression lines are plotted separately using the common slope and separate intercepts for each group (SZ: red; HC: blue) to show the relationship between paradigms for PLF (partial r (controlling for group) = 0.326, p = 0.018) and total power (partial r (controlling for group) = 0.254, p = 0.069). (For color figures, please refer to the color figures in last section of the book.)

they do not appear to provide unique information about auditory gamma oscillation phase consistency or magnitude abnormalities in schizophrenia.

In many respects, our independent ASSR and GBR results are consistent with other studies in the literature. Like most (Light et al., 2006; Spencer et al., 2008b, 2009; Teale et al., 2008; Krishnan et al., 2009), but not all (Hamm et al., 2011), prior reports, we found a reduction in the PLF, or phase consistency across trials, of the 40 Hz ASSR in SZ patients. We also found reduced auditory GBR

PLF, consistent with our prior report (Roach and Mathalon, 2008) from a patient sample that partially overlapped with the current sample, and replicating some (Hirano et al., 2008; Hall et al., 2009; Leicht et al., 2010), but not all (Spencer et al., 2008a; Teale et al., 2008; Krishnan et al., 2009), prior studies. Further, reduced total power in SZ relative to HC in both the 40 Hz ASSR and GBR measures replicates the findings of Krishnan et al. (2009).

A few prior studies have simultaneously examined the 40 Hz ASSR and transient auditory GBR in the same patient sample, and of those that have (Teale et al., 2008; Krishnan et al., 2009), none have directly compared their sensitivity to the SZ effect. We predicted that 40 Hz ASSR power and phase measures would better differentiate SZ from HC than auditory GBR, in part based on the stronger signal (i.e., greater phase synchrony across trials and greater magnitude) associated with the ASSR relative to the GBR paradigm. However, our results failed to support this hypothesis, instead showing the schizophrenia effect sizes to be statistically equivalent for the 40 Hz ASSR and GBR measures. Moreover, although the GBR and 40 Hz ASSR measures were only modestly related for PLF and total power measures, controlling for their shared variance eliminated the significant schizophrenia group difference in the 40 Hz ASSR phase and magnitude. This suggests that it is the physiological mechanisms shared by the GBR and 40 Hz ASSR, rather than the independent aspects of their underlying physiology, that are compromised in schizophrenia.

The relatively small correlation between the GBR and 40 Hz ASSR measures is not consistent with the view, originally proposed by Galambos et al. (1981), that the 40 Hz steady-state response consists of nothing more than overlapping phase synchronized auditory GBRs (also referred to in the time domain as middle-latency responses; MLRs), or similarly, that the 40 Hz ASSR can be constructed by superimposition of MLRs evoked by auditory stimuli spaced roughly 25 ms apart (Bohorquez and Özdamar, 2008). However,

the small correlation between the ASSR and GBR is consistent with other lines of evidence suggesting that the measures are not equivalent. This evidence includes observations that the 40 Hz ASSR takes about 200 ms to plateau and is disrupted for multiple cycles when perturbed with irregular stimulation in the middle of an amplitude-modulated steady-state tone (Ross et al., 2005; Krishnan et al., 2009). Furthermore, even studies of deconvolved and synthetically constructed 40 Hz ASSRs have documented unpredictable onset characteristics in the response that must be further explored (Presacco et al., 2010). Additional evidence of distinct processes contributing to the GBR and ASSR comes from source localization studies implicating different generators of each response in the primary auditory cortex (Pantev et al., 1993; Ross et al., 2002) or ASSR-specific subcortical generators, such as bilateral posterolateral portions of the cerebellar hemispheres (Pastor et al., 2002). In addition, differences in task features in our study may have weakened any intrinsic correlation between the GBR and ASSR measures. Bottom-up modulation of the GBR has been demonstrated by manipulating stimulus intensity (Schadow et al., 2007), raising the possibility that differences between the physical characteristics of the auditory stimuli used in our GBR and ASSR paradigms may have attenuated the correlation between them. Specifically, because of the tonotopic organization of the auditory cortex, the broadband white noise clicks used to elicit ASSRs would be expected to activate a larger neural population than the pure tones used to elicit the GBRs, resulting in greater phase consistency across trials and larger event-related increases in power. Further attenuation of the relationship between the measures could have arisen from the top-down attentional processes directed toward the auditory stream during the oddball task used to assess the GBR, processes that would not have been engaged during the passive presentation of click trains used to assess the ASSR.

Yet another factor that may have attenuated the relationship between the GBR and ASSR is the presence of more noise in the GBR signal relative to the ASSR, which benefits from enhanced signal-to-noise due to the overlapping MLRs. The literature on test–retest reliability of ASSR is limited to clinical studies of hearing levels in audiology research (Kaf et al., 2006), or frequency-based fast Fourier transformation measurements of evoked power (Van Deursen et al., 2011). However, reliability of evoked power and phase consistency across repeated test sessions has been demonstrated in the visual domain (Frund et al., 2007). Future studies are needed to assess test–retest reliability of the PLF and total power of 40 Hz ASSR and GBR since unreliability of one or both measures may account for their modest correlation. Moreover, establishing that these measures are reliable in schizophrenia patients is a prerequisite for using them to track treatment response or illness progression.

A prior study of the 40 Hz ASSR that specifically compared SAD patients to SZ patients and HC found that while SZ patients had abnormally reduced PLF, SAD patients had normal PLF and, further, had greater 40 Hz evoked power than both HC and SZ (Reite et al., 2010). Examining the sub-group of SAD patients included in our patient sample ($n = 10$), we failed to replicate this pattern of results. In our sample, the SAD patients showed significant reductions in both 40 Hz ASSR and GBR PLF relative to HC. Similar effects were observed for the total power measures. In no case did the SAD and SZ patient sub-groups differ from each other. In both the current study and the prior report by Reite et al. (2010), the number of SAD patients was relatively small, suggesting that sampling error may account for the conflicting results between the two studies. However, our results in SAD patients are broadly consistent with reports of 40 Hz ASSR reductions in patients with affective psychoses (Spencer et al., 2008b) and bipolar disorder (O'Donnell et al., 2004), suggesting that disturbances in gamma

oscillations may be associated with psychotic syndromes across the schizophrenia-affective disorder spectrum.

In addition to gamma oscillations in response to auditory stimuli, EEG gamma activity has been implicated in registration of stimuli in other sensory modalities, as well as in higher order cognitive processes like perceptual binding (Tallon-Baudry et al., 1997) and cognitive control (Cho et al., 2006; Lewis et al., 2008; Minzenberg et al., 2010). It remains unclear whether the 40 Hz ASSR and auditory GBR measures of gamma oscillations assessed in the current study are correlated with the gamma activity elicited by stimuli presented in other sensory modalities or during more cognitively demanding tasks. If visual, olfactory and somatosensory GBRs, as well as gamma responses elicited by higher order cognitive tasks, correlate with the auditory GBR, the hypothesis that gamma oscillations measured by EEG reflect ubiquitous pan-cortical assemblies of similar local circuits, such as interneuron–pyramidal cell networks, would be supported. This might suggest that auditory gamma-band measures could serve as proxies for measures of gamma activity across cortical regions, regardless of the sensory system or cognitive process engaged. Arguing against this possibility are the roles attention (Ross et al., 2004; Skosnik et al., 2007) and arousal (Griskova et al., 2007) play in modulating the phase consistency of the 40 Hz ASSR across trials and its event-related change in power. Skosnik et al. (2007) used 20 and 40 Hz steady-state stimuli as frequent and infrequent stimuli in an oddball paradigm, revealing 40 Hz ASSR PLF and evoked power enhancement on 40 Hz targets relative to 40 Hz standards even after matching the trial numbers for each stimulus type. These results support the literature showing gamma-band ASSR enhancement with increased attention (Ross et al., 2004; Bidet-Caulet et al., 2007; Saupe et al., 2009a,b). Thus, if ASSRs or GBRs are a proxy for other methods of eliciting gamma-band responses, attention must be controlled. Krishnan et al. (2009) used a visual task to address potential differences in attention between patient and control groups during passive listening and found phase-locking and power reductions in SZ similar to those described here and elsewhere (Kwon et al., 1999; Brenner et al., 2003; Light et al., 2006; Spencer et al., 2008b, 2009), despite the failure to control attention with a visual distracter task in these latter studies. However, to our knowledge, there have been no studies comparing the ASSR between SZ and HC while explicitly directing subject attention to the auditory stimuli by making them task relevant. Thus, it remains uncertain whether the schizophrenia deficits in the 40 Hz ASSR can be ameliorated by enhancing attention to the auditory stimuli.

All patients in our study were on either typical, atypical, or a combination of typical and atypical antipsychotic medications, creating a medication confound for the patient vs. control comparisons. Prior literature addressing the role of antipsychotic medication in modulating gamma oscillations is sparse and equivocal. One study of 40 Hz ASSR showed enhanced evoked power in SZ on atypical antipsychotics relative to both SZ on typical antipsychotics and HC (Hong et al., 2004). However, these differences were not replicated in a larger sample (Light et al., 2006).

In conclusion, patients with schizophrenia show deficits across time-frequency decompositions of gamma oscillations in both steady-state and oddball paradigms. Both phase and power measures of 40 Hz ASSR and GBR seem to be sensitive to the same pathophysiological process in schizophrenia, despite only being modestly correlated. Indeed, results from our study suggest that each paradigm provides essentially the same information about auditory gamma-band abnormalities in schizophrenia, despite the overall enhancement of both phase-resetting and event-related changes in power in the 40 Hz ASSR relative to the GBR. Thus, collecting both paradigms appears to offer little or no advantage relative to using just one of the paradigms, an important consideration when developing an EEG/ERP battery for schizophrenia studies.

References

Başar, E. (1972) A study of the time and frequency characteristics of the potentials evoked in the acoustical cortex. *Kybernetik*, 10: 61–64.

Başar, E., Rosen, B., Başar-Eroğlu, C. and Greitschus, F. (1987) The associations between 40 Hz EEG and the middle latency response of the auditory evoked potential. *Int. J. Neurosci.*, 33: 103–117.

Bidet-Caulet, A., Fischer, C., Besle, J., Aguera, P.E., Giard, M.H. and Bertrand, O. (2007) Effects of selective attention on the electrophysiological representation of concurrent sounds in the human auditory cortex. *J. Neurosci.*, 27: 9252–9261.

Bohorquez, J. and Özdamar, Ö. (2008) Generation of the 40-Hz auditory steady-state response (ASSR) explained using convolution. *Clin. Neurophysiol.*, 119: 2598–2607.

Brenner, C.A., Sporns, O., Lysaker, P.H. and O'Donnell, B.F. (2003) EEG synchronization to modulated auditory tones in schizophrenia, schizoaffective disorder, and schizotypal personality disorder. *Am. J. Psychiatry*, 160: 2238–2240.

Brenner, C.A., Krishnan, G.P., Vohs, J.L., Ahn, W.Y., Hetrick, W.P. and Morzorati, S.L. (2009) Steady state responses: electrophysiological assessment of sensory function in schizophrenia. *Schizophr. Bull.* 35: 1065–1077.

Buszáki, G. and Draguhn, A. (2004) Neuronal oscillations in cortical networks. *Science*, 304: 1926–1929.

Cho, R.Y., Konecky, R.O. and Carter, C.S. (2006) Impairments in frontal cortical gamma synchrony and cognitive control in schizophrenia. *Proc. Natl. Acad. Sci. USA*, 103: 19878–19883.

Clementz, B.A., Blumenfeld, L.D. and Cobb, S. (1997) The gamma band response may account for poor P50 suppression in schizophrenia. *NeuroReport*, 8: 3889–3893.

Coyle, J.T., Tsai, G. and Goff, D. (2003) Converging evidence of NMDA receptor hypofunction in the pathophysiology of schizophrenia. *Ann. NY Acad. Sci.*, 1003: 318–327.

Debener, S., Herrmann, C.S., Kranczioch, C., Gembris, D. and Engel, A.K. (2003) Top-down attentional processing enhances auditory evoked gamma band activity. *Neuroreport*, 14: 683–686.

Deng, C. and Huang, X.F. (2006) Increased density of $GABA_A$ receptors in the superior temporal gyrus in schizophrenia. *Exp. Brain Res.*, 168: 587–590.

Doheny, H.C., Faulkner, H.J., Gruzelier, J.H., Baldeweg, T. and Whittington, M.A. (2000) Pathway-specific habituation of induced gamma oscillations in the hippocampal slice. *NeuroReport*, 11: 2629–2633.

Dutton, R.C., Smith, W.D., Rampil, I.J., Chortkoff, B.S. and Eger, E.I. 2nd (1999) Forty Hertz midlatency auditory evoked potential activity predicts wakeful response during desflurane and propofol anesthesia in volunteers. *Anesthesiology*, 91: 1209–1220.

First, M.B. and Frances, A. (1995) *DSM-IV Handbook of Differential Diagnosis.* American Psychiatric Press, Washington, DC.

Ford, J.M., Roach, B.J., Hoffman, R.S. and Mathalon, D.H. (2008) The dependence of P300 amplitude on gamma synchrony breaks down in schizophrenia. *Brain Res.*, 1235: 133–142.

Frund, I., Schadow, J., Busch, N.A., Korner, U. and Herrmann, C.S. (2007) Evoked gamma oscillations in human scalp EEG are test–retest reliable. *Clin. Neurophysiol.*, 118: 221–227.

Galambos, R., Makeig, S. and Talmachoff, P.J. (1981) A 40-Hz auditory potential recorded from the human scalp. *Proc. Natl. Acad. Sci. USA*, 78: 2643–2647.

Gandal, M.J., Edgar, J.C., Klook, K. and Siegel, S.J. (2012) Gamma synchrony: towards a translational biomarker for the treatment-resistant symptoms of schizophrenia. *Neuropharmacology*, 62: 1504–1518.

Gonzalez-Burgos, G. and Lewis, D.A. (2008) GABA neurons and the mechanisms of network oscillations: implications for understanding cortical dysfunction in schizophrenia. *Schizophr. Bull.*, 34: 944–961.

Gratton, G., Coles, M.G. and Donchin, E. (1983) A new method for off-line removal of ocular artifact. *Electroencephalogr. Clin. Neurophysiol.*, 55: 468–484.

Gray, C.M. and Singer, W. (1989) Stimulus-specific neuronal oscillations in orientation columns of cat visual cortex. *Proc. Natl. Acad. Sci. USA*, 86: 1698–1702.

Griskova, I., Morup, M., Parnas, J., Ruksenas, O. and Arnfred, S.M. (2007) The amplitude and phase precision of 40 Hz auditory steady-state response depend on the level of arousal. *Exp. Brain Res.*, 183: 133–138.

Hall, M.H., Taylor, G., Sham, P., Schulze, K., Rijsdijk, F., Picchioni, M. et al. (2009) The early auditory gamma-band response is heritable and a putative endophenotype of schizophrenia. *Schizophr. Bull.*, 37: 778–787.

Hall, M.H., Taylor, G., Salisbury, D.F. and Levy, D.L. (2011) Sensory gating event-related potentials and oscillations in schizophrenia patients and their unaffected relatives. *Schizophr. Bull.*, 37: 1187–1199.

Hamm, J.P., Gilmore, C.S., Picchetti, N.A., Sponheim, S.R. and Clementz, B.A. (2011) Abnormalities of neuronal oscillations and temporal integration to low- and high-frequency auditory stimulation in schizophrenia. *Biol. Psychiatry*, 69 (10): 989–996.

Hashimoto, T., Volk, D.W., Eggan, S.M., Mirnics, K., Pierri, J.N., Sun, Z., Sampson, A.R. and Lewis, D.A. (2003) Gene expression deficits in a subclass of GABA neurons in the prefrontal cortex of subjects with schizophrenia. *J. Neurosci.*, 23: 6315–6326.

Hirano, S., Hirano, Y., Maekawa, T., Obayashi, C., Oribe, N., Kuroki, T., Kanba, S. and Onitsuka, T. (2008) Abnormal neural oscillatory activity to speech sounds in schizophrenia: a magnetoencephalography study. *J. Neurosci.*, 28: 4897–4903.

Hong, L.E., Summerfelt, A., McMahon, R., Adami, H., Francis, G., Elliott, A., Buchanan, R.W. and Thaker, G.K. (2004) Evoked gamma band synchronization and the liability for schizophrenia. *Schizophr. Res.*, 70: 293–302.

Impagnatiello, F., Guidotti, A.R., Pesold, C., Dwivedi, Y., Caruncho, H., Pisu, M.G. et al. (1998) A decrease of reelin expression as a putative vulnerability factor in schizophrenia. *Proc. Natl. Acad. Sci. USA*, 95: 15718–15723.

Kaf, W.A., Sabo, D.L., Durrant, J.D. and Rubinstein, E. (2006) Reliability of electric response audiometry using 80 Hz auditory steady-state responses. *Int. J. Audiol.*, 45: 477–486.

Kay, S.R., Fiszbein, A. and Opler, L.A. (1987) The positive and negative syndrome scale (PANSS) for schizophrenia. *Schizophr. Bull.*, 13: 261–276.

Krishnan, G.P., Hetrick, W.P., Brenner, C.A., Shekhar, A., Steffen, A.N. and O'Donnell, B.F. (2009) Steady state and induced auditory gamma deficits in schizophrenia. *Neuroimage*, 47: 1711–1719.

Krystal, J.H., Anand, A. and Moghaddam, B. (2002) Effects of NMDA receptor antagonists: implications for the pathophysiology of schizophrenia. *Arch. Gen. Psychiatry*, 59: 663–664.

Kwon, J.S., O'Donnell, B.F., Wallenstein, G.V., Greene, R.W., Hirayasu, Y., Nestor, P.G. et al. (1999) Gamma frequency-range abnormalities to auditory stimulation in schizophrenia. *Arch. Gen. Psychiatry*, 56: 1001–1005.

Leicht, G., Kirsch, V., Giegling, I., Karch, S., Hantschk, I., Möller, H.J., Pogarell, O., Hegerl, U., Rujescu, D. and Mulert, C. (2010) Reduced early auditory evoked gamma-band response in patients with schizophrenia. *Biol. Psychiatry*, 67: 224–231.

Leicht, G., Karch, S., Karamatskos, E., Giegling, I., Möller, H.J., Hegerl, U., Pogarell, O., Rujescu, D. and Mulert, C. (2011) Alterations of the early auditory evoked gamma-band response in first-degree relatives of patients with schizophrenia: hints to a new intermediate phenotype. *J. Psychiatry. Res.*, 45: 699–705.

Lenz, D., Fischer, S., Schadow, J., Bogerts, B. and Herrmann, C.S. (2011) Altered evoked gamma-band responses as a neurophysiological marker of schizophrenia? *Int. J. Psychophysiol.*, 79: 25–31.

Lewis, D.A., Hashimoto, T. and Volk, D.W. (2005) Cortical inhibitory neurons and schizophrenia. *Nat. Rev. Neurosci.*, 312–324.

Lewis, D.A., Cho, R.Y., Carter, C.S., Eklund, K., Forster, S., Kelly, M.A. and Montrose, D. (2008) Subunit-selective modulation of GABA type A receptor neurotransmission and cognition in schizophrenia. *Am. J. Psychiatry*, 165: 1585–1593.

Light, G.A., Hsu, J.L., Hsieh, M.H., Meyer-Gomes, K., Sprock, J., Swerdlow, N.R. and Braff, D.L. (2006) Gamma band oscillations reveal neural network cortical coherence dysfunction in schizophrenia patients. *Biol. Psychiatry*, 60: 1231–1240.

Mathalon, D.H., Hoffman, R.E., Watson, T.D., Miller, R.M., Roach, B.J. and Ford, J.M. (2010) Neurophysiological distinction between schizophrenia and schizoaffective disorder. *Front. Hum. Neurosci.*, 3: 70.

Minzenberg, M.J., Firl, A.J., Yoon, J.H., Gomes, G.C., Reinking, C. and Carter, C.S. (2010) Gamma oscillatory power is impaired during cognitive control independent of medication status in first-episode schizophrenia. *Neuropsychopharmacology*, 35: 2590–2599.

O'Donnell, B.F., Hetrick, W.P., Vohs, J.L., Krishnan, G.P., Carroll, C.A. and Shekhar, A. (2004) Neural synchronization deficits to auditory stimulation in bipolar disorder. *NeuroReport*, 15: 1369–1372.

Pantev, C., Makeig, S., Hoke, M., Galambos, R., Hampson, S. and Gallen, C. (1991) Human auditory evoked gamma-band magnetic fields. *Proc. Natl. Acad. Sci. USA*, 88: 8996–9000.

Pantev, C., Elbert, T., Makeig, S., Hampson, S., Eulitz, C. and Hoke, M. (1993) Relationship of transient and steady-state auditory evoked fields. *Electroencephalogr. Clin. Neurophysiol.*, 88: 389–396.

Pastor, M.A., Artieda, J., Arbizu, J., Marti-Climent, J.M., Penuelas, I. and Masdeu, J.C. (2002) Activation of human cerebral and cerebellar cortex by auditory stimulation at 40 Hz. *J. Neurosci.*, 22: 10501–10506.

Plourde, G. (2006) Auditory evoked potentials. *Best Pract. Res. Clin. Anaesthesiol.*, 20: 129–139.

Plourde, G. and Villemure, C. (1996) Comparison of the effects of enflurane/N2O on the 40-Hz auditory steady-state response versus the auditory middle-latency response. *Anesth. Analg.*, 82: 75–83.

Presacco, A., Bohorquez, J., Yavuz, E. and Özdamar, Ö. (2010) Auditory steady-state responses to 40-Hz click trains: relationship to middle latency, gamma band and beta band responses studied with deconvolution. *Clin. Neurophysiol.*, 121: 1540–1550.

Reite, M., Teale, P., Collins, D. and Rojas, D.C. (2010) Schizoaffective disorder—a possible MEG auditory evoked field biomarker. *Psychiatry Res.*, 182: 284–286.

Roach, B.J. and Mathalon, D.H. (2008) Event-related EEG time-frequency analysis: an overview of measures and an analysis of early gamma band phase locking in schizophrenia. *Schizophr. Bull.*, 34: 907–926.

Roopun, A.K., Cunningham, M.O., Racca, C., Alter, K., Traub, R.D. and Whittington, M.A. (2008) Region-specific changes in gamma and beta$_2$ rhythms in NMDA receptor dysfunction models of schizophrenia. *Schizophr. Bull.*, 34: 962–973.

Ross, B., Picton, T.W. and Pantev, C. (2002) Temporal integration in the human auditory cortex as represented by the development of the steady-state magnetic field. *Hear. Res.*, 165: 68–84.

Ross, B., Picton, T.W., Herdman, A.T. and Pantev, C. (2004) The effect of attention on the auditory steady-state response. *Neurol. Clin. Neurophysiol.*, 2004: 22.

Ross, B., Herdman, A.T. and Pantev, C. (2005) Stimulus induced desynchronization of human auditory 40-Hz steady-state responses. *J. Neurophysiol.*, 94: 4082–4093.

Santarelli, R., Maurizi, M., Conti, G., Ottaviani, F., Paludetti, G. and Pettorossi, V.E. (1995) Generation of human auditory steady-state responses (SSRs). II. Addition of responses to individual stimuli. *Hear. Res.*, 83: 9–18.

Saupe, K., Schroger, E., Andersen, S.K. and Muller, M.M. (2009a) Neural mechanisms of intermodal sustained selective attention with concurrently presented auditory and visual stimuli. *Front. Hum. Neurosci.*, 3: 58.

Saupe, K., Widmann, A., Bendixen, A., Muller, M.M. and Schroger, E. (2009b) Effects of intermodal attention on the auditory steady-state response and the event-related potential. *Psychophysiology*, 46: 321–327.

Schadow, J., Lenz, D., Thaerig, S., Busch, N.A., Frund, I. and Herrmann, C.S. (2007) Stimulus intensity affects early sensory processing: sound intensity modulates auditory evoked gamma-band activity in human EEG. *Int. J. Psychophysiol.*, 65: 152–161.

Skosnik, P.D., Krishnan, G.P. and O'Donnell, B.F. (2007) The effect of selective attention on the gamma-band auditory steady-state response. *Neurosci. Lett.*, 420: 223–228.

Sohal, V.S., Zhang, F., Yizhar, O. and Deisseroth, K. (2009) Parvalbumin neurons and gamma rhythms enhance cortical circuit performance. *Nature (Lond.)*, 459: 698–702.

Spencer, K.M., Niznikiewicz, M.A., Shenton, M.E. and McCarley, R.W. (2008a) Sensory-evoked gamma oscillations in chronic schizophrenia. *Biol. Psychiatry*, 63: 744–747.

Spencer, K.M., Salisbury, D.F., Shenton, M.E. and McCarley, R.W. (2008b) Gamma-band auditory steady-state responses are impaired in first episode psychosis. *Biol. Psychiatry*, 64: 369–375.

Spencer, K.M., Niznikiewicz, M.A., Nestor, P.G., Shenton, M.E. and McCarley, R.W. (2009) Left auditory cortex gamma synchronization and auditory hallucination symptoms in schizophrenia. *BMC Neurosci.*, 10: 85.

Tallon-Baudry, C., Bertrand, O., Delpuech, C. and Permier, J. (1997) Oscillatory gamma-band (30–70 Hz) activity induced by a visual search task in humans. *J. Neurosci.*, 17: 722–734.

Teale, P., Collins, D., Maharajh, K., Rojas, D.C., Kronberg, E. and Reite, M. (2008) Cortical source estimates of gamma band amplitude and phase are different in schizophrenia. *Neuroimage*, 42: 1481–1489.

Tiitinen, H., Sinkkonen, J., Reinikainen, K., Alho, K., Lavikainen, J. and Näätänen, R. (1993) Selective attention enhances the auditory 40-Hz transient response in humans. *Nature (Lond.)*, 364: 59–60.

Van Deursen, J.A., Vuurman, E.F., Van Kranen-Mastenbroek, V.H., Verhey, F.R. and Riedel, W.J. (2011) 40-Hz steady state response in Alzheimer's disease and mild cognitive impairment. *Neurobiol. Aging*, 32: 24–30.

Vierling-Claassen, D., Siekmeier, P., Stufflebeam, S. and Kopell, N. (2008) Modeling GABA alterations in schizophrenia: a link between impaired inhibition and altered gamma and beta range auditory entrainment. *J. Neurophysiol.*, 99: 2656–2671.

Wilson, T.W., Hernandez, O.O., Asherin, R.M., Teale, P.D., Reite, M.L. and Rojas, D.C. (2008) Cortical gamma generators suggest abnormal auditory circuitry in early-onset psychosis. *Cereb. Cortex*, 18: 371–378.

Application of Brain Oscillations in Neuropsychiatric Diseases
(Supplements to Clinical Neurophysiology, Vol. 62)
Editors: E. Başar, C. Başar-Eroğlu, A. Özerdem, P.M. Rossini, G.G. Yener

Chapter 12

Connectivity and local activity within the fronto-posterior brain network in schizophrenia

Anuradha Sharma[a,*], Matthias Weisbrod[a,b] and Stephan Bender[a,c]

[a]*Department of General Psychiatry, Centre for Psychosocial Medicine, University of Heidelberg, D-69115 Heidelberg, Germany*
[b]*Psychiatric Department, SRH Klinikum Karlsbad-Langensteinbach, D-76307 Karlsbad, Germany*
[c]*Child and Adolescent Psychiatry, Section for Clinical Neurophysiology and Multimodal Neuroimaging, Technical University of Dresden, D-01307 Dresden, Germany*

ABSTRACT

Background: Fronto-posterior networks have been implicated in cognitive control and understanding the detailed functional dynamics within this network is important to understand the pathophysiology of cognitive deficits in schizophrenia. In a previous study (Sharma et al., 2011), we found reduced event-related coherence between frontal and posterior electrode sites in delta and theta frequencies during cognitive control in schizophrenia. The current study aimed to look at the relationship between locally evoked frontal and posterior activity (measured by event-related potentials (ERPs)) and long-range coherence within the fronto-posterior network in healthy controls and patients with schizophrenia.
Methods: 16 schizophrenic/schizoaffective patients and 20 age-matched healthy controls performing a choice reaction task took part in the study. We examined ERPs occurring at frontal and posterior sites between 100 and 250 ms (overlapping with the time period where coherence deficits were previously found) for differences between patients and controls. ERPs examined were P1a/P2a and N1/N2b components occurring simultaneously during 100–200/200–250 ms post stimulus at the frontal (F5′/F6′) and posterior (P7′/P8′) sites, respectively. We further looked at group difference in event-related delta and theta fronto-posterior coherence in the exact same time windows as the ERPs and calculated the correlation between ERP amplitudes and simultaneous event-related delta and theta coherence for both hemispheres and time periods. Bonferroni correction was applied to correct for multiple correlations.
Results: We found a significant reduction in schizophrenia patients of the posterior N2b and a trend for reduction for the frontal P2a which are implicated in target-related information processing while the earlier frontal P1a and posterior N1 associated with more general sensory processing were relatively spared. However, the event-related coherence between the frontal and posterior areas was reduced in patients compared to controls during both the early and late time windows, indicating connectivity deficits to be a more consistent impairment in schizophrenia. There was limited linear correlation between fronto-posterior coherence and frontal and posterior ERP amplitudes but uncorrected correlation coefficients showed coherence in delta frequency to be correlated with P2a amplitude in both hemispheres and with P1a only in the left hemisphere in healthy controls. In the patients, however, this correlation was disrupted in the left hemisphere for both early and later stage evoked activity, whereas they showed a similar degree of correlation as healthy controls between P2a and delta coherence in the right hemisphere. Coherence in theta frequency showed no significant correlation with ERPs nor did N1/N2b show any significant correlation with coherence.

---

[*]*Correspondence to:* Dr. Anuradha Sharma, Section for Experimental Psychopathology and Neurophysiology, Department of General Psychiatry, Center for Psychosocial Medicine, University of Heidelberg, Voßstrasse 4, D-69115 Heidelberg, Germany.
Tel.: +49-6221-56-36071; Fax: +49-6221-56-8094;
E-mail: Anuradha.Sharma@med.uni-heidelberg.de

Conclusions: Impaired cognitive control in schizophrenia might be driven by disrupted communication between the frontal and posterior brain areas, long-range connectivity being a more consistent deficit in schizophrenia as compared to locally evoked activity. Event-related fronto-posterior coherence and locally evoked frontal and posterior ERP amplitudes seem to reflect independent aspects of information processing in the brain although some linear relationship may exist between local frontal activity and fronto-posterior coherence in the delta frequency, implicating this frequency in frontal top-down control of information processing. A disruption of this relationship specifically in the left hemisphere is consistent with previously reported disturbances of the left hemisphere in schizophrenia. Connectivity measures may add important information as markers of cognitive pathophysiology in schizophrenia and may represent a fundamental impairment underlying cognitive control deficits in schizophrenia.

KEYWORDS

Schizophrenia; Cognitive deficits; Fronto-posterior brain network; Connectivity impairment; Cognition

12.1. Introduction

It has become clear lately that the brain is not a compartmentalized organ with different areas acting independently, but rather connectivity between brain areas is essential to cognition. There have been many studies recently that have aimed at investigating connectivity impairments in schizophrenia to explain cognitive deficits.

One of the most important brain networks, the fronto-posterior network, which is the network formed when the frontal and posterior brain areas connect with each other, has been consistently implicated in control cognitive processes such as attention, executive control, and working memory (Posner and Dehaene, 1994; Banich et al., 2000; Mitchell et al., 2005; Buschman and Miller, 2007). The frontal part of the network, especially the pre-frontal cortex, is thought to be involved in the active maintenance of information over time and executive/top-down part of control cognitive processes, where responses are mediated by task-specific, goal-oriented constraints (Posner and Dehaene, 1994). The posterior part of the network consisting of occipital, temporal, and parietal association areas is, on the other hand, responsible for processing incoming sensory information and generation of perceptual representations with different areas known to be involved in different aspects of sensory/perceptual processing. Together, these areas are thought to be responsible for the salience-driven/bottom-up

part of information processing during cognition (Buschman and Miller, 2007).

Given the impairments in control cognitive processes in schizophrenia (Green, 2006; Kerns et al., 2008), it is not surprising that both structural (Gaser et al., 2004; Spoletini et al., 2009) and functional (Lawrie et al., 2002; Schlösser et al., 2003; Ford and Mathalon, 2005; Bob et al., 2008; Yoon et al., 2008; Kim et al., 2009) abnormalities in the fronto-posterior network have been repeatedly shown in patients with schizophrenia. However, a related aspect that is not so well investigated is the relation between long-range fronto-posterior connectivity and the local brain activity in the frontal and posterior areas. In a recent study (Sharma et al., 2011), we were able to show that abnormal functional connectivity in the fronto-posterior brain network in schizophrenia is not necessarily characterized by a global reduction of connectivity, but can be either increased (during rest) or decreased (during cognitive control) depending on the stage of the task. In this paper, we extend the previous analysis to look at how the fronto-posterior connectivity relates to local evoked activity in frontal and posterior areas during cognitive control in healthy controls and schizophrenia patients, and whether patients showed similar deficits in both connectivity and local evoked activity. Studying the detailed dynamics of this important functional network can have important implications in elucidating the pathophysiology of cognitive deficits in schizophrenia.

12.2. Materials and Methods

12.2.1. Subjects

Sixteen schizophrenic/schizoaffective patients (9 schizoaffective, 4 paranoid, 2 disorganized, 1 undifferentiated) age matched to 20 young healthy adults were included in the study. Diagnosis was established according to DSM-IV by the structured clinical interview (SCID) (Wittchen et al., 1997). Patients were recruited from the University Hospital Heidelberg (in-patients) and were recorded after (partial) remission of positive symptoms so that they could well accomplish the choice reaction task. Patients were on stable medication and most of them received atypical antipsychotics. More details of the patient sample can be found in Sharma et al. (2011). Exclusion criteria were neurological comorbidity and other psychiatric diseases. First- and second-grade relatives of controls were not allowed to have a record of axis I psychiatric diagnosis. All subjects were right-handed according to the Edinburgh Handedness Inventory (Oldfield, 1971), had German as their mother language, and provided written informed consent. The study was approved by the local ethics committee and conducted according to the Declaration of Helsinki. Controls received 20 € for their participation. All subjects passed a test of color vision.

12.2.2. Task

The emotional Stroop task that was employed in the current study is a modified version of the classical Stroop task, involving the presentation of emotional words in different colors and reporting of colors by the subjects. The emotional Stroop task has been traditionally used to demonstrate and assess attentional biases to emotional stimuli in various emotional disorders (Williams et al., 1996). However, since word reading is a more pre-potent/automatized process as compared to color naming (MacLeod, 1991), this task involves similar control cognitive processes as the classical Stroop task, though with a lesser degree of conflict and, therefore, can also be used to investigate these processes. In the current version of the emotional Stroop task, subjects were presented with 48 emotional words (16 neutral, 16 negative, 16 positive) in 4 different colors (red, yellow, green, or blue) for 150 ms on a computer screen at 60 cm distance (Gentask; Stim software package; Neuroscan, Texas, USA). We do not give further details about the emotional valence of the words as we found no effect of valence on the reaction times and on the EEG measures that we analyzed (see Section 12.3 and Sharma et al. (2011) for more details). Subjects were instructed to attend to the color and indicate the presented color by pressing the corresponding button on a response pad as fast as possible. The sequence of button presses according to the assignment of color was randomized and each color appeared with equal probability. The inter-stimulus interval was 2000–2400 ms (pseudorandomized, 100 ms steps). Every color/word combination was presented twice, so that 384 trials were performed, half of them requiring right-hand button presses and half requiring left-hand button presses. Directly before the words, a fixation cross was shown for 700 ms in the middle of the screen to mark the start of a trial in order to reduce eye movement artifacts. Subjects were given 100 trials for practice before the recordings.

12.2.3. Recordings

Recordings were performed with a 64-channel continuous DC-EEG by Neuroscan Synamps amplifiers with a sampling rate of 250 Hz with a low-pass 70 Hz anti-aliasing filter (Brain Vision Analyzer, Brain Products GmbH, Munich, Germany) applied during recordings. 64 sintered silver/silver chloride electrodes were fixed using equidistant electrode caps (Easycap, FMS, Herrsching, Germany) according to head size. Electrodes were named after the equivalent positions in the extended international 10–20 system.

184

Small deviations are indicated by primes ('). Vertical and horizontal electrooculograms (VEOG and HEOG) were also recorded from electrodes attached 1 cm above and below the left eye (VEOG) and next to the outer canthi (HEOG). Electrode impedances were kept below 5 kΩ. Data were recorded against a reference near Cz, and offline, the data were transformed to the average reference. Recordings took place during the mornings.

12.2.4. Data processing

Data were low-pass filtered with a 30 Hz zero-phase Butterworth filter (Brain Vision Analyzer, Brain Products GmbH, Munich, Germany) for the ERP analysis and segmented around stimulus triggers into epochs of 1500 ms (–200 to 1300 ms post stimulus). Only epochs with correct responses between 200 and 1300 ms post stimulus were included. Epochs were baseline corrected with the first 200 ms of the epoch as the baseline interval. Eye movements and blinks were corrected using Gratton and Coles algorithm (Gratton et al., 1983) as implemented in Brain Vision Analyzer. Segments containing major artifacts were removed manually by an experienced person. Artifacts exceeding 100 µV were rejected automatically. Trials for all emotional valences were pooled together for further analysis but a parallel ERP analysis was carried out also only with trials containing neutral words in order to assess any emotional valence effects on the ERP results. The average number of trials that entered the analysis showed a trend for difference between the two groups ($t(34) = 2.0; p = 0.06$), the average number of trials being 344 for healthy controls and 319 for patients.

12.2.5. Frontal and posterior event-related potentials

Event-related potentials (ERPs) are generated by averaging EEG signals over many trials. The averaging process cancels out EEG activity from the ongoing processes in the brain that are not strictly time and phase locked to the experimental events and, therefore, ERPs represent EEG activity tightly time and phase locked to the experimental events. In order to look at the local neuronal activity elicited by control cognitive processes in the current experiment in the frontal and posterior brain areas, we chose to look at the following ERPs that have been localized to the frontal and posterior areas during sensory and control information processing:

• *Posterior N1 and N2b.* The occipito-temporal N1 occurring between 100 and 200 ms post stimulus has been reported for visually presented stimuli and has been found related to the processing of general features of the stimuli (Harter and Guido, 1980; Potts et al., 1996) and to general arousal, being larger for both targets and non-targets during tasks that require a motor response (Potts, 2004). The posterior N2b occurring around 200 ms post stimulus, that follows the N1 and has a similar topography, has been found related to the selection and perceptual processing of task-relevant features of the stimuli, that is to stimulus-specific processes enhanced by attention (Harter and Guido, 1980; Potts et al., 1996; O'Donnell et al., 1997). The consecutive posterior negative potentials (N1 and N2b), with a similar topography, have been found to reflect a progressive change in the differential processing of relevant features of the stimuli, with N1 reflecting the processing of the general characteristics and N2b reflecting the processing on the basis of specific task-relevant characteristics of the stimulus (Harter and Guido, 1980; Potts et al., 1996; Potts and Tucker, 2001).
• *Frontal P1a and P2a.* Two consecutive anterior positive deflections, P1a (early frontal positivity) and P2a, having a similar time course as N1 and N2b have been reported for visual tasks requiring controlled processing. The P1a, like the N1, has been

associated with general arousal being larger to both targets and non-targets during tasks requiring a motor response (Potts, 2004). However, further functional significance of P1a as well as its distinction from N1 are yet ambiguous (Potts et al., 1996). The P2a has been associated with control processes in the frontal lobes involved in the evaluation of task relevance of the stimuli (more enhanced to target stimuli and in blocks requiring a response, both overt and covert) (Potts et al., 1996; Potts, 2004).

Although the N2b and the P2a have a similar time course, they have been shown to have different properties (Potts et al., 1996, 2008) and source localizations (Potts, 2004) and therefore are not likely to be two poles of the same source. Rather, the concurrent activation of N2b and P2a at the posterior and frontal sites, respectively, may point to connectivity between the underlying areas.

12.2.5.1. ERP electrode sites
Previous studies that have looked at the visual N1/N2b and P1a/P2a ERPs have located these components to occipito-temporal (Harter and Guido, 1980; Potts et al., 1996; O'Donnell et al., 1997; Bender et al., 2008) and frontal brain areas (Potts et al., 1996, 2002; Doniger et al., 2002; Potts, 2004), respectively. In agreement with these studies and obtained topographic maps (Fig. 1) of grand averages, we chose F5′ and F6′ electrodes overlying the pre-frontal brain regions for looking at P1a/P2a, and P7′ and P8′ electrodes overlying the occipito-temporal brain regions for looking at N1/N2b components.

12.2.5.2. ERP time windows
According to the previous literature (Harter and Guido, 1980; Potts et al., 1996; O'Donnell et al., 1997; Bentin et al., 1999) and in agreement with the obtained grand-averaged ERP waveforms (Fig. 2, see also Section 12.3), a time window of 100–200 ms was chosen for N1 analysis. As N2b reflects the processing of task-relevant characteristics of

visual stimuli, depending on the exact type of stimulus and task, previous studies have used different time windows for N2b analysis, varying between 200 and 400 ms with a clear emphasis between 200 and 300 ms (O'Donnell et al., 1997; Potts et al., 2002; Bender et al., 2008). In line with these studies and the obtained grand-averaged ERP waveforms, we measured N2b as the mean amplitude between 200 and 250 ms. Similarly, since previous studies (Potts et al., 1996, 2002; Doniger et al., 2002) have reported a temporally coincidental occurrence of the frontal positive potentials with N1 and N2b, the frontal ERPs were analyzed using the same time windows as for N1 and N2b, that is 100–200 ms for P1a and 200–250 ms for P2a, respectively. Grand-averaged ERP waveforms confirmed this choice of time window for both groups. Mean amplitudes for the ERPs were extracted for the selected time windows and electrodes.

12.2.6. Fronto-posterior coherence

Fronto-posterior connectivity was measured by calculating linear coherence between frontal and posterior electrode sites that were used for ERP analysis, separately for the right (F5′–P7′) and the left (F6′–P8′) hemisphere. For this analysis, the 30 Hz low-pass filter was not applied to the data and, therefore, only the 70 Hz anti-aliasing filter applied during the recordings restricted the frequency range of the signal. To keep the coherence measures comparable to the earlier study (Sharma et al., 2011), epochs of 1800 ms (–1000 to 800 ms post stimulus) were retained for this analysis and frequency- and time-resolved linear coherence was calculated by applying a short time Fourier Transform (STFT) using the function "newcrossf" of the EEGLAB software (Delorme and Makeig, 2004), based on MATLAB (The MathWorks, USA). The length of the STFT sliding window used was 512 ms. Analysis gave a time resolution of 8.42 ms (200 sliding windows from –944 to 740 ms) and a frequency resolution of 0.97 Hz (1–49.8 Hz). The coherence between frontal and posterior

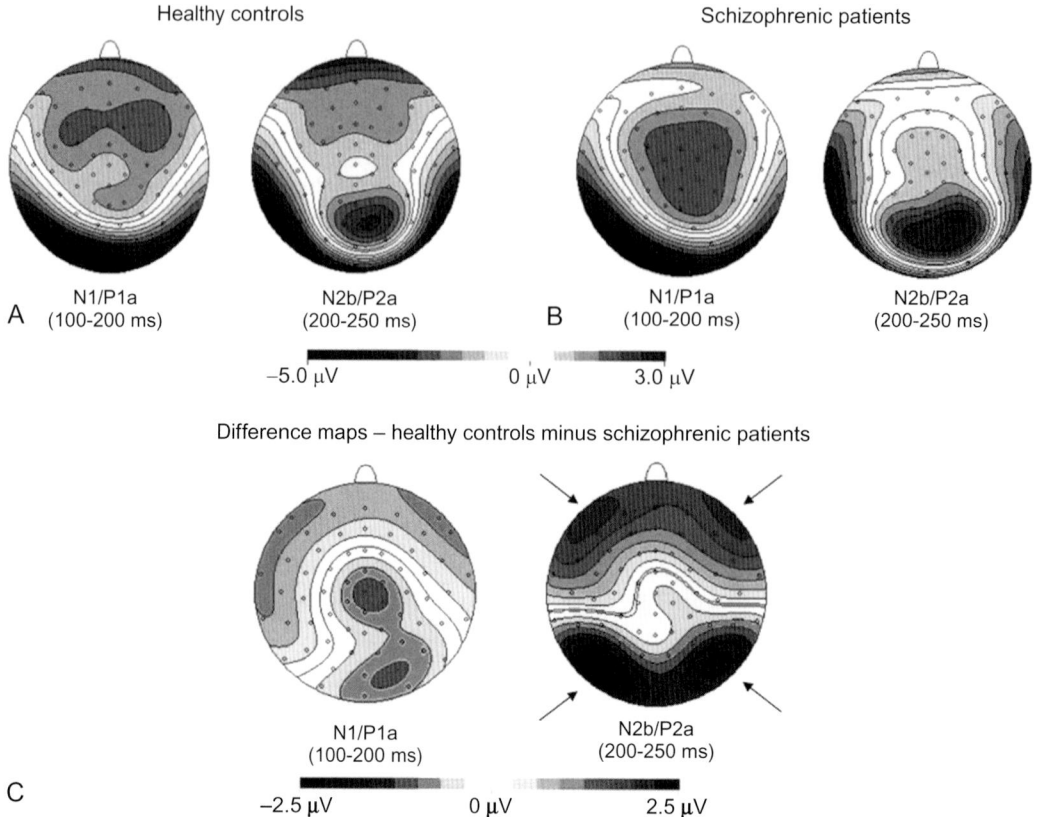

Fig. 1.   Voltage topography maps for the early and late ERPs. (A) Voltage maps for healthy controls during the early (100–200 ms) and late (200–250 ms) ERP time intervals. Maps confirm the frontal positive and occipito-temporal negative distribution of brain electrical activity during the examined time intervals. (B) Voltage maps for schizophrenia patients during the same intervals which show a distribution of activity during the early interval similar to healthy controls but during the later time interval there is a reduced frontal positive and posterior negative activity as compared to healthy controls. (C) Voltage maps for difference waves (healthy controls minus schizophrenia patients). Patients show a greater reduction in the frontal positive and posterior negative activity in the later time interval. (For color figures, please refer to the color figures in last section of the book.)

electrodes was calculated for every time and frequency point, and event-related coherence was obtained after baseline correction (by calculating absolute coherence for every frequency point averaged across the inter-trial time interval from −944 to −800 ms and subtracting it from the coherence values for the corresponding frequencies across all time-points in the post-baseline time intervals).

In order to explore the relationship between frontal and posterior ERPs (local evoked activity) and the connectivity between these areas, and to compare these different measures of brain activity, event-related coherence was calculated for the 100–200- and 200–250-ms time intervals separately. We chose to look at event-related coherence for the delta and theta frequencies only, because we found significant increases with respect to baseline in healthy controls and significant group differences during task-related cognitive control for these two frequencies only in the previous study (Sharma et al., 2011; Fig. 3).

12.2.7. Statistical analysis

For looking at group differences for the examined ERPs, repeated-measures ANOVA was performed.

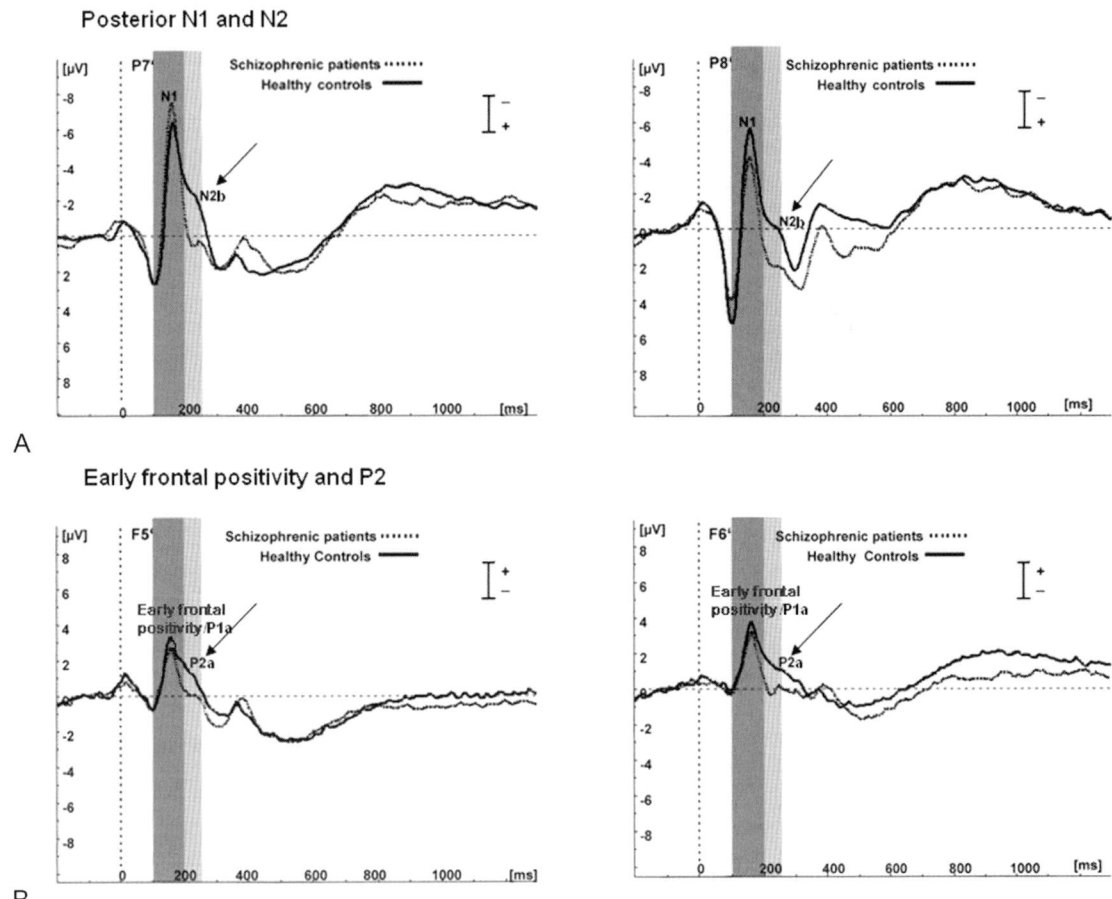

Fig. 2. Grand-averaged waveforms showing early and late ERP components in the posterior and frontal areas. (A) Group-averaged EEG waveforms for occipito-temporal electrodes, P7′ and P8′. Patients show a differential reduction of N2b (200–250 ms post stimulus) which is related to target-relevant processing as compared to N1 (100–200 ms post stimulus) which is associated with more general sensory processing. (B) Group-averaged EEG waveforms for frontal electrodes, F5′ and F6′. Patients show a trend for reduced P2a (200–250 ms post stimulus) which is related to frontal processes involved in the evaluation of task relevance of stimuli, while there was no significant group difference for P1a (100–200 ms post stimulus), the functional significance of which is ambiguous. 0 ms refers to the onset of the word stimulus.

Post-hoc tests (Newman–Keuls) were calculated when the main effects or interactions reached significance. In order to see how the frontal and the posterior ERP components differed between the two groups, an ANOVA for the four ERP components (N1/P1a/N2b/P2a) together was performed on the mean voltage values, with group (patients, controls) as a between-subjects factor and location (frontal for F5′–F6′, posterior for P7′–P8′), hemisphere

(left, right), and interval (100–200 ms for N1/P1a, 200–250 ms for N2b/P2a) as within-subject factors.

In order to make sure that the pattern of results obtained was independent of the emotional valence, we verified the results with a similar ANOVA on ERPs calculated with only the neutral trials.

To compare the ERP results with that of coherence, an ANOVA similar to that for the ERPs

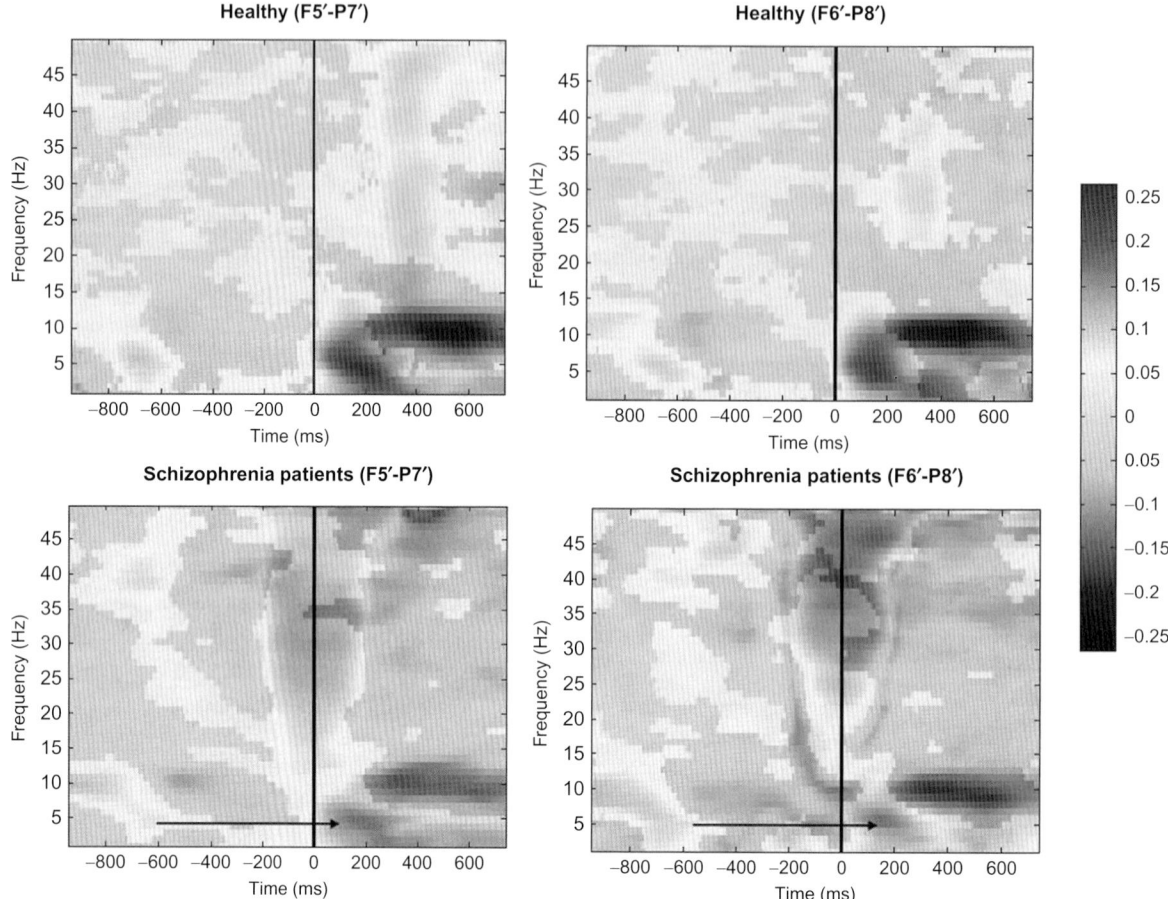

Fig. 3. Grand-averaged plots of event-related fronto-posterior coherence changes. Reproduced from Sharma et al. (2011). Time- and frequency-resolved coherence related to the task is shown for healthy controls and patients separately for the left (F5′–P7′) and right (F6′–P8′) hemispheres. 0 ms refers to the onset of the word stimulus. With respect to baseline, fronto-posterior coherence was significantly increased between 0 and 250 ms post stimulus in both hemispheres for healthy controls for the delta and theta frequencies. This coherence increase was significantly less in patients as compared to healthy controls and is indicated by arrows in the figure. The increased event-related coherence in patients during the pre-stimulus interval (–200 to –0 ms) seen in the plot, turned out to be due to one patient showing an extremely high value of coherence (30 times the standard deviation) for the beta and gamma frequencies during this time interval. Even-related coherence analysis specifically for 100–200 ms and 200–250 ms time intervals revealed group differences across both time intervals. (For color figures, please refer to the color figures in last section of the book.)

was conducted for event-related fronto-posterior coherence with group (patients, controls) as a between-subjects factor and hemisphere (left, right), frequency (delta, theta), and time interval (100–200, 200–250 ms) as within-subject factors.

For examining the linear relationship between fronto-posterior coherence (signifying long distance connectivity between frontal and posterior areas) and temporally coincident local evoked potential measures (signifying local neuronal activity in the frontal and posterior areas) in the frontal and posterior areas, exploratory correlation analyses were conducted. Correlation between the event-related delta and theta coherence during the 100–200- and 200–250-ms time intervals and the corresponding ERPs (N1, P1a and N2b, P2a), amplitudes was calculated separately for the two hemispheres. These correlations were calculated separately for healthy controls and patients. Bonferroni correction was applied to correct for multiple tests. Since 16 correlations were made for each group, the corrected alpha level was 0.003.

12.3. Results

12.3.1. Behavioral measures

A t test revealed that the patient group responded significantly slower than healthy controls (t (34) = 2.8; $p = 0.007$). Average reaction time for healthy controls was 652 ± 113 ms and for patients 794 ± 173 ms. The number of errors was not significantly different between the two groups.

12.3.2. Event-related potential differences across groups

The amplitude of N2b and P2a was reduced in patients (Figs. 1 and 2). N2b and P2a appeared as a prolongation of N1 and P1a rather than a clearly separated peak in our paradigm and sample. N2b was more pronounced on the left side. The ANOVA for mean voltages (Table 1) revealed a significant three fold interaction between group, location, and time interval (F (1, 34) = 5.8; $p = 0.02$), indicating a stronger group difference

for one of the time intervals and locations. The four fold interaction between group, location, time, and hemisphere showed only a trend for statistical significance (F (1, 34) = 3.3; $p = 0.08$). Post-hoc analysis with the Newman–Keuls test for the four fold interaction revealed significant group differences for N2b with patients, showing a less negative N2b as compared to healthy controls for both the right ($p = 0.004$) and the left hemisphere ($p = 0.0004$). Similarly the post-hoc test for P2a showed a trend for being less positive in patients for both the right ($p = 0.09$) and the left ($p = 0.09$) hemisphere. Among the earlier components, although N1 at the right hemisphere showed a trend for being lower in patients ($p = 0.10$), P1a (right hemisphere, $p = 0.72$; left hemisphere, $p = 0.84$) did not show any difference between the groups and there was even a non-significant elevation in schizophrenic patients of N1 at the left hemisphere ($p = 0.25$).

ANOVA for ERPs calculated with only neutral trials also revealed a pattern similar to that for ERPs calculated with all trials pooled together. A significant three fold interaction between group, location, and time interval (F (1, 34) = 5.9; $p = 0.02$) was obtained indicating a stronger group difference for one of the time intervals and locations. Post-hoc analysis with the Neuman–Keuls test revealed significant differences only for the later time interval, being more pronounced for N2b ($p = 0.0001$) than for P2a ($p = 0.04$).

TABLE 1

EARLY AND LATE ERP AMPLITUDES FOR THE FRONTAL AND POSTERIOR ELECTRODE SITES — MEAN (S.D.) IN μV

p values for differences between the two groups are shown in parentheses below the patient group for the significant and trend-level differences. n.s. = not significant.

ERP	N1		P1a		N2b		P2a	
Hemisphere	Right	Left	Right	Left	Right	Left	Right	Left
Schizophrenia patients	−0.7 (2.8) ($p = 0.10$)	−3.1 (2.2) (n.s.)	1.6 (1.0) (n.s.)	1.2 (1.0) (n.s.)	1.9 (3.3) ($p = 0.004$)	0.2 (3.0) ($p < 0.001$)	0.01 (1.8) ($p = 0.09$)	0.08 (1.5) ($p = 0.09$)
Healthy controls	−1.5 (3.2)	−2.5 (2.2)	2.1 (1.4)	1.7 (1.2)	−0.3 (2.4)	−2.4 (2.1)	1.4 (1.6)	1.2 (1.6)

12.3.3. Coherence differences across groups

Consistent with our previous analysis (Sharma et al., 2011; Fig. 3), ANOVA for mean event-related coherence (Table 2) yielded a significant main effect of group (F (1, 34) = 8.7; p = 0.005) and none of the interactions with the factor group reached significance, indicating that the patients had significantly reduced event-related coherence during both early (100–200 ms) and late (200–250 ms) time intervals for both frequencies and hemispheres, even though the early ERPs in frontal and posterior sites were spared in the patient group.

We already showed in the previous study (Sharma et al., 2011) that there was no effect of emotional valence on the coherence pattern.

12.3.4. Relation between coherence and event-related potentials

None of the correlations between event-related coherence and simultaneous ERPs were significant at the Bonferroni-corrected alpha level indicating limited linear relationship between ERPs and coherence measures. However, since Bonferroni correction can be overly conservative (Pernger, 1998), we also report the non-corrected results. These results revealed that in healthy controls, fronto-posterior coherence in the delta frequency during 200–250 ms correlated with later stage frontal evoked activity (P2a) in the left as well as right hemisphere and delta coherence during 100–200 ms correlated with early-stage frontal evoked activity (P1a) only in the left hemisphere. In the patients however, this correlation was non-significant in the left hemisphere for both early and later stage activity, whereas they showed a similar degree of correlation as healthy controls between P2a and simultaneous delta coherence in the right hemisphere. Coherence in the theta frequency showed no significant correlation with ERPs for any of the hemispheres and time intervals, nor did N1 and N2b show any significant correlation with coherence. The results of this correlation analysis are shown in Tables 3 and 4 for the control and the patients groups, respectively.

12.4. Discussion

The main results of the study were

- Patients showed significantly reduced later task-relevant ERPs (200–250 ms) as compared to earlier ERPs (100–200 ms) related to more general sensory processing. This reduction was more pronounced for posterior as compared to frontal areas.

TABLE 2

FRONTO-POSTERIOR COHERENCE FOR EARLY (100–200 MS) AND LATER (200–250 MS) TIME INTERVALS — MEAN (S.D.)

ANOVA for mean event-related coherence yielded a significant main effect of group (F (1, 34) = 8.7; p = 0.005) and none of the interactions with the factor group reached significance, indicating that the patients had significantly reduced event-related coherence during both early (100–200 ms) and late (200–250 ms) time intervals for both frequencies and hemispheres.

Coherence	Early delta		Early theta		Late delta		Late theta	
Hemisphere	Right	Left	Right	Left	Right	Left	Right	Left
Schizophrenia	0.08	0.09	0.10	0.08	0.08	0.11	0.08	0.06
patients	(0.07)	(0.11)	(0.11)	(0.11)	(0.07)	(0.11)	(0.09)	(0.09)
Healthy controls	0.11	0.16	0.19	0.16	0.10	0.19	0.13	0.10
	(0.09)	(0.07)	(0.10)	(0.11)	(0.11)	(0.09)	(0.09)	(0.11)

TABLE 3

LINEAR CORRELATION BETWEEN ERPS AND SIMULTANEOUS EVENT-RELATED COHERENCE IN DELTA AND THETA FREQUENCY FOR HEALTHY CONTROLS — CORRELATION COEFFICIENTS (p values)

Hemisphere	Right				Left			
Frequency	Delta	Theta	Delta	Theta	Delta	Theta	Delta	Theta
Right hemisphere								
N1	0.11 ($p = 0.64$)	0.40 ($p = 0.08$)						
P1a	0.11 ($p = 0.65$)	0.09 ($p = 0.71$)						
N2b			0.24 ($p = 0.30$)	0.16 ($p = 0.49$)				
P2a			**0.44** (**$p = 0.05$**)	0.04 ($p = 0.86$)				
Left hemisphere								
N1					0.27 ($p = 0.24$)	0.09 ($p = 0.69$)		
P1a					**0.57** (**$p = 0.008$**)	0.28 ($p = 0.23$)		
N2b							0.07 ($p = 0.75$)	0.10 ($p = 0.68$)
P2a							**0.56** (**$p = 0.01$**)	0.16 ($p = 0.49$)

Bold indicates significant correlations at uncorrected alpha level. Corrected alpha for 16 comparisons was 0.003

TABLE 4

LINEAR CORRELATION BETWEEN ERPS AND SIMULTANEOUS EVENT-RELATED COHERENCE IN DELTA AND THETA FREQUENCY FOR SCHIZOPHRENIA PATIENTS — CORRELATION COEFFICIENTS (p values)

Hemisphere	Right				Left			
Frequency	Delta	Theta	Delta	Theta	Delta	Theta	Delta	Theta
Right hemisphere								
N1	0.04 ($p = 0.87$)	0.11 ($p = 0.69$)						
P1a	0.22 ($p = 0.42$)	0.07 ($p = 0.81$)						
N2b			0.31 ($p = 0.25$)	0.27 ($p = 0.30$)				
P2a			**0.50** (**$p = 0.05$**)	0.28 ($p = 0.29$)				
Left hemisphere								
N1					0.08 ($p = 0.76$)	0.14 ($p = 0.60$)		
P1a					0.09 ($p = 0.73$)	0.20 ($p = 0.46$)		
N2b							0.14 ($p = 0.60$)	0.01 ($p = 0.97$)
P2a							0.24 ($p = 0.38$)	0.07 ($p = 0.79$)

Bold indicates significant correlations at uncorrected alpha level. Corrected alpha for 16 comparisons was 0.003

- Event-related fronto-posterior coherence was reduced in patients during the early (100–200 ms) time interval even though the early simultaneous ERPs in the frontal and posterior sites were relatively spared.
- For results corrected for multiple comparisons, there was no significant correlation between coherence and ERPs. For uncorrected results, event-related fronto-posterior coherence in the delta frequency correlated with early (P1a) as well as later frontal evoked activity (P2a) in the left hemisphere and only with the P2a in the right hemisphere in healthy controls. In patients, this correlation failed to reach significance in the left hemisphere for both early and later evoked activity, whereas they showed a significant correlation between P2a and delta coherence in the right hemisphere.

Our ERP results indicate that in schizophrenia patients, the sensory and frontal areas showed reduced evoked activity only during the time intervals associated with the later, more task-relevant processing while the evoked activity during the earlier, more general sensory processing was relatively spared. Given the implication of N2b component in the perceptual level processing of specific task-relevant stimulus features and of N1 in the processing of more general stimulus features (Harter and Guido, 1980; Potts et al., 1996; O'Donnell et al., 1997), our results indicate that the evoked activity in the posterior association cortex during later target evaluation and perceptual processes is more strongly reduced in schizophrenia. Although the group difference for P2a did not reach statistical significance, it revealed a trend for a decreased frontal P2a in patients while the frontal P1a was preserved. As P2a has been associated with frontal processes involved in the evaluation of the task relevance of stimuli (Potts et al., 1996), this result again indicated that the evoked activity in frontal areas was differentially reduced during the utilization of task-specific information to guide the specific processing of task-relevant features. The previous evidence for differential reduction of the N2b and P2a components in schizophrenia is mixed. While some studies have shown differential reduction of visual N2b in schizophrenia as compared to N1 (Ford et al., 1994; Wood et al., 2006), others have found a reduction in both components (Bruder et al., 1998). Studies that have looked at these components separately have reported a reduction in the visual N2b and P2a in schizophrenia (Potts et al., 2002) but an intact visual N1 (Doniger et al., 2002). These different results could be explained by different task demands operating in different studies. Similarly, the higher reduction of the posterior evoked activity as compared to frontal evoked activity in patients in the present study could be explained by task demands, as in the current task, the demand on the frontal control may not have been as high as in other studies with tasks involving higher conflict.

However, the most interesting result of the study was that the fronto-posterior coherence was reduced in patients during the early examined time intervals, even when the early ERPs were preserved, and differentiated the two groups as early as 100 ms which corresponds to the time point in controlled information processing when frontal and posterior areas have been shown to connect with each other (Barcelo et al., 2000; Foxe and Simpson, 2002; Yago et al., 2004). These results indicate that connectivity disturbances may be a more fundamental deficit in schizophrenia and may manifest very early on during cognitive control. This may also have an implication for the later local evoked activity, where connectivity impairments which are manifested earlier could drive impairments in the later local activity. While both local and connectivity impairments in frontal and posterior cortices in schizophrenia have been widely reported (see Meyer-Lindenberg, 2010, for a review), to our knowledge this is the first study that demonstrates that connectivity deficits in the fronto-posterior network may manifest earlier and more persistently during the time course of cognitive control as compared to local activity in the frontal and posterior areas. This is an important result pointing to the central role of connectivity deficits in explaining cognitive impairments in schizophrenia. This pattern of results also highlights the advantage of single-trial analysis which captures dimensions of information processing in the brain that are not strictly time locked to the stimulus (Makeig et al., 2004).

At the corrected alpha level, a limited linear relationship between ERPs and coherence indicated that the long-distance event-related coherence measures added important new information to traditional ERP analysis. However, our results do not exclude the possibility of non-linear and complex modulation of local neuronal activity by long-distance information flow. This has indeed shown to be the case by simulation studies (Cohen et al., 1990; Jaramillo and Pearlmutter, 2007). Therefore, even though the present study found only a limited linear relationship between long distance connectivity and local neuronal activity, given the complexity of long range connections and local neuronal architecture, modulation of one by the other in a more complex non-linear manner cannot be ruled out.

The uncorrected results from the correlation analysis, however, indicated that in healthy controls, especially for the left hemisphere (and to a lesser extent for the right hemisphere), event-related coherence in the delta range might be connected in a linear manner to evoked frontal activity, whereas the theta coherence was not linearly connected to evoked activity in the frontal or the posterior areas. These results are consistent with the reports of both pre-frontal cortex (Barbas and Zikopoulos, 2007; Walther et al., 2010) and delta frequency (Harmony et al., 1996; Başar et al., 2001) in the inhibition of non-relevant stimuli and distinguishing target from non-target stimuli and point to modulation of delta oscillations as a possible mechanism for top-down control in the prefrontal cortex.

Interestingly, in the patients, for the uncorrected results, the correlation between delta coherence and P1a/P2a in the left hemisphere did not reach significance even though they showed a significant correlation between P2a and delta coherence in the right hemisphere. The connection between local and long-range connectivity in the brain is not been very well examined, even less in schizophrenia. However, one earlier study (Spoletini et al., 2009) has looked at the relation between white matter and gray matter abnormalities in schizophrenia and while they reported extensive white matter abnormalities (reduced fractional anisotropy) in white fiber tracts connecting frontal and posterior brain areas in both hemispheres, they found the white matter fractional anisotropy to be correlated with frontal gray matter density only in the right hemisphere in the patients. Our results show a similar pattern on a functional level, with a preserved correlation between local activity and long-range connectivity only in the right hemisphere in schizophrenia. Previous studies have reported abnormalities in both right (Mitchell and Crow, 2005) and left hemisphere (Angrilli et al., 2009) in schizophrenia. The results from the current study provide evidence for local and network deficits in both hemispheres but also point to a possible disruption of the relationship between local and network aspects specifically in the left hemisphere. However, it should be noted that the linear correlation between ERPs and coherence examined in the current study is only a very simple measure of the interplay of the two aspects which was rendered non-significant after correction for multiple testing. Therefore, any generalizations should be made with caution and future studies with more power should employ both linear and non-linear measures to study the relationship between local ERP amplitudes and connectivity measures and to examine this in the context of schizophrenia.

References

Angrilli, A., Spironelli, C., Elbert, T., Crow, T.J., Marano, G. and Stegagno, L. (2009) Schizophrenia as failure of left hemispheric dominance for the phonological component of language. *PLoS One*, 4(2): e4507.

Banich, M.T., Milham, M.P., Atchley, R., Cohen, N.J., Webb, A., Wszalek, T., Kramer, A.F., Liang, Z.P., Wright, A., Shenker, J. and Magin, R. (2000) fMRI studies of Stroop tasks reveal unique roles of anterior and posterior brain systems in attentional selection. *J. Cogn. Neurosci.*, 12(6): 988–1000.

Barbas, H. and Zikopoulos, B. (2007) The prefrontal cortex and flexible behavior. *Neuroscientist*, 13(5): 532–545.

Barcelo, F., Suwazono, S. and Knight, R.T. (2000) Prefrontal modulation of visual processing in humans. *Nat. Neurosci.*, 3(4): 399–403.

Başar, E., Schurmann, M., Demiralp, T., Başar-Eroğlu, C. and Ademoğlu, A. (2001) Event-related oscillations are 'real brain responses'—wavelet analysis and new strategies. *Int. J. Psychophysiol.*, 39(2–3): 91–127.

Bender, S., Oelkers-Ax, R., Hellwig, S., Resch, F. and Weisbrod, M. (2008) The topography of the scalp-recorded visual N700. *Clin. Neurophysiol.*, 119(3): 587–604.

Bentin, S., Mouchetant-Rostaing, Y., Giard, M.H., Echallier, J.F. and Pernier, J. (1999) ERP manifestations of processing printed words at different psycholinguistic levels: time course and scalp distribution. *J. Cogn. Neurosci.*, 11(3): 235–260.

Bob, P., Palus, M., Susta, M. and Glaslova, K. (2008) EEG phase synchronization in patients with paranoid schizophrenia. *Neurosci. Lett.*, 447(1): 73–77.

Bruder, G., Kayser, J., Tenke, C., Rabinowicz, E., Friedman, M., Amador, X., Sharif, Z. and Gorman, J. (1998) The time course of visuospatial processing deficits in schizophrenia: an event-related brain potential study. *J. Abnorm. Psychol.*, 107(3): 399–411.

Buschman, T.J. and Miller, E.K. (2007) Top-down versus bottom-up control of attention in the prefrontal and posterior parietal cortices. *Science*, 315(5820): 1860–1862.

Cohen, J.D., Dunbar, K. and McClelland, J.L. (1990) On the control of automatic processes: a parallel distributed processing account of the Stroop effect. *Psychol. Rev.*, 97(3): 332–361.

Delorme, A. and Makeig, S. (2004) EEGLAB: an open source toolbox for analysis of single-trial EEG dynamics including independent component analysis. *J. Neurosci. Meth.*, 134: 9–21.

Doniger, G.M., Foxe, J.J., Murray, M.M., Higgins, B.A. and Javitt, D.C. (2002) Impaired visual object recognition and dorsal/ventral stream interaction in schizophrenia. *Arch. Gen. Psychiatry*, 59(11): 1011–1020.

Ford, J.M. and Mathalon, D.H. (2005) Corollary discharge dysfunction in schizophrenia: can it explain auditory hallucinations? *Int. J. Psychophysiol.*, 58(2–3): 179–189.

Ford, J.M., White, P.M., Csernansky, J.G., Faustman, W.O., Roth, W.T. and Pfefferbaum, A. (1994) ERPs in schizophrenia: effects of antipsychotic medication. *Biol. Psychiatry*, 36: 153–170.

Foxe, J.J. and Simpson, G.V. (2002) Flow of activation from V1 to frontal cortex in humans. A framework for defining "early" visual processing. *Exp. Brain Res.*, 142(1): 139–150.

Gaser, C., Nenadic, I., Volz, H.P., Buchel, C. and Sauer, H. (2004) Neuroanatomy of "hearing voices": a frontotemporal brain structural abnormality associated with auditory hallucinations in schizophrenia. *Cereb. Cortex*, 14(1): 91–96.

Gratton, G., Coles, M.G. and Donchin, E. (1983) A new method for off-line removal of ocular artifact. *Electroenceph. Clin. Neurophysiol.*, 55: 468–484.

Green, M.F. (2006) Cognitive impairment and functional outcome in schizophrenia and bipolar disorder. *J. Clin. Psychiatry*, 67(Suppl. 9): 3–8, discussion 36–42.

Harmony, T., Fernandez, T., Silva, J., Bernal, J., Diaz-Comas, L., Reyes, A., Marosi, E. and Rodriguez, M. (1996) EEG delta activity: an indicator of attention to internal processing during performance of mental tasks. *Int. J. Psychophysiol.*, 24(1–2): 161–171.

Harter, R.M. and Guido, W. (1980) Attention to pattern orientation: negative cortical potentials, reaction time, and the selection process. *Electroenceph. Clin. Neurophysiol.*, 49: 461–475.

Jaramillo, S. and Pearlmutter, B.A. (2007) Optimal coding predicts attentional modulation of activity in neural systems. *Neural Comput.*, 19(5): 1295–1312.

Kerns, J.G., Nuechterlein, K.H., Braver, T.S. and Barch, D.M. (2008) Executive functioning component mechanisms and schizophrenia. *Biol. Psychiatry*, 64(1): 26–33.

Kim, D.I., Mathalon, D.H., Ford, J.M., Mannell, M., Turner, J.A., Brown, G.G., Belger, A., Gollub, R., Lauriello, J., Wible, C., O'Leary, D., Lim, K., Toga, A., Potkin, S.G., Birn, F. and Calhoun, V.D. (2009) Auditory oddball deficits in schizophrenia: an independent component analysis of the fMRI multisite function BIRN study. *Schizophr. Bull.*, 35(1): 67–81.

Lawrie, S.M., Buechel, C., Whalley, H.C., Frith, C.D., Friston, K.J. and Johnstone, E.C. (2002) Reduced frontotemporal functional connectivity in schizophrenia associated with auditory hallucinations. *Biol. Psychiatry*, 51(12): 1008–1011.

MacLeod, C.M. (1991) Half a century of research on the Stroop effect: an integrative review. *Psychol. Bull.*, 109(2): 163–203.

Makeig, S., Debener, S., Onton, J. and Delorme, A. (2004) Mining event-related brain dynamics. *Trends Cogn. Sci.*, 8(5): 204–210.

Meyer-Lindenberg, A. (2010) From maps to mechanisms through neuroimaging of schizophrenia. *Nature (Lond.)*, 468(7321): 194–202.

Mitchell, R.L. and Crow, T.J. (2005) Right hemisphere language functions and schizophrenia: the forgotten hemisphere? *Brain*, 128(5): 963–978.

Mitchell, T.V., Morey, R.A., Inan, S. and Belger, A. (2005) Functional magnetic resonance imaging measure of automatic and controlled auditory processing. *NeuroReport*, 16(5): 457–461.

O'Donnell, B.F., Swearer, J.M., Smith, L.T., Hokama, H. and McCarley, R.W. (1997) A topographic study of ERPs elicited by visual feature discrimination. *Brain Topogr.*, 10(2): 133–143.

Oldfield, R.C. (1971) The assessment and analysis of handedness: the Edinburgh inventory. *Neuropsychologia*, 9(1): 97–113.

Pernger, T.V. (1998) What's wrong with Bonferroni adjustments. *Br. Med. J.*, 316(7139): 1236–1237.

Posner, M.I. and Dehaene, S. (1994) Attentional networks. *Trends Neurosci.*, 17(2): 75–79.

Potts, G.F. (2004) An ERP index of task relevance evaluation of visual stimuli. *Brain Cogn.*, 56(1): 5–13.

Potts, G.F. and Tucker, D.M. (2001) Frontal evaluation and posterior representation in target detection. *Cogn. Brain Res.*, 11(1): 147–156.

Potts, G.F., Liotti, M., Tucker, D.M. and Posner, M.I. (1996) Frontal and inferior temporal cortical activity in visual target detection: evidence from high spatially sampled event-related potentials. *Brain Topogr.*, 9(1): 3–14.

Potts, G.F., O'Donnell, B.F., Hirayasu, Y. and McCarley, R.W. (2002) Disruption of neural systems of visual attention in schizophrenia. *Arch. Gen. Psychiatry*, 59: 418–424.

Potts, G.F., Wood, S.M., Kothmann, D. and Martin, L.E. (2008) Parallel perceptual enhancement and hierarchic relevance evaluation in an audio-visual conjunction task. *Brain Res.*, 1236: 126–139.

Schlösser, R., Gesierich, T., Kaufmann, B., Vucurevic, G., Hunsche, S., Gawehn, J. and Stoeter, P. (2003) Altered effective connectivity during working memory performance in schizophrenia: a study with fMRI and structural equation modelling. *Neuroimage*, 19: 751–763.

Sharma, A., Weisbrod, M., Kaiser, S., Markela-Lerenc, J. and Bender, S. (2011) Deficits in fronto-posterior interactions point to inefficient resource allocation in schizophrenia. *Acta Psychiatr. Scand.*, 123(2): 125–135.

Spoletini, I., Cherubini, A., Di Paola, M., Banfi, G., Rusch, N., Martinotti, G., Bria, P., Rubino, I.A., Siracusano, A., Caltagirone, C. and Spalletta, G. (2009) Reduced fronto-temporal connectivity is associated with frontal gray matter density reduction and neuropsychological deficit in schizophrenia. *Schizophr. Res.*, 108(1–3): 57–68.

Walther, S., Goya-Maldonado, R., Stippich, C., Weisbrod, M. and Kaiser, S. (2010) A supramodal network for response inhibition. *NeuroReport*, 21(3): 191–195.

Williams, J.M., Mathews, A. and MacLeod, C. (1996) The emotional Stroop task and psychopathology. *Psychol. Bull.*, 120(1): 3–24.

Wittchen, H.U., Zaudig, M. and Fydrich, T. (1997) *Strukturiertes Klinisches Interview für DSM-IV (SKID), Achse I und II.* Hogrefe, Göttingen.

Wood, S.M., Potts, G.F., Hall, J.F., Ulanday, J.B. and Netsiri, C. (2006) Event-related potentials to auditory and visual selective attention in schizophrenia. *Int. J. Psychophysiol.*, 60(1): 67–75.

Yago, E., Duarte, A., Wong, T., Barcelo, F. and Knight, R.T. (2004) Temporal kinetics of prefrontal modulation of the extrastriate cortex during visual attention. *Cogn. Affect. Behav. Neurosci.*, 4(4): 609–617.

Yoon, J.H., Minzenberg, M.J., Ursu, S., Ryan Walter, B.S., Wendelken, C., Ragland, J.D. and Carter, C.S. (2008) Association of dorsolateral prefrontal cortex dysfunction with disrupted coordinated brain activity in schizophrenia: relationship with impaired cognition, behavioral disorganization, and global function. *Am. J. Psychiatry*, 165(8): 1006–1014.

Application of Brain Oscillations in Neuropsychiatric Diseases
(Supplements to Clinical Neurophysiology, Vol. 62)
Editors: E. Başar, C. Başar-Eroğlu, A. Özerdem, P.M. Rossini, G.G. Yener

Chapter 13

Neurophysiological findings in patients with bipolar disorder

Toshiaki Onitsuka*, Naoya Oribe and Shigenobu Kanba

Department of Neuropsychiatry, Graduate School of Medical Sciences, Kyushu University, Fukuoka 812-8582, Japan

ABSTRACT

The present article reviews findings from measuring evoked and event-related responses, neural oscillation and synchronization, and near-infrared spectroscopy (NIRS) studies in patients with bipolar disorder. Studies of evoked responses have indicated that the P50 suppression deficits may be related to the generation of psychosis and may constitute an endophenotype of bipolar disorder patients with psychotic features. The N100 may be intact in patients with bipolar disorder, and the N100 might be a biological index to distinguish bipolar disorder and schizophrenia. In studies of event-related responses, bipolar disorder patients appear to exhibit P300 abnormalities to some extent. In addition, some bipolar disorder patients may have preattentive dysfunction, indexed by abnormal mismatch negativities.

Recent studies of neural oscillations suggest that bipolar disorder may be characterized by deficits in the auditory steady-state response. Moreover, bipolar patients may have altered gamma band responses, as well as abnormal beta and alpha activities perhaps related to deficits of fronto-temporal–parietal functional connectivity. NIRS studies of bipolar disorder have indicated hypofrontality during a verbal fluency task, and altered NIRS responses compared with those of patients with major depressive disorder or healthy subjects.

In future studies, these techniques may be used to elucidate the neurophysiological abnormalities in patients with bipolar disorder. Moreover, neurophysiological approaches may reveal appropriate biological indices to distinguish bipolar disorder and schizophrenia, aiding the development of more effective medication at the early stages of illness.

KEYWORDS

Neurophysiology; Neural oscillation; Electroencephalography; Magnetoencephalography; Bipolar disorder; Schizophrenia

13.1. Introduction

Kraepelin (1913) conceptualized the psychological disorders "manische-depressive Irresein" and "Dementia praecox," which were subsequently

---
*Correspondence to: Dr. Toshiaki Onitsuka, Department of Neuropsychiatry, Graduate School of Medical Sciences, Kyushu University, 3-1-1 Maidashi, Higashiku, Fukuoka 812-8582, Japan.
Tel.: +81 92 642-5627; Fax: +81 92 642-5644;
E-mail: toshiaki@npsych.med.kyushu-u.ac.jp

categorized as bipolar disorder and schizophrenia, respectively, in the DSM-IV (American Psychiatric Association, 2000). There is evidence that several common susceptibility genes exist between the two groups, indicated by epidemiological characteristics, family studies, and overlaps in the confirmed linkages of bipolar disorder and schizophrenia (Berrettini, 2004). It is important to determine whether bipolar disorder and schizophrenia are the clinical outcomes of distinct or shared causative processes. Neuroanatomical and functional studies are essential to determine the similarities and differences between these disorders. Therefore, in each section, the present article will address neurophysiological findings discriminating schizophrenia and bipolar disorder.

Bipolar disorder is a chronic illness presenting with recurrent manic and depressive episodes, and a prevalence of at least 1%. The manic state is characterized by persistently elevated, expansive, or irritable mood. Other symptoms include inflated self-esteem, decreased need for sleep, increased talkativeness, flight of ideas, distractibility, and excessive involvement in pleasurable activities with a high potential for painful consequences. In contrast, the depressive state is characterized by depressed mood throughout most of the day, as well as diminished interest or pleasure, significant weight loss, insomnia or hypersomnia, psychomotor agitation or retardation, fatigue or loss of energy, feelings of worthlessness or excessive or inappropriate guilt, diminished ability to think or concentrate, indecisiveness, recurrent thoughts of death, and suicidal ideation (American Psychiatric Association, 2000). There is accumulating evidence suggesting that patients with bipolar disorder exhibit brain morphometric abnormalities (Hajek et al., 2005), and magnetic resonance imaging (MRI) has been useful in revealing subtle structural brain differences compared to healthy subjects. However, neurophysiological studies of bipolar disorder have received less attention. In neurophysiology research, evoked potentials and event-related potentials (or magnetic fields) are commonly used to assess certain neurofunctional aspects of psychiatric diseases using electroencephalography (EEG) and magnetoencephalography (MEG). These methods are capable of examining brain activity with high temporal resolution.

The present article first presents an overview of the findings of studies measuring evoked and event-related responses in patients with bipolar disorder. Second, we review studies reporting abnormalities in neural oscillation and synchronization, highlighting recent developments in their methods of analysis. Finally, we present findings

of near-infrared spectroscopy (NIRS) studies in patients with bipolar disorder.

13.2. Auditory P50 suppression

Human middle latency auditory evoked potentials (MLAEPs) are elicited by click or tone burst stimuli in the 10–80 ms latency range. The P50 is a positive potential occurring at around 50 ms. This potential is elicited by auditory stimuli and can be used to assess the auditory sensory gating system. The auditory gating is indexed by P50 suppression to the second auditory stimulus with a paired-click paradigm, and the gating ratio is defined as the response to the second stimulus divided by the response to the first stimulus in a paired-click paradigm (Adler et al., 1982; Potter et al., 2006). The P50 component is one of the MLAEPs and has attracted clinical interest in examining patients with various psychiatric disorders (Adler et al., 1982; Freedman et al., 1983; Buchwald et al., 1989, 1992; Neylan et al., 1999; Jessen et al., 2001). For example, Adler et al. (1982) reported that patients with schizophrenia exhibited deficits in sensory gating indexed by decreased P50 inhibition to a second auditory stimulus. Moreover, the P50 gating ratio is reported to be a stable and reliable indicator of sensory gating dysfunction in schizophrenia patients (Bramon et al., 2004) and is thought to be generated in or near the primary auditory cortex (Mäkelä et al., 1994; Onitsuka et al., 2000; Godey et al., 2001).

In a study of bipolar disorder, Olincy and Martin (2005) reported P50 suppression deficits in bipolar disorder with a lifetime history of psychosis, while no deficits of P50 suppression were observed in bipolar disorder without a history of psychosis. Sánchez-Morla et al. (2008) demonstrated P50 gating deficits in euthymic bipolar disorder patients with a lifetime history of psychosis compared with healthy subjects. Schulze et al. (2007) reported that patients with bipolar disorder, who had experienced psychotic symptoms, and their unaffected relatives both exhibited P50 suppression deficits.

On the other hand, these studies reported that patients with bipolar disorder without psychotic features showed no deficits in P50 sensory gating (Olincy and Martin, 2005; Sánchez-Morla et al., 2008). Therefore, the P50 suppression deficits may be related to the generation of psychosis and may constitute an endophenotype of bipolar disorder patients with psychotic features. However, to the best of our knowledge, all existing studies on P50 suppression deficits in bipolar disorder have used a cross-sectional design, meaning that the deficit remains to be confirmed by longitudinal studies.

13.3. Auditory N100

The N100 is a negative evoked potential occurring at around 100 ms after the onset of a stimulus. This potential consists of a component generated in the supratemporal auditory cortex and a number of other components consisting of complex potentials (Wolpaw and Penry, 1975). The N100 is elicited by any discernible auditory stimulus, and the amplitude is influenced by several factors, including inter-stimulus interval, stimulus intensity, arousal level, and subjects' attention. Reductions of the N100 have been consistently reported in patients with schizophrenia (Rosburg et al., 2008; Salisbury et al., 2010). N100 amplitude reduction has been proposed as a marker of functional brain abnormalities related to the genetic predisposition to schizophrenia (Ahveninen et al., 2006). O'Donnell et al. (2004b) evaluated the N100 in bipolar disorder patients in a manic or mixed state, patients with schizophrenia, and healthy subjects. The results revealed reduced N100 amplitude in patients with schizophrenia, but not in bipolar disorder patients (O'Donnell et al., 2004b). Using a dichotic listening paradigm, Force et al. (2008) conducted a target discrimination task and recorded electrophysiological responses in schizophrenia patients, first-degree biological relatives of schizophrenia patients, bipolar disorder patients, first-degree biological relatives of bipolar disorder patients, and healthy subjects. They reported that schizophrenia patients and their relatives exhibited N100 reductions, while no reductions were observed in bipolar disorder patients or their relatives (Force et al., 2008). Fridberg et al. (2009) investigated the N100 in euthymic bipolar disorder patients, symptomatic bipolar disorder patients, and healthy subjects. They reported no significant differences in N100 amplitudes and latencies among groups. Overall, it seems that the N100 may be intact in patients with bipolar disorder, and the N100 might be a biological index for distinguishing bipolar disorder and schizophrenia.

13.4. Auditory P300

The P300 is a positive event-related potential elicited by infrequent and task-relevant stimuli during an oddball paradigm, peaking at around 300 ms. This potential is thought to reflect a variety of cognitive processes elicited by a change in the sensory environment, such as attention, the contextual updating of working memory, and the attribution of salience to a deviant stimulus. P300 amplitude reduction and prolonged P300 latency have been reported repeatedly in patients with schizophrenia (Turetsky et al., 2007). In a study of bipolar disorder patients, O'Donnell et al. (2004b) recorded the P300 in patients with mixed or manic bipolar disorder, patients with schizophrenia, and healthy subjects. They reported that both bipolar disorder and schizophrenia patients exhibited reduced P300 amplitude and prolonged P300 latency (O'Donnell et al., 2004b). Schulze et al. (2008) reported that bipolar disorder patients with a history of psychosis and their unaffected relatives showed significantly delayed P300 latency compared with healthy subjects. However, no significant differences in P300 amplitude were observed between patients with bipolar disorder and healthy subjects. Salisbury et al. (1999) reported that P300 amplitude was reduced in both bipolar disorder patients with psychotic mania and schizophrenia patients, compared to healthy subjects, while bipolar disorder patients showed no delay in P300 latency. In addition, the authors reported that schizophrenia patients showed left temporal scalp area reductions in P300, whereas lateralized topographic abnormalities were not present in bipolar patients. Overall, bipolar disorder patients appear to exhibit P300 abnormalities to some extent. However, the precise nature of P300 deficits in bipolar disorder remains unclear, and further research will be needed to clarify this issue.

13.5. Auditory mismatch negativity

Mismatch negativity (MMN) is the negative component of a waveform obtained by subtracting event-related potential responses to a frequent stimulus (standard) from those to a rare stimulus (deviant) (Garrido et al., 2009), with interstimulus intervals of approximately 500–1000 ms. The MMN can be elicited regardless of whether the subject is paying attention to the sequence, and it reflects the function of auditory sensory memory. The MMN is thought to reflect an automatic process that detects a difference between an incoming stimulus and the sensory memory trace of preceding stimuli. The scalp MMN consists of the component from Heschl's gyrus and the frontal lobe. In patients with schizophrenia, the attenuated MMN amplitude constitutes a robust neurophysiological abnormality (Näätänen and Kähkönen, 2009). There have been a small number of studies of MMN in patients with bipolar disorder. Although some studies have reported no significant differences in MMN amplitude and latency between bipolar disorder patients and healthy subjects (Catts et al., 1995; Hall et al., 2007), Andersson et al. (2008) demonstrated a significantly prolonged MMN latency and frontal MMN reduction in patients with bipolar disorder II. To the best of our knowledge, only one MEG study has been conducted to investigate MMNm (the magnetic counterpart of MMN) in bipolar disorder patients (Takei et al., 2010). The authors reported significantly prolonged MMNm latency in the right hemisphere of bipolar disorder patients. Some bipolar disorder patients may exhibit preattentive dysfunction, indexed by abnormal MMN. However, the nature of MMN dysfunction in bipolar disorder remains unclear.

13.6. Neural oscillations

Neural oscillations and synchronization may reflect variable signals underlying flexible communication within and between cortical areas (Uhlhaas, 2011). In particular, neural oscillations in the gamma band frequency (30–80 Hz) are thought to play a crucial role in information processing in cortical networks (Uhlhaas et al., 2011). Two types of neural oscillations exist: evoked neural oscillations, in which phases are locked to the stimulus onset, and induced neural oscillations, which are not strictly locked to the stimulus onset, but are related to the stimulus. The auditory steady-state response (ASSR) is one of the evoked neural oscillations and can be well recorded by presenting click trains of 40–Hz frequency (Picton et al., 2003). Although the ASSR itself may not reflect cognitive processes, the resonant frequencies of the ASSR suggest that basic neural circuits predominantly oscillate at 40 Hz, and that the ASSR may shed light on the neural circuit functions of auditory-evoked and cognition-related gamma band oscillations.

In patients with schizophrenia, a reduced 40 Hz ASSR has been consistently reported. For example, Kwon et al. (1999) reported a reduced 40 Hz ASSR and delayed phase synchronization/desynchronization in response to a click train in schizophrenia. Light et al. (2006) reported reduction in both evoked power and phase synchronization in response to 30 and 40 Hz ASSR in schizophrenia. Moreover, Spencer et al. (2008) reported that reduced 40 Hz ASSR phase locking was more pronounced over the left hemisphere in first-episode schizophrenia. Hong et al. (2004) reported that relatives with schizophrenia spectrum personality symptoms had reduced 40 Hz ASSR power. Our group reported a reduced 40 Hz MEG ASSR in patients with chronic schizophrenia (Tsuchimoto et al., 2011).

For patients with bipolar disorder, Spencer et al. (2008) reported that first-episode psychotic bipolar disorder patients exhibited a reduced 40 Hz ASSR. Rass et al. (2010) reported reduced ASSR power at 40 Hz and reduced ASSR synchronization at 40 and 50 Hz stimulation in bipolar disorder patients. O'Donnell et al. (2004a) reported reduced 20, 30, 40, and 50 Hz ASSR in bipolar disorder patients. In summary, bipolar disorder patients appear to demonstrate reduced ASSR power to some extent; however, the study of ASSR has received less attention in bipolar disorder than in schizophrenia.

Özerdem et al. (2008) demonstrated altered beta and alpha oscillatory response patterns to target stimuli with a visual odd-ball paradigm in bipolar disorder patients during a manic episode. In addition, they reported that hyper beta band event-related neural oscillations in response to visual target stimuli were normalized after valproate monotherapy in bipolar disorder (Özerdem et al., 2008). Subsequently, the authors investigated long-distance event-related gamma (28–48 Hz) coherence in patients with bipolar disorder and reported a disturbance in functional long-range connectivity in euthymic and manic bipolar disorder patients (Özerdem et al., 2010, 2011). The authors proposed that the coherence of gamma band oscillation may provide a candidate biomarker for bipolar disorder. Meanwhile, Hall et al. (2011) examined whether or not gamma band oscillations constitute endophenotypes of bipolar disorder by testing bipolar disorder patients, monozygotic bipolar disorder twins, unaffected relatives, and healthy subjects using the auditory oddball task and the paired-click paradigm. Patients with bipolar disorder exhibited reduced gamma band power, while the deficits were not observed in clinically unaffected relatives. The authors concluded that these responses do not appear to satisfy criteria for being endophenotypes of bipolar disorder (Hall et al., 2011). Lee et al. (2010) recorded event-related MEG signals in healthy subjects, patients with bipolar disorder, and patients with major depressive disorder during an implicit emotional task with face stimuli,

examining the results using time–frequency analysis. The authors reported that gamma oscillation decreased in the frontal regions in both bipolar disorder and major depressive disorder patients. In addition, gamma oscillation increased in the bilateral temporal regions of patients with major depressive disorder, while alpha and beta oscillations increased in bipolar disorder patients (Lee et al., 2010). The authors concluded that bipolar disorder patients exhibited more widely distributed increases in neural oscillatory activity in the fronto-parieto-occipital regions compared to major depressive disorder patients.

Palva et al. (2002) reported different MEG patterns of evoked neural oscillations at 20–45 Hz between speech and non-speech sounds, suggesting the existence of a fast mechanism for identifying speech sounds in healthy subjects. Based on this finding, researchers in our laboratory recently investigated evoked neural oscillations at 20–45 Hz (Oribe et al., 2010). We hypothesized that the evoked neural oscillation to speech sounds would differentiate bipolar disorder and schizophrenia patients. The study produced three major findings: (1) subjects with bipolar disorder exhibited greater power in evoked neural oscillations in response to speech sounds compared to healthy subjects and schizophrenia subjects (see Fig. 1); (2) schizophrenia patients exhibited delayed evoked neural oscillation peak- and phase-locking to speech sounds (see Fig. 2); and (3) no significant differences were observed in the response to pure tones among the three groups. This study indicated that the evoked neural oscillation to speech sounds provides a useful index to distinguish bipolar disorder from schizophrenia.

Taken together, the research discussed in this section suggests that bipolar disorder may be characterized by some deficits in neural oscillations. Moreover, bipolar patients may have altered gamma band responses, as well as abnormal beta and alpha activities perhaps related to deficits of fronto-temporal-parietal functional connectivity. Recent advances in the analysis of neural oscillations have produced a new field in neuroscience,

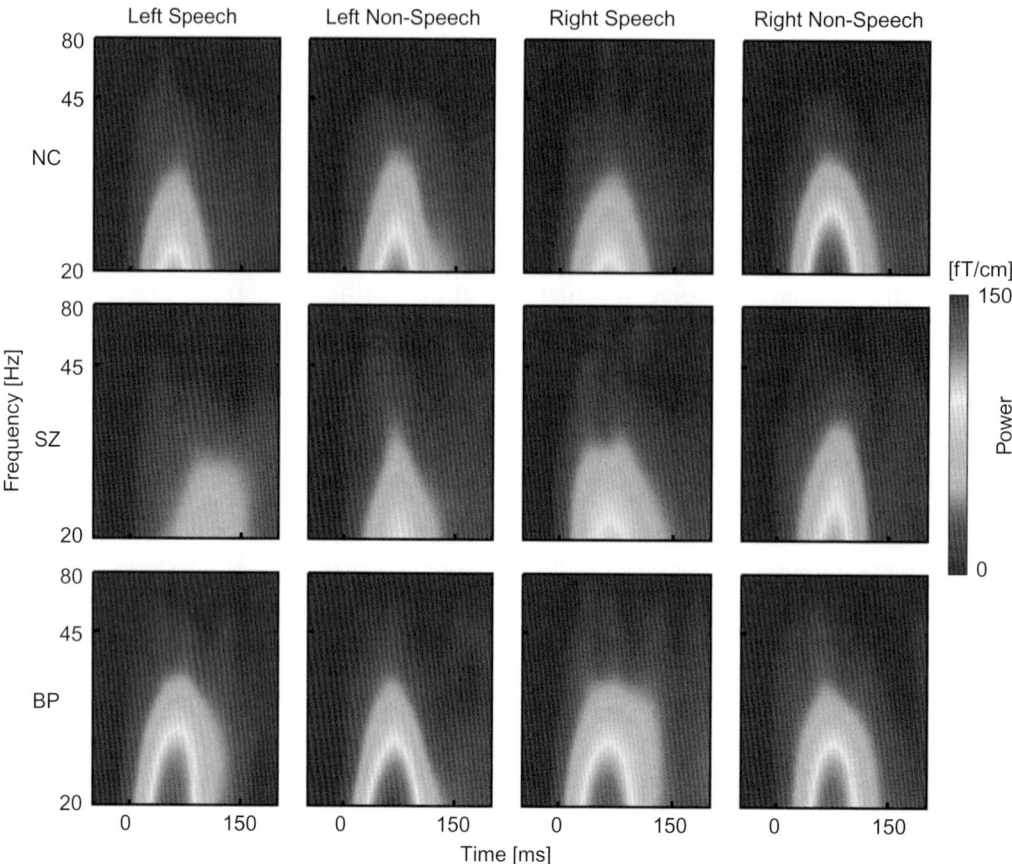

Fig. 1. Overall average time–frequency maps of evoked neural oscillation power to speech sounds and pure tones in patients with bipolar disorder (BP), patients with schizophrenia (SZ), and normal controls (NC). The color scale represents the evoked neural oscillation power. (Adapted from Oribe et al., 2010.) (For color figures, please refer to the color figures in last section of the book.)

and studies of neural oscillations have just begun. Neurophysiological abnormalities in bipolar disorder patients should be further elucidated using these techniques in future studies.

13.7. Near-infrared spectroscopy (NIRS)

It is generally assumed that neuronal activity itself produces neurovascular coupling and increases blood flow volume (Warach et al., 1996). NIRS can detect changes in oxygenated hemoglobin (oxy-Hb) and deoxygenated hemoglobin (deoxy-Hb) in micro-blood vessels on the brain surface (Yamamoto and Kato, 2002). When a certain brain region becomes activated, oxy-Hb increases

due to the dilation of the blood vessels and the acceleration of cerebral blood velocity. Simultaneously, deoxy-Hb decreases since the increase in cerebral blood volume is greater than that of the oxygen consumption in the activated region (Gsell et al., 2000; Matsuo et al., 2007).

Matsuo et al. (2004) measured hemodynamic responses in the prefrontal cortex during verbal fluency and hyperventilation tasks in patients with bipolar disorder and healthy subjects. It was found that increases of oxy-Hb and total-Hb in bipolar disorder patients were significantly smaller than those in healthy subjects during the verbal fluency task. In addition, the total-Hb response during hyperventilation was found to be weaker in the

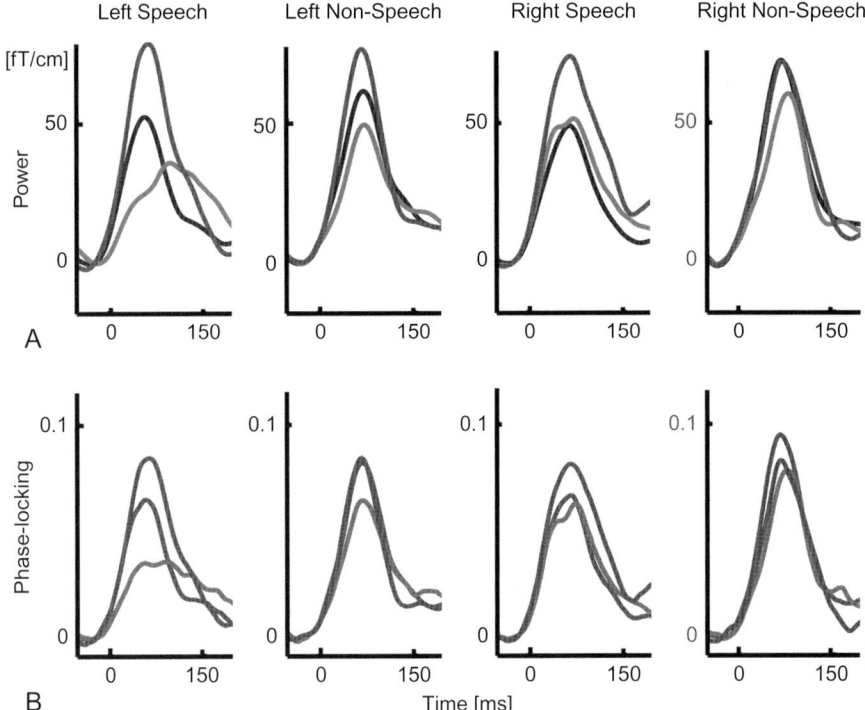

| Left Speech | Left Non-Speech | Right Speech | Right Non-Speech |

Fig. 2.   (A) The overall average of the evoked neural oscillation power waveforms across 20–45 Hz. (B) grand average evoked neural oscillation phase-locking waveforms of schizophrenia (red), bipolar disorder (green), and normal control subjects (blue). (Adapted from Oribe et al., 2010.) (For color figures, please refer to the color figures in last section of the book.)

bipolar patient group compared to the healthy control group. Taken together, these findings suggest that remitted subjects with bipolar disorder exhibit bilateral hypofrontality during a cognitive task, which may be related to vascular function, as measured by the response to hyperventilation. Kameyama et al. (2006) measured changes in oxy-Hb during a verbal fluency task using frontal and temporal probes of two 24-channel NIRS machines in patients with bipolar disorder, patients with major depressive disorder, and healthy subjects. It was reported that oxy-Hb increases in bipolar disorder were reduced compared to those in healthy subjects during the early period of the verbal fluency task, and larger than those in major depressive disorder patients and healthy subjects during the late period of the task. Matsuo et al. (2007) recorded NIRS responses during a verbal fluency task and during 5% CO_2

inhalation to measure alterations of oxy- and deoxy-Hb. The results suggested the existence of functional hypoactivation of the prefrontal lobe during cognitive load in bipolar disorder patients while they were in a euthymic state. The mechanism of this hypoactivation appears to differ from that of vascular regulation in response to a physiological stimulus. Overall, NIRS studies of bipolar disorder have indicated hypofrontality during a verbal fluency task, and altered NIRS responses compared to patients with major depressive disorder and healthy subjects.

13.8. Conclusions

The present article reviewed major neurophysiological findings in patients with bipolar disorder. The research discussed above suggests that P50 suppression deficits may be related to the generation of bipolar psychosis and constitutes a candidate end-ophenotype of psychotic bipolar disorder. The N100 appears to remain intact in bipolar disorder patients. Patients with bipolar disorder appear to show some abnormalities in the P300 and MMN; however, the precise nature of these deficits remains unclear. Although appropriate methods and analyses for examining neural oscillations and NIRS responses have been developed relatively recently, they have revealed a range of novel findings. Neurophysiological abnormalities in patients with bipolar disorder may be further elucidated using these techniques in future studies.

Future investigations should examine whether the findings described here are associated with post-onset course of illness, or whether they are neurodevelopmental in origin, or a combination of both. In addition, it will be important to investigate the specificity of certain neurophysiological abnormalities to bipolar disorder, to determine both the similarities and differences between bipolar disorder and schizophrenia. Investigating the biological substrates of bipolar disorder I and II is another important aim for research. Longitudinal studies of patients during both manic and depressive mood phases will be needed to further elucidate the pathophysiology of bipolar disorder. In the future, it will be necessary to conduct cross-sectional electrophysiological studies with more homogenous patient groups (drug-free vs. medicated), and prospective investigations before and after a certain medication, to control for the illness state, eliminate potential medication effects, and to understand the role of oscillatory activity in assessing treatment response. Neurophysiological approaches may reveal appropriate biological indices to distinguish bipolar disorder and schizophrenia, aiding the development of more effective medication at the early stages of illness.

Acknowledgments

This work was supported in part by a grant-in-aid for Scientific Research from the Ministry of Education, Culture, Sports, Science and Technology, Japan (B19390306 to S.K., C23591712 to T.O.); and a Research Grant from the Ministry of Health, Labor and Welfare, Japan (17B-2 for Nervous and Mental Disorders to T.O., H18 kokoro-ippan-012 to S.K.).

References

Adler, L.E., Pachtman, E., Franks, R.D., Pecevich, M., Waldo, M.C. and Freedman, R. (1982) Neurophysiological evidence for a defect in neuronal mechanisms involved in sensory gating in schizophrenia. *Biol. Psychiatry*, 17: 639–654.

Ahveninen, J., Jääskeläinen, I.P., Osipova, D., Huttunen, M.O., Ilmoniemi, R.J., Kaprio, J., Lönnqvist, J., Manninen, M., Pakarinen, S., Therman, S., Näätänen, R. and Cannon, T.D. (2006) Inherited auditory cortical dysfunction in twin pairs discordant for schizophrenia. *Biol. Psychiatry*, 60: 612–620.

American Psychiatric Association (2000) *Diagnostic and Statistical Manual of Mental Disorders, IVth Edition Text Version (DSM-IV-TR)*. American Psychiatric Association, New York.

Andersson, S., Barder, H.E., Hellvin, T., Løvdahl, H. and Malt, U.F. (2008) Neuropsychological and electrophysiological indices of neurocognitive dysfunction in bipolar II disorder. *Bipolar Disord.*, 10: 888–899.

Berrettini, W. (2004) Bipolar disorder and schizophrenia: convergent molecular data. *Neuromolecular Med.*, 5: 109–117.

Bramon, E., Rabe-Hesketh, S., Sham, P., Murray, R.M. and Frangou, S. (2004) Meta-analysis of the P300 and P50 waveforms in schizophrenia. *Schizophr. Res.*, 70: 315–329.

Buchwald, J.S., Erwin, R.J., Read, S., Van Lancker, D. and Cummings, J.L. (1989) Midlatency auditory evoked responses: differential abnormality of P1 in Alzheimer's disease. *Electroenceph. Clin. Neurophysiol.*, 74: 378–384.

Buchwald, J.S., Erwin, R.J., Van Lancker, D., Gutherie, D., Schwafel, J. and Tanguay, P. (1992) Midlatency auditory evoked responses: P1 abnormalities in adult autistic subjects. *Electroenceph. Clin. Neurophysiol.*, 84: 164–171.

Catts, S.V., Shelley, A.M., Ward, P.B., Liebert, B., McConaghy, N., Andrews, S. and Michie, P.T. (1995) Brain potential evidence for an auditory sensory memory deficit in schizophrenia. *Am. J. Psychiatry*, 152: 213–219.

Force, R.B., Venables, N.C. and Sponheim, S.R. (2008) An auditory processing abnormality specific to liability for schizophrenia. *Schizophr. Res.*, 103: 298–310.

Freedman, R., Adler, L.E., Waldo, M.C., Pachtman, E. and Franks, R.D. (1983) Neurophysiological evidence for a detect in inhibitory pathways in schizophrenia: comparison of medicated and drug-free patients. *Biol. Psychiatry*, 18: 537–551.

Fridberg, D.J., Hetrick, W.P., Brenner, C.A., Shekhar, A., Steffen, A.N., Malloy, F.W. and O'Donnell, B.F. (2009) Relationships between auditory event-related potentials and mood state, medication, and comorbid psychiatric illness in patients with bipolar disorder. *Bipolar Disord.*, 11: 857–866.

Garrido, M.I., Kilner, J.M., Stephan, K.E. and Friston, K.J. (2009) The mismatch negativity: a review of underlying mechanisms. *Clin. Neurophysiol.*, 120: 453–463.

Godey, B., Schwartz, D., De Graaf, J.B., Chauvel, P. and Liégeois-Chauvel, C. (2001) Neuromagnetic source localization of auditory evoked fields and intracerebral evoked potentials: a comparison of data in the same patients. *Clin. Neurophysiol.*, 112: 1850–1859.

Gsell, W., De Sadeleer, C., Marchalant, Y., MacKenzie, E.T., Schumann, P. and Dauphin, F. (2000) The use of cerebral blood flow as an index of neuronal activity in functional neuroimaging: experimental and pathophysiological considerations. *J. Chem. Neuroanat.*, 20: 215–224.

Hajek, T., Carrey, N. and Alda, M. (2005) Neuroanatomical abnormalities as risk factors for bipolar disorders. *Bipolar Disord.*, 7: 393–403.

Hall, M.H., Rijsdijk, F., Kalidindi, S., Schulze, K., Kravariti, E., Kane, F., Sham, P., Bramon, E. and Murray, R.M. (2007) Genetic overlap between bipolar illness and event-related potentials. *Psychol. Med.*, 37: 667–678.

Hall, M.H., Spencer, K.M., Schulze, K., McDonald, C., Kalidindi, S., Kravariti, E., Kane, F., Murray, R.M., Bramon, E., Sham, P. and Rijsdijk, F. (2011) The genetic and environmental influences of event-related gamma oscillations on bipolar disorder. *Bipolar Disord.*, 13: 260–271.

Hong, L.E., Summerfelt, A., McMahon, R., Adami, H., Francis, G., Elliott, A., Buchanan, R.W. and Thaker, G.K. (2004) Evoked gamma band synchronization and the liability for schizophrenia. *Schizophr. Res.*, 70: 293–302.

Jessen, F., Kucharski, C., Fries, T., Papassotiropoulos, A., Hoenig, K., Maier, W. and Heun, R. (2001) Sensory gating deficit expressed by a disturbed suppression of the P50 event-related potential in patients with Alzheimer's disease. *Am. J. Psychiatry*, 158: 1319–1321.

Kameyama, M., Fukuda, M., Yamagishi, Y., Sato, T., Uehara, T., Ito, M., Suto, T. and Mikuni, M. (2006) Frontal lobe function in bipolar disorder: a multichannel near-infrared spectroscopy study. *Neuroimage*, 29: 172–184.

Kraepelin, E. (1913) *Compendium der Psychiatrie zum Gebrauche für Studierende und Ärzte*. Von Krosigk, Berlin.

Kwon, J.S., O'Donnell, B.F., Wallenstein, G.V., Greene, R.W., Hirayasu, Y., Nestor, P.G., Hasselmo, M.E., Potts, G.F., Shenton, M.E. and McCarley, R.W. (1999) Gamma frequency-range abnormalities to auditory stimulation in schizophrenia. *Arch. Gen. Psychiatry*, 56: 1001–1005.

Lee, P.S., Chen, Y.S., Hsieh, J.C., Su, T.P. and Chen, L.F. (2010) Distinct neuronal oscillatory responses between patients with bipolar and unipolar disorders: a magnetoencephalographic study. *J. Affect. Disord.*, 123: 270–275.

Light, G.A., Hsu, J.L., Hsieh, M.H., Meyer-Gomes, K., Sprock, J., Swerdlow, N.R. and Braff, D.L. (2006) Gamma band oscillations reveal neural network cortical coherence dysfunction in schizophrenia patients. *Biol. Psychiatry*, 60: 1231–1240.

Mäkelä, J.P., Hämäläinen, M., Hari, R. and McEvoy, L. (1994) Whole-head mapping of middle-latency auditory evoked magnetic fields. *Electroenceph. Clin. Neurophysiol.*, 92: 414–421.

Matsuo, K., Watanabe, A., Onodera, Y., Kato, N. and Kato, T. (2004) Prefrontal hemodynamic response to verbal-fluency task and hyperventilation in bipolar disorder measured by multichannel near-infrared spectroscopy. *J. Affect. Disord.*, 82: 85–92.

Matsuo, K., Kouno, T., Hatch, J.P., Seino, K., Ohtani, T., Kato, N. and Kato, T. (2007) A near-infrared spectroscopy study of prefrontal cortex activation during a verbal fluency task and carbon dioxide inhalation in individuals with bipolar disorder. *Bipolar Disord.*, 9: 876–883.

Näätänen, R. and Kähkönen, S. (2009) Central auditory dysfunction in schizophrenia as revealed by the mismatch negativity (MMN) and its magnetic equivalent MMNm: a review. *Int. J. Neuropsychopharmacol.*, 12: 125–135.

Neylan, T.C., Fletcher, D.J., Lenoci, M., McCallin, K., Weiss, D.S., Schoenfeld, F.B., Marmar, C.R. and Fein, G. (1999) Sensory gating in chronic posttraumatic stress disorder: reduced auditory P50 suppression in combat veterans. *Biol. Psychiatry*, 46: 1656–1664.

O'Donnell, B.F., Hetrick, W.P., Vohs, J.L., Krishnan, G.P., Carroll, C.A. and Shekhar, A. (2004a) Neural synchronization deficits to auditory stimulation in bipolar disorder. *Neuroreport*, 15: 1369–1372.

O'Donnell, B.F., Vohs, J.L., Hetrick, W.P., Carroll, C.A. and Shekhar, A. (2004b) Auditory event-related potential abnormalities in bipolar disorder and schizophrenia. *Int. J. Psychophysiol.*, 53: 45–55.

Olincy, A. and Martin, L. (2005) Diminished suppression of the P50 auditory evoked potential in bipolar disorder subjects with a history of psychosis. *Am. J. Psychiatry*, 162: 43–49.

Onitsuka, T., Ninomiya, H., Sato, E., Yamamoto, T. and Tashiro, N. (2000) The effect of interstimulus intervals and between-block rests on the auditory evoked potential and magnetic field: is the auditory P50 in humans an overlapping potential? *Clin. Neurophysiol.*, 111: 237–245.

Oribe, N., Onitsuka, T., Hirano, S., Hirano, Y., Maekawa, T., Obayashi, C., Kasai, K., Ueno, T. and Kanba, S. (2010) Differentiation between bipolar disorder and schizophrenia revealed by neural oscillation to speech sounds: a MEG study. *Bipolar Disord.*, 12: 804–812.

Özerdem, A., Güntekin, B., Tunca, Z. and Başar, E. (2008) Brain oscillatory responses in patients with bipolar disorder manic episode before and after valproate treatment. *Brain Res.*, 1235: 98–108.

Özerdem, A., Güntekin, B., Saatçi, E., Tunca, Z. and Başar, E. (2010) Disturbance in long distance gamma coherence in bipolar disorder. *Prog. Neuropsychopharmacol. Biol. Psychiatry*, 34: 861–865.

Özerdem, A., Güntekin, B., Atagun, I., Turp, B. and Başar, E. (2011) Reduced long distance gamma (28–48 Hz) coherence in euthymic patients with bipolar disorder. *J. Affect. Disord.*, 132: 325–332.

Palva, S., Palva, J.M., Shtyrov, Y., Kujala, T., Ilmoniemi, R.J., Kaila, K. and Näätänen, R. (2002) Distinct gamma-band evoked responses to speech and non-speech sounds in humans. *J. Neurosci.*, 22: RC211.

Picton, T.W., John, M.S., Dimitrijevic, A. and Purcell, D. (2003) Human auditory steady-state responses. *Int. J. Audiol.*, 42: 177–219.

Potter, D., Summerfelt, A., Gold, J. and Buchanan, R.W. (2006) Review of clinical correlates of P50 sensory gating abnormalities in patients with schizophrenia. *Schizophr. Bull.*, 32: 692–700.

Rass, O., Krishnan, G., Brenner, C.A., Hetrick, W.P., Merrill, C.C., Shekhar, A. and O'Donnell, B.F. (2010) Auditory steady state response in bipolar disorder: relation to clinical state, cognitive performance, medication status, and substance disorders. *Bipolar Disord.*, 12: 793–803.

Rosburg, T., Boutros, N.N. and Ford, J.M. (2008) Reduced auditory evoked potential component N100 in schizophrenia—a critical review. *Psychiatry Res.*, 161: 259–274.

Salisbury, D.F., Shenton, M.E. and McCarley, R.W. (1999) P300 topography differs in schizophrenia and manic psychosis. *Biol. Psychiatry*, 45: 98–106.

Salisbury, D.F., Collins, K.C. and McCarley, R.W. (2010) Reductions in the N1 and P2 auditory event-related potentials in first-hospitalized and chronic schizophrenia. *Schizophr. Bull.*, 36: 991–1000.

Sánchez-Morla, E.M., García-Jiménez, M.A., Barabash, A., Martínez-Vizcaíno, V., Mena, J., Cabranes-Díaz, J.A., Baca-Baldomero, E. and Santos, J.L. (2008) P50 sensory gating deficit is a common marker of vulnerability to bipolar disorder and schizophrenia. *Acta Psychiatr. Scand.*, 117: 313–318.

Schulze, K.K., Hall, M.-H., McDonald, C., Marshall, N., Walshe, M., Murray, R.M. and Bramon, E. (2007) P50 auditory evoked potential suppression in bipolar disorder patients with psychotic features and their unaffected relatives. *Biol. Psychiatry*, 62: 121–128.

Schulze, K.K., Hall, M.-H., McDonald, C., Marshall, N., Walshe, M., Murray, R.M. and Bramon, E. (2008) Auditory P300 in patients with bipolar disorder and their unaffected relatives. *Bipolar Disord.*, 10: 377–386.

Spencer, K.M., Salisbury, D.F., Shenton, M.E. and McCarley, R.W. (2008) Gamma-band auditory steady-state responses are impaired in first episode psychosis. *Biol. Psychiatry*, 64: 369–375.

Takei, Y., Kumano, S., Maki, Y., Hattori, S., Kawakubo, Y., Kasai, K., Fukuda, M. and Mikuni, M. (2010) Preattentive dysfunction in bipolar disorder: a MEG study using auditory mismatch negativity. *Prog. Neuropsychopharmacol. Biol. Psychiatry*, 34: 903–912.

Tsuchimoto, R., Kanba, S., Hirano, S., Oribe, N., Ueno, T., Hirano, Y., Nakamura, I., Oda, Y., Miura, T. and Onitsuka, T. (2011) Reduced high and low frequency gamma synchronization in patients with chronic schizophrenia. *Schizophr. Res.*, 133: 99–105.

Turetsky, B.I., Calkins, M.E., Light, G.A., Olincy, A., Radant, A.D. and Swerdlow, N.R. (2007) Neurophysiological endophenotypes of schizophrenia: the viability of selected candidate measures. *Schizophr. Bull.*, 33: 69–94.

Uhlhaas, P.J. (2011) High-frequency oscillations in schizophrenia. *Clin. EEG Neurosci.*, 42: 77–82.

Uhlhaas, P.J., Pipa, G., Neuenschwander, S., Wibral, M. and Singer, W. (2011) A new look at gamma? High (>60 Hz) gamma-band activity in cortical networks: function, mechanisms and impairment. *Prog. Biophys. Mol. Biol.*, 105: 14–28.

Warach, S., Ives, J.R., Schlaug, G., Patel, M.R., Darby, D.G., Thangaraj, V., Edelman, R.R. and Schomer, D.L. (1996) EEG-triggered echo-planar functional MRI in epilepsy. *Neurology*, 47: 89–93.

Wolpaw, J.R. and Penry, J.K. (1975) A temporal component of the auditory evoked response. *Electroencephalogr. Clin. Neurophysiol.*, 39: 609–620.

Yamamoto, T. and Kato, T. (2002) Paradoxical correlation between signal in functional magnetic resonance imaging and deoxygenated haemoglobin content in capillaries: a new theoretical explanation. *Phys. Med. Biol.*, 47: 1121–1141.

Chapter 14

Brain oscillations in bipolar disorder in search of new biomarkers

Ayşegül Özerdem[a,b,c,d,*], Bahar Güntekin[d], M. İlhan Atagün[e]
and Erol Başar[d]

[a]Department of Psychiatry, Dokuz Eylül University Medical School, Narlidere, 35340 Izmir, Turkey
[b]Department of Neuroscience, Dokuz Eylül University Health Sciences Institute, 35340 Izmir, Turkey
[c]Multidisciplinary Brain Dynamics Research Center, Dokuz Eylül University, 35340 Izmir, Turkey
[d]Brain Dynamics, Cognition, and Complex Systems Research Center, Istanbul Kultur University, 35340
Istanbul, Turkey
[e]Bakirkoy Research and Training Hospital for Psychiatry and Neurology, 34145 Istanbul, Turkey

ABSTRACT

This report presents six cardinal results obtained with methods of oscillatory brain dynamics in euthymic and manic bipolar patients in comparison to healthy controls. Measurements include changes in oscillatory response activities in the theta, alpha, beta, and gamma frequency ranges. The analysis shows that spontaneous and response activities in the alpha range are highly reduced in euthymic and manic patients, respectively; conversely, beta responses are increased in euthymic and manic patients. Lithium use seems to be associated with further and significant increase in the beta frequency range in euthymic patients. Theta responses to auditory target stimulus during odd-ball paradigm appeared in two different frequency bands (4–6 and 6–8 Hz) in healthy participants. However, only fast theta responses were highly reduced under cognitive load in drug-free euthymic patients.

The analysis of connectivity was performed by assessment of long-distance coherence function in the gamma frequency range. Both manic and euthymic patients presented significantly decreased fronto-temporal coherence function during visual odd-ball task, indicating a selective reduction in connectivity during cognitive processing.

The present report also discusses that these six oscillatory parameters may serve as an ensemble of biomarkers for diagnostic purposes and tracking treatment response in bipolar disorder.

KEYWORDS

Brain oscillations; Bipolar disorder; Biomarkers; Brain imaging; Delta; Theta; Alpha; Beta; Gamma; Coherence; Evoked coherence; Event-related coherence; Lithium; Valproate; Event-related oscillation; Evoked oscillation; Odd-ball paradigm

14.1. Introduction

*Correspondence to: Dr. Ayşegül Özerdem, M.D., Ph.D., Department of Psychiatry, Dokuz Eylül University Medical School, Narlidere, 35340 Izmir, Turkey.
Tel.: +90 232 412 4152; Fax: +90 232 412 4169;
E-mail: aysegul.ozerdem@deu.edu.tr

The last decade witnessed a substantial increase in the utilization of the concept and methods of oscillatory brain dynamics in different neuropsychiatric disorders (O'Donnell et al., 2004; Herrmann and Demiralp, 2005; Başar and Güntekin, 2008;

Spencer et al., 2008; Uhlhaas et al., 2008), including bipolar disorder (BP) (Bhattacharya, 2001; O'Donnell et al., 2004; Chen et al., 2008; Spencer et al., 2008; Lee et al., 2010; Rass et al., 2010; Hall et al., 2011).

Findings from assessment of brain oscillatory activity in neuropsychiatric disorders indicate a high potential for an alternative functional imaging method. The aim of the present paper is to explore emerging biomarkers of spontaneous EEG oscillations, and event-related as well as sensory evoked oscillatory responses in BP. As the data derived from euthymic drug-free patients show a break of spontaneous alpha oscillatory activity (Başar et al., 2012), both manic and euthymic drug-free patients display a substantial event-related decrease in long-distance gamma coherence (Özerdem et al., 2010, 2011). The latter can be referred to as "differential connection deficit," as it appears prominently in fronto-temporal location in both cases. Increase in event-related beta activity in patients treated only with lithium in comparison to drug-free patients indicates a treatment effect through oscillatory responses in patients (Tan et al., 2011). This issue of whether this effect is a sign of treatment response or a side effect remains to be further explored. We also emphasize that a review or a mini review related to oscillatory dynamics in bipolar patients is not yet possible, since these types of analysis are seldom encountered in the literature and are mostly limited to the results of our research team. Therefore, this report can be defined as a first survey on published and, as yet, unpublished but statistically significant results. We do not intend to present a systematic and detailed description of topological changes; rather, the reader will be introduced to evidence for a number of promising oscillatory biomarkers, an "ensemble of biomarkers" or "efficient collective biomarkers," as we call them. More detailed analysis, including the topology of these event-related responses, can be found in previous papers from our group.

14.2. What is bipolar disorder?

Bipolar disorder is a chronic illness with an unpredictable relapsing and remitting course. Relapses are manic or depressive or mixed in nature. Bipolar disorder is one of the most debilitating illnesses worldwide (Murray and Lopez, 1996). The prevalence of BD types I and II together reaches 4.4% of the population (Merikangas et al., 2007), which is considerably higher than the 1% prevalence of another severe psychiatric disorder, schizophrenia. Poor clinical and functional outcome is a common feature of BP type I and is associated with a serious economic burden (Baldessarini and Tondo, 2003). The risk of suicide in BD is high (Valtonen et al., 2005). The serious problem of delayed initiation of appropriate treatment and a consequent poor prognosis (Bowden, 2001, 2005) is caused mainly by misdiagnosis, which is quite frequent, ranging between 30% and 69% (Hirschfeld et al., 2003; Baca-Garcia et al., 2007).

Symptoms in both manic and depressive phases of bipolar disorder involve a wide range of areas such as mood, energy, motor activity, sleep, appetite, thought, and cognition. A subtle chronic course between the full-blown mood episodes with residual symptoms, sleep and circadian rhythm disturbances, emotional disregulation, and cognitive impairment has been found to be more common than initially thought (Leboyer and Kupfer, 2010).

Neurocognition has been shown to be largely disturbed in bipolar disorder. In depression, patients suffer from attentional and memory deficits, impairment in verbal recall and fine motor skills, and disturbance of sustained attention. Manic patients also display signs of dysfunction in attentional measures, complex processing, and memory as well as emotional processing (Goldberg and Chengappa, 2009). Cognitive deficits in euthymia involve response inhibition, set-shifting, executive function, verbal memory, sustained attention, processing speed, visual memory, and verbal fluency (Bora et al., 2009).

The underlying mechanism of the wide range of cognitive problems in bipolar disorder involves neural circuits, with projections connecting pre-frontal to striatal structures with further projections to thalamic nuclei (Vawter et al., 2000). These functional systems regulate cognitive, emotional, and social behavior and represent an interface between the cognitive and affective systems in BD. Based on existing evidence from fronto-temporal- and fronto-limbic-related cognitive impairments, Bora et al. (2009) recently defined a cognitive end-ophenotype for bipolar disorder.

14.3. What is the importance of biomarkers in BD?

The identification of endophenotypes (Thaker, 2008) is an important strategy, recently developed to facilitate identification of the neurobiological and genetic underpinnings of BD. A first step toward developing an endophenotype is the dis-covery of biological markers that are specific and/or consistent in BD. Biomarkers play an important role in early diagnosis and initiation of proper treatment of BD, and can also be used in tracking treatment response. The brain is a com-plex structure that remains to be largely explored. Owing to current limited knowledge at the molec-ular and the circuitry level, it would be over-optimistic to expect a single biomarker in bipolar disorder. However, recent findings concentrate on cognitive dysfunction and corresponding imaging findings as candidate biomarkers in bipolar disor-der (Pavuluri, 2010). From an electrophysiological perspective, sensory gating has been characterized as an endophenotype for schizophrenia (Thaker, 2008). Sensory gating is a measure of the integrity of the brain's inhibitory function. It is measured by using the amplitude of the evoked potential at 50 ms to the first of two paired clicks, divided by the response to the second. Currently, no such bio-logical marker exists for bipolar disorder. One study suggested P85 gating ratio as a new marker, specific to bipolar disorder (Patterson et al., 2009), but the finding needs replication.

14.4. Research challenges in discovery of bipolar disorder biomarkers

Bipolar disorder is a challenging illness for discovery of the underlying mechanisms. Changes in the state of the brain along with fluctuations in mood state between mania, depression, and euthymia are con-founding factors affecting research on brain func-tionality, with further interference due to the medication state. Evidence points to a possible med-ication effect in electrophysiology (Özerdem et al., 2008, 2010) and in other imaging findings (Lyoo et al., 2010) in bipolar disorder. There is currently insufficient evidence to differentiate between the effects of monotherapy and polypharmacy other than the notion that polypharmacy may add further complexity to the interpretation of findings.

14.5. Brain oscillations as candidate biomarkers in bipolar disorder: findings from our group

14.5.1. Methods applied

Studying event-related oscillations provides us with detailed assessment of the brain's instant activity in a given condition, or its reactivity to a given stimu-lus, by filtering the recording into delta (0.5–3.5 Hz), theta (4–7 Hz), alpha (9–13 Hz), beta (18–30 Hz), and gamma (28–48 Hz) oscillations. The methods of analyzing EEG data follow an algo-rithm that begins with power spectrum analysis of spontaneous EEG, followed by analysis of evoked and event-related oscillatory responses. The latter can be done by analyzing amplitude changes, and through coherence analysis. Within this context, the findings in BD will be presented accordingly.

Recording of the evoked or event-related oscil-latory responses requires application of a task. In our studies, in order to analyze evoked oscillations, participants were presented both visual and audi-tory sensory stimulations. A visual and auditory odd-ball paradigm was used as the cognitive task to analyze event-related oscillatory responses.

In this task, participants are instructed to focus on the target stimuli, which were embedded randomly within a series of standard stimuli. The task was to count the number of target stimuli and report it at the end of the session, the aim being to assess focused attention and working memory. The following section presents findings from both auditory and visual stimulation types.

Given the above-mentioned confounding factors originating either from the nature of bipolar disorder, or from the medication condition, we focused on either euthymic or manic patients to date, each being compared to healthy controls. Considering the medication effect, our patients were either drug-free or, if medicated, they were on monotherapy, either with lithium or with valproate. Thus, we were able to provide as homogenous sets of patients as possible. In principle, data from each set of patients were first screened for the most prominent frequency band in the power spectra and further exploration was completed on evoked and event-related oscillations.

14.5.2. Results

14.5.2.1. Power spectrum analysis of spontaneous EEG
Alpha frequency range-related changes: Although these power spectra are also called "resting state," the recording is actually far from being "resting" in terms of the brain's baseline activity and provides an excellent source for predicting how the brain would respond when exposed to a sensory or cognitive stimulation.

In a recently published study from our group (Başar et al., 2012), we studied spontaneous EEG activity (4 min eyes closed, 4 min eyes open) in 18 drug-free DSM-IV euthymic bipolar patients (bipolar I $n = 15$, bipolar II $n = 3$) in comparison to 18 healthy controls. The digital FFT-based power spectrum analysis was performed for spontaneous eyes-closed and eyes-open conditions. Spontaneous EEG alpha

(8–13 Hz) power of healthy subjects was significantly higher than the spontaneous EEG alpha power of euthymic patients. Fig. 1 shows significantly reduced alpha power in bipolar patients in the right and left occipital region at the eyes-closed condition.

Berger (1929) was the first to observe alpha rhythm. It was initially considered as the "brain's idling rhythm." Later, several authors stated that EEG was not noise and that selectively synchronized alpha oscillations in the mammalian and human brain are part of the fundamental functional signaling of the central nervous system (Başar, 1980; Lehmann, 1989; Klimesch, 1999; Başar et al., 2001a,b; Nunez et al., 2001). In one study prior to ours (Başar et al., 2012), alpha activity was found to be reduced in bipolar patients with psychotic characteristics and in patients with schizophrenia when compared to healthy controls (Clementz et al., 1994). Several years later, the replication of a reduced alpha activity in bipolar disorder, this time in drug-free euthymic patients, demonstrated that the reduction is neither associated with psychosis or any mood-related symptom, nor it can be explained by medication effect.

14.5.2.2. Power spectrum of the evoked and event-related oscillatory responses
Alpha (8–13 Hz) frequency range-related changes: This is a helpful step to determine the behavior of a given oscillation upon application of a stimulus. In the same study population presented in the previous section (Başar et al., 2012), analysis of evoked alpha response upon application of simple visual stimuli showed significantly higher evoked alpha power in the healthy controls compared to euthymic patients.

14.5.2.3. Event-related oscillatory responses: analysis of amplitude changes
Alpha (8–13 Hz) frequency range-related changes: This assessment was completed in a group of drug-free manic patients ($n = 10$) in comparison to healthy controls ($n = 10$) (Özerdem et al.,

Grand Average of Eyes Closed Spontaneous EEG

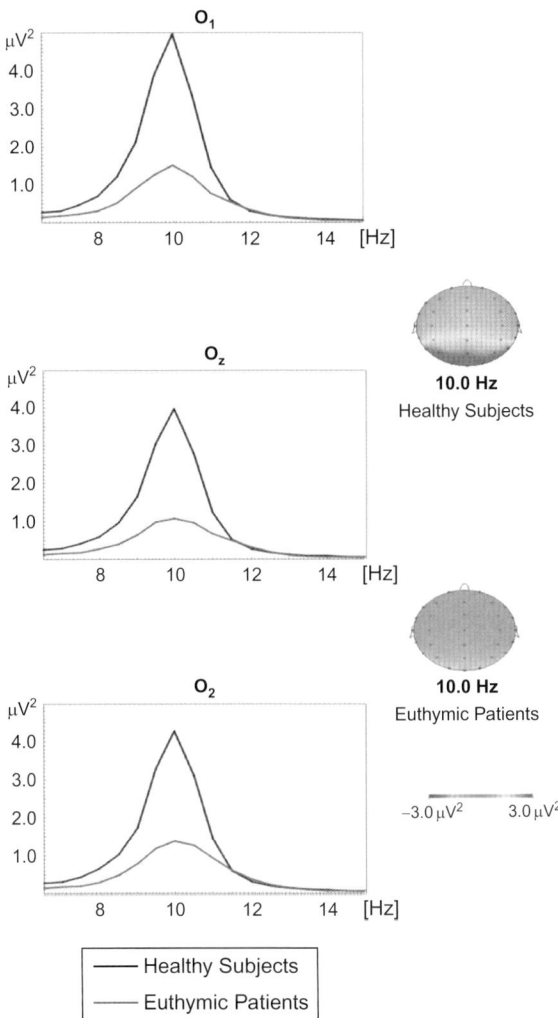

Fig. 1. Grand averages of power spectra of 18 healthy and 18 euthymic subjects for the eyes-closed condition. The locations presented are from top to bottom: top (O_1), central (O_z), and bottom (O_2) electrodes. The black line is the grand average of power spectra of evoked response in healthy participants. The red line is the grand average of power spectra of evoked response in euthymic participants. (For color figures, please refer to the color figures in last section of the book.)

2008). Significantly larger alpha responses in the posterior temporal, parietal, and occipital locations over frontal and anterior temporal locations of the control group were not present in the patient group. This was due to lower occipital alpha response in the presence of similar frontal alpha activity in the patients compared to controls. After 6 weeks of valproate monotherapy, patients showed either unchanged or reduced alpha responses in general.

Beta (15–30 Hz) frequency range-related changes: We ran comparative assessments of event-related oscillations in response to visual target stimuli during an odd-ball task in drug-free manic (Özerdem et al., 2008) and, later, in euthymic patients. Preliminary results of the latter study were presented at the Ninth International Conference on Bipolar Disorder (Tan et al., 2011). In both studies, there was a medication involvement. In the manic group ($n = 10$), the drug-free baseline assessment was followed by a second assessment after 6 weeks of valproate monotherapy (prospective design), whereas euthymic drug-free patients ($n = 16$) were compared to lithium-treated euthymic patients ($n = 13$) cross-sectionally. Both studies had a control group of sex- and age-matched healthy volunteers. Euthymic patients were required to be in this state for at least 6 months. Both valproate and lithium were given as monotherapy. The maximum peak-to-peak amplitudes were measured for each participant's averaged beta (15–30 Hz) response in the 0–300-ms time window. Patients in manic state showed a significantly higher occipital beta response compared to healthy controls at baseline, which reduced significantly after 6 weeks of valproate monotherapy and became similar to controls. In the second study, both drug-free euthymic patients and patients on lithium monotherapy had higher beta responses compared to healthy controls. However, the highest responses were from the lithium-treated patients, which were significantly higher than both drug-free patients and healthy controls. Fig. 2 depicts grand averages of event-related beta responses in left (F_3) and right (F_4) frontal electrode sites in (from top to bottom) healthy controls, euthymic drug-free patients, and in patients under lithium monotherapy.

Lithium is known to have a neuroprotective effect through changes in the activity of pro- and

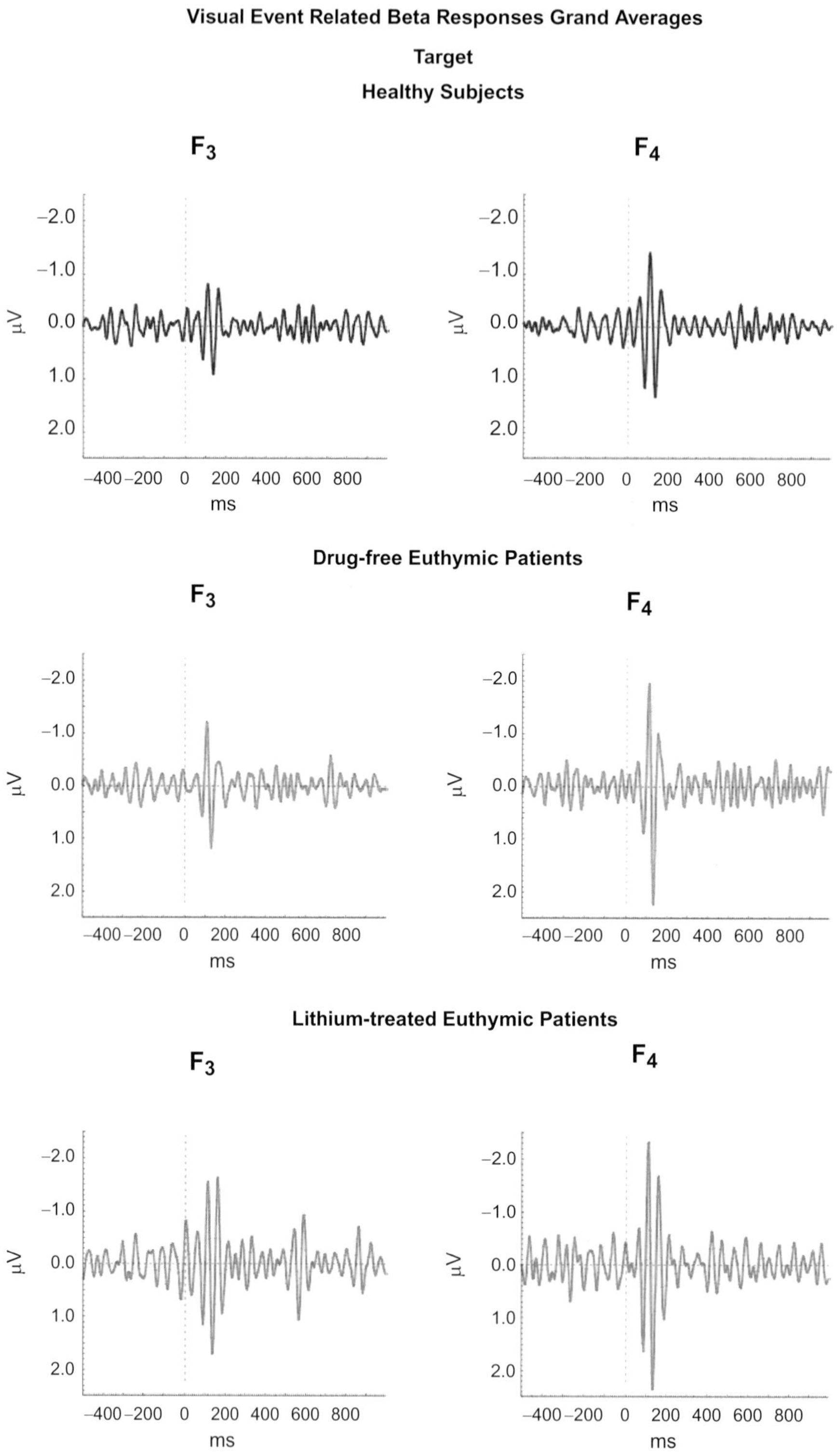

Visual Event Related Beta Responses Grand Averages

Target

Healthy Subjects

Drug-free Euthymic Patients

Lithium-treated Euthymic Patients

Fig. 2. Grand averages of event-related beta responses in left (F_3) and right (F_4) frontal electrode sites in (from top to bottom) healthy controls, untreated euthymic patients, and in patients under lithium monotherapy. (For color figures, please refer to the color figures in last section of the book.)

anti-apoptotic proteins (Machado-Vieira et al., 2009). This finding is important from the point of view that these are lithium-responsive patients and this lithium sensitivity of beta responses may be of crucial importance in tracking treatment response in patients with bipolar disorder.

Theta (4–6 and 6–8 Hz) frequency range-related changes: Theta rhythm is considered to be the fingerprint of all limbic structures. It is most prominent in the hippocampal formation (Lopes da Silva et al., 1990). Numerous structures in frontal (e.g., Gevins et al., 1997; Onton et al., 2005) and medial temporal regions (Başar-Eroğlu et al., 1992; Kahana et al., 1999; Raghavachari et al., 2001) generate cognition-related theta oscillations. Theta activity reflects functional integration of the above-mentioned structures into coherent neurocognitive networks (Başar et al., 1998, 2001a,b; Klimesch, 1999; Von Stein and Sarnthein, 2000).

Our group studied evoked and event-related slow and fast theta oscillations in response to auditory stimulus in 22 euthymic, drug-free patients with bipolar I ($n = 19$) or bipolar II ($n = 3$) diagnoses in comparison to sex, age, and education-matched healthy controls. Preliminary results of the latter study were presented at the Ninth International Conference on Bipolar Disorder (Atagün et al., 2011). Slow (4–6 Hz) and fast (6–8 Hz) theta responses behaved differently during odd-ball paradigm in patients with bipolar disorder. Slow theta (4–6 Hz) responses were significantly lower compared to healthy controls upon simple auditory stimulation and compared to the target stimuli at bilateral frontal (F_3 and F_4), central (C_3, C_4), right temporal (T_8), and right parietal (P_4) regions (Fig. 3A), whereas 6–8 Hz responses showed significant reductions in the same locations only upon target stimulus (Fig. 3B). Fast theta response seems to be more specific to target stimuli, meaning a selective response under cognitive load.

Auditory processing disturbances occurring during auditory cognitive activity may be indicative of defective synchronization. Reduced theta response to auditory challenge is confirmatory for synchronization deficits in bipolar disorder previously reported from our group (Özerdem et al., 2010, 2011).

14.5.2.4. Evoked/event-related oscillatory response — coherence analysis

Gamma (28–48 Hz) frequency range-related changes: EEG coherence describes the coupling of, or relationship between, signals in a given frequency band. Varying degrees of spatial coherence occur over long distances as parallel processing (Başar, 1980; Miltner et al., 1999; Schürmann et al., 2000). EEG coherence is considered to be an important large-scale measure of functional relationships or synchronized functioning between pairs of cortical regions, and therefore represents the brain's functional connectivity (Rappelsberger et al., 1982; Nunez, 1997; Petsche and Etlinger, 1998). Synchronous neural gamma oscillations are critical for cortico-cortical communication and the large-scale integration of distributed sets of neurons for integrated cognitive functioning (Rodriguez et al., 1999).

We studied the cortico-cortical connectivity by examining sensory evoked coherence (EC) and event-related coherence (ERC) values for the gamma frequency band during simple light stimulation and visual odd-ball paradigm in euthymic drug-free patients. The study group consisted of 20 drug-free euthymic bipolar patients and 20 sex- and age-matched healthy controls. Groups were compared for the coherence values of the left (F_3–T_3, F_3–TP_7, F_3–P_3, F_3–O_1) and right (F_4–T_4, F_4–TP_8, F_4–P_4, F_4–O_2) intra-hemispheric electrode pairs and showed bilaterally diminished long-distance gamma coherence between frontal and temporal as well as between frontal and temporo-parietal regions compared to healthy controls. However, no significant reduction in sensory evoked coherence was recorded in the patient group compared to the healthy controls. The decrease in event-related coherence differed topologically and ranged between 28.85% (right fronto-temporal location)

214

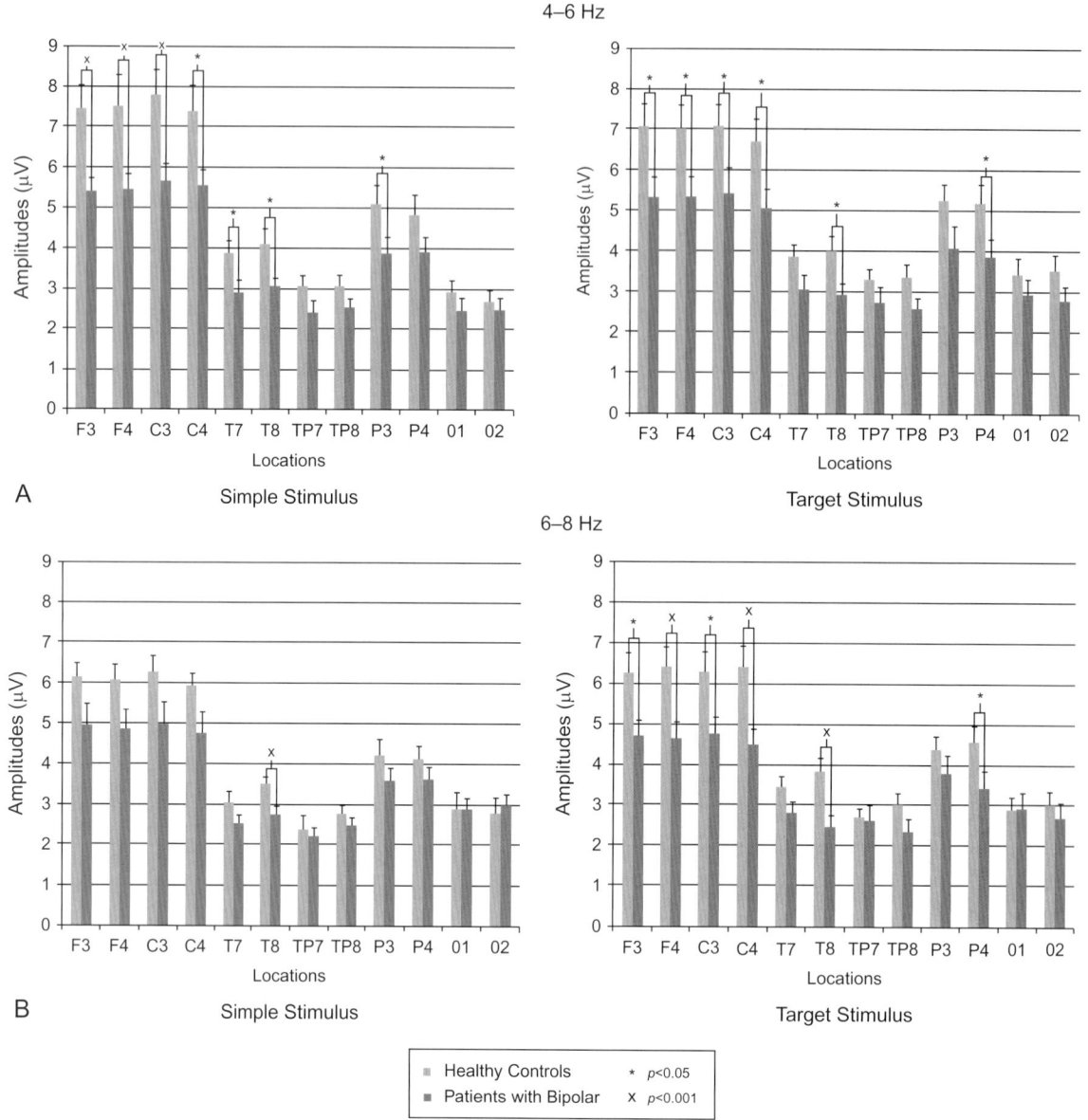

Fig. 3. (A) Mean amplitudes of patients with bipolar disorder and healthy controls in 4–6 Hz frequency range. Red bars represent patients with bipolar disorder and blue bars represent healthy controls. * p values lower than 0.05; $^\times$ p values lower than 0.001. (B) Mean amplitudes of patients with bipolar disorder and healthy controls in 6–8 Hz frequency range. Red bars represent patients with bipolar disorder and blue bars represent healthy controls. * p values lower than 0.05; $^\times$ p values lower than 0.001. (For color figures, please refer to the color figures in last section of the book.)

and 44.44% (left fronto-temporo-parietal location) (Fig. 4A, B, and C). Fig. 5A and B depicts the grand average of visual event-related coherence in gamma frequency (28–48 Hz) band in response to target stimuli between the right (F_4–T_8) and left (F_3–T_7) fronto-temporal electrode pairs in euthymic bipolar patients ($n = 20$) compared with healthy controls ($n = 20$) (Özerdem et al., 2011).

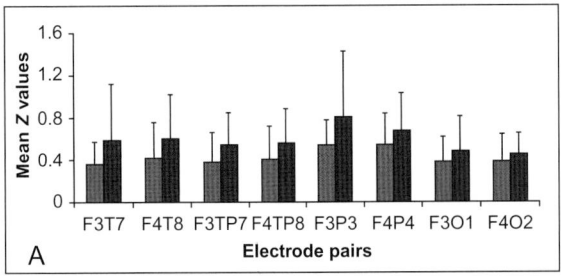

Event-related Gamma (28-48 Hz) Coherence in Response to Simple Sensory Stimuli

A

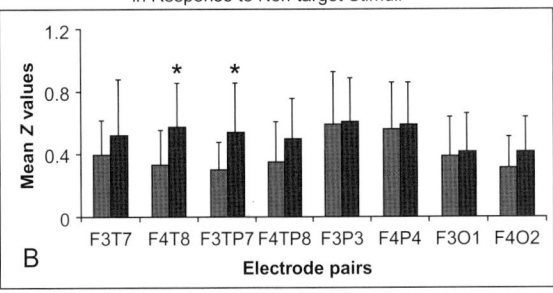

Event-related Gamma (28-48 Hz) Coherence in Response to Non-target Stimuli

B

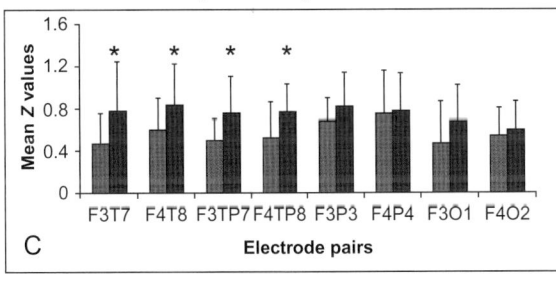

Event-related Gamma (28-48 Hz) Coherence in Response to Target Stimuli

C

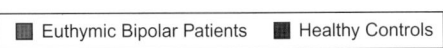

Euthymic Bipolar Patients   Healthy Controls

Fig. 4. A, B, and C: mean Z values for sensory evoked (A), for event-related non-target (B), and target (C) coherence in response to visual stimuli at all electrode pairs. * $p < 0.005$. (For color figures, please refer to the color figures in last section of the book.)

Similarly, assessment of drug-free manic patients ($n = 10$) showed a significantly reduced right-sided long-distance gamma coherence in response to both target and non-target stimuli. Target and non-target coherence values increased after 6 weeks of

Visual Event-related Target Coherence

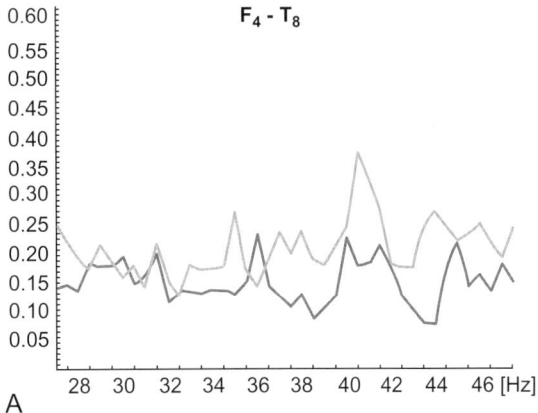

$F_4 - T_8$

A

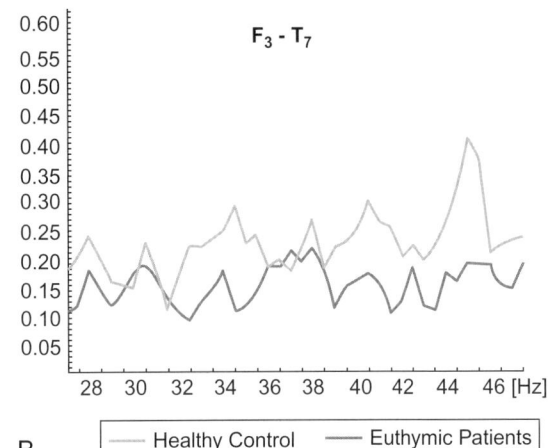

$F_3 - T_7$

B

Healthy Control   Euthymic Patients

Fig. 5. Visual event-related target coherence between the right fronto-temporal (A) and left fronto-temporal (B) locations in euthymic drug-free and healthy controls. Red line represents patients and blue line represents healthy controls. The EEG coherence function is shown along the ordinate (numerical value) and the frequency (Hz) is shown along the abscissa. (For color figures, please refer to the color figures in last section of the book.)

valproate monotherapy, although the change was statistically non-significant (Özerdem et al., 2010).

Oscillatory responses to both target and non-target stimuli are manifestations of working memory processes. Therefore, the coherence decrease in response to both stimuli points to inadequate connectivity between different parts of the brain under cognitive load.

14.6. Brain oscillations as candidate biomarkers in bipolar disorder: findings from other groups

There have been a relatively limited number of earlier electrophysiology studies of bipolar disorder covering both symptomatic and euthymic states (Muir et al., 1991; Bruder et al., 1992; Souza et al., 1995; Salisbury et al., 1998, 1999). Despite different stimulus modalities, mostly being auditory, the common finding was of prolonged P300 latency and reduced P300 amplitude, which was equivocal, mostly found to be related to psychosis, and suggested to have an association with an underlying frontal lobe pathology (Salisbury et al., 1999).

The degree of resting state long-range synchrony was significantly reduced in manic patients compared to healthy controls in all frequency bands (Bhattacharya, 2001). Chen et al. (2008) showed frontally located increased delta and decreased beta synchronization in euthymic medicated patients.

In one of the very few studies addressing neural synchronization in bipolar disorder, patients in the manic or mixed state were shown to have deficits in auditory EEG synchronization in beta (20 Hz) and gamma (30, 40, 50 Hz) range activity during click entrainment paradigm (O'Donnell et al., 2004). Spencer et al. (2008) reported significantly reduced phase locking and reduced evoked power at 30 and 40 Hz stimulation as well as at 40 Hz harmonic of the 20 Hz auditory steady-state responses in first-episode schizophrenia and affective psychosis patients compared to healthy controls. Although Hall et al. (2011) did not detect evoked gamma band response defect to auditory stimulus in a mixed group of symptomatic and euthymic bipolar patients, another recent study reported reduced gamma oscillation in the frontal regions of a mixed population of depressed and euthymic medicated patients with bipolar disorder in response to negative emotion context (Lee et al., 2010).

It is clear that existing data from other groups consist of heterogeneous patient populations, from the perspectives of both medication and illness state. Also, there is no standardization in either the tasks applied during recording or in methods of analyzing recordings. However, synchronization deficits in bipolar disorder seem to localize in frontal and temporal regions and to be dominated by gamma and beta band deficits.

14.7. Brain oscillations as candidate biomarkers differentiating bipolar disorder from schizophrenia

We have limited this discussion mainly to alpha and gamma activity, given that existing data in other pathologies often focused on these two frequencies.

Specificity of reduced alpha activity: A number of previous studies showed decreased EEG alpha activity (Itil et al., 1972, 1974; Iacono, 1982; Miyauchi et al., 1990; Sponheim et al., 1994, 2000; Alfimova and Uvarova, 2008) and reduced alpha response in schizophrenia (Ford et al., 2008; Başar-Eroğlu et al., 2009); this reduction once was shown to be up to 15% (Başar-Eroğlu et al., 2009). However, the amount of reported alpha activity reduction in patients with schizophrenia does not correspond to the magnitude we have measured in patients with bipolar disorder.

Specificity of reduced gamma coherence to bipolar disorder: Gamma responses to various stimulus modalities have been studied extensively in different pathologies. Previous investigators reported alterations in gamma activity in schizophrenia (Gallinat et al., 2004; Light et al., 2006; Yeragani et al., 2006; Başar-Eroğlu et al., 2007; Ford and Mathalon, 2008). Başar-Eroğlu et al. (2007) reported increased gamma activity during a working memory task in patients with schizophrenia. In another study that assessed first-episode psychosis patients with schizophrenia and affective disorder, gamma band auditory steady-state responses (ASSR) were found to be impaired in both patient groups compared to healthy controls (Spencer et al., 2008). The impairment had different patterns of expression in schizophrenia and affective disorder patients. The findings were attributed to the possibility that both conditions shared some common neural circuits and that different aspects of psychosis were common denominators of both conditions. Oribe et al. (2010) showed different patterns of evoked neural oscillations in the 20–45 Hz frequency range to speech sounds in patients with bipolar disorder and schizophrenia and in healthy controls. Bipolar patients who had no psychotic symptoms exhibited larger evoked neural oscillatory power to speech sounds compared to normal controls and patients with schizopohrenia. Authors suggested that the evoked neural oscillatory power to speech sounds in the left hemisphere would be a potential index to distinguish bipolar disorder and schizophrenia. Another recent study by Reite et al. (2009) showed diminished left–right hemisphere asymmetry of the primary, but not the secondary, auditory cortex, in response to steady-state (SS) gamma band eliciting stimuli in euthymic bipolar patients. Overall, the results indicated shared and non-shared features of auditory cortical disruption between schizophrenia and bipolar disorder and functional disorganization that help explain previously reported decreases in amplitude and phase synchrony of SS gamma band responses in bipolar subjects. Our findings from drug-free patients in euthymia (Özerdem et al., 2011), as well as from patients in mania (Özerdem et al., 2010), provide clear evidence of a gamma response dysfunction in bipolar disorder in response to visual stimuli. Despite existing data, the question of whether gamma response alteration is specific to bipolar disorder still remains to be answered. Comparative studies are needed that include both patient groups with bipolar disorder and schizophrenia in the absence of psychotic symptoms.

14.8. Comments related to methodology

Electrophysiological assessment of the brain's functions in bipolar disorder using different evaluation approaches (such as power spectra, coherence analysis, etc.) reveals state-, task-, and treatment-dependent changes in a complex network of different neurons that are topographically distributed over the brain. Determining the nature of these neural interactions may help improve our understanding of underlying pathology and medication effects in the way of discovering biomarkers.

From a methodological point of view, it is crucial that any given assessment in bipolar disorder needs special care for the homogeneity of the targeted patient population with regard to illness state and medication status. Up to date, only one study (Rass et al., 2010), assessing the impact of clinical features and medication use, showed that medication status may affect auditory steady-state responses and that clinical features, including mood state, psychotic features, cognitive performance, smoking, or history of substance use disorder, were unrelated to parameters measuring response magnitude and phase synchronization. In the light of such limited data, it is still important to include as homogeneous patient populations as possible with regard to illness state and psychotrop use. If this is not possible, a large sample size may be necessary to delineate responses from subgroups of symptomatic and non-symptomatic patients and for robust statistical analysis. For the medication effect, the ideal design would be prospective, consisting of euthymic patients. Another approach is to run cross-sectional assessments in medicated and non-medicated groups of patients in comparison to healthy controls during long-lasting euthymia. Because the collection of altered oscillatory activity we have presented during recent years was from homogeneous groups of patients in comparison to matched controls, we are able to consider these oscillatory changes as biomarkers. However, the specifity of these proposed biomarkers still remains to be explored.

14.9. Concluding remarks

(1) A good example for the above-mentioned points is the occurrence of large gamma coherence decrease only under cognitive load, but not in response to simple sensory stimuli in the drug-free euthymic patients. It is a major reflection of the well-documented cognitive

dysfunction across all states of bipolar disorder (Martínez-Arán et al., 2004).

(2) A selective decrease of the fast theta response to cognitive load in the presence of a non-specific decrease in the slow theta response to both sensory and cognitive challenges also shows the importance of choosing an appropriate frequency range for the assessment of any given function. We suggest that decrease in the fast theta response under cognitive load can also be a biomarker for the cognitive decline in bipolar disorder.

(3) A major break of alpha, which is beyond the alpha reduction already shown in other neuropsychiatric disorders, is also a striking finding, indicating an important deficit in the main operator of the central nerve system in bipolar disorder.

(4) A further increase in beta activity in lithium-responsive patients in comparison to unmedicated euthymic patients, who show higher beta activity than normal controls, is an intriguing finding with regard to the expectation that treatment response would be associated with a reversal in the already increased response compared to healthy controls. However, we do not yet know whether any given alteration in oscillatory activity after treatment should be related to treatment response, as it may be indicative of an adverse effect of the medication under study. In this case, the further increase in the beta response in lithium-responsive patients would be a sign of the adverse effect of lithium on cognitive function (Goldberg and Chengappa, 2009).

Up to this point, we have underlined five different potential electrophysiological biomarkers in bipolar disorder, which were obtained in different frequency ranges and by applying different signal analysis methods, as shown in Table 1. All of these

TABLE 1

SUMMARY OF POTENTIAL ELECTROPHYSIOLOGICAL BIOMARKERS IN BIPOLAR DISORDER

The table depicts results obtained by application of different signal analysis methods. All presented increases and decreases are in comparison to healthy controls. Wide arrows represent significant differences compared to healthy controls, whereas narrow arrows represent non-significant results; vertical arrows represent being similar to healthy controls.

Illness state / Method	Euthymic								Manic							
	Drug-free				Lithium treated				Drug-free				Valproate treated			
	θ	α	β	γ	θ	α	β	γ	θ	α	β	γ	θ	α	β	γ
Power spectrum																
Spontaneous EEG		⬇														
Sensory evoked		↓														
Coherence																
Event related				⬇							⬇					↓
Evoked				↓							↓					↓
Event-related oscillatory response	⬇	↑					⬆		⬇	⬆			⬇	↔		

electrophysiological markers can be considered as relevant tools to describe changes in bipolar patients in comparison to healthy subjects. Furthermore, in future, these markers could serve to elucidate cognitive processes under study and to further reveal the association between oscillations and neurotransmitters. These four different electrophysiological markers could be also grouped as oscillatory response changes in separate structures and may also be used as an indicator of connectivity changes between distant brain structures. Accordingly, the joint application of local and connectivity-related oscillatory assessment provides a more general understanding of normal and defective brain functionality.

Although each individual oscillatory finding presented as a candidate biomarker in this report is significant enough, we recommend that these electrophysiological markers should not be used separately. Instead, a constellation of these electrophysiological markers should be considered to be more appropriate for diagnostic and response-tracking purposes in bipolar disorder. This approach can provide a more solid basis for application of oscillatory assessments and a substantial reduction in potential errors when assessing diagnosis and medication response. It is to note that analyses of euthymic bipolar patients are not yet exhausted. We expect that at least four or five additional candidate biomarkers may be discovered in future studies by application of these methods.

References

Alfimova, M.V. and Uvarova, L.G. (2008) Changes in EEG spectral power on perception of neutral and emotional words in patients with schizophrenia, their relatives, and healthy subjects from the general population. *Neurosci. Behav. Physiol.*, 38: 533–540.

Atagün, M.I., Özerdem, A., Güntekin, B. and Başar, E. (2011) Theta oscillations are diminished in medication-free euthymic patients with bipolar disorder. Paper presented at the Ninth International Conference on Bipolar Disorder. *Bipolar Disord.*, 13(Suppl. 1): 28.

Baca-Garcia, E., Perez-Rodriguez, M.M., Basurte-Villamor, I., López-Castromán, J., Fernandez del Moral, A.L., Jimenez-Arriero, M.A., Gronzalez de Rivera, J.L., Saiz-Ruiz, J., Leiva-Murillo, J.M., De Prado-Cumplido, M., Santiago-Mozos, R., Artés-Rodríguez, A., Oquendo, M.A. and De Leon, J. (2007) Diagnostic stability and evolution of bipolar disorder in clinical practice: a prospective cohort study. *Acta Psychiatr. Scand.*, 115(6): 473–480.

Baldessarini, R.J. and Tondo, L. (2003) Suicide risk and treatments for patients with bipolar disorder. *J. Am. Med. Ass.*, 290: 1517–1519.

Başar, E. (1980) *EEG–Brain Dynamics. Relation between EEG and Brain Evoked Potentials.* Elsevier, Amsterdam, 412 pp.

Başar, E. and Güntekin, B. (2008) A review of brain oscillations in cognitive disorders and the role of neurotransmitters. *Brain Res.*, 1235: 172–193.

Başar, E., Rahn, E., Demiralp, T. and Schürmann, M. (1998) Spontaneous EEG theta activity controls frontal visual evoked potential amplitudes. *Electroenceph. Clin. Neurophysiol.*, 108(2): 101–109.

Başar, E., Schürmann, M. and Sakowitz, O. (2001a) The selectively distributed theta system: functions. *Int. J. Psychophysiol.*, 39(2–3): 197–212.

Başar, E., Başar-Eroğlu, C., Karakas, S. and Schürmann, M. (2001b) Gamma, alpha, delta, and theta oscillations govern cognitive processes. *Int. J. Psychophysiol.*, 39: 241–248.

Başar, E., Güntekin, B., Atagün, İ., Turp, B., Tülay, E. and Özerdem, A. (2012) Brain's alpha activity is highly reduced in euthymic bipolar disorder patients. *Cogn. Neurodyn.* 6(1): 11–20.

Başar-Eroğlu, C., Başar, E., Demiralp, T. and Schürmann, M. (1992) P300 response: possible psychophysiological correlates in delta and theta frequency channels. A review. *Int. J. Psychophysiol.*, 13: 161–179.

Başar-Eroğlu, C., Brand, A., Hildebrandt, H., Kedzior, K.K., Mathes, B. and Schmiedt, C. (2007) Working memory related gamma oscillations in schizophrenia patients. *Int. J. Psychophysiol.*, 64(1): 39–45.

Başar-Eroğlu, C., Schmiedt Fehr, C., Mathes, B., Zimmermann, J. and Brand, A. (2009) Are oscillatory brain responses generally reduced in schizophrenia during long sustained attentional processing? *Int. J. Psychophysiol.*, 71: 75–83.

Berger, H. (1929) Über das Elektroenkephalogramm des Menschen. I. Bericht. *Arch. Psychiatr. Nervenkrankh.*, 87: 527–570.

Bhattacharya, J. (2001) Reduced degree of long-range phase synchrony in pathological human brain. *Acta Neurobiol. Exp.*, 61: 309–318.

Bora, E., Yucel, M. and Pantelis, C. (2009) Cognitive endophenotypes of bipolar disorder: a meta-analysis of neuropsychological deficits in euthymic patients and their first-degree relatives. *J. Affect. Disord.*, 113: 1–20.

Bowden, C.L. (2001) Strategies to reduce misdiagnosis of bipolar depression. *Psychiatr. Serv.*, 52: 51–55.

Bowden, C.L. (2005) A different depression: clinical distinctions between bipolar and unipolar depression. *J. Affect. Disord.*, 84: 117–125.

Bruder, G.E., Stewart, J.W., Towey, J.P., Fredman, D., Tekne, C.E., Voglmaier, M.M., Leite, P., Cohen, P. and Quitkin, F.M. (1992) Abnormal cerebral laterality in bipolar depression: convergence of behavioral and brain event-related potential findings. *Biol. Psychiatry*, 32: 3–47.

220

Chen, S.S., Tu, P.C., Su, T.P., Hsieh, J.C., Lin, Y.C. and Chen, L.F. (2008) Impaired frontal synchronization of spontaneous magnetoencephalographic activity in patients with bipolar disorder. *Neurosci. Lett.*, 445: 174–178.

Clementz, B.A., Sponheim, S.R. and Iacono, W.G. (1994) Resting EEG in first-episode schizophrenia patients, bipolar psychosis patients and their first degree relatives. *Psychophysiology*, 31: 486–494.

Ford, J.M. and Mathalon, D.H. (2008) Neural synchrony in schizophrenia. *Schizophr. Bull.*, 34(5): 904–906.

Ford, J.M., Roach, B., Hoffman, R.S. and Mathalon, D.H. (2008) The dependence of P300 amplitude on gamma synchrony breaks down in schizophrenia. *Brain Res.*, 1235: 133–142.

Gallinat, J., Winterer, G., Herrmann, C.S. and Senkowski, D. (2004) Reduced oscillatory gamma-band responses in unmedicated schizophrenic patients indicate impaired network processing. *Clin. Nurophysiol.*, 115: 1863–1874.

Gevins, A., Smith, M.E., McEvoy, L. and Yu, D. (1997) High-resolution EEG mapping of cortical activation related to working memory: effects of task difficulty, type of processing, and practice. *Cereb. Cortex*, 7(4): 374–385.

Goldberg, J.F. and Chengappa, K.N.R. (2009) Identifying and treating cognitive impairment in bipolar disorder. *Bipolar Disord.*, 11(Suppl. 2): 123–137.

Hall, M.H., Spencer, K.M., Schulze, K., McDonald, C., Kalidindi, S., Kravariti, E., Kane, F., Murray, R.M., Bramon, E., Sham, P. and Rijsdijk, F. (2011) The genetic and environmental influences of event-related gamma oscillations on bipolar disorder. *Bipolar Disord.*, 13(3): 260–271.

Herrmann, C.S. and Demiralp, T. (2005) Human EEG gamma oscillations in neuropsychiatric disorders. *Clin. Neurophysiol.*, 116(12): 2719–2733.

Hirschfeld, R.M., Calabrese, J.R., Weissman, M.M., Reed, M., Davies, M.A., Frye, M.A., Keck, P.E., Jr., Lewis, L., McElroy, S.L., McNulty, J.P. and Wagner, K.D. (2003) Screening for bipolar disorder in the community. *J. Clin. Psychiatry*, 64(1): 53–59.

Iacono, W.G. (1982) Bilateral electrodermal habituation–dishabituation and resting EEG in remitted schizophrenics. *J. Nerv. Ment. Dis.*, 170: 91–101.

Itil, T.M., Saletu, B. and Davis, S. (1972) EEG findings in chronic schizophrenics based on digital computer period analysis and analog power spectra. *Biol. Psychiatry*, 5: 1–13.

Itil, T.M., Saletu, B., Davis, S. and Allen, M. (1974) Stability studies in schizophrenics and normals using computer-analyzed EEG. *Biol. Psychiatry*, 8: 321–335.

Kahana, M.J., Sekuler, R., Caplan, J.B., Kirschen, M. and Madsen, J.R. (1999) Human theta oscillations exhibit task dependence during virtual maze navigation. *Nature (Lond.)*, 399(6738): 781–784.

Klimesch, W. (1999) EEG alpha and theta oscillations reflect cognitive and memory performance: a review and analysis. *Brain Res. Rev.*, 29(2–3): 169–195.

Leboyer, M. and Kupfer, D. (2010) Bipolar disorder: new perspectives in health care and prevention. *J. Clin. Psychiatry*, 71(12): 1689–1695.

Lee, P.S., Chen, Y.S., Hsieh, J.C., Su, T.P. and Chen, L.F. (2010) Distinct neuronal oscillatory responses between patients with bipolar and unipolar disorders: a magnetoencephalographic study. *J. Affect. Disord.*, 123: 270–275.

Lehmann, D. (1989) From mapping to the analysis and interpretation of EEG/EP maps. In: K. Maurer (Ed.), *Topographic Brain Mapping of EEG and Evoked Potentials*. Springer, Berlin, pp. 53–75.

Light, G.A., Hsu, J.L., Hsieh, M.H., Meyer-Gomes, K., Sprock, J., Swerdlow, N.R. and Braff, D.L. (2006) Gamma band oscillations reveal neuronal network cortical coherence dysfunction in schizophrenia patients. *Biol. Psychiatry*, 60: 1231–1240.

Lopes da Silva, F.H., Witter, M.P., Boeijinga, P.H. and Lohman, A.H. (1990) Anatomic organization and physiology of the limbic cortex. *Physiol. Rev.*, 70(2): 453–511.

Lyoo, I.K., Dager, S.R., Kim, J.E. et al. (2010) Lithium-induced gray matter volume increase as a neural correlate of treatment response in bipolar disorder: a longitudinal brain imaging study. *Neuropsychopharmacology*, 35: 1743–1750.

Machado-Vieira, R., Manji, H.K. and Zarate, C.A., Jr. (2009) The role of lithium in the treatment of bipolar disorder: convergent evidence for neurotrophic effects as a unifying hypothesis. *Bipolar Disord.*, 11(Suppl. 2): 92–109.

Martínez-Arán, A., Vieta, E., Reinares, M., Colom, F., Torrent, C., Sánchez-Moreno, J., Benabarre, A., Goikolea, J.M., Comes, M. and Salamero, M. (2004) Cognitive function across manic or hypomanic, depressed, and euthymic states in bipolar disorder. *Am. J. Psychiatry*, 161: 262–270.

Merikangas, K.R., Akiskal, H.S., Angst, J. et al. (2007) Lifetime and 12/month prevalence of bipolar spectrum disorder in the National Comorbidity Survey replication. *Arch. Gen. Psychiatry*, 64(5): 543–552.

Miltner, W., Braun, C., Arnold, M., Witte, H. and Taub, E. (1999) Coherence of gamma-band EEG activity as a basis for associative learning. *Nature (Lond.)*, 397: 434–436.

Miyauchi, T., Tanaka, K., Hagimoto, H., Miura, T., Kishimoto, H. and Matsushita, M. (1990) Computerized EEG in schizophrenic patients. *Biol. Psychiatry*, 28: 488–494.

Muir, W.J., St. Clair D.M. and Blackwood, D.H.R. (1991) Long latency auditory event-related potentials in schizophrenia and in bipolar and unipolar affective disorder. *Psychol. Med.*, 21: 867–879.

Murray, C. and Lopez, A. (1996) *The Global Burden of Disease, a Comprehensive Assessment of Morbidity and Disability from Diseases, Injuries and Risk Factors in 1990 and Projected to 2020.* Harvard University Press, Cambridge, MA.

Nunez, P.L. (1997) EEG coherence measures in medical and cognitive science: a general overview of experimental methods, computer algorithms, and accuracy. In: M. Eselt, U. Swiener and H. Witte (Eds.), *Quantitative and Topological EEG and MEG Analysis*. Universitätsverlag Druckhaus Mayer, Jena.

Nunez, P.L., Wingeier, B.M. and Silberstein, R.B. (2001) Spatial-temporal structures of human alpha rhythms: theory, microcurrent sources, multiscale measurements, and global binding of local networks. *Hum. Brain Mapp.*, 13: 125–164.

O'Donnell, B.F., Hetrick, W.P., Vohs, J.L., Krishnan, G.P., Carroll, C.A. and Shekhar, A. (2004) Neural synchronization deficits to auditory stimulation in bipolar disorder. *Neuroreport*, 15: 1369–1372.

Onton, J., Delorme, A. and Makeig, S. (2005) Frontal midline EEG dynamics during working memory. *Neuroimage*, 15: 341–356.

Oribe, N., Onitsuka, T., Hirano, S., Hirano, Y., Maekawa, T., Obayashi, C., Ueno, T., Kasai, K. and Kanba, S. (2010) Differentiation between bipolar disorder and schizophrenia revealed by neural oscillation to speech sounds: a MEG study. *Bipolar Disord.*, 12: 804–812.

Özerdem, A., Güntekin, B., Tunca, Z. and Başar, E. (2008) Brain oscillatory responses in patients with bipolar disorder manic episode before and after valproate treatment. *Brain Res.*, 1235: 98–108.

Özerdem, A., Güntekin, B., Saatçi, E., Tunca, Z. and Başar, E. (2010) Disturbance in long-distance gamma coherence in bipolar disorder. *Prog. Neuropsychopharmacol. Biol. Psychiatry*, 34(6): 861–865.

Özerdem, A., Güntekin, B., Atagün, I., Turp, B. and Başar, E. (2011) Reduced long-distance gamma (28–48 Hz) coherence in euthymic patients with bipolar disorder. *J. Affect. Disord.*, 132(3): 325–332.

Patterson, J.V., Sandman, C.A., Ring, A., Jin, Y. and Bunney, W.E., Jr. (2009) An initial report of a new biological marker for bipolar disorder: P85 evoked brain potential. *Bipolar Disord.*, 11: 596–609.

Pavuluri, M.N. (2010) Effects of early intervention on the course of bipolar disorder: theories and realities. *Curr. Psychiatry Rep.*, 12: 490–498.

Petsche, H. and Etlinger, S.C. (1998) *EEG and Thinking: Power and Coherence Analysis of Cognitive Processes.* Verlag der Österreichischen Akademie der Wissenschaften, Vienna.

Raghavachari, S., Kahana, M.J., Rizzuto, D.S., Caplan, J.B., Kirschen, M.P., Bourgeois, B., Madsen, J.R. and Lisman, J.E. (2001) Gating of human theta oscillations by a working memory task. *J. Neurosci.*, 21(9): 3175–3183.

Rappelsberger, P., Pockberger, H. and Petsche, H. (1982) The contribution of the cortical layers to the generation of the EEG: field potential and current source density analyses in the rabbit's visual cortex. *Electroeneph. Clin. Neurophysiol.*, 53(3): 254–269.

Rass, O., Krishnan, G., Brenner, C.A., Hetrick, W.P., Merrill, C.C., Shekhar, A. and O'Donnell, B.F. (2010) Auditory steady state response in bipolar disorder: relation to clinical state, cognitive performance, medication status, and substance disorders. *Bipolar Disord.*, 12(8): 793–803.

Reite, M., Teale, P., Rojas, D.C., Reite, E., Asherin, R. and Hernandez, O. (2009) MEG auditory evoked fields suggest altered structural/functional asymmetry in primary but not secondary auditory cortex in bipolar disorder. *Bipolar Disord.*, 11(4): 371–381.

Rodriguez, E., George, N., Lachaux, J.P., Martinerie, J., Renault, B. and Varela, F.J. (1999) Perception's shadow: long-distance synchronization of human brain activity. *Nature (Lond.)*, 397: 430–433.

Salisbury, D.F., Shenton, M.E., Sherwood, A.R., Fischer, I.A., Yurgelun-Todd, D.A., Tohen, M. and McCarley R.W.

(1998) First-episode schizophrenic psychosis differs from first-episode affective psychosis and controls in P300 amplitude over left temporal lobe. *Arch. Gen. Psychiatry*, 55: 173–180.

Salisbury, D.F., Shenton, M.E. and McCarley, R.W. (1999) P300 topography differs in schizophrenia and manic depressive psychosis. *Biol. Psychiatry*, 45: 98–106.

Schürmann, M., Demiralp, T., Başar, E. and Başar-Eroğlu, C. (2000) Electroencephalogram alpha (8–15 Hz), responses to visual stimuli in cat cortex, thalamus, and hippocampus: a distributed alpha network? *Neurosci. Lett.*, 292: 175–178.

Souza, V.B., Muir, W.J., Walker, M.T., Glabus, M.F., Roxborough, H.M., Sharp, C.W., Dunan, J.R. and Blackwood, D.H.R. (1995) Auditory P300 event-related potentials and neuropsychological performance in schizophrenia and bipolar affective disorder. *Biol. Psychiatry*, 37: 300–310.

Spencer, K.M., Salisbury, D.F., Shenton, M.E. and McCarley, R.W. (2008) Gamma-band auditory steady-state responses are impaired in first episode psychosis. *Biol. Psychiatry*, 64: 369–375.

Sponheim, S.R., Clementz, B.A., Iacono, W.G. and Beiser, M. (1994) Resting EEG in first-episode and chronic schizophrenia. *Psychophysiology*, 31: 37–43.

Sponheim, S.R., Clementz, B.A., Iacono, W.G. and Beiser, M. (2000) Clinical and biological concomitants of resting state EEG power abnormalities in schizophrenia. *Biol. Psychiatry*, 48: 1088–1097.

Tan, D., Özerdem, A., Güntekin, B., Atagün, I., Tülay, E., Karadağ, F. and Başar, E. (2011) Lithium monotherapy increases beta oscillatory responses in euthymic patients with bipolar disorder. Paper presented at the Ninth International Conference on Bipolar Disorder. *Bipolar Disord.*, 13 (Suppl. 1): 98.

Thaker, G.K. (2008) Neurophysiological endophenotypes across bipolar and schizophrenia psychosis. *Schizophr. Bull.*, 34: 760–773.

Uhlhaas, P.J., Haenschel, C., Nikolić, D. and Singer, W. (2008) The role of oscillations and synchrony in cortical networks and their putative relevance for the pathophysiology of schizophrenia. *Schizophr. Bull.*, 34(5): 927–943.

Valtonen, H., Suominen, K., Mantere, O., Leppamaki, S., Arvilommi, P. and Isometsa, E.T. (2005) Suicidal ideation and attempts in bipolar I and II disorders. *J. Clin. Psychiatry*, 66: 1456–1462.

Vawter, M.P., Freed, W.J. and Kleinman, J.E. (2000) Neuropathology of bipolar disorder. *Biol. Psychiatry*, 48(6): 486–504.

Von Stein, A. and Sarnthein, J. (2000) Different frequencies for different scales of cortical integration: from local gamma to long range alpha/theta synchronization. *Int. J. Psychophysiol.*, 38(3): 301–313.

Yeragani, V.K., Cashmere, D., Miewald, J., Tancer, M. and Keshavan, M.S. (2006) Decreased coherence in higher frequency ranges (beta and gamma) between central and frontal EEG in patients with schizophrenia: a preliminary report. *Psychiatry Res.*, 141(1): 53–60.

Application of Brain Oscillations in Neuropsychiatric Diseases
(Supplements to Clinical Neurophysiology, Vol. 62)
Editors: E. Başar, C. Başar-Eroğlu, A. Özerdem, P.M. Rossini, G.G. Yener

Chapter 15

Resting state cortical EEG rhythms in Alzheimer's disease: toward EEG markers for clinical applications: a review

Fabrizio Vecchio[a], Claudio Babiloni[b,c,*], Roberta Lizio[c],
Fabrizio De Vico Fallani[d], Katarzyna Blinowska[e], Giulio Verrienti[f],
Giovanni Frisoni[g] and Paolo M. Rossini[c,h]

[a]*A.Fa.R., Dipartimento di Neuroscienze, Ospedale Fatebenefratelli, Isola Tiberina, 00186 Rome, Italy*
[b]*Department of Clinical and Experimental Medicine, University of Foggia, 71100 Foggia, Italy*
[c]*IRCCS San Raffaele Pisana, 00163 Rome, Italy*
[d]*IRCCS "Fondazione Santa Lucia", 00142 Rome, Italy*
[e]*Department of Biomedical Physics, Warsaw University, 00-927 Warsaw, Poland*
[f]*Department of Neurology, University "Campus Biomedico", 00128 Rome, Italy*
[g]*IRCCS "S. Giovanni di Dio-Fatebenefratelli", 25125 Brescia, Italy*
[h]*Department of Neurology, Policlinic A. Gemelli, Catholic University, 00186 Rome, Italy*

ABSTRACT

The human brain contains an intricate network of about 100 billion neurons. Aging of the brain is characterized by a combination of synaptic pruning, loss of cortico-cortical connections, and neuronal apoptosis that provoke an age-dependent decline of cognitive functions. Neural/synaptic redundancy and plastic remodeling of brain networking, also secondary to mental and physical training, promote maintenance of brain activity and cognitive status in healthy elderly subjects for everyday life. However, age is the main risk factor for neurodegenerative disorders such as Alzheimer's disease (AD) that impact on cognition. Growing evidence supports the idea that AD targets specific and functionally connected neuronal networks and that oscillatory electromagnetic brain activity might be a hallmark of the disease. In this line, digital electroencephalography (EEG) allows noninvasive analysis of cortical neuronal synchronization, as revealed by resting state brain rhythms. This review provides an overview of the studies on resting state eyes-closed EEG rhythms recorded in amnesic mild cognitive impairment (MCI) and AD subjects. Several studies support the idea that spectral markers of these EEG rhythms, such as power density, spectral coherence, and other quantitative features, differ among normal elderly, MCI, and AD subjects, at least at group level. Regarding the classification of these subjects at individual level, the most previous studies showed a moderate accuracy (70–80%) in the classification of EEG markers relative to normal and AD subjects. In conclusion, resting state EEG makers are promising for large-scale, low-cost, fully noninvasive screening of elderly subjects at risk of AD.

KEYWORDS

Electroencephalography (EEG) marker; Alzheimer's disease (AD); Diagnostic accuracy

Correspondence to: Prof. Claudio Babiloni, Ph.D., Department of Clinical and Experimental Medicine, University of Foggia, Viale Pinto 7, 71100 Foggia, Italy. Tel.: +39 0881 713276; Fax: +39 0881 711716; E-mail: c.babiloni@unifg.it

15.1. Introduction

Alzheimer's disease (AD) is the most common cause of dementia in geriatric patients and is characterized by loss of intellectual (especially memory) and behavioral abilities that interfere with daily functioning. The incidence of AD tends to increase with age, affecting 30–50% of the population by the age of 85 (Graves and Kukull, 1994; Vicioso, 2002).

In brain aging, including prodromal AD, neural/synaptic redundancy and plastic remodeling of brain networking guarantee functional maintenance, so that neuronal death and synaptic loss can occur in the absence of cognitive symptoms for several years. These neuroprotective mechanisms are facilitated by mental and physical training and constitute a form of "cognitive or brain reserve."

The lack of objective cognitive impairment at the earlier stages of prodromal AD motivates the use of instrumental markers of AD in association with standard assessment of cognitive functions with "paper and pencil" neuropsychological batteries (Dubois et al., 2007). Some instrumental markers are already mature for clinical applications, such as dosing of $A\beta$ amyloid and tau proteins in cerebrospinal fluid, magnetic resonance imaging (MRI) of hippocampus volume, and positron emission tomography (PET) of brain glucose metabolism/regional cerebral blood flow (rCBF) or PIB ligand (Wolf et al., 2003; Dubois et al., 2007). Of note, these markers are costly, not available in any memory clinic, and/or partially invasive, making them unsuitable for wide screening use in large populations of elderly subjects at risk of AD. In contrast, electroencephalographic (EEG) markers are cheap, largely available, and fully noninvasive, in line with the ideal characteristics of daily clinical routines (Rossini et al., 2007).

Standard EEG techniques are characterized by low spatial resolution (several centimeters) when compared to structural MRI and PET techniques producing relatively noninvasive views of "in vivo" brain anatomy (millimeters to a few centimeters). However, structural MRI does not provide functional information about the brain, and PET scan of brain glucose metabolism/rCBF is limited in its temporal resolution (i.e., seconds to minutes for PET) compared to EEG (i.e., milliseconds; Rossini and Dal Forno, 2004). It should be noted that high temporal resolution of EEG is crucial for the study of an emerging property of brain activity, namely the spontaneous and event-related oscillatory gross electromagnetic activity at different frequency ranges, categorized as 1–4 Hz (delta), 4–8 Hz (theta), 8–13 Hz (alpha), 13–30 Hz (beta), and >30 Hz (gamma). Any EEG frequency band conveys particular physiological information on brain functional state during sleep and awake periods (Nunez et al., 1999).

In recent years, great attention has been focused on the evaluation of quantitative EEG (qEEG) and/or event-related potentials (ERPs) as clinical markers of the early stages of AD (Celesia et al., 1987; Rossini et al., 2007; Yener et al., 2008, 2009; Rossini, 2009; Vecchio and Määttä, 2011). In this regard, the recording of resting state eyes-closed cortical EEG rhythms represents a fully standardized procedure that may be carried out easily and rapidly in a clinical environment. In contrast to ERPs, the use of resting state EEG rhythms does not require stimulation devices or registration of a subject's behavior and is not prone to fatigue and anxiety typically associated with task performance. This is ideal when EEG recordings are performed in elderly subjects. Furthermore, resting state cortical EEG rhythms can be recorded in highly comparable experimental conditions in normal subjects, individuals with subjective memory complaints, objective mild cognitive impairment (MCI), and overt AD (Rossini et al., 2007).

The following review of the field literature outlines the impact of resting state eyes-closed EEG markers for the instrumental assessment of AD. Its major goal is to highlight the emerging neurophysiological findings to determine whether markers derived by resting state eyes-closed EEG rhythms provide potentially useful information as candidate markers for clinical applications in individual AD patients (i.e., early diagnosis, prognosis, and disease monitoring).

15.2. Resting state eyes-closed cortical EEG rhythms along physiological aging and AD

15.2.1. Comparison of resting state EEG power among AD and control groups

Resting state eyes-closed cortical EEG rhythms typically change with physiological aging, with gradual modifications observable as variation of EEG power density spectrum computed at scalp electrodes or in mathematically estimated cortical sources (Rossini et al., 2007). The majority of the following studies addressed these EEG changes at group level. Compared to healthy young subjects, healthy elderly subjects were characterized by a marked decrease of alpha power (8–13 Hz) (Dujardin et al., 1994, 1995; Klass and Brenner, 1995; Klimesch, 1999). Such changes in alpha power were confirmed in a large sample of healthy subjects ($n = 215$, 18–85 years), showing an age-dependent power decrement of posterior low-frequency alpha (alpha$_1$; 8–10.5 Hz) and delta rhythms with physiological aging (Babiloni et al., 2006a). The present results support those of several studies showing a shift of alpha activity toward frontal brain regions in resting state EEG of Alzheimer patients (Dierks et al., 1993), as well as during cognitive processes in physiological aging (Yordanova et al., 1996, 1998; Kolev et al., 2002; Başar, 2010). Of note, parieto-occipital alpha rhythms presumably reflect the dominant oscillatory activity of brain networks in the resting state eyes-closed condition as a result of massive synchronization of cortical pyramidal neurons (Pfurtscheller and Lopes da Silva, 1999). This activity is modulated by thalamo-cortical and cortico-cortical interactions facilitating/inhibiting the transmission of sensorimotor information and the retrieval of semantic information from cortical storage (Steriade and Llinás, 1988; Brunia, 1999; Pfurtscheller and Lopes da Silva, 1999). In the condition of awake resting state, low-frequency alpha rhythms (about 8–10 Hz) can be observed in widely distributed brain networks and reflect

the general brain arousal and subject's global attentional readiness (Steriade and Llinás, 1988; Rossini et al., 1991; Klimesch, 1996, 1997; Klimesch et al., 1998). The power of these rhythms also reflects intelligent quotient, memory, and global cognition status (Klimesch, 1999). In parallel, high-frequency alpha rhythms (about 10–12 Hz) reflect the oscillation of more selective neural systems for the elaboration of sensorimotor or semantic information (Klass and Brenner, 1995; Klimesch, 1996, 1997). Of note, it is be remarked that topology-related frequencies should be carefully taken into account; the differentiation of 8–10 and 10–12 Hz is not an overall phenomenon and can be completely different in anterior and posterior areas, as reported in several experiments in both humans and animals (Schürmann et al., 2000; Başar, 2010).

At the group level, resting state eyes-closed cortical EEG rhythms present topographical and frequency differences in the EEG power spectra of healthy normal elderly (Nold), MCI, cerebrovascular dementia (CVD), Parkinson disease with dementia (PDD), and AD subjects. When compared to Nold subjects, AD subjects showed a power increase of topographically widespread delta and theta rhythms and a power decrease of posterior alpha (8–13 Hz) and/or beta (13–30 Hz) rhythms (Dierks et al., 2000; Huang et al., 2000; Ponomareva et al., 2003; Babiloni et al., 2004a; Jeong, 2004; Prichep, 2005). Posterior alpha rhythms were lower in power in AD than CVD and PDD subjects, whereas topographically widespread theta rhythms were higher in power in CVD and PDD than AD subjects (Babiloni et al., 2004a, 2013).

Resting state EEG power density differed between AD patients and amnesic MCI subjects, who were considered to be at high risk to suffer from prodromal AD. There was an "intermediate" power of low-frequency alpha rhythms (8–10.5 Hz) in parietal and occipital regions in MCI compared to mild AD and Nold subjects (Babiloni et al., 2006b). Furthermore, maximum alpha and beta power shifted more anteriorly in AD patients compared to Nold and MCI subjects (Huang et al., 2000). Moreover, longitudinal studies have shown that increased delta or theta power, decreased alpha and beta power, and slowing of mean EEG frequency were in some way predictors of the progression from MCI to dementia at about 1-year follow-up (Jelic et al., 1996, 2000; Huang et al., 2000; Grunwald et al., 2001; Kwak, 2006; Rossini et al., 2006). High power of posterior alpha rhythms also predicted a stable global cognitive function in MCI subjects at 1-year follow-up (Babiloni et al., 2011b).

Some EEG studies assessed changes in resting state eyes-closed EEG rhythms with disease progression, namely during the period from "baseline" to "follow-up" at about 1 year or longer. In MCI subjects, the EEG markers of disease progression included a power increase of theta and delta rhythms in temporal and occipital regions as well as a power decrease of beta rhythms in temporal and occipital regions (Jelic et al., 2000). AD patients were characterized by a power increase of parieto-occipital theta and delta rhythms as well as by a power reduction of alpha and beta rhythms in parieto-occipital regions (Coben et al., 1985). Furthermore, AD patients showed a power increase of theta and delta rhythms in temporal–occipital regions (Soininen et al., 1989, 1991).

15.2.2. Relationships of resting state EEG rhythms with markers of neurodegeneration and global cognitive status in Nold, MCI, and AD subjects

Resting state eyes-closed EEG rhythms were found to be related to objective markers of neurodegeneration in AD subjects, as revealed by rCBF or glucose hypometabolism. An early study showed the first evidence of a relationship among autopsy findings, visual features of resting state EEG rhythms, and rCBF in AD subjects. AD subjects were characterized by fronto-temporal cortical degeneration and parietal/temporal loss of neurons, visual EEG abnormalities, and reduction of parietal rCBF, as revealed by intra-arterial ^{133}Xenon clearance technique (Jóhannesson et al., 1977). A majority of subsequent studies compared the power of resting state eyes-closed EEG rhythms and SPECT perfusion (^{99}mTc HMPAO) in AD subjects. It was shown that AD subjects were correctly classified on the basis of an association among clinical diagnosis, rating of resting state EEG rhythms, and rCBF (Sloan et al., 1995). In AD subjects, a global decrease in rCBF was associated with a shift in the topographical maximum alpha power in the posterior direction; in addition, alpha and beta power were positively correlated with cognitive status as measured by Syndrome–Kurz test, whereas delta and theta power inversely correlated with minimental state evaluation (MMSE) score (Müller et al., 1997). Further evidence showed that topographically widespread delta and theta power, lower alpha power, and lower alpha peak frequency characterized AD patients compared to control subjects, while SPECT perfusion was reduced in all regions, with special emphasis in temporal and parietal areas (Passero et al., 1995). Moreover, there was a close relationship between rCBF and certain qEEG parameters in AD patients, mainly the power of theta and delta rhythms (Passero et al., 1995). In AD patients, widely distributed delta and alpha power were also correlated with SPECT perfusion level in the parietal regions, the delta power being also correlated with SPECT perfusion level in the right hippocampus (Rodriguez et al., 1999). Based on these SPECT and EEG variables, 88% of AD subjects (sensitivity) and 89% of Nold subjects (specificity) were classified correctly (Rodriguez et al., 1998). A correlation was also observed between parieto-occipital alpha power and SPECT perfusion in early AD subjects, namely lower power of parieto-occipital alpha rhythms was related to lower rCBF in temporal and parietal regions (Claus et al., 2000). Compared to frontal lobe dementia patients, AD subjects were denoted by more severe EEG abnormalities, less severe reduction of frontal rCBF, and more severe reduction of parietal rCBF, as revealed by SPECT perfusion (Julin et al., 1995). The above SPECT findings were corroborated by PET evidence showing a reduced parieto-temporal hypometabolism, increased widely distributed delta and theta power, and reduced parieto-temporal alpha power (Buchan et al., 1997). Consistent localization of PET brain hypometabolism and abnormal power of EEG rhythms was confirmed by further investigations in AD patients (Dierks et al., 2000). There was also a significant negative correlation between a slow-to-fast EEG activity ratio indexing the degree of slowing of the EEG rhythms and the regional metabolic rate for oxygen in parietal and temporal regions (Buchan et al., 1997).

A relationship between the power of resting state eyes-closed EEG rhythms and rCBF or brain glucose hypometabolism of neurodegeneration also emerged in studies testing the effects of pharmacological treatments in AD subjects. Beneficial effects of estrogen on female AD patients (6 weeks) were observed as increased SPECT perfusion level in right frontal regions, reduction of delta and theta power in bilateral frontal regions, and improved dementia rating score (Ohkura et al., 1994). Citicoline (i.e., an endogenous intermediate in the biosynthesis of structural membrane phospholipids and brain acetylcholine) was given for a 2-week period of treatment versus a 2-week period of placebo in AD patients with the important genetic risk factor of dementia called epsilon 4 allele of the ApoE (Alvarez et al., 1999). There was an increase of the cerebrovascular function, as revealed by transcranial Doppler, in association with an increase of occipital alpha power and a topographically widespread decrease of delta power, especially in left temporal regions (Alvarez et al. 1999). On the other hand, the effects of acetylcholinesterase inhibitors such as tetrahydroaminoacridine and donepezil were tested. A medium-term period of tetrahydroaminoacridine (6 weeks) therapy showed different clinical effects in the recruited AD patients, the

responders to the therapy being characterized by pre-treatment rCBF and increased post-treatment beta power (Minthon et al., 1993). A long-term period of donepezil in AD patients (about 1 year) showed a small area of SPECT perfusion increase in right occipital cuneus and left lingual gyrus but no remarkable change of EEG power associated with rCBF (Rodriguez et al., 2004). In addition, a correlation was observed between the mean frequency of EEG power and rCBF in posterior parietal cortex irrespective of the effects of the therapy (Rodriguez et al., 2004). As an innovative therapeutic approach, AD patients received a continuous, deep electrical stimulation of memory circuits over 12 months, including entorhinal areas, hippocampus, fornix, and hypothalamus with no serious adverse events (Laxton et al., 2010). PET scans showed an early and striking reversal of the impaired glucose utilization in temporal and parietal regions that was maintained after 12 months of continuous deep-brain stimulation, while MMSE score suggested possible improvements and/or slowing in the rate of cognitive decline at 6 and 12 months in some patients. Changes in cortical EEG rhythms were also mapped.

Power of resting state eyes-closed EEG rhythms was correlated to brain atrophy in the typical track of AD neurodegeneration, as revealed by structural MRI. In AD patients with global cognitive impairment, hippocampal atrophy was associated with increased power of delta and theta rhythms in temporal and parietal regions (Helkala et al., 1996), in line with recent magnetoencephalographic evidence (Fernandez et al., 2003). Furthermore, volume decrement of hippocampus was related to decreased power of alpha rhythms in temporal, parietal, and occipital regions in MCI and AD subjects (Babiloni et al., 2009a). The same was true for the relationship between the power of resting state eyes-closed EEG rhythms and volumetric changes of subcortical white (i.e., connection pathways to and from the cerebral cortex) and cortical gray matter. The total volume of frontal white matter was negatively correlated to the frontal delta power in AD patients; namely, the higher the white matter volume, the lower the (pathological) delta power, thus suggesting that reduced modulation/regulatory inputs to frontal cortex through white matter might disinhibit the intrinsic delta oscillations of cerebral cortex (Babiloni et al., 2006d). Furthermore, global delta and alpha power were related to the total amount of atrophy of cortical gray matter in amnesic MCI and AD subjects, as revealed by MRI voxel-to-voxel volumetry of lobar brain volume; the higher the total gray matter volume, the lower the global delta power and the higher the global alpha power (Babiloni et al., 2013). Of note, these modifications of delta and alpha power in MCI and AD subjects were not merely due to vascular brain lesions of white matter (Babiloni et al., 2008a,b, 2011c). Keeping in mind the above findings, it can be speculated that posterior delta/theta and alpha power of resting state eyes-closed EEG rhythms reflect neurodegenerative processes along the time course of AD, at least at group level.

The power of resting state eyes-closed EEG rhythms was repeatedly found to be correlated to cognitive status in MCI and AD subjects. It has been shown that posterior alpha power was positively correlated to global cognitive status, as measured by ADAS-cog in MCI and AD subjects; namely, the lower the alpha power, the lower the cognitive status (Luckhaus et al., 2008). This relationship can be extended to cognitive health condition. Furthermore, posterior delta and alpha power were correlated to MMSE score in Nold, MCI, and AD subjects; namely, the lower the alpha power, the higher the delta power and the lower the cognitive status (Babiloni et al., 2006b). Moreover, lower cognitive performance, as revealed by CAMCOG scores, was associated with lower alpha power in parieto-occipital and fronto-central regions in AD subjects (Claus et al., 2000).

These findings suggest that EEG markers at delta and alpha rhythms may be used alone or in combination with structural MRI, SPECT, and PET markers to corroborate and support the standard clinical and neuropsychological assessment of MCI and AD subjects. In this line, a first important study has combined EEG, structural MRI, and PET markers using an ensemble of classifiers based on a decision-fusion approach, in order to determine whether a strategic combination of these different modalities can improve the diagnostic accuracy over any of the individual data sources when used with an automated classifier (Polikar et al., 2010). The results showed an improvement of up to 10–20% using this approach, compared to the classification performance obtained when using each individual data source (Polikar et al., 2010).

15.2.3. Longitudinal studies on resting state EEG rhythms in AD subjects

Few longitudinal studies have evaluated resting state eyes-closed EEG rhythms to determine the changes in the baseline EEG makers that may be able to predict a cognitive decline at follow-up. It has been shown that, in MCI subjects, the markers of disease progression included an increase in the power of theta and delta activity in the temporal and occipital lobes as well as the reduction of beta power in the temporal and occipital lobes (Jelic et al., 2000). AD patients were characterized by an increase in the power of theta and delta activity and by the reduction of alpha and beta activity in the parieto-occipital lobes (Coben et al., 1985). Furthermore, half of the AD patients showed an increase in the power of theta and delta activity in a temporal–occipital lead (Soininen et al., 1989).

15.2.4. Functional coupling of resting state EEG rhythms in Nold, MCI, and AD subjects

The above results on resting state eyes-closed EEG power and neuroimaging of the structural and functional brain organization in MCI and AD subjects have led to the widely supported hypothesis that neuronal networks of temporally coordinated brain activity across different regional brain structures underpin cognitive function and denote AD neurodegeneration. In this vein, failure of integration within a network may lead to cognitive dysfunction in prodromal and manifest AD. In this sense, AD can be viewed, at least in part, as a disconnection syndrome (Bokde et al., 2009). In this theoretical framework, EEG power spectrum per se may not fully capture the impairment of functional neural connectivity. Promising markers of functional neural connectivity derive from the measurement of the functional coupling of resting state eyes-closed EEG rhythms between pairs of electrodes. Linear components of such coupling, functional coordination, and mutual information exchange can be evaluated by the analysis of spectral coherence (Thatcher et al., 1986; Rappelsberger and Petsche, 1988; Gerloff et al., 1998; Gevins et al., 1998). Spectral coherence is a normalized value that quantifies the temporal synchronization of two EEG time series between pairs of electrodes in the frequency domain and can be derived by Fast Fourier Transform (FFT; Rappelsberger and Petsche, 1988; Pfurtscheller and Andrew, 1999). Its basic theoretical assumption is that, when the oscillatory activity of two cortical areas is functionally coordinated, the EEG rhythms of these cortical areas show linear correlation and high spectral coherence. In general, decreased coherence reflects reduced linear functional coupling and information transfer (i.e., functional uncoupling or unbinding following) among cortical areas or the reduced modulation of common areas by a third region. In contrast, an increase in the coherence values is interpreted as an enhancement of the linear functional connections and information transfer (i.e., functional coupling or binding), which reflects the interaction of different cortical structures for a given task. Indeed, it has been repeatedly demonstrated that perceptive, cognitive, and motor processes are associated with enhanced EEG spectral coherence in the cortical regions involved in intensive task-related information processing (Sauseng et al., 2005; Babiloni et al., 2006c; Vecchio et al., 2007, 2010, 2012) as a function of the extension and type of the neural networks engaged (Pfurtscheller and Lopes da Silva, 1999; Von Stein and Sarnthein, 2000). In addition, spectral coherence may reflect the integrity of cortical neural pathways (Locatelli et al., 1998).

At the group level, functional coupling of resting state, eyes-closed cortical EEG rhythms differs among Nold, MCI, and AD subjects. The majority of previous EEG studies have reported a prominent decrease of coherence at alpha rhythms in AD compared to Nold subjects (Leuchter et al., 1987, 1992; Cook and Leuchter, 1996; Jelic et al., 1997, 2000; Locatelli et al., 1998; Wada et al., 1998a,b; Knott et al., 2000; Almkvist et al., 2001; Adler et al., 2003). This effect was found to be associated with ApoE genetic risk, which is hypothesized to be mediated by cholinergic deficit (Jelic et al., 1997). On the other hand, some previous studies have shown contradictory results, with either a decrease or an increase of low-band EEG coherence at delta and theta rhythms (Leuchter et al., 1987; Locatelli et al., 1998; Adler et al., 2003; Brunovsky et al., 2003). A recent study has reconciled these conflicting results by computing "total coherence," obtained by averaging the EEG spectral coherence across all combinations of electrode pairs (Babiloni et al., 2011a). The latter may better take into account, frequency band-by-frequency band, the global impairment of brain networks and cognition along the AD process, which is presumed to affect the functional integration within cerebral neural networks supporting cognition. Recently, one such study reported that delta total coherence was higher in AD than MCI subjects and in MCI than Nold subjects (Babiloni et al., 2011a). Furthermore, the low-frequency alpha total coherence was lower in AD than in MCI and Nold subjects. Of note, these EEG coherence values were negatively correlated to (moderate to high) cholinergic lesion across the MCI subjects (Babiloni et al., 2011a). Unpublished data of our group indicated that spectral delta coherence was higher in the AD than MCI and Nold subjects, while spectral alpha coherence was lower in the AD than MCI and Nold subjects.

Spectral coherence is a linear measurement of the functional coupling of EEG rhythm. Instead, the so-called synchronization likelihood is an index capturing both linear and nonlinear dimensions of this coupling. It has been shown that, compared with the Nold subjects, patients with vascular dementia and mild AD presented a marked reduction of synchronization likelihood at both fronto-parietal (delta–alpha) and interhemispherical (delta–beta) electrode pairs (Babiloni et al., 2004b). The feature distinguishing patients with mild AD with respect to patients with VaD groups was a more prominent reduction of synchronization likelihood at fronto-parietal alpha rhythms, suggesting that mild AD is characterized by an abnormal fronto-parietal coupling of the dominant human alpha rhythms (Babiloni et al., 2004b). Furthermore, synchronization likelihood was lower in MCI than Nold subjects and in AD than MCI subjects at midline and right fronto-parietal electrodes (Babiloni et al., 2006c). The same was found for the likelihood of delta synchronization at the right fronto-parietal electrodes. For these EEG bands, the synchronization likelihood correlated with global cognitive status, as measured by the MMSE protocol.

Spectral coherence and synchronization likelihood do not allow the determination of the directional flux of information in the fronto-parietal coupling of resting state EEG rhythms. This dimension can be explored by a technique called direct transfer function (DTF; Kaminski and Blinowska, 1991; Blinowska et al., 2010; Blinowska, 2011; Blinowska and Zygierewicz, 2011; Brzezicka et al., 2011). DTF has been shown to be reliable for the determination of directional information flux within linear EEG functional coupling, as an intrinsic feature of cerebral functional connectivity (Kaminski et al., 1997; Korzeniewska et al., 1997). Kaminski et al. (1997) reported that, in the eyes-closed resting state, EEG activity propagates mainly from posterior regions. This finding may be a reference point for assessment of changes in propagation for demented patients.

Across pathological aging, it has been shown that a reduction of parietal-to-frontal directional information flux within the functional coupling of alpha and beta rhythms is stronger in normal controls than in MCI and/or AD subjects (Babiloni et al., 2009b), in line with the idea of a common pathophysiological background linking these subjects, at least at group level (Babiloni et al., 2009b; Vecchio and Babiloni, 2011). It is noteworthy that such a direction of the fronto-parietal functional coupling is relatively preserved in amnesic MCI subjects in whom the cognitive decline is mainly explained by extent of white-matter vascular disease, supporting the additive model, according to which MCI state would result from the combination of cerebrovascular and neurodegenerative lesions (Babiloni et al., 2008b).

15.3. Resting state eyes-closed cortical EEG rhythms along physiological aging and AD: classification of MCI and AD individuals based on EEG markers toward clinical applications

In the previous section, the review of the literature shows that, at group level, MCI and AD subjects are characterized by abnormal power of delta/theta and alpha rhythms in temporal, parietal, and occipital regions as well as by abnormal fronto-parietal coupling of these rhythms. In this section, we revise resting state eyes-closed EEG studies, testing the hypothesis that features of resting state eyes-closed EEG studies can be used to classify single individuals toward diagnostic and prognostic clinical applications.

In the classification of Nold, MCI, and AD subjects, it has been shown that spectral EEG coherence and other EEG features contributed to the differentiation of Nold from mild AD with 89–45% success, from MCI to AD with 92–78% success, and the conversion of MCI subjects to AD with 87–60% success (Nuwer, 1997; Claus et al., 1999; Huang et al., 2000; Jelic et al., 2000;

Bennys et al., 2001; Adler et al., 2003; Brassen et al., 2004; Missonnier et al., 2006; Buscema et al., 2007; Lehmann et al., 2007).

Concerning the progression from MCI to AD status, it has been shown that a multiple logistic regression of theta power (3.5–7.5 Hz), mean frequency, and interhemispheric coherence were able to predict the decline from MCI to AD at long term with an overall predictive accuracy of about 90% (Prichep et al., 2006). Furthermore, spectral coherence and power of EEG rhythms in 69 MCI cases were evaluated at baseline and at a follow-up after 14 months (Rossini et al., 2006). At follow-up, 45 subjects were classified as stable MCI (MCI stable), whereas the remaining 24 subjects converted to AD (MCI "converted"). The results showed that, at baseline, fronto-parietal midline coherence as well as delta (temporal), theta (parietal, occipital, and temporal), and low-frequency alpha (central, parietal, occipital, temporal, and limbic) power were stronger in MCI "converted" than MCI "stable" subjects (Rossini et al., 2006). Cox regression modeling showed low midline coherence and weak temporal source were associated with 10% annual rate of AD conversion, while this rate increased up to 40% and 60% when strong temporal delta source and high midline gamma coherence were observed, respectively (Rossini et al., 2006). This outcome indicated that resting state EEG markers can contribute to the prediction of the progression from MCI to AD at about 1-year follow-up.

These findings encourage confirmatory studies aimed at testing the prognostic and, perhaps, diagnostic value of resting state eyes-closed EEG markers. These confirmatory studies are mandatory due to the great variability of the EEG variables and classifiers used in previous studies. In the reviewed studies, EEG variables for classification purposes were the simple voltage of ongoing resting state eyes-closed EEG spatial distributions used as an input to artificial neural networks (Buscema et al., 2007; Rossini et al., 2008). Alternatively, they were derived from linear spectral procedures such as power density and coherence spectra used as inputs to linear and nonlinear classifiers (Gueguen et al., 1991; Szelies et al., 1992; Rodriguez et al., 1998; Huang et al., 2000; Ihl et al., 2000; Bennys et al., 2001; Adler et al., 2003; Rossini et al., 2006; Abásolo et al., 2008; Knyazeva et al., 2010). In other cases, the input EEG variables were obtained by nonlinear procedures typically inspired by Chaos theory (Pritchard et al., 1994).

15.4. Conclusions

Keeping in mind the present review of the literature, it can be concluded that resting state eyes-closed cortical delta/theta and alpha rhythms, as indexed by posterior source power, fronto-parietal coherence, and DTF, were abnormal in amnesic MCI and AD subjects, at least at group level. These EEG markers may reflect an abnormal synchronization of cortical pyramidal neurons and a functional disconnection among cortical areas along the AD process. Indeed, power and local functional coupling of delta and theta rhythms reflect a cortical disconnection from subcortical structures, while power and local functional coupling of alpha rhythms reflect an effective global synchronization of default cortical networks in the awake, resting state eyes-closed condition (Spiegel et al., 2006).

The present review of the literature also showed encouraging results in the moderate accuracy (around 70–80% on average), achieved in the classification of individual EEG datasets in Nold and AD subjects, although a variety of methodologies were applied. This accuracy level may be useful for the preliminary screening of large populations of elderly subjects at risk of AD, such as subjects with subjective memory impairment or people with genetic risk of AD. Furthermore, the resting state eyes-closed EEG markers may be used alone or in combination with structural MRI, SPECT, and PET markers to corroborate and support the standard clinical and neuropsychological assessment of MCI and AD subjects in the diagnostic process. Each of these approaches has shown some promising outcomes; however, a comprehensive data fusion analysis should be performed to investigate whether these different modalities provide complementary information. If affirmative, they can be combined to provide a more accurate analysis, taking into account important variables such as costs, invasiveness, and local availability of the procedures.

Acknowledgments

This chapter was developed within the framework of the project "Diagnostic Enhancement of Confidence by an International Distributed Environment" (DECIDE; FP7 ICT "infrastructure" 2010–2012), in order to review the resting state EEG markers most promising for the early diagnosis of Alzheimer's disease on the basis of the extant literature. These EEG markers were candidates to be implemented in the DECIDE GRID-based diagnostic service. This chapter is presented on behalf of the DECIDE Consortium. Complete information about the Consortium and the principal investigators is available at www.eu-decide.eu.

References

Abásolo, D., Hornero, R., Escudero, J. and Espino, P. (2008) A study on the possible usefulness of detrended fluctuation analysis of the electroencephalogram background activity in Alzheimer's disease. *IEEE Trans. Biomed. Eng.*, 55(9): 2171–2179.

Adler, G., Brassen, S. and Jajcevic, A. (2003) EEG coherence in Alzheimer's dementia. *J. Neural Transm.*, 110(9): 1051–1058.

Almkvist, O., Jelic, V., Amberla, K., Hellström-Lindahl, E., Meurling, L. and Nordberg, A. (2001) Responder characteristics to a single oral dose of cholinesterase inhibitor: a double-blind placebo-controlled study with tacrine in Alzheimer patients. *Dement. Geriatr. Cogn. Disord.*, 12: 22–32.

Alvarez, X.A., Mouzo, R., Pichel, V., Pérez, P., Laredo, M., Fernández-Novoa, L., Corzo, L., Zas, R., Alcaraz, M., Secades, J.J., Lozamo, R. and Cacabelos, R. (1999) Double-blind placebo-controlled study with citicoline in ApoE genotyped Alzheimer's disease patients. Effects on cognitive performance, brain bioelectrical activity and cerebral perfusion. *Meth. Find. Exp. Clin. Pharmacol.*, 21(9): 633–644.

Babiloni, C., Binetti, G., Cassetta, E., Cerboneschi, D., Dal Forno, G., Del Percio, C., Ferreri, F., Ferri, R., Lanuzza, B., Miniussi, C., Moretti, D.V., Nobili, F., Pascual-Marqui, R.D., Rodriguez, G., Romani, G.L., Salinari, S., Tecchio, F., Vitali, P., Zanetti, O.,

Zappasodi, F. and Rossini, P.M. (2004a) Mapping distributed sources of cortical rhythms in mild Alzheimer's disease. A multicentric EEG study. *Neuroimage*, 22: 57–67.

Babiloni, C., Ferri, R., Moretti, D.V., Strambi, A., Binetti, G., Dal Forno, G., Ferreri, F., Lanuzza, B., Bonato, C., Nobili, F., Rodriguez, G., Salinari, S., Passero, S., Rocchi, R., Stam, C.J. and Rossini, P.M. (2004b) Abnormal fronto-parietal coupling of brain rhythms in mild Alzheimer's disease: a multicenter EEG study. *Eur. J. Neurosci.*, 19(9): 2583–2590.

Babiloni, C., Binetti, G., Cassarono, A., Dal Forno, G., Del Percio, C., Ferreri, F., Ferri, R., Frisoni, G., Galderisi, S., Hirata, K., Lanuzza, B., Miniassi, C., Mucci, A., Nobili, F., Rodriguez, G., Romani, G.L. and Rossini, P.M. (2006a) Sources of cortical rhythms in adults during physiological aging: a multicenter EEG study. *Hum. Brain Mapp.*, 27(2): 162–172.

Babiloni, C., Binetti, G., Cassetta, E., Dal Forno, G., Del Percio, C., Ferreri, F., Ferri, R., Frisoni, G., Hirata, K., Lanuzza, B., Miniussi, C., Moretti, D.V., Nobili, F., Rodriguez, G., Romani, G.L., Salinari, S. and Rossini, P.M. (2006b) Sources of cortical rhythms change as a function of cognitive impairment in pathological aging: a multicenter study. *Clin. Neurophysiol.*, 117: 252–268.

Babiloni, C., Ferri, R., Binetti, G., Cassarino, A., Forno, G.D., Ercolani, M., Ferreri, F., Frisoni, G.B., Lanuzza, B., Miniussi, C., Nobili, F., Rodriguez, G., Rundo, F., Stam, C.J., Musha, T., Vecchio, F. and Rossini, P.M. (2006c) Fronto-parietal coupling of brain rhythms in mild cognitive impairment: a multicentric EEG study. *Brain Res. Bull.*, 69: 63–73.

Babiloni, C., Frisoni, G., Steriade, M., Bresciani, L., Binetti, G., Del Percio, C., Geroldi, C., Miniussi, C., Nobili, F., Rodriguez, G., Zappasodi, F., Carfagna, T. and Rossini, P.M. (2006d) Frontal white matter volume and delta EEG sources negatively correlate in awake subjects with mild cognitive impairment and Alzheimer's disease. *Clin. Neurophysiol.*, 117(5): 1113–1129.

Babiloni, C., Frisoni, G.B., Pievani, M., Toscano, L., Del Percio, C., Geroldi, C., Eusebi, F., Miniussi, C. and Rossini, P.M. (2008a) White-matter vascular lesions correlate with alpha EEG sources in mild cognitive impairment. *Neuropsychologia*, 46(6): 1707–1720.

Babiloni, C., Frisoni, G.B., Pievani, M., Vecchio, F., Infarinato, F., Geroldi, C., Salinari, S., Ferri, R., Fracassi, C., Eusebi, F. and Rossini, P.M. (2008b) White matter vascular lesions are related to parietal-to-frontal coupling of EEG rhythms in mild cognitive impairment. *Hum. Brain Mapp.*, 29(12): 1355–1367.

Babiloni, C., Frisoni, G.B., Pievani, M., Vecchio, F., Lizio, R., Buttiglione, M., Geroldi, C., Fracassi, C., Eusebi, F., Ferri, R. and Rossini, P.M. (2009a) Hippocampal volume and cortical sources of EEG alpha rhythms in mild cognitive impairment and Alzheimer disease. *Neuroimage*, 44(1): 123–135.

Babiloni, C., Ferri, R., Binetti, G., Vecchio, F., Frisoni, G.B., Lanuzza, B., Miniussi, C., Nobili, F., Rodriguez, G., Rundo, F., Cassarino, A., Infarinato, F., Cassetta, E., Salinari, S., Eusebi, F. and Rossini, P.M. (2009b)

Directionality of EEG synchronization in Alzheimer's disease subjects. *Neurobiol. Aging*, 30(1): 93–102.

Babiloni, C., Frisoni, G.B., Vecchio, F., Lizio, R., Pievani, M., Cristina, G., Fracassi, C., Vernieri, F., Rodriguez, G., Nobili, F., Ferri, R. and Rossini, P.M. (2011a) Stability of clinical condition in mild cognitive impairment is related to cortical sources of alpha rhythms: an electroencephalographic study. *Hum. Brain Mapp.*, 32(11): 1916–1931.

Babiloni, C., De Pandis, M.F., Vecchio, F., Buffo, P., Sorpresi, F., Frisoni, G.B. and Rossini, P.M. (2011b) Cortical sources of resting state electroencephalographic rhythms in Parkinson's disease related dementia and Alzheimer's disease. *Clin. Neurophysiol.*, 122(12): 2355–2364.

Babiloni, C., Lizio, R., Carducci, F., Vecchio, F., Redolfi, A., Marino, S., Tedeschi, G., Montella, P., Guizzaro, A., Esposito, F., Bozzao, A., Giubilei, F., Orzi, F., Quattrocchi, C.C., Soricelli, A., Salvatore, E., Baglieri, A., Bramanti, P., Boccardi, M., Ferri, R., Cosentino, F., Ferrara, M., Mundi, C., Grilli, G., Pugliese, S., Gerardi, G., Parisi, L., Vernieri, F., Triggiani, A.I., Pedersen, J.T., Hårdemark, H.G., Rossini, P.M. and Frisoni, G.B. (2011c) Resting state cortical electroencephalographic rhythms and white matter vascular lesions in subjects with Alzheimer's disease: an Italian multicenter study. *J. Alzheimer's. Dis.*, 26(2): 331–346.

Babiloni, C., Carducci, F., Lizio, R., Vecchio, F., Baglieri, A., Bernardini, S., Boccardi, M., Bozzao, A., Buttinelli, C., Esposito, F., Giubilei, F., Guizzaro, A., Marino, S., Montella, P., Quattrocchi, C.C., Redolfi, A., Soricelli, A., Tedeschi, G., Ferri, R., Rossi-Fedele, G., Parisi, L., Vernieri, F., Pedersen, J.T., Hårdemark, H., Rossini, P.M. and Frisoni, G.B. (2013) Resting state cortical electroencephalographic rhythms are related to gray matter volume in subjects with mild cognitive impairment and Alzheimer's disease. *Hum. Brain Mapp.*, 123(2), in press.

Başar, E. (2010) *Brain–Body–Mind in the Nebulous Cartesian System. A Holistic Approach by Oscillations.* Springer, Berlin.

Bennys, K., Rondouin, G., Vergnes, C. and Touchon, J. (2001) Diagnostic value of quantitative EEG in Alzheimer disease. *Neurophysiol. Clin.*, 31: 153–160.

Blinowska, K.J. (2011) Review of the methods of determination of directed connectivity from multichannel data. *Med. Biol. Eng. Comput.*, 49(5): 521–529.

Blinowska, K.J. and Zygierewicz, J. (2011) *Practical Biomedical Signal Analysis Using MATLAB.* CRC Press, Boca Raton, FL.

Blinowska, K., Kus, R., Kaminski, M. and Janiszewska, J. (2010) Transmission of brain activity during cognitive task. *Brain Topogr.*, 23(2): 205–213.

Bokde, A.L., Ewers, M. and Hampel, H. (2009) Assessing neuronal networks: understanding Alzheimer's disease. *Prog. Neurobiol.*, 89(2): 125–133.

Brassen, S., Braus, D.F., Weber-Fahr, W., Tost, H., Moritz, S. and Adler, G. (2004) Late-onset depression with mild cognitive deficits: electrophysiological evidences for a preclinical dementia syndrome. *Dement. Geriatr. Cogn. Disord.*, 18: 271–277.

Brunia, C.H. (1999) Neural aspects of anticipatory behavior. *Acta Psychol. (Amst.)*, 101: 213–242.

Brunovsky, M., Matoušek, M., Edman, A., Cervena, K. and Krajca, V. (2003) Objective assessment of the degree of dementia by means of EEG. *Neuropsychobiology*, 48: 19–26.

Brzezicka, A., Kamiński, M., Kamiński, J. and Blinowska, K. (2011) Information transfer during a transitive reasoning task. *Brain Topogr.*, 24(1): 1–8.

Buchan, R.J., Nagata, K., Yokoyama, E., Langman, P., Yuya, H., Hirata, Y., Hatazawa, J. and Kanno, I. (1997) Regional correlations between the EEG and oxygen metabolism in dementia of Alzheimer's type. *Electroencephalogr. Clin. Neurophysiol.*, 103(3): 409–417.

Buscema, M., Rossini, P., Babiloni, C. and Grossi, E. (2007) The IFAST model, a novel parallel nonlinear EEG analysis technique, distinguishes mild cognitive impairment and Alzheimer's disease patients with high degree of accuracy. *Artif. Intell. Med.*, 40(2): 127–1241.

Celesia, G.G., Kaufman, D. and Cone, S. (1987) Effects of age and sex on pattern electroretinograms and visual evoked potentials. *Electroencephalogr. Clin. Neurophysiol.*, 68: 161–171.

Claus, J.J., Strijers, R.L., Jonkman, E.J., Ongerboer de Visser, B.W., Jonker, C., Walstra, G.J., Scheltens, P. and Van Gool, W.A. (1999) The diagnostic value of electroencephalography in mild senile Alzheimer's disease. *Clin. Neurophysiol.*, 110: 825–832.

Claus, J.J., Ongerboer de Visser, B.W. et al. (2000) Determinants of quantitative spectral electroencephalography in early Alzheimer's disease: cognitive function, regional cerebral blood flow, and computed tomography. *Dement. Geriatr. Cogn. Disord.*, 11: 81–89.

Coben, L.A., Danziger, W. and Storandt, M. (1985) A longitudinal EEG study of mild senile dementia of Alzheimer type: changes at 1 year and at 2.5 years. *Electroencephalogr. Clin. Neurophysiol.*, 61: 101–112.

Cook, I.A. and Leuchter, A.F. (1996) Synaptic dysfunction in Alzheimer's disease: clinical assessment using quantitative EEG. *Behav. Brain Res.*, 78. 15–23.

Dierks, T., Ihl, R., Frölich, L. and Maurer, K. (1993) Dementia of the Alzheimer type: effects on the spontaneous EEG described by dipole sources. *Psychiatry Res.*, 50(3): 151–162.

Dierks, T., Jelic, V., Pascual-Marqui, R.D., Wahlund, L., Julin, P., Linden, D.E., Maurer, K., Winblad, B. and Nordberg, A. (2000) Spatial pattern of cerebral glucose metabolism (PET) correlates with localization of intracerebral EEG generators in Alzheimer's disease. *Clin. Neurophysiol.*, 111: 1817–1824.

Dubois, B., Feldman, H.H., Jacova, C., Dekosky, S.T., Barberger-Gateau, P., Cummings, J., Delacourte, A., Galasko, D., Gauthier, S., Jicha, G., Meguro, K., O'Brien, J., Pasquier, F., Robert, P., Rossor, M., Salloway, S., Stern, Y., Visser, P.J. and Scheltens, P. (2007) Research criteria for the diagnosis of Alzheimer's disease: revising the NINCDS-ADRDA criteria. *Lancet Neurol.*, 6: 734–746.

Dujardin, K., Bourriez, J.L. and Guieu, J.D. (1994) Event-related desynchronization (ERD) patterns during verbal memory tasks: effect of age. *Int. J. Psychophysiol.*, 16: 17–27.

Dujardin, K., Bourriez, J.L. and Guieu, J.D. (1995) Event-related desynchronization (ERD) patterns during memory processes: effects of aging and task difficulty. *Electroencephalogr. Clin. Neurophysiol.*, 96: 169–182.

Fernandez, A., Arrazola, J., Maestu, F., Amo, C., Gil-Gregorio, P., Wienbruch, C. and Ortiz, T. (2003) Correlations of hippocampal atrophy and focal low frequency magnetic activity in Alzheimer disease: volumetric MR imaging magnetoencephalographic study. *Am. J. Neuroradiol.*, 24: 481–487.

Gerloff, C., Richard, J., Hadley, J., Schulman, A.E., Honda, M. and Hallett, M. (1998) Functional coupling and regional activation of human cortical motor areas during simple, internally paced and externally paced finger movements. *Brain*, 121(8): 1513–1531.

Gevins, A., Smith, M.E., Leong, H., McEvoy, L., Whitfield, S., Du, R. and Rush, G. (1998) Monitoring working memory load during computer-based tasks with EEG pattern recognition methods. *Hum. Factors*, 40(1): 79–91.

Graves, A.B. and Kukull, W.A. (1994) The epidemiology of dementia. In: J.C. Morris (Ed.), *Handbook of Dementing Illnesses*. Marcel Dekker, New York, pp. 23–69.

Grunwald, M., Busse, F., Hensel, A., Kruggel, F., Riedel-Heller, S., Wolf, H., Arendt, T. and Gertz, H.J. (2001) Correlation between cortical theta activity and hippocampal volumes in health, mild cognitive impairment, and mild dementia. *J. Clin. Neurophysiol.*, 18: 178–184.

Gueguen, B., Derouesné, C., Bourdel, M.C., Guillou, S., Landre, E., Gaches, J., Hossard, H., Ancri, D. and Mann, M. (1991) Quantified EEG in the diagnosis of Alzheimer's type dementia. *Neurophysiol. Clin.*, 21(5–6): 357–371.

Helkala, E.L., Hanninen, T., Hallikainen, M., Kononen, M., Laakso, M.P., Hartikainen, P., Soininen, H., Partanen, J., Partanen, K., Vainio, P. and Riekkinen, Sr., P. (1996) Slow-wave activity in the spectral analysis of the electroencephalogram and volumes of hippocampus in subgroups of Alzheimer's disease patients. *Behav. Neurosci.*, 110: 1235–1243.

Huang, C., Wahlund, L., Dierks, T., Julin, P., Winblad, B. and Jelic, V. (2000) Discrimination of Alzheimer's disease and mild cognitive impairment by equivalent EEG sources: a cross-sectional and longitudinal study. *Clin. Neurophysiol.*, 111: 1961–1967.

Ihl, R., Brinkmeyer, J., Jänner, M. and Kerdar, M.S. (2000) A comparison of ADAS and EEG in the discrimination of patients with dementia of the Alzheimer type from healthy controls. *Neuropsychobiology*, 41(2): 102–107.

Jelic, V., Shigeta, M., Julin, P., Almkvist, O., Winblad, B. and Wahlund, L.O. (1996) Quantitative electroencephalography power and coherence in Alzheimer's disease and mild cognitive impairment. *Dementia*, 7: 314–323.

Jelic, V., Julin, P., Shigeta, M., Nordberg, A., Lannfelt, L., Winblad, B. and Wahlund, L.O. (1997) Apolipoprotein E epsilon4 allele decreases functional connectivity in Alzheimer's disease as measured by EEG coherence. *J. Neurol. Neurosurg. Psychiatry*, 63: 59–65.

Jelic, V., Johansson, S.E., Almkvist, O., Shigeta, M., Julin, P., Nordberg, A., Winblad, B. and Wahlund, L.O. (2000) Quantitative electroencephalography in mild cognitive impairment: longitudinal changes and possible prediction of Alzheimer's disease. *Neurobiol. Aging*, 21: 533–540.

Jeong, J. (2004) EEG dynamics in patients with Alzheimer's disease. *Clin. Neurophysiol.*, 115: 1490–1505.

Jóhannesson, G., Brun, A., Gustafson, I. and Ingvar, D.H. (1977) EEG in presenile dementia related to cerebral blood flow and autopsy findings. *Acta Neurol. Scand.*, 56(2): 89–103.

Julin, P., Wahlund, L.O., Basun, H., Persson, A., Måre, K. and Rudberg, U. (1995) Clinical diagnosis of frontal lobe dementia and Alzheimer's disease: relation to cerebral perfusion, brain atrophy and electroencephalography. *Dementia*, 6(3): 142–147.

Kaminski, M.J. and Blinowska, K.J. (1991) A new method of the description of the information flow in the structures. *Biol. Cybern.*, 65: 203–210.

Kaminski, M.J., Blinowska, K.J. and Szclenberger, W. (1997) Topographic analysis of coherence and propagation of EEG activity during sleep and wakefulness. *Electroencephalogr. Clin. Neurophysiol.*, 102: 216–227.

Klass, D.W. and Brenner, R.P. (1995) Electroencephalography of the elderly. *J. Clin. Neurophysiol.*, 12: 116–131.

Klimesch, W. (1996) Memory processes, brain oscillations and EEG synchronization. *Int. J. Psychophysiol.*, 24: 61–100.

Klimesch, W. (1997) EEG-alpha rhythms and memory processes. *Int. J. Psychophysiol.*, 26: 319–340.

Klimesch, W. (1999) EEG alpha and theta oscillations reflect cognitive and memory performance: a review and analysis. *Brain Res. Rev.*, 29: 169–195.

Klimesch, W., Doppelmayr, M., Russegger, H., Pachinger, T. and Schwaiger, J. (1998) Induced alpha band power changes in the human EEG and attention. *Neurosci. Lett.*, 244(2): 73–76.

Knott, V., Mohr, E., Mahoney, C. and Ilivitsky, V. (2000) Electroencephalographic coherence in Alzheimer's disease: comparisons with a control group and population norms. *J. Geriatr. Psychiatry Neurol.*, 13: 1–8.

Knyazeva, M.G., Jalili, M., Brioschi, A., Bourquin, I., Fornari, E., Hasler, M., Meuli, R., Maeder, P. and Ghika, J. (2010) Topography of EEG multivariate phase synchronization in early Alzheimer's disease. *Neurobiol. Aging*, 31(7): 1132–1144.

Kolev, V., Yordanova, J., Başar-Eroglu, C. and Başar, E. (2002) Age effects on visual EEG responses reveal distinct frontal alpha networks. *Clin. Neurophysiol.*, 113(6): 901–910.

Korzeniewska, A., Kasicki, S., Kaminski, M. and Blinowska, K.J. (1997) Information flow between hippocampus and related structures during various types of rat's behavior. *J. Neurosci. Meth.*, 73: 49–60.

Kwak, Y.T. (2006) Quantitative EEG findings in different stages of Alzheimer's disease. *J. Clin. Neurophysiol.*, 23: 456–461.

Laxton, A.W., Tang-Wai, D.F., McAndrews, M.P., Zumsteg, D., Wennberg, R., Keren, R., Wherrett, J., Naglie, G., Hamani, C., Smith, G.S. and Lozano, A.M. (2010) A phase I trial of deep brain stimulation of memory circuits in Alzheimer's disease. *Ann. Neurol.*, 68(4): 521–534.

Lehmann, C., Koenig, T., Jelic, V., Prichep, L., John, R.E., Wahlund, L.O., Dodge, Y. and Dierks, T. (2007) Application and comparison of classification algorithms for recognition of Alzheimer's disease in electrical brain activity (EEG). *J. Neurosci. Meth.*, 161: 342–350.

Leuchter, A.F., Spar, J.E., Walter, D.O. and Weiner, H. (1987) Electroencephalographic spectra and coherence in the diagnosis of Alzheimer's-type and multi-infarct dementia. A pilot study. *Arch. Gen. Psychiatry*, 44: 993–998.

Leuchter, A.F., Newton, T.F., Cook, I.A., Walter, D.O., Rosenberg-Thompson, S. and Lachenbruch, P.A. (1992) Changes in brain functional connectivity in Alzheimer-type and multi-infarct dementia. *Brain*, 115: 1543–1561.

Locatelli, T., Cursi, M., Liberati, D., Franceschi, M. and Comi, G. (1998) EEG coherence in Alzheimer's disease. *Electroencephalogr. Clin. Neurophysiol.*, 106: 229–237.

Luckhaus, C., Grass-Kapanke, B., Blaeser, I., Ihl, R., Supprian, T., Winterer, G., Zielasek, J. and Brinkmeyer, J. (2008) Quantitative EEG in progressing vs stable mild cognitive impairment (MCI): results of a 1-year follow-up study. *Int. J. Geriatr. Psychiatry*, 23(11): 1148–1155.

Minthon, L., Gustafson, L., Dalfelt, G., Hagberg, B., Nilsson, K., Risberg, J., Rosén, I., Seiving, B. and Wendt, P.E. (1993) Oral tetrahydroaminoacridine treatment of Alzheimer's disease evaluated clinically and by regional cerebral blood flow and EEG. *Dementia*, 4(1): 32–42.

Missonnier, P., Gold, G., Herrmann, F.R., Fazio-Costa, L., Michel, J.P., Deiber, M.P., Michon, A. and Giannakopoulos, P. (2006) Decreased theta event-related synchronization during working memory activation is associated with progressive mild cognitive impairment. *Dement. Geriatr. Cogn. Disord.*, 22: 250–259.

Müller, T.J., Thome, J., Chiaramonti, R., Dierks, T., Maurer, K., Fallgatter, A.J., Frölich, L., Scheubeck, M. and Strik, W.K. (1997) A comparison of qEEG and HMPAO-SPECT in relation to the clinical severity of Alzheimer's disease. *Eur. Arch. Psychiatry Clin. Neurosci.*, 247(5): 259–263.

Nunez, P.L., Silberstein, R.B., Shi, Z., Carpenter, M.R., Srinivasan, R., Tucker, D.M., Doran, S.M., Cadusch, P.J. and Wijesinghe, R.S. (1999) EEG coherency. II. Experimental comparisons of multiple measures. *Clin. Neurophysiol.*, 110(3): 469–486.

Nuwer, M. (1997) Assessment of digital EEG, quantitative EEG and brain mapping: report of the American Clinical Neurophysiology Society. *Neurology*, 49: 277–292.

Ohkura, T., Isse, K., Akazawa, K., Hamamoto, M., Yaoi, Y. and Hagino, N. (1994) Evaluation of estrogen treatment in female patients with dementia of the Alzheimer type. *Endocr. J.*, 41(4): 361–371.

Passero, S., Rocchi, R., Vatti, G., Burgalassi, L. and Battistini, N. (1995) Quantitative EEG mapping, regional cerebral blood flow, and neuropsychological function in Alzheimer's disease. *Dementia*, 6(3): 148–156.

Pfurtscheller, G. and Andrew, C. (1999) Event-related changes of band power and coherence: methodology and interpretation. *J. Clin. Neurophysiol.*, 16(6): 512–519.

Pfurtscheller, G. and Lopes da Silva, F.H. (1999) Event-related EEG/MEG synchronization and desynchronization: basic principles. *Clin. Neurophysiol.*, 110(11): 1842–1857.

Polikar, R., Tilley, C., Hillis, B. and Clark, C.M. (2010) Multimodal EEG, MRI and PET data fusion for Alzheimer's disease diagnosis. *Proc. IEEE Eng. Med. Biol. Soc.*, 2010: 6058–6061.

Ponomareva, N.V., Selesneva, N.D. and Jarikov, G.A. (2003) EEG alterations in subjects at high familial risk for Alzheimer's disease. *Neuropsychobiology*, 48: 152–159.

Prichep, L.S. (2005) Use of normative databases and statistical methods in demonstrating clinical utility of qEEG: importance and cautions. *Clin. EEG Neurosci.*, 36: 82–87.

Prichep, L.S., John, E.R., Ferris, S.H., Rausch, L., Fang, Z., Cancro, R., Torossian, C. and Reisberg, B. (2006) Prediction of longitudinal cognitive decline in normal elderly with subjective complaints using electrophysiological imaging. *Neurobiol. Aging*, 27: 471–481.

Pritchard, W.S., Duke, D.W., Coburn, K.L., Moore, N.C., Tucker, K.A., Jann, M.W. and Hostetler, R.M. (1994) EEG-based, neural-net predictive classification of Alzheimer's disease versus control subjects is augmented by non-linear EEG measures. *Electroencephalogr. Clin. Neurophysiol.*, 91(2): 118–130.

Rappelsberger, P. and Petsche, H. (1988) Probability mapping: power and coherence analyses of cognitive processes. *Brain Topogr.*, 1(1): 46–54.

Rodriguez, G., Nobili, F., Rocca, G., De Carli, F., Gianelli, M.V. and Rosadini, G. (1998) Quantitative electroencephalography and regional cerebral blood flow: discriminant analysis between Alzheimer's patients and healthy controls. *Dement. Geriatr. Cogn. Disord.*, 9(5): 274–283.

Rodriguez, G., Nobili, F., Copello, F., Vitali, P., Gianelli, M.V., Taddei, G., Catsafados, E. and Mariani, G. (1999) 99mTc-HMPAO regional cerebral blood flow and quantitative electroencephalography in Alzheimer's disease: a correlative study. *J. Nucl. Med.*, 40(4): 522–529.

Rodriguez, G., Vitali, P., Canfora, M., Calvini, P., Girtler, N., De Leo, C., Piccardo, A. and Nobili, F. (2004) Quantitative EEG and perfusional single photon emission computed tomography correlation during long-term donepezil therapy in Alzheimer's disease. *Clin. Neurophysiol.*, 115(1): 39–49.

Rossini, P.M. (2009) Implications of brain plasticity to brain–machine interfaces operation: a potential paradox? A review. *Int. Rev. Neurobiol.*, 86: 81–90.

Rossini, P.M. and Dal Forno, G. (2004) Integrated technology for evaluation of brain function and neural plasticity. *Phys. Med. Rehabil. Clin. N. Am.*, 15(1): 263–306.

Rossini, P.M., Desiato, M.T., Lavaroni, F. and Caramia, M.D. (1991) Brain excitability and electroencephalographic activation: non-invasive evaluation in healthy humans via transcranial magnetic stimulation. *Brain Res.*, 13567(1): 111–119.

Rossini, P.M., Del Percio, C., Pasqualetti, P., Cassetta, E., Binetti, G., Dal Forno, F., Ferreri, F., Frisoni, G., Chiovenda, P., Miniussi, C., Parisi, L., Tombini, M., Vecchio, F. and Babiloni, C. (2006) Conversion from mild cognitive impairment to Alzheimer's disease is predicted by sources and coherence of brain electroencephalography rhythms. *Neuroscience*, 143: 793–803.

Rossini, P.M., Rossi, S., Babiloni, C. and Polich, J. (2007) Clinical neurophysiology of aging brain: from normal aging to neurodegeneration. *Prog. Neurobiol.*, 83(6): 375–400.

Rossini, P.M., Buscema, M., Capriotti, M., Grossi, E., Rodriguez, G., Del Percio, C. and Babiloni, C. (2008) Is it possible to automatically distinguish resting EEG data of normal elderly vs. mild cognitive impairment subjects with high degree of accuracy? *Clin. Neurophysiol.*, 119(7): 1534–1545.

Sauseng, P., Klimesch, W., Schabus, M. and Doppelmayr, M. (2005) Fronto-parietal EEG coherence in theta and upper alpha reflect central executive functions of working memory. *Int. J. Psychophysiol.*, 57(2): 97–103.

Schürmann, M., Demiralp, T., Başar, E. and Başar-Eroğlu, C. (2000) Electroencephalogram alpha (8–15 Hz) responses to visual stimuli in cat cortex, thalamus, and hippocampus: a distributed alpha network? *Neurosci. Lett.*, 292(3): 175–178.

Sloan, E.P., Fenton, G.W., Kennedy, N.S. and MacLennan, J.M. (1995) Electroencephalography and single photon emission computed tomography in dementia: a comparative study. *Psychol. Med.*, 25(3): 631–638.

Soininen, H., Partanen, J., Laulumaa, V., Helkala, E.L., Laakso, M. and Riekkinen, P.J. (1989) Longitudinal EEG spectral analysis in early stage of Alzheimer's disease. *Electroencephalogr. Clin. Neurophysiol.*, 72(4): 290–297.

Soininen, H., Partanen, J., Pääkkönen, A., Koivisto, E. and Riekkinen, P.J. (1991) Changes in absolute power values of EEG spectra in the follow-up of Alzheimer's disease. *Acta Neurol. Scand.*, 83(2): 133–136.

Spiegel, A., Tonner, P.H. and Renna, M. (2006) Altered states of consciousness: processed EEG in mental disease. *Best Pract. Res. Clin. Anaesthesiol.*, 20: 57–67.

Steriade, M. and Llinás, R.R. (1988) The functional states of the thalamus and the associated neuronal interplay. *Physiol. Rev.*, 68: 649–742.

Szelies, B., Grond, M., Herholz, K., Kessler, J., Wullen, T. and Heiss, W.D. (1992) Quantitative EEG mapping and PET in Alzheimer's disease. *J. Neurol. Sci.*, 110(1–2): 46–56.

Thatcher, R.W., Krause, P.J. and Hrybyk, M. (1986) Cortico-cortical associations and EEG coherence: a two-compartmental model. *Electroencephalogr. Clin. Neurophysiol.*, 64(2): 123–143.

Vecchio, F. and Babiloni, C. (2011) Direction of information flow in Alzheimer's disease and MCI patients. *Int. J. Alzheimer's. Dis.*, 2011(7): 214580.

Vecchio, F. and Määttä, S. (2011) The use of auditory event-related potentials in Alzheimer's disease diagnosis. *Int. J. Alzheimer's. Dis.*, 2011: 653173.

Vecchio, F., Babiloni, C., Ferreri, F., Curcio, G., Fini, R., Del Percio, C. and Rossini, P.M. (2007) Mobile phone emission modulates interhemispheric functional coupling of EEG alpha rhythms. *Eur. J. Neurosci.*, 25(6): 1908–1913.

Vecchio, F., Babiloni, C., Ferreri, F., Buffo, P., Cibelli, G., Curcio, G., Van Dijkman, S., Melgari, J.M., Giambattistelli, F. and Rossini, P.M. (2010) Mobile phone emission modulates inter-hemispheric functional coupling of EEG alpha rhythms in elderly compared to young subjects. *Clin. Neurophysiol.*, 121(2): 163–171.

Vecchio, F., Buffo, P., Sergio, S., Iacoviello, D., Rossini, P.M. and Babiloni, C. (2012) Mobile phone emission modulates event-related desynchronization of alpha rhythms and cognitive-motor performance in healthy humans. *Clin. Neurophysiol.*, 123(1): 121–128.

Vicioso, B.A. (2002) Dementia: when is it not Alzheimer disease? *Am. J. Med. Sci.*, 324: 84–95.

Von Stein, A. and Sarnthein, J. (2000) Different frequencies for different scales of cortical integration: from local gamma to long range alpha/theta synchronization. *Int. J. Psychophysiol.*, 38(3): 301–313.

Wada, Y., Nanbu, Y., Kikuchi, M., Koshino, Y., Hashimoto, T. and Yamaguchi, N. (1998a) Abnormal functional connectivity in Alzheimer's disease: intrahemispheric EEG coherence during rest and photic stimulation. *Eur. Arch. Psychiatry Clin. Neurosci.*, 248: 203–208.

Wada, Y., Nanbu, Y., Koshino, Y., Yamaguchi, N. and Hashimoto, T. (1998b) Reduced interhemispheric EEG coherence in Alzheimer disease: analysis during rest and photic stimulation. *Alzheimer's. Dis. Ass. Disord.*, 12: 175–181.

Wolf, H., Jelic, V., Gertz, H.J., Nordberg, A., Julin, P. and Wahlund, L.O. (2003) A critical discussion of the role of neuroimaging in mild cognitive impairment. *Acta Neurol. Scand. Suppl.*, 179: 52–76.

Yener, G., Güntekin, B. and Başar, E. (2008) Event-related delta oscillatory responses of Alzheimer patients. *Eur. J. Neurol.*, 15(6): 540–547.

Yener, G.G., Güntekin, B., Tülay, E. and Başar, E. (2009) A comparative analysis of sensory visual evoked oscillations with visual cognitive event related oscillations in Alzheimer's disease. *Neurosci. Lett.*, 462(3): 193–197.

Yordanova, J., Kolev, V. and Başar, E. (1996) Evoked brain rhythms are altered markedly in middle-aged subjects: single-sweep analysis. *Int. J. Neurosci.*, 85(1–2): 155–163.

Yordanova, J.Y., Kolev, V.N. and Başar, E. (1998) EEG theta and frontal alpha oscillations during auditory processing change with aging. *Electroencephalogr. Clin. Neurophysiol.*, 108(5): 497–505.

Application of Brain Oscillations in Neuropsychiatric Diseases
(Supplements to Clinical Neurophysiology, Vol. 62)
Editors: E. Başar, C. Başar-Eroğlu, A. Özerdem, P.M. Rossini, G.G. Yener

Chapter 16

Biomarkers in Alzheimer's disease with a special emphasis on event-related oscillatory responses

Görsev G. Yener[a,b,c,d,*] and Erol Başar[d]

[a]*Brain Dynamics Multidisciplinary Research Center, Dokuz Eylül University, Izmir 35340, Turkey*
[b]*Department of Neurosciences, Dokuz Eylül University, Izmir 35340, Turkey*
[c]*Department of Neurology, Dokuz Eylül University Medical School, Izmir 35340, Turkey*
[d]*Brain Dynamics, Cognition and Complex Systems Research Center, Istanbul Kultur University, Istanbul 34156, Turkey*

ABSTRACT

Alzheimer's disease (AD) is a devastating neurodegenerative dementing illness. Early diagnosis at the prodromal stage is an important topic of current research. Significant advances were recently made in the validation process of several biomarkers, including structural/amyloid imaging, cerebrospinal fluid measurements, and glucose positron emission tomography. Nevertheless, there remains a need to develop an efficient, low cost, potentially portable, noninvasive biomarker in the diagnosis, course, or treatment of AD. There is also a great need for a biomarker that would reflect functional brain dynamic changes within a very short time period, such as milliseconds, to provide information about cognitive deficits. Electrophysiological methods have the highest time resolution for reflecting brain dynamics in cognitive impairments. There are several strategies available for measuring cognitive changes, including spontaneous electroencephalography (EEG), sensory-evoked oscillations (SEOs), and event-related oscillations (EROs). The term "sensory evoked" (SE) implies responses elicited upon simple sensory stimulation, whereas "event-related" (ER) indicates responses elicited upon a cognitive task, generally an oddball paradigm. Further selective connectivity deficit in sensory or cognitive networks is reflected by coherence measurements. When simple sensory stimulus is used, a sensory network becomes activated, whereas an oddball task initiates an activation in a sensory network and additionally in a related cognitive network.

In AD, spontaneous activity reveals a topographically changed pattern of oscillations. In addition, the most common finding in spontaneous EEG of AD is decrease of fast and increase of slow frequencies. The hyperexcitability of motor and sensory cortices in AD has been demonstrated in many studies. The motor cortex hyperexcitability has been shown by transcranial magnetic stimulation studies. Also, the SEOs reflecting sensory network indicate a visual sensory cortex hyperexcitability in AD, as demonstrated by increased responses over posterior regions of the hemispheres. On the other hand, ERO studies reflecting activation of a cognitive network imply decreased responses in fronto-central regions of the brain in delta and theta frequencies. Coherence studies show the connectivity between different parts of the brain. Studies of SE coherence in mild AD subjects imply almost intact connectivity in all frequency ranges, whereas ER coherence is decreased in wide connections in alpha, theta, and delta frequency ranges. Moreover, alpha ER coherence seems to be sensitive to cholinergic treatment in AD.

In further research in a search of AD biomarkers, multimodal methods should be introduced to electrophysiology in order to validate these methods. Standardization and harmonization of user-friendly acquisition and analysis protocols in larger cohort populations are also needed in order to incorporate electrophysiology as a part of the clinical criteria of AD.

Correspondence to: Dr. Görsev G. Yener, M.D., Ph.D,
Department of Neurology, Dokuz Eylül University
Medical School, Balçova, Izmir 35340, Turkey.
Tel.: +90 232 412 4050; Fax: +90 232 277 7721;
E-mail: gorsev.yener@deu.edu.tr

KEYWORDS

EEG; Brain oscillation; P300; Oddball; Event-related; Evoked potential; Dementia; Alzheimer; Biomarker

16.1. Introduction

As the most common cause of dementias, Alzheimer's disease (AD) is one of the most intensively researched subjects in neuroscience. In this paper, we review and investigate possible electrophysiological biomarkers in AD. The status of many biomarker techniques is reviewed, focusing on brain oscillatory responses in AD.

This paper is outlined as follows. We start by reviewing: (1) signal processing methods to detect perturbations in brain dynamics; (2) changes of spontaneous EEG and event-related (ER) potentials in AD; (3) the major effects of AD on brain sensory-evoked (SE) or event-related oscillatory (ERO) responses and their changes in AD subjects on cholinergic medication; (4) perturbations in synchrony: (a) SE coherences and (b) ER coherences in AD. In previous studies of spontaneous electroencephalography (EEG), AD patients had increased delta and theta, and decreased alpha rhythms compared to healthy controls and/or amnesic mild cognitive impairment (MCI) subjects (Dierks et al., 2000; Huang et al., 2000; Jelic et al., 2000; Jeong, 2004; Babiloni et al., 2006a, 2010). For a review of spontaneous EEG and/or ERP, the reader is referred to Rossini et al. (2007), Jackson and Snyder (2008), Lizio et al. (2011), Vecchio et al. (2013, in this issue). For a review of evoked/ER oscillations, see Başar-Eroğlu et al. (2001), Başar and Güntekin (2008), Başar et al. (2010), Dauwels et al. (2010a,b), Güntekin and Başar, (2010), Yener and Başar, (2010, 2013, in this issue). The reader is also referred to many studies on the spontaneous EEG by Babiloni et al. At the end of this paper, we offer some concluding remarks.

AD is the most common and devastating cause of degenerative dementias and is generally found in people aged over 65. Approximately 24 million people worldwide have dementia, of which two-thirds are due to AD (Ferri et al., 2005). Clinical signs of AD are characterized by progressive cognitive deterioration, together with declining activities in daily life, and by neuropsychiatric symptoms. Although the ultimate cause of AD is unknown, genetic factors are clearly indicated, as dominant mutations in three different genes have been identified (Waldemar et al., 2007). Diagnosis of MCI and AD is important for several reasons. Diagnosis gives the patients and their caregivers time to make decisions related to life and to plan for the future. Early diagnosis of AD allows the use of medications when they are most useful and reduces the cost of the disease, it also delays institutionalization, and electrophysiological biomarkers may be used in early diagnosis (Dauwels et al., 2010a,b).

Neuropathological characteristics of AD are intracellular neurofibrillary tangles due to accumulation of phosphorylated tau protein and extracellular amyloid plaque due to amyloid beta (Aß) deposition. The commonly used NINCDS-ADRDA (McKhann et al., 1984) and DSM-IV-TR (American Psychiatric Association, 2000) criteria for AD assessments detect AD at a relatively late stage of the disease. The pathophysiological process of AD is thought prior to eventual diagnosis of AD dementia. This long "preclinical" phase of AD would provide a critical opportunity for therapeutic intervention; however, there is a need to elucidate the link between the pathological cascade of AD and the emergence of clinical symptoms (Sperling et al., 2011). This notion calls for the definition of procedures for early diagnosis/prognosis of AD in the preclinical condition called MCI (Petersen et al., 2001) or very early phase of AD. In the majority of cases, amnestic MCI is a precursor of AD with an annual conversion rate of approximately 15% per year (Petersen et al., 2001; Rasquin et al., 2005; Alexopoulos et al., 2006) that may be predicted from hippocampal atrophy rates in magnetic resonance images (Jack et al., 2005). Furthermore, the pathological deposits in AD may affect certain oscillatory networks; as Adaya-Villanueva et al. (2010) demonstrated, kainate-induced beta-like hippocampal network activity is differentially affected by amyloid β1–42 and relatively shorter and soluble peptide amyloid β25–35. However, it remains unclear which particular evoked oscillatory activity is sensitive to amyloid deposition.

Although it is very important to have reliable and validated markers for MCI-to-AD progression or for MCI/AD diagnosis, these are not yet available (McKhann et al., 2011). Potential biomarkers should be noninvasive, inexpensive, and potentially portable in order to screen large population samples of elderly subjects at risk of AD.

The National Institute on Aging and the Alzheimer's Association convened an international workgroup to review the biomarker, epidemiological, and neuropsychological evidence, and to develop recommendations to determine the factors that best predict the risk of progression from "normal" cognition to MCI and AD dementia. A conceptual framework and operational research criteria were recommended to test and refine these models with longitudinal clinical research studies. These recommendations are only intended for research purposes and do not have any clinical implications at this time (Sperling et al., 2011). Recent AD criteria (Dubois et al., 2007; McKhann et al., 2011) support the hypothesis that early diagnosis and prognosis of AD/MCI might be facilitated by an appropriate combination of multimodal biomarkers of biological (genomics, proteomics), structural neuroimaging (i.e., structural magnetic resonance imaging, MRI), and functional neuroimaging (positron emission tomography, PET), but neurophysiological methods are not similarly emphasized. As Jackson and Snyder (2008) quoted, a neuroimaging tool that is relatively inexpensive, potentially portable, and capable of providing high-density spatial resolution, electrophysiological methods can offer a noninvasive, rapid, and replicable method for assessing age-related and disease-related neurophysiologic changes. The electrophysiological methods combined with other multimodal measurements are potential candidates in the search for such a biomarker.

16.2. Methods of medical diagnosis and determination of biomarkers

In terms of public health, disease prevention is one of the main foci. Three levels of prevention can be discerned: (1) primary prevention before development of the disease; (2) secondary prevention during asymptomatic stage; (3) tertiary prevention that takes place after clinical symptoms appear and where the aims are preventing further deterioration, slowing progression, or reducing complications (Fig. 1) (Wright et al., 2009).

The National Institute of Health defines a biomarker as any "characteristic that is objectively measured and evaluated as an indicator of normal biological processes, pathogenic processes, or pharmacologic responses to a therapeutic intervention." The National Institute on Aging (NIA) Working Group on Molecular and Biochemical Markers of Alzheimer's Disease (1998) stated that "the ideal biomarker ... should detect a fundamental feature of the neuropathology and be validated in neuropathologically confirmed cases; it should have a sensitivity of >80% for detecting AD and a specificity of >80% for distinguishing other dementias; it should be reliable, non-invasive, simple to perform, and inexpensive" (Wright et al., 2009).

The global cost of dementia in 2005 was estimated to be over 300 billion USD per year (Wimo et al., 2006). As there is a rise in age-specific incidence of dementia (Matthews et al., 2006) and aging global population, a biomarker for dementia becomes a central topic for brain research.

Medical diagnosis of AD can be easily dismissed even by specialist centers at a rate of 10–15% (Knopman, 2001). Diagnosis is usually made by extensive neuropsychological testing, the results of which depend on many heterogeneous social and cultural factors. As aging is the most

240

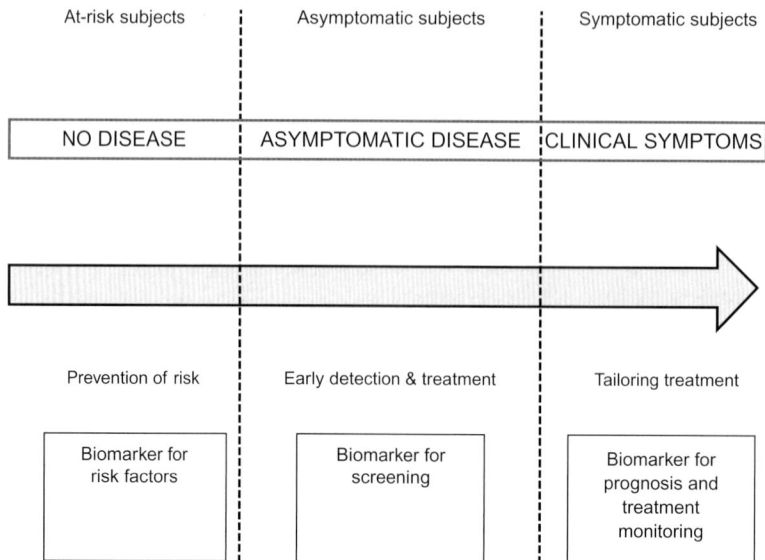

At-risk subjects | Asymptomatic subjects | Symptomatic subjects

| NO DISEASE | ASYMPTOMATIC DISEASE | CLINICAL SYMPTOMS |

Prevention of risk | Early detection & treatment | Tailoring treatment

Biomarker for risk factors | Biomarker for screening | Biomarker for prognosis and treatment monitoring

Fig. 1.   Biomarkers are needed for screening the risk factors, early detection or for tailoring the treatment. (Modified from Wright et al., 2009.)

important risk factor for development of dementia, the rapidly aging populations, especially in developing countries (Keskinoğlu, et al., 2006) within recent decades, cause AD to become an important public health problem. There is increasing evidence implying that pathological development of AD starts several decades before the appearance of clinical symptoms (Price and Morris, 1999). Interventions to pathological course, as early as possible, may be more effective than at any other time period.

For these reasons, there is an increasing need for a biomarker derived from blood tests, spinal fluid, imaging or neurophysiological techniques.

16.2.1. Imaging

16.2.1.1. Structural magnetic resonance imaging
Until recently, the role of imaging was the exclusion of other pathologies, including hydrocephalus, vascular infarcts or lacunes, or tumors. Recently, the use of specialized magnetic resonance imaging (MRI) methods allows pathologies to be

determined. For example, new microbleeds that are indicative of amyloid deposits on a vascular bed are caught by susceptibility-weighted images in MRI, or the hyperintensities of putamen, cortex, or pulvinar in diffusion-weighted images can be used in diagnosis of Jakob–Creutzfeldt disease (Vitali et al., 2011). Patterns of atrophy also offer important clues about several degenerative pathologies. Semantic dementia can be diagnosed by severe asymmetrical anterior temporal atrophy on T1-weighted coronal images, indicating ubiquitin-positive, tau-negative neuronal inclusions; a behavioral variant FTD is characterized by bifrontal severe atrophy (Rabinovici and Miller, 2010), and primary progressive aphasia is characterized by left perisylvian atrophy (Yener et al., 2010). Recent publications offer a wealth of evidence that the presence of hippocampal atrophy, detectable either by visual assessment or by volumetric measurement, is proportional to the severity of the disease (Jack et al., 2011a,b) and furthermore it can predict the conversion from MCI to AD (De Carli et al., 2007). Even visual rating of one coronal slice of MRI for differentiating MCI from controls showed sensitivity and specificity rates of 80% and 85% (Duara et al., 2008). In the light of these neuroimaging findings, the new diagnostic criteria for AD propose to incorporate the presence of temporal lobe atrophy.

16.2.1.2. Single photon emission tomography

Single photon emission tomography (SPECT) measures regional blood flow, whereas fluorodeoxyglucose positron emission tomography (FDG-PET) examines glucose metabolism in the brain. The deficit pattern in posterior cingulate, posterior precuneus and temporal lobe regions helps to differentiate AD from controls with a sensitivity and specificity rate of 90% and 70%, respectively (Jagust et al., 2007).

Neurotransmitters can also be traced by neuroimaging techniques. Dopamine transport loss in SPECT provided good separation between dementia with Lewy body (DLB) and AD. Transporter loss in DLBs was of similar magnitude to that seen in Parkinson's disease. The significant reductions in transporter loss binding occurred in the caudate and anterior and posterior putamens in subjects with DLB compared with subjects with AD and controls (O'Brien et al., 2004).

16.2.1.3. Fluorodeoxyglucose positron emission tomography

Substantial impairment of FDG uptake in temporo-parietal association cortices in PET emerges as a predictor of rapid progression to dementia in MCI patients. Frontal and temporo-parietal metabolic impairment is closely related to disease progression in longitudinal studies, and multicenter studies suggest its utility as an outcome parameter to increase the efficiency of therapeutic trials (Herholz, 2010), in a study comparing hypometabolic convergence index (HCI) in FDG-PET for the assessment of AD to other biological, cognitive, and clinical measures, and it shows potential as a predictor of clinical decline in (MCI) patients. HCIs were significantly different in the probable AD, MCI converter, MCI stable and normal control groups and were correlated with clinical disease severity. MCI patients with either higher HCIs or smaller hippocampal volumes had the highest hazard ratios (HRs) for an 18 month progression to probable AD (7.38 and 6.34, respectively), and those when both had an even higher HR (36.72; Chen et al., 2011). In another study comparing CSF, MRI, and PET, all biomarkers were found sensitive to a diagnostic group. Combining MR morphometry and CSF biomarkers improved diagnostic classification (controls vs. AD). For MRI, hippocampal volume, entorhinal and retrosplenial thickness yielded an overall classification accuracy of 85.0%. For FDG-PET, entorhinal, retrosplenial, and lateral orbitofrontal metabolism gave an overall classification accuracy of 82.5. For CSF, the ratio of total tau protein T-tau/amyloid β42 peptide (Aβ42) as the single unique predictor produces an overall classification accuracy of 81.2%. In the final model, when hippocampal volume, retrosplenial thickness, and T-tau/Aβ42-ratio were included as predictors, an overall classification accuracy of 88.8% was achieved (Walhovd et al., 2010). MR morphometry and PET were largely overlapping in value for discrimination, as also shown by Karow et al. (2010). The only study using multimodal ERO responses, MRI and PET data fusion comes from Polikar et al. (2010) who included 37 AD and 36 healthy elderly subjects. The accuracy rates when the top 15 classifiers were used were 80% for ERO + MRI, 81% for ERO + PET, 80% for MRI + PET, and 86% for ERO + MRI + PET.

16.2.1.4. Pittsburgh compound-B positron emission tomography

One of the current favorable explanations for AD pathogenesis is the amyloid cascade hypothesis. According to this hypothesis, accumulation of toxic amyloid beta peptides initiates AD pathogenesis, which in turn results in the formation of phospho-tau (P-tau) filaments (Hardy and Selkoe, 2002). Amyloid imaging has improved our understanding of timing in the pathological process. C-labeled Pittsburgh compound-B (PIB) PET allows amyloid deposits to become evident in vivo one to two decades before the symptoms appear. This became complicated when nondemented elderly subjects were reported to display amyloid burden. However, recent publications report that high amyloid burden is a risk for progression to dementia (Mathis et al., 2005; Villemagne et al., 2008). Amyloid burden does not correlate with glucose metabolism in AD, yet it is congruent with CSF amyloid by 91% (Jagust et al., 2009). However, it still shows an increasing level among normal controls, MCI or AD subjects (Quigley et al., 2011). In another study using a combination of three methods (MRI, FDG-PET, and CSF) for classifying AD from healthy controls, a classification accuracy of 93.2% (with a sensitivity of 93% and a specificity of 93.3%), and only 86.5% were achieved when using even the best individual modality of biomarkers. Similarly, in classifying MCI from healthy controls, a classification accuracy of 76.4% (with a sensitivity of 81.8% and a specificity of 66%) for the combined method, and 72% using the best individual modality of biomarkers were found. Further analysis on MCI sensitivity of the combined method indicated that 91.5% of MCI converters and 73.4% of MCI nonconverters were correctly classified. In that study, the most discriminative markers were MR and FDG-PET features (Zhang et al., 2011).

Future preventive studies of at-risk populations will address many fundamental questions by means of multimodal use of these techniques.

16.2.2. Cerebrospinal fluid and plasma biomarkers

As today, the core diagnostic cerebrospinal fluid (CSF) markers for AD are Aβ42, T-tau, and P-tau. Low levels of Aβ42 together with high levels of either P- or T-tau identify AD with a sensitivity and specificity rate of over 80% (Blennow et al., 2010). Various laboratories have developed cut-off criteria for defining the "low" Aβ42 and "high" tau from autopsy series or large cohorts (Mattsson et al., 2009; Shaw et al., 2009; Visser et al., 2009).

The lower level of Aβ42 is explained by the deposition of the peptide in plaques in AD. Beta-secretase (BACE-1) activity in CSF is increased in AD and MCI patients that are often considered as prodromal AD by many. CSF Aβ42 and tau are quite stable over time and are therefore not considered as valuable markers for progression (Blennow et al., 2007). However, a later report states that a reduction in the CSF Aβ42 level denotes a pathophysiological process that significantly departs from normality (i.e., becomes dynamic) early, whereas the CSF total tau level and the adjusted hippocampal volume are biomarkers of downstream pathophysiological processes. The CSF total tau level becomes dynamic before the adjusted hippocampal volume, but the hippocampal volume is more dynamic in the clinically symptomatic MCI and AD dementia phases of the disease than is the CSF total tau level (Jack et al., 2011b). In MCI subjects, the combination of greater learning impairment and increased atrophy are associated with highest risk (hazard ratio of 29.0): 85% of patients with both risk factors converted to AD within 3 years versus 5% of those with neither. The presence of medial temporal atrophy was associated with shortest median dementia-free survival (15 months) (Heister et al., 2011).

Recent quantitative multiplex proteomics approach to identify AD achieved a diagnostic accuracy of 90% and 81% over a 7-year follow-up for AD and MCI, respectively (Ray et al., 2007). However, later reports repeating these tests in larger series yielded lower accuracy (Soares et al., 2009).

16.2.3. Genetic biomarkers

The amyloid precursor protein (APP), presenilin-1 (PSEN1), and presenilin-2 (PSEN 2) are currently accepted as susceptibility genes for early onset AD. Sortilin-related receptor (SORL1) is involved in trafficking APP from the cell surface to the Golgi–endoplasmic reticulum complex (Reitz and Mayeux, 2009). Underexpression of SORL1 leads to overexpression of Aβ42 and an increased risk of AD (Rogaeva, 2007). Besides the well-known risk increase in ApoE4 allele carriers in late onset AD (Hyman et al.,1996), urokinase-type plasminogen activator (PLAU) gene (Ertekin-Taner et al., 2005) and insulin degrading enzyme mapping (Ertekin-Taner et al., 2004) were found to be related to Aβ42 levels.

Despite promising developments in imaging and CSF biomarkers, there are limitations to their widespread use. PET technologies are not widely available and involve high cost. Collection of CSF is not common in many centers for the diagnosis of dementia and is also an invasive method. The accessibility of MRI is good in many countries; however, the lack of standard algorithms currently limits its applicability as a biomarker. There is a great need for low-cost and noninvasive screening. We suggest a set of candidate electrophysiological biomarkers for AD. Table 1 illustrates the current possible biomarkers for AD.

16.3. Signal processing methods

Spontaneous EEG is routinely used in clinical applications, mostly for epilepsy. Within the past 30 years, it was also used in understanding cognition or related brain dynamics. Electroencephalography or ER potentials are proposed by several authors as possible biomarkers in AD (for reviews, see Herrmann and Demiralp, 2005; Uhlhaas and Singer, 2006; Jackson and Snyder, 2008; Başar et al., 2010; Lizio et al., 2011). However, the full potential of electrophysiological methods in helping to predict (Cichocki et al., 2005; Rossini et al., 2006), to diagnose (Yener et al., 1996; Polich and Herbst, 2000; Jeong, 2004; Babiloni et al., 2006a; Karrasch et al., 2006), and to monitor either treatment or progress (Jelic et al., 2000; Babiloni et al., 2006b) in AD patients has not been incorporated into routine clinical practice. The term "event-related" refers to a potential elicited after an event including a cognitive task. The word "evoked" is used when the potential is elicited by simple sensory stimulation. The term "oscillations" imply rhythm of specific time interval.

EROs in various frequency bands may reflect different aspects of information processing (Başar, 1980, 2004).

In this paper, we review recent progress in investigating AD using methods such as EEG, event-related potential (ERP), and derived oscillatory responses. Studies have shown that AD-related changes in EEG (Rossini et al., 2006, 2007), ERP, or brain oscillatory responses (for a review, see Başar et al., 2010; Yener and Başar, 2010) can be summarized as: (1) slowing of the spontaneous EEG; (2) reductions in amplitude or increase in latency of ERP; (3) reductions in amplitude or phase-locking of ERO activity in slow frequency ranges over fronto-central regions; (4) amplitude increments of visual sensory-evoked oscillatory (SEO) activities over primary sensory cortical regions; (5) reductions in EEG or ERO synchrony, such as (a) conspicuous decrement of ER coherences (i.e., elicited upon a cognitive task) between frontal and all other parts of the brain in many frequency ranges; and (b) less prominent SE coherence (i.e., elicited upon simple sensory stimuli) decrement between frontal and modality-specific primary sensory cortical regions.

Those perturbations, however, are not always detectable on an individual basis, as there tends to be large variability among AD patients. This finding implies that none of these methods alone is currently suitable as a biomarker for early AD or MCI. However, many recent studies have investigated how to improve the sensitivity of EEG or brain oscillatory responses to understand brain dynamics in AD. The changes observed in this disorder may also provide clues to understanding the healthy brain. This paper reviews the progress reported in such studies.

16.3.1. Spontaneous EEG

To date, many signal-processing techniques were utilized to reveal pathological changes in spontaneous EEG associated with AD (Jeong, 2004). A number of studies have been published related

TABLE 1

BIOLOGICAL MARKERS USED IN AD AND/OR MCI, AND THEIR USAGE OR ADVANTAGES

AD markers	For diagnosis	For progression	For drug effects	Noninvasiveness	Low cost
Amyloid PET	+	−	−	+	−
FDG-PET	+	+	+	+	−
CSF	+	±	−	−	−
Structural MRI	+	+	−	+	−
Electrophysiology	+	+	+	+	+

AD: Alzheimer's disease; FDG-PET: fluorodeoxyglucose positron emission tomography; CSF: cerebrospinal fluid; MRI: magnetic resonance imaging.

to the analysis of oscillatory dynamics in MCI and AD patients, and several groups have published core results on EEG rhythms in MCI patients (see Vecchio et al., in this issue). EEG is one of the tools widely used in functional brain studies due to its high temporal resolution and low cost. Previous EEG studies have shown an increased power of low frequencies (delta (0.5–4 Hz) and theta (4–8 Hz) bands) and decreased power of high frequencies (alpha (8–13 Hz) and beta (15–30 Hz) bands) over posterior regions in AD patients compared with healthy subjects (Yener et al., 1996; Besthorn et al., 1997; Van der Hiele et al., 2007; Bhattacharya et al., 2011) and related to cognitive profile (Smits et al., 2011). Generally the "slowing" of the EEG rhythms has been correlated with severity of dementia. In particular, significant decrease of cortical alpha$_1$ (8–10.5 Hz) power in central, parietal, temporal, and limbic areas is observed in AD patients (Babiloni et al., 2004). However, the age of AD onset seems to change this benchmark. Early onset AD subjects more often display focal or diffuse EEG abnormalities than those with late onset (De Waal et al., 2011). Patients with amnestic MCI (aMCI) have also shown reduction of alpha$_1$ band power in parieto-occipital and temporal areas. The evaluation of the LORETA solutions indicates a correlation with hippocampal volumes in the MCI/AD spectrum (Babiloni et al., 2009a). In MCI subjects, the

EEG markers of disease progression included a power increase of theta and delta rhythms in temporal and occipital regions and a power decrease of beta rhythms in temporal and occipital regions (Soininen et al., 1991; Jelic et al., 2000) or power decrease of alpha rhythms in temporal–occipital regions (Coben et al., 1985). An entropy study reported irregular magnetoencephalographic (MEG) activity among AD patients and a significantly higher variability than controls. The method achieved both specificity and sensitivity rates of 85% (Poza et al., 2008). Lehmann et al. (2007) compared resting EEG in 116 mild AD cases with 45 elderly controls and reported sensitivity and specificity of 85% and 78%, respectively.

Osipova et al. (2005) also reported a shift of alpha from parieto-occipital regions to temporal regions in AD. Recent studies found that frontal delta and occipital theta sources of amnesic MCI patients were greater than those of healthy controls (Babiloni et al., 2010). A negative correlation was also found between frontal delta sources with global cognitive status (MMSE) and the volume of frontal white matter (Babiloni et al., 2006c). Furthermore, increased power of delta and theta activity in temporal and parietal regions (Helkala et al., 1996) and decreased alpha power in temporal, parietal, and occipital regions were associated with hippocampal atrophy (Babiloni et al., 2009a). Thus, spontaneous EEG rhythm abnormalities observed in MCI and AD patients might reflect the pathology of cortical information processing within distributed cortical networks. It is speculated that alterations of spontaneous EEG rhythms are affected in MCI (Babiloni et al., 2009b) and AD patients (Yener et al., 1996), mainly due to the loss of cholinergic basal forebrain neurons projecting to the hippocampus and fronto-parietal connections. Furthermore, spontaneous EEG has been suggested as a useful predictive technique in patients with MCI who will later develop AD (Cichocki et al., 2005). A longitudinal study evaluated the baseline EEG markers for predicting a cognitive decline at follow-up. However, Osipova et al. (2006) did not find any difference between MEG activity of MCI subjects and controls in resting state. Another meta-analysis of resting EEG has indicated that classification accuracies between AD and controls ranged between 2.3 and 38.5, and diagnostic odds ratios consequently showed large variations between 7 and 219 (Jelic and Kowalski, 2009). The best results distinguishing between MCI stable and MCI/AD achieved up to 86% sensitivity by using a computational model compressing the temporal sequence of EEG data into spatial invariants (Buscema et al., 2010). Despite the wealth of published research and reported high indexes of diagnostic accuracy of EEG in individual studies, evidence of diagnostic utility of resting EEG in dementia and MCI is still not sufficient to establish this method for routine initial clinical evaluation of subjects with cognitive impairment. In that sense, temporal summation of EEG responses after stimulation is expected to give more accurate results in evaluation of AD (Polich and Herbst, 2000).

16.3.2. Motor-evoked potentials

An earlier pathology study indicated relatively spared primary sensory or motor areas in AD (Braak et al., 1993). A transcranial magnetic stimulation (TMS) study found reduced TMS-evoked P30 in AD over ipsilateral temporo-parietal areas, and contralateral fronto-central cortex corresponding to the sensorimotor network, and decrease in the N100 amplitude in the MCI subjects when compared with the control subjects (Julkunen et al., 2008). Ferreri et al. (2003) showed that motor cortex excitability was increased in AD, and the center of gravity of motor cortical output, as represented by excitable scalp sites, showed a frontal and medial shift. This finding may indicate a functional reorganization, possibly after the neuronal loss in motor areas. The authors concluded that hyperexcitability might be caused by a disregulation of the intra-cortical GABAergic inhibitory circuitries and selective alteration of glutamatergic neurotransmission, and the method might supplement traditional methods to assess the effects of therapy. The hyperexcitability in motor areas, as shown by Ferreri et al. (2003), is congruent with the findings of hyperexcitable visual sensory areas in mild AD subjects as shown by Yener et al. (2009). In their study, simple SEO responses resulted in increased theta responses over parietal and occipital regions where primary and secondary visual areas were located, whereas cognitive tasks elicited decreased theta phase-locking and delta responses over fronto-central regions. Decreased cortico-cortical connectivity between frontal and parieto-occipital areas has also been demonstrated by means of diminished coherence (Başar et al., 2010). Therefore, brain oscillatory responses indicate a decreased modulation of frontal lobes on the posterior parts of the brain where sensory visual cortices are located, possibly resulting in an increased response upon a simple sensory stimulation in AD.

16.3.3. P300 or event-related potentials

The target response of the applied P300 oddball paradigm is considered to be activated by four basic cognitive functions: "perception," "focused attention," "learning," and "working memory" (Başar-Eroğlu and Başar, 1991; Halgren et al., 2002; Rektor et al., 2004; Klimesch et al., 2006). These potentials are obtained after averaging EEG after application of a cognitive task in a time-locked and phase-locked way. The basic P300 is elicited by the oddball paradigm (Hillyard and Kutas, 1983), where rare "target" stimuli are randomly embedded in a sequence of standard stimuli. The P300 is named after a positive voltage maximum at about 300 ms response to the oddball stimulus. An oddball discrimination paradigm involves responding to stimuli that are dissimilar to the majority of stimuli presented. The subject is instructed to count target stimuli mentally. By means of this paradigm, subjects have to first perceive and then compare the stimuli with the one they were taught, to decide whether the stimulus is a target or not and, finally, to keep a mental count of the total number of target stimuli. These processes involve activation of many intriguing cognitive networks that last about 1 s, starting at about 50 ms, and peaking within the first 600-ms time window. Polich (1997) showed that the P300 of healthy subjects is affected by many factors including age and sex. The scalp topographic distribution of P300 amplitude was affected by the group factor, such that AD produced appreciably less frontal-to-parietal increase across task difficulty. P300 latency was relatively unaffected by scalp topography other than the usual increase from the frontal-to-parietal electrodes. Thus, at the group level, P300 can discriminate between AD and healthy controls (Rossini et al., 2006).

In recent years, studies have shown increase in P300 latency (Lai et al., 2010) and N200 latency (Missonnier et al., 2007) and decrease in N200 amplitude (Papaliagkas et al., 2008) in MCI or AD. Increase in P300 correlated with baseline cognitive scores (Papaliagkas et al., 2011a), and MCI subjects who progressed to AD had significantly lower Aβ42 levels (Papaliagkas et al., 2009), significantly higher N200 latencies and their P300 latency correlated with age (Papaliagkas et al., 2011b). Similar changes were also reported in somatosensory modality (Stephen et al., 2010). In patients with MCI with abnormal/reduced N400 or P600, word repetition effects had an

87–88% likelihood of dementia within 3 years (Olichney et al., 2008).

Genetically, AD mutation carriers without dementia showed less positivity in frontal regions and more positivity in occipital regions, compared to controls. These differences were more pronounced during the 200–300 ms period. Discriminant analysis at this time interval showed promising sensitivity (72.7%) and specificity (81.8%) (Quiroz et al., 2011). Another study on familial AD mutation carriers found significantly longer latencies of the N100, P200, N200, and P300 components, and smaller slow wave amplitudes (Golob et al., 2009). In another study comparing symptomatic carriers with asymptomatic carriers and noncarriers, the asymptomatic and noncarrier groups showed similar N400 amplitudes, whereas those of symptomatic carriers were significantly lower. However, N400 topography differed in mutation carrier groups with respect to the noncarriers. Intracranial source analysis evidenced that the presymptomatic carriers presented a decrease of N400 generator strength in right inferior-temporal and medial cingulate areas and increased generator strength in the left hippocampus and parahippocampus compared to the noncarrier controls (Bobes et al., 2010). Bennys et al. (2007) used prolonged P300 and N200 latencies to differentiate AD, MCI, and controls. The sensitivity rates were 87–95% for the differentiation of AD patients from MCI and control subjects, using prolonged P3 latencies (specificity 90–95%), whereas sensitivity when using N2 prolonged latencies was 70–75% (specificity 70–90%). Moreover, in the MCI group, N200 latencies strongly differentiated MCI from control subjects, with 90% sensitivity and 70% specificity; and correctly categorized 80% of MCI subjects against 73% for P300. In a visual pattern and motion onset EPs study, AD pathology in visual cortex was predicted (Fernandez et al., 2007). Ahiskali et al. (2009) introduced an approach using an ensemble of classifiers to combine ERP obtained from different electrode locations in the early diagnosis of AD.

It seems that late rather than earlier cognitive components in P300 show decreased amplitude, as reported by many groups, to differentiate between normal aging and AD (Polich and Corey-Bloom, 2005) by an accuracy rate of 92% (Chapman et al., 2007). ERPs have important predictive power in measuring conversion from MCI to AD (Missonnier et al., 2005, 2007; Olichney et al., 2008, 2011) by an accuracy rate of 79% (Chapman et al., 2011). In a study comparing AD and dementia with Lewy bodies, P300 latency was found to be delayed and its amplitude was lower with a different topography in DLB compared to AD groups (Bonanni et al., 2010).

16.3.4. Sensory evoked and event-related oscillations

The analysis of working memory has been one of major subjects of the major studies in neurophysiology. In the last few years, analysis of the oddball-P300 paradigm has become one the most commonly used methods in this context. Its underlying assumption is that the ERP response is evoked by the cognitive task (i.e., oddball paradigm in most cases), and can then be detected by averaging. The evoked responses increase the signal-to-noise ratio (SNR) in the average signal reflecting cognitive processes (Tallon-Baudry and Bertrand, 1999). EROs are elicited by digital filtering of "event-related potential" or "P300" in certain frequency bands, such as delta, theta, alpha, beta, and gamma. ERO responses can provide additional information about sensory and cognitive functions during stimulus and task evaluation (Başar, 1992; Başar et al., 1997). The first studies of brain oscillatory dynamics in P300 included those of Başar et al. (1984), Başar and Stampfer (1985), Stampfer and Başar (1985), Başar-Eroğlu et al. (1992, 2001), and Schürmann et al. (2001). Another series of studies on local oscillatory dynamics showed that the major operating rhythms of P300 are mainly the delta and theta oscillations (Başar-Eroğlu et al., 1992; Kolev et al., 1997; Demiralp et al., 1999; Spencer and Polich, 1999;

Karakaş et al., 2000; Yordanova et al., 2000; Başar et al., 2001). The prolongation of theta, delta, and alpha oscillations was described for the target stimuli in comparison to standard stimuli (Stampfer and Başar, 1985; Başar-Eroğlu et al., 1992; Yordanova and Kolev, 1998; Demiralp and Ademoğlu, 2001; Öniz and Başar, 2009). The methods described in the referenced studies were mainly amplitude and latency measures of averaged filtered responses, spectral power of target response, wavelet decomposition, and phase-locking factor of target and nontarget responses.

16.3.4.1. Sensory evoked oscillatory SEO responses

SEO responses can be elicited upon application of simple sensory stimuli without any cognitive load by digital filtering of "evoked potential" in certain frequency bands. Interpretation of differing cognitive and sensory networks might be possible by comparing the SEO responses with ERO responses upon application of a cognitive task.

Haupt et al. (2008) studied visual evoked oscillatory responses in AD, MCI, and healthy controls. They found dominant gamma and beta$_2$ bands in elderly controls in all significantly different brain areas. In addition, MCI and AD subjects differed from controls in current density distribution with a movement from the right hemisphere toward the left hemisphere in AD/MCI.

In a visual SEO study (Yener et al., 2009), it was shown that, when a stimulus does not contain a cognitive load, the differences between AD and healthy control groups were not as prominent as those observed for cognitive tasks. Furthermore, contra-intuitively, parieto-occipital theta-evoked oscillations were higher in untreated AD subjects than both controls and treated AD groups. This finding, showing a hyperexcitable visual sensory cortex, is congruent with a TMS study by Ferreri et al. (2003), indicating hyperexcitable motor cortex in AD. This is an understandable result, since the neuropathological changes at the mild stage of AD do not involve the primary sensory or motor areas (Fig. 2, Braak et al., 1993; Yener et al., 2009).

248

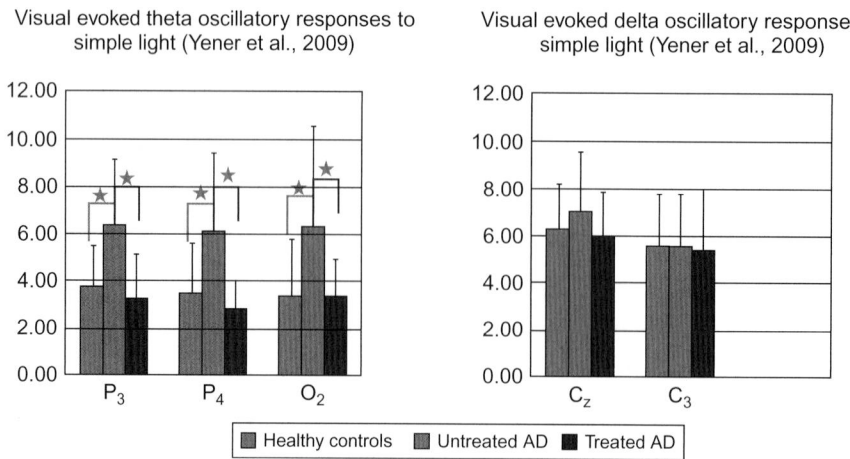

Fig. 2. Visual SEO responses are increased contra-intuitively in AD, indicating a hyperexcitability in primary and secondary visual sensory areas. (Modified from Yener et al., 2009.) (For color figures, please refer to the color figures in last section of the book.)

Osipova et al. (2006) analyzed 40 Hz auditory steady-state responses in AD patients. They showed that the amplitudes were significantly increased in AD compared to controls. Another steady-state-evoked study by Van Deursen et al. (2011) indicated a significant increase of 40 Hz (in gamma frequency range) SSR power in the AD group compared to MCI and controls. Furthermore a moderate correlation between 40 Hz SSR power and cognitive performance was shown, as measured by ADAS-cog. During early visual processing, Haupt et al. (2008) showed topological differences between AD patients and healthy controls upon application of LORETA analysis and increased $beta_2$ and gamma power in AD. The results of Osipova et al. (2006), Haupt et al. (2008), Yener et al. (2009), and Van Deursen et al. (2011) showed that SEOs were higher in AD subjects upon application of sensory stimuli. This could be due to the lack of frontal modulation on sensory cortical areas in AD patients. Earlier work of Sauseng et al. (2005) indicated the control of posterior cortical activation by anterior brain areas. An increase of prefrontal EEG alpha amplitudes, which is accompanied by a decrease at posterior sites, may thus not be interpreted in terms of idling or "global" inhibition but may enable a tight

functional coupling between prefrontal cortical areas and, thereby, allows the control of the execution of processes in primary visual brain regions. As Yener and Başar (2010) stated, decreased inhibition of cortical visual sensory processing, possibly due to decreased prefrontal activity, may lead to increased SE cortical responses in AD (Fig. 2).

16.3.4.2. ERO responses
Event-related synchronization is elicited by EEG recording during a cognitive task. It gives an induced response that is time-locked, but not phase-locked. The major change seen in spontaneous EEG of AD is "slowing" over posterior hemispheres (Vecchio et al., in this issue). Missonnier et al. (2006a,b) conducted a longitudinal study and analyzed ERS in MCI patients upon application of N-back working memory task. Their results showed that progressive MCI subjects demonstrated lower theta synchronization in comparison to stable MCI subjects with a sensitivity rate of 87% and a specificity rate of 60%. The same group's longitudinal study on progressive and stable MCI subjects during the N-back task showed that progressive MCI cases displayed significantly higher gamma fractal dimension values compared

to stable MCI cases (Missonnier et al., 2010). A similar increase in gamma band was also found by Van Deursen et al. (2008, 2011). Also, EEG functional coupling for alpha and beta rhythms was stronger in normal elderly than in MCI and/or AD patients (Karrasch et al., 2006). In an event-related synchronization (ERS) study, MCI and control subjects were examined longitudinally by an N-back paradigm (Deiber et al., 2009). In that study, induced theta response described as time-locked, but not phase-locked, activity was decreased over frontal regions in MCI. The results demonstrated that an early decrease of induced theta amplitude occurs in progressive MCI cases; in contrast, induced theta amplitude in stable MCI cases did not differ from elderly controls. Deiber et al. (2007) compared the results of working memory tasks to passive tasks and showed that induced frontal theta activity was related to focused attention to the stimulus. Global theta activity during a visual cognitive task, on the other hand, did not differ between healthy controls and progressive or stable MCI groups. The authors stated that primary cortical processing of visual stimulus was not affected in MCI. The ERD/ERS results, presented by Missonnier et al. (2006a,b), indicate that a decrease in the early phasic theta power during working memory activation may predict cognitive decline in MCI. This phenomenon is not related to working memory load, but may reflect the presence of early deficits in directed, attention-related neural circuits in patients with MCI. Grunwald et al. (2002) reported decreased theta reactivity during haptic tasks over parieto-occipital regions in MCI, while Van der Hiele et al. (2007) suggested a loss of attentional resources during memory that not only memory but also impaired attention is encountered at the earliest stages of the disease (Perry and Hodges, 1999).

Babiloni et al. (2005) evaluated MEG upon application of visual delayed choice reaction time task in AD, vascular dementia, young and elderly healthy control subjects. Their analysis of event-related alpha desynchronization showed that the alpha ERD peak was stronger in amplitude in the demented patients than in the normal subjects. Cummins et al. (2008) evaluated event-related theta oscillations in MCI patients and elderly controls during performance of a modified Sternberg word recognition task. Their results demonstrated that MCI subjects exhibited lower recognition interval power than controls at left fronto-central electrodes.

Caravaglios et al. (2010) analyzed single-trial theta ERO responses in two time windows (0–250 ms; 250–500 ms) and compared the results to prestimulus theta power during both target tone and standard tone processing in AD patients and in elderly controls. They indicated that AD patients had an increased prestimulus theta response, but did not show a significant poststimulus theta power increase upon both target and nontarget stimulus processing. On the other hand, the healthy aged controls showed enhanced early and late theta responses in comparison to the prestimulus baseline only during auditory oddball paradigm.

Zervakis et al. (2011) analyzed event-related inter-trial coherence in mild probable AD patients and elderly controls upon stimulation of an auditory oddball paradigm. The authors reported that the theta band in AD patients is reflected in slightly more energy than in controls and the absence of nonphase-locked late alpha activity. They commented that the increase of theta responses in AD patients could be due to cholinesterase inhibitors, which all their AD subjects were taking.

According to the few published event-related oscillation studies (Yener et al., 2007, 2008, 2012; Caravaglios et al., 2008, 2010), frontal delta ERO responses are decreased in AD either in visual or auditory modality. In these studies, it was clearly demonstrated that the most affected frequency bands upon the application of the oddball paradigms were in theta and delta bands (Yener et al., 2007, 2008; Caravaglios et al., 2008, 2010). Theta oscillatory responses displayed lower values of phase-locking in frontal area in AD (Fig. 3; Yener et al., 2007). Delta oscillatory

250

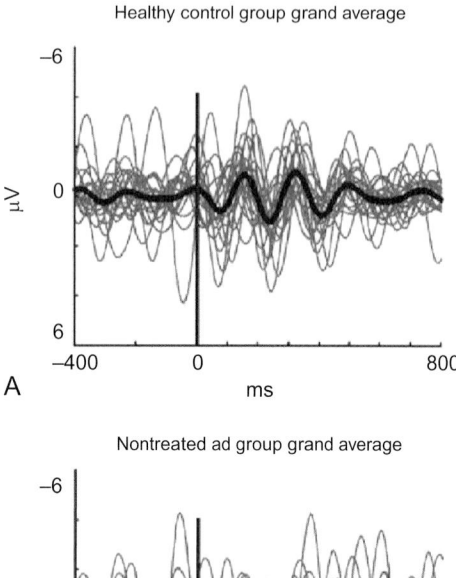

F_3

Healthy control group grand average

A

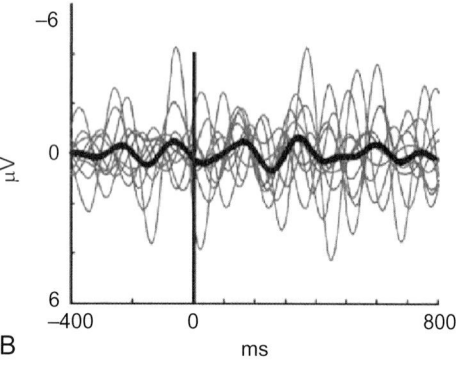

Nontreated ad group grand average

B

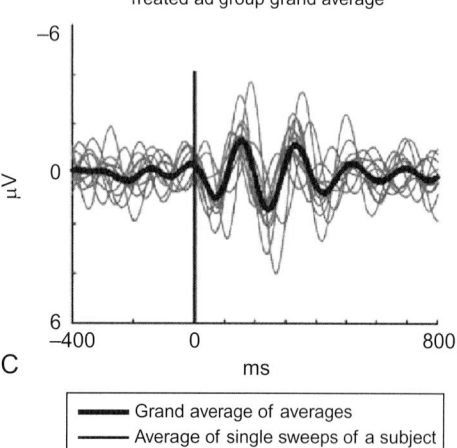

Treated ad group grand average

C

—— Grand average of averages
— Average of single sweeps of a subject

Fig. 3. Decreased visual ER theta phase-locking in AD. (Modified from Yener et al., 2007.)

response amplitudes, both upon application of visual (Fig. 4; Yener et al., 2008) and auditory odd-ball paradigms (Caravaglios et al., 2008; Yener et al., 2012) were decreased in fronto-central regions (Fig. 5). A gradual decrease of auditory delta oscillatory response amplitudes was seen among healthy control (HC), MCI, and AD groups (Yener et al., 2011, unpublished data), indicating a continuum between MCI and AD (Fig. 6). Caravaglios et al. (2008) found that neither pre-stimulus nor poststimulus delta ERO activity differed from controls in an AD group of 21 subjects. However, they showed that the reactivity of delta upon stimulus processing reduces over frontal regions. Yener et al. (2008) similarly found reduced amplitude in auditory delta ERO activity over central regions.

This reduction of frontal activity can be explained by Fuster's (1990) findings, showing anticipatory activation in frontal neurons in time delay tasks in monkeys. Although earlier anatomical studies indicate less prominent pathologic involvement of frontal lobes (Braak et al., 1993), the latest findings on in vivo amyloid imaging in MCI subjects who convert to AD imply that amyloid deposits accumulate in lateral frontal lobes (Koivunen et al., 2011). Many different methods have shown that strong connections of frontal lobe and limbic and heteromodal cortical areas are also affected in early AD, resulting in decreased frontal lobe function (Leuchter et al., 1992; Grady et al., 2001; Delatour et al., 2004).

Phase-locking is a manifestation of synchronization between individual neurons of neural populations upon application of a sensory or cognitive stimulation. The sensory or cognitive inputs can originate from external physical signals or can also be triggered from internal sources. Several publications report phase-locking of theta oscillatory responses as a result of cognitive load in P300 target paradigm (Başar-Eroğlu et al., 1992; Demiralp et al., 1994; Klimesch et al., 2004). Healthy subjects show strong theta phase-locking in the frontal area in visual ERO responses (Fig. 3). The principle of superposition describes

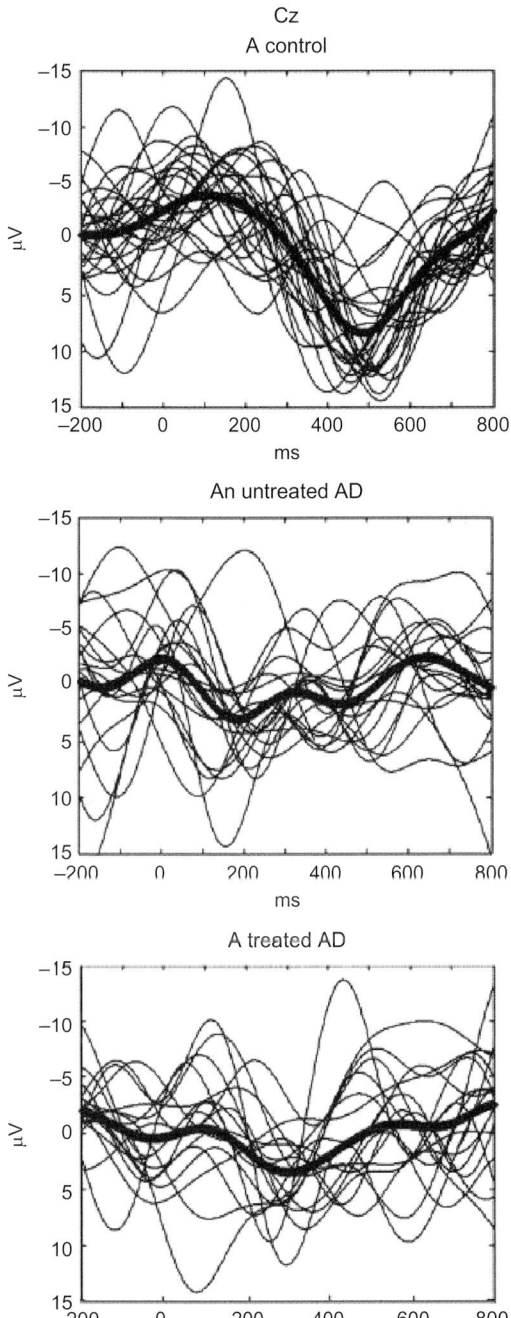

Cz
A control

An untreated AD

A treated AD

Fig. 4. Decreased visual ER delta oscillatory responses in AD over the central area. (Modified from Yener et al., 2008.)

integration over the temporal axis, consisting of a relationship between the amplitude and phases of oscillations in various frequency bands. In a pilot study (Yener et al., 2007) describing the phase-locking of event-related oscillations, unmedicated patients with AD showed weaker phase-locking than both healthy controls and AD subjects treated with cholinergic drugs. In the medicated AD patients and the controls, phase-locking following target stimulation was two times higher in comparison to the responses of the unmedicated patients (Fig. 3). The findings implied that the theta oscillatory responses at the frontal region are highly unstable in unmedicated mild AD patients, and that cholinergic agents may modulate event-related theta oscillatory activities.

It seems as though in slower frequency ranges (delta, theta), peak amplitudes following cognitive stimulus are decreased over frontal-central regions in AD, regardless of sensory modality (auditory or visual) (Figs. 4 and 5). Also, there is a continuum between the AD and MCI subjects' event-related responses, observed as decreased delta amplitudes and delay in the latency of delta peak (Fig. 6; Yener et al., 2011).

16.3.4.3. Comparison of SEO and ERO responses
Amplitude analysis of digitally filtered SEO or ERO responses provides the opportunity to explore sensory or cognitive neurodynamics. Yener et al. (2009) compared SEOs and EROs of patients with AD using a visual oddball paradigm. Significant decreases in delta event-related oscillatory activity over central regions were seen in AD, whereas increased delta visual SEO responses were recorded at parieto-occipital regions where primary and secondary sensory areas were located (Fig. 7). For further information on methodological issues, the reader is referred to reviews by Başar et al. (2010) and by Güntekin and Başar (2010). Similar to these findings, by means of auditory oscillatory responses, Caravaglios et al. (2008) found significant enhancement in delta responses in healthy controls when compared to Alzheimer's subjects (especially at

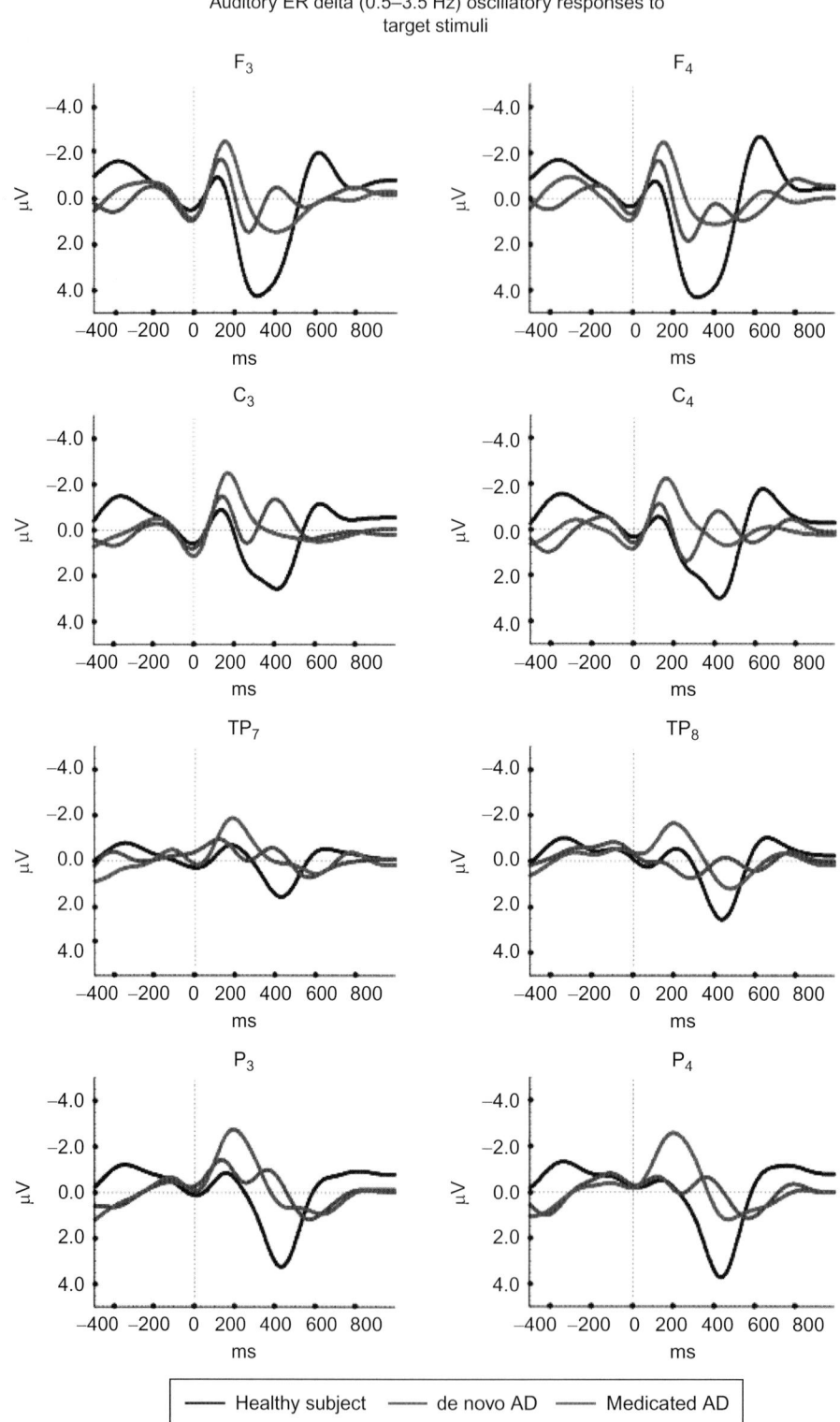

Fig. 5. Auditory delta ERO responses are decreased in frontal regions in AD. (Modified from Yener et al., 2012.) (For color figures, please refer to the color figures in last section of the book.)

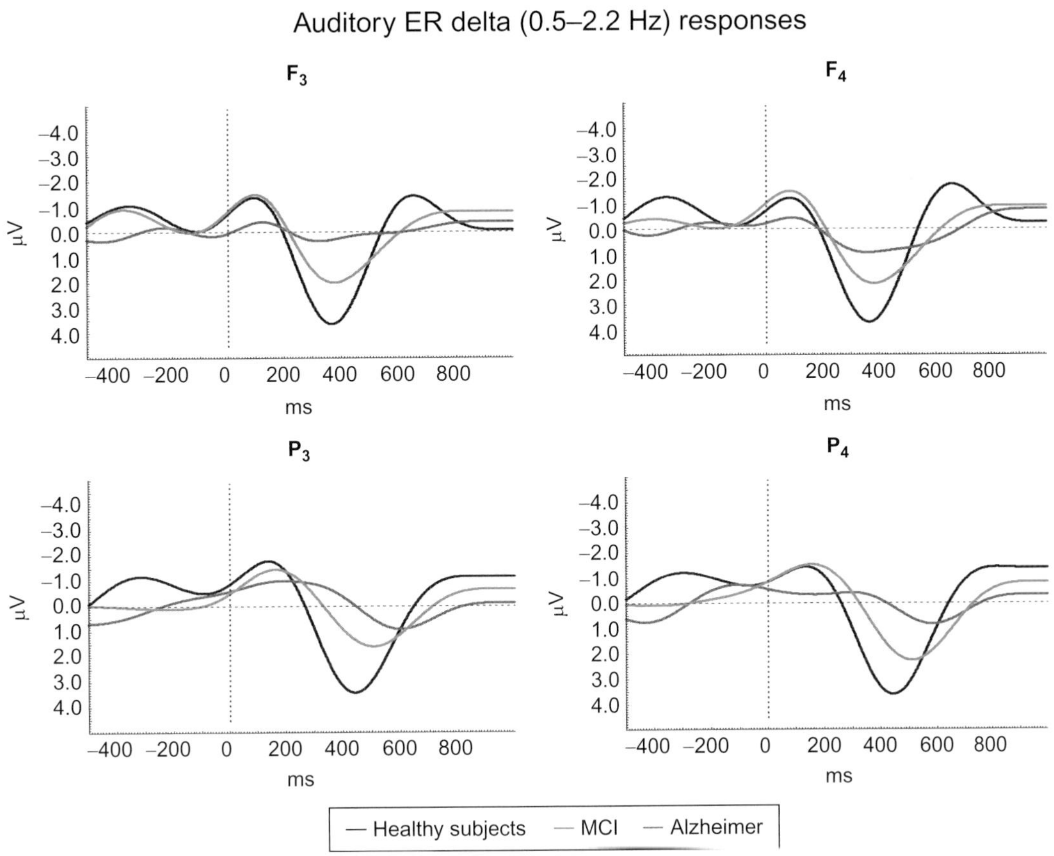

Auditory ER delta (0.5–2.2 Hz) responses

Fig. 6. MCI and AD continuity is prominent in auditory ER delta oscillatory activity, showing gradually decreasing delta amplitudes and delayed delta peak responses among healthy subjects, MCI, and mild Alzheimer subjects. (Modified from Yener et al., 2011.) (For color figures, please refer to the color figures in last section of the book.)

frontal locations). The lack of frontal delta responses, irrespective of stimulus modality, implies a decision-making impairment and decreased frontal functioning in mild AD.

Table 2 shows the latest studies of brain oscillations in AD.

16.3.5. Coherence

Coherence is a measure of synchrony between separate structures and it was first used five decades ago by Adey et al. (1960), as a pioneering work on theta rhythms of the cat limbic system during conditioning. Coherence (Gardner, 1992) or phase-locking statistics (Lachaux et al., 2002) are some of the common techniques used to evaluate relationships between neural populations. Coherence values range between 0 and 1, with higher values indicating better connectivity between two structures.

Adey et al. (1960) used spectral analysis and coherence functions to investigate how the rhythmic potentials of the cat brain were related to behavior. The use of the coherence function in comparing EEG activity in various nuclei of the cat brain was one of the essential steps in refuting the view that the EEG was an epiphenomenon. Accordingly, the induced theta rhythm and the task-relevant increase of coherence in the limbic

254

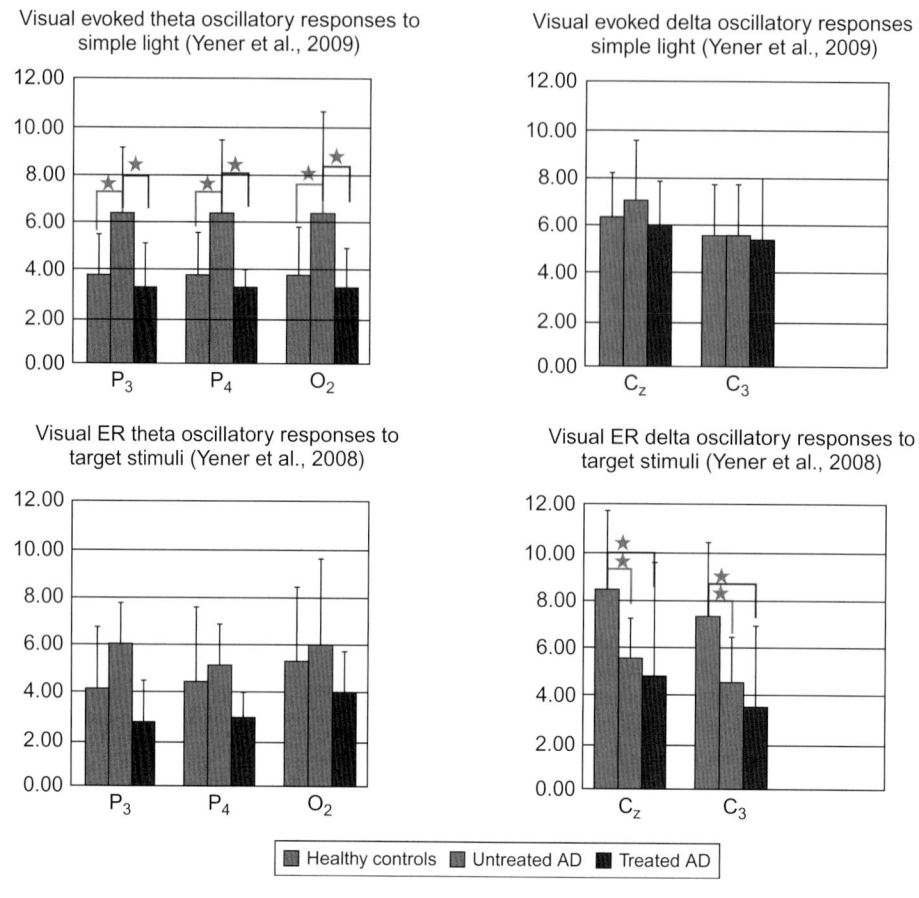

Fig. 7.   Comparison of visual evoked and ER oscillatory activity in AD. (Modified from Yener et al., 2009.) (For color figures, please refer to the color figures in last section of the book.)

system is a milestone in EEG research. When carrying out a behavioral task, the cat hippocampal activity exhibits a transition from irregular activity to coherent, induced rhythms. Sauseng et al. (2005) calculated the coherence function during a visuospatial working memory task in a group of healthy subjects. Their findings indicated that the involvement of prefrontal areas in executive functions are reflected in a decrease of anterior upper alpha short-range connectivity and a parallel increase of fronto-parietal long distance coherence, mirroring the activation of a fronto-parietal network.

Many studies reported the successful use of EEG coherence to measure functional connectivity (Lopes da Silva et al., 1980; Rappelsberger et al.,

1982). According to these studies, EEG coherence may be regarded as an indispensable large-scale measure of functional relationships between pairs of cortical regions (Nunez, 1997). It is also important to mention the studies of T.H. Bullock's research group (Bullock et al., 1995), which clearly showed that the connectivity (coherence) between neural groups is a main factor for the evolution of cognitive processes (Başar et al., 2010). According to Bullock and Başar (1988) and Bullock et al. (1995), no significant coherences were found in the neural networks of invertebrates, in contrast to the higher coherences between distant structures that were recorded in mammalian and human brains. The highest coherences were found in the subdural structures of the human brain (Bullock,

TABLE 2

THE EVOKED, AND EVENT-RELATED OSCILLATION STUDIES IN AD/MCI IN RECENT YEARS

Studies on MCI/AD subjects	Modality and paradigms	Subjects	Methods	Results
Evoked oscillatory activity				
Kikuchi et al. (2002)	Visual photic stimulation	AD	Evoked coherence	Decreased interhemispheric coherence in AD in alpha frequencies
Hogan et al. (2003)	Visual photic	AD	Evoked coherence	Reduced upper alpha coherence in AD
Zheng-yan (2005)	Visual photic	AD	Evoked coherence	Reduced upper alpha coherence inter and intrahemispheric coherences in AD
Osipova et al. (2006)	Auditory steady state	AD	40 Hz SSR	A significant increase of 40 Hz SSR power in AD
Haupt et al. (2008)	Visual checkerboard stimulation	AD/MCI	Evoked oscillatory response	Mild AD and MCI were more active for beta$_2$ and gamma band. The asymmetry seen in healthy elderly people moved from the right hemisphere to the left hemisphere in MCI and AD
Başar et al. (2010)	Visual evoked	AD	Evoked coherence	Decreased delta SE coherence in left fronto-occipital connection only
Yener et al. (2009)	Visual evoked	AD	Evoked oscillatory response	A significant theta response increase in parieto-occipital regions
Van Deursen et al. (2011)	Auditory steady state	AD/MCI	40 Hz SSR	A significant increase of 40 Hz SSR power in the AD group compared to MCI and controls
ER oscillatory activity				
Babiloni et al. (2005)	Simple delayed response tasks	VaD/AD	MEG ERD	The alpha ERD peak was stronger in amplitude in the demented patients than in the normal subjects
Karrasch et al. (2006)	Auditory Sternberg word test	MCI/AD	ERD/ERS	Alpha and beta ERD (7–17 Hz) frequencies was absent in the AD group particularly in anterior and left temporal electrode locations
Missonnier et al. (2007)	N-back test	MCI/AD	ERD/ERS	Decreased beta ERS in progressive MCI and AD compared with controls and stable MCI cases in the 1000–1700 ms time window

Continued

TABLE 2

THE EVOKED, AND EVENT-RELATED OSCILLATION STUDIES IN AD/MCI IN RECENT
YEARS — CONT'D

Studies on MCI/AD subjects	Modality and paradigms	Subjects	Methods	Results
Zheng et al. (2007)	Three-level working memory test	MCI	Inter–and intra-hemispheric coherence	Interhemispheric coherence is increased more than intra-hemispheric coherence in MCI
Yener et al. (2007)	Visual oddball	AD	Event-related phase-locking	Decreased theta phase-locking at the left frontal in untreated AD in comparison to controls and cholinergically treated AD
Polikar et al. (2007)	Auditory oddball	AD	ERO response	1–2 and 2–4 Hz at P_z, C_z, 4–8 Hz at F_z provide the most discriminatory information for automated classification
Cummins et al. (2008)	Auditory Sternberg word test	MCI	ERD/ERS	Lower theta in all significantly different areas
Yener et al. (2008)	Visual oddball	AD	ERO response	Decreased delta oscillatory peak-to-peak amplitudes at central electrodes
Güntekin et al. (2008)	Visual oddball	AD	Event-related coherence	Decreased alpha, theta, delta event-related coherence between frontal and all connections
Van Deursen et al. (2008)	Music and story listening, visual task	MCI/AD	ERS	A significant increase of gamma band power in AD cases compared to healthy controls and MCI cases
Caravaglios et al. (2008)	Auditory oddball	AD	ERO response	Decreased enhancement of the delta response in single sweep maximal peak-to-peak amplitude especially at the frontal location in AD
Deiber et al. (2009)	N-back paradigm	MCI	ERS	Decreased induced theta activity in progressive MCI than stable MCI or controls
Missonnier et al. (2010)	Visual N-back task	MCI	ERO response	Progressive MCI cases displayed higher gamma values and reduced theta than stable MCI cases
Caravaglios et al. (2010)	Auditory oddball	AD	ERO response	Increased prestimulus theta power, and lack of poststimulus theta power in AD. Healthy controls had a frontal dominance of theta power
Polikar et al. (2010)	Auditory oddball	AD	ERO response	The ERO+MRI parameters together show as high accuracy rates (80%) as PET+MRI parameters for classification of AD

TABLE 2

THE EVOKED, AND EVENT-RELATED OSCILLATION STUDIES IN AD/MCI IN RECENT
YEARS — CONT'D

Studies on MCI/AD subjects	Modality and paradigms	Subjects	Methods	Results
Yener et al. (2011)	Auditory oddball	MCI/AD	ERO response	Across groups (controls, MCI, and AD), there is a gradual decrease of delta responses and increase of delta peak latency, respectively
Zervakis et al. (2011)	Auditory oddball	AD	ER inter-trial coherence	Theta energy increase in AD possibly due to cholinergic medication
Yener et al. (2012)	Auditory oddball	AD	ERO response	Decreased delta oscillatory peak-to-peak amplitudes at the right frontal site

2006). Since coherence is, in essence, a correlation coefficient per frequency band, it is used to describe the coupling or relationship between signals for a certain frequency band. According to Bullock et al. (2003), increased coherence between two structures, namely A and B, can be caused by the following processes: (1) structures A and B are driven by the same generator; (2) structures A and B can mutually drive each other; and (3) one of the structures, A or B, drives the other (Fig. 8). There are several synchrony measures studied in AD diagnosis, including the correlation coefficient, mean square, phase coherence, Granger causality, phase synchrony indices, information theoretic divergence measures, state–space-based measures, and stochastic event synchrony measures. Among these, Granger causality and stochastic event synchrony measures were used to distinguish MCI from healthy controls, achieving an accuracy of 83% (Dauwels et al., 2010b).

16.3.5.1. SE coherences

EEG coherence globally describes the coupling of, or relationship between, signals in a given frequency band. The term "sensory evoked (SE) coherence" reflects the property of sensory networks activated by a simple sensory stimulation without a cognitive

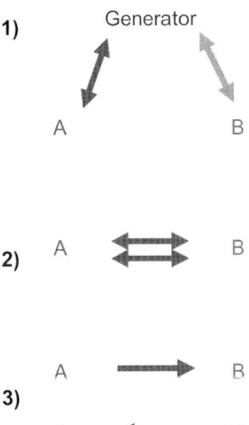

Fig. 8.   Bullock's electrophysiological driving sources. (For color figures, please refer to the color figures in last section of the book.)

load, whereas "event-related (ER) coherence" manifests coherent activity of sensory and cognitive networks triggered by a cognitive task, i.e., oddball paradigm (Fig. 9). According to Başar et al. (2010) the results of SE coherence show that the coherence values in all frequency ranges do not exceed 0.35 (Fig. 10), whereas ER coherence values elicited upon a cognitive paradigm reach 0.7. Thus, the comparison of ER and SE coherences demonstrates that sensory signal elicits only negligible coherence values in comparison to the results of a cognitive task.

Rossini et al. (2006) measured the spontaneous EEG coherences in healthy controls and two groups of MCI (progressive and stable) and found that progression to conversion is faster in patients with high coherence in delta and gamma frequency bands. Later Babiloni et al. (2010) demonstrated that total coherence of alpha$_1$ rhythms was highest in the healthy elderly, intermediate in the MCI subjects with no cholinergic white matter lesion, and lowest in the MCI with cholinergic lesion. Furthermore, damage to the cholinergic system is associated with alterations of the functional global coupling of resting alpha rhythms.

The topography of changed connectivity in AD upon visual simple sensory stimulation is not straightforward. Hogan et al. (2003) examined memory-related EEG power and coherence over

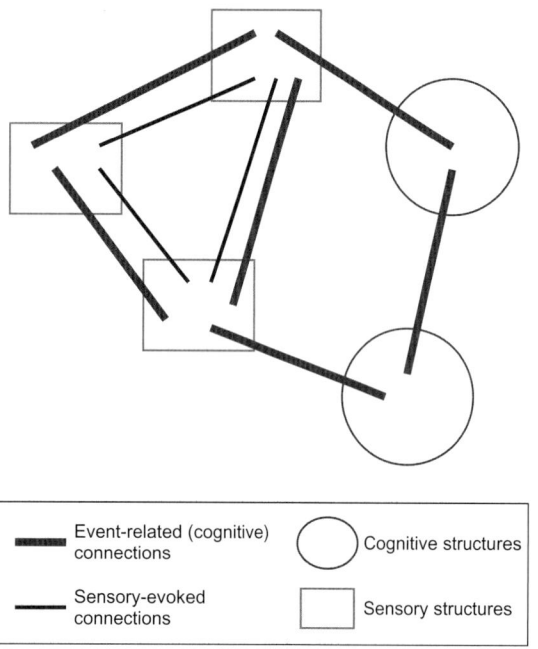

Fig. 9.   Neural assemblies involved in sensory and cognitive networks. Cognitive networks (here shown by magenta lines) probably contain sensory neural elements, but also involve additional neural assemblies as shown by magenta circles. Sensory network elements are illustrated by blue squares and connections by blue lines. It is expected that sensory signals trigger activation of sensory areas, whereas cognitive stimulation would evoke both neural groups reacting to sensory and cognitive inputs. (For color figures, please refer to the color figures in last section of the book.)

temporal and central recording sites in patients with early AD and normal controls. While the behavioral performance of very mild AD patients did not differ significantly from that of normal controls, when compared with normal controls, the AD patients had reduced upper alpha coherence between the central and right temporal cortex. Zheng-yan (2005) stated that during photic stimulation, inter- and intrahemispheric EEG coherences of the AD patients showed lower values in the alpha (9.5–10.5 Hz) band than those of the control group.

Taken together, these results indicate that the sensory network is affected in AD; however, the severity of dysfunction does not seem to be as high as that in the cognitive network (Figs. 10 and 11).

16.3.5.2. ER coherences

ER coherences manifest coherent activity of sensory and cognitive networks triggered by attending to a cognitive task. Accordingly, the cognitive response coherences comprehend activation of a greater number of neural networks that are most possibly not activated, or less activated than the spontaneous EEG or SE coherences (Fig. 9). Therefore, ER coherence merits special attention. Particularly in AD patients with strong cognitive impairment, it is relevant to analyze whether medical treatment (drug application) selectively acts upon sensory and cognitive networks manifested in topologically different areas and in different frequency windows. Such an observation may provide a deeper understanding of distributed functional networks and, in turn, the possibility of determining biomarkers for medical treatment. According to the statements above, there are new steps and newly emerging questions. Güntekin et al. (2008) investigated ER coherence of patients with mild AD using a visual oddball paradigm. The AD group was divided into unmedicated and the medicated (cholinergic) subgroups. The authors found that the control group showed higher ER coherence in the "delta," "theta," and "alpha" bands compared to the unmedicated AD group (Fig. 12; Başar et al., 2010). Alpha ER coherence values were higher in the medicated AD subjects than

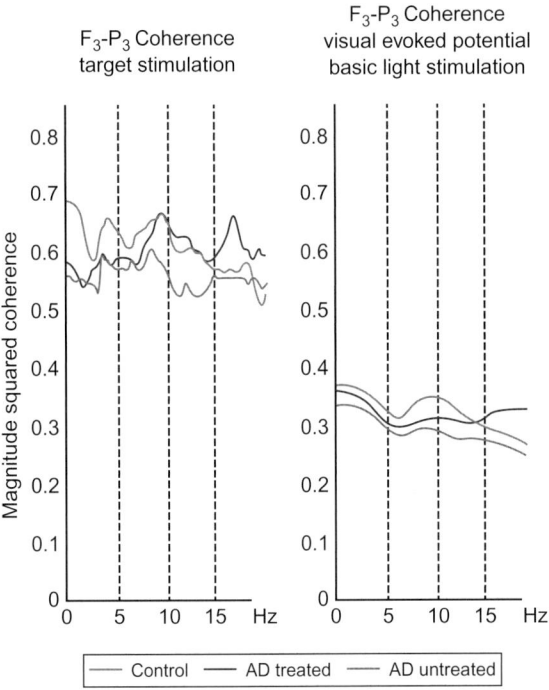

F₃-P₃ Coherence target stimulation

F₃-P₃ Coherence visual evoked potential basic light stimulation

— Control — AD treated — AD untreated

Fig. 10.   Coherences of brain oscillations upon a cognitive task (i.e., target stimulus in classical visual oddball paradigm) reach higher values than those elicited upon simple sensory visual stimuli (i.e., basic light stimulation). Coherence, which reflects functional connectivity between fronto-parietal regions, is higher in controls than in (AD) subjects. Coherence values in alpha ranges are greater in the cholinergically treated subgroup than those with no treatment. (Modified from Yener et al., 2010.) (For color figures, please refer to the color figures in last section of the book.)

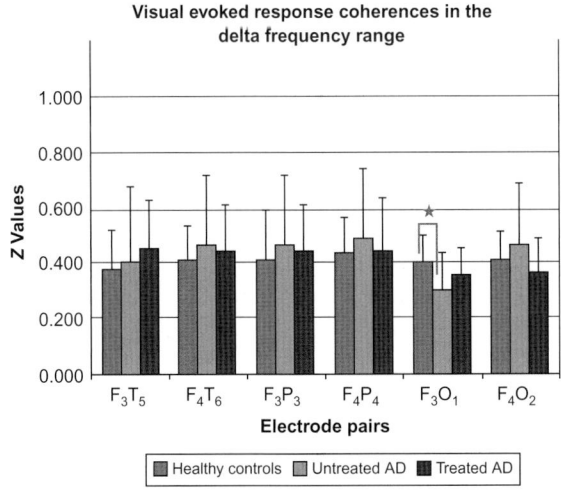

Fig. 11.   Visual SEO responses in AD are not that different from that of controls with the exception of a mild decrease in delta band between the left frontal and occipital regions. (Modified from Başar et al., 2010.) (For color figures, please refer to the color figures in last section of the book.)

in the unmedicated group. This finding implies better connectivity with the use of cholinergic drugs in AD.

16.3.5.3. Comparison of SE and ER coherences
Coherence values range between 0 (lowest) and 1 (highest). Upon application of an oddball paradigm, the ER coherences between left fronto-parietal (F₃ and P₃) locations could show significant coherences of up to 0.7 in the theta, delta, and alpha frequencies in healthy subjects (Fig. 10). Unmedicated AD subjects showed a reduction of 30–40% in theta, delta, and alpha frequency ranges compared with both the controls and the medicated AD subjects. In the medicated group, the coherence of alpha frequency was restored, whereas in theta and delta ranges the cholinergic medication did not cause any change in coherence. It should be emphasized that values in the range of 0.6–0.7

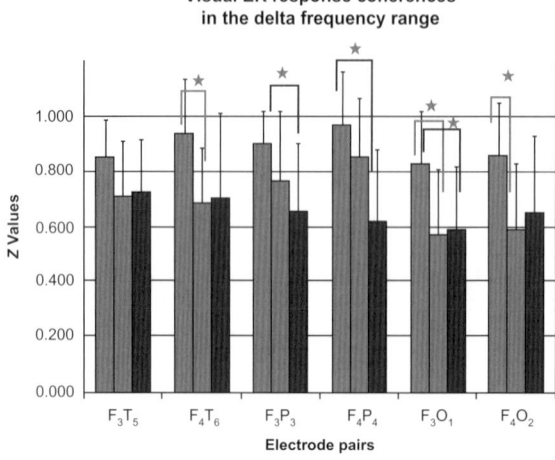

Visual ER response coherences in the delta frequency range

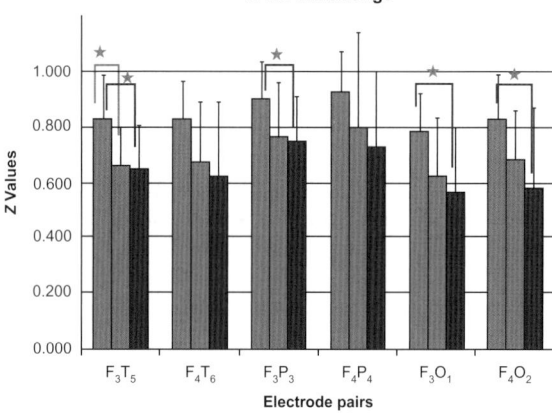

Visual ER response coherences in the theta range

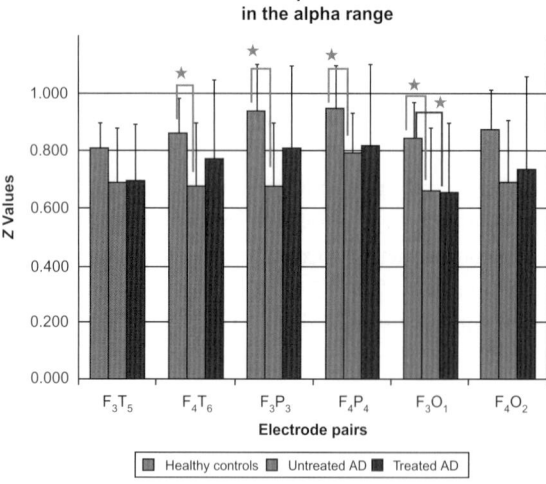

Visual ER response coherences in the alpha range

■ Healthy controls ■ Untreated AD ■ Treated AD

Fig. 12. Visual ER coherences are decreased in slower frequencies (delta, theta, alpha bands) over a wide range of connections in AD. (Modified from Başar et al., 2010.) (For color figures, please refer to the color figures in last section of the book.)

indicate significantly high coherence values, because of the long distance between frontal and parietal location. According to Güntekin et al. (2008), the results emphasized that left fronto-parietal connections are highly affected by AD pathology, occurring primarily within the fronto-parietal limbic regions during the early stages of the disease. Fig. 10 compares SE coherences and event-related coherence following target stimulation at F3-P3 electrode pairs during an oddball paradigm.

Zheng-yan (2005) reported that, during photic stimulation, AD patients showed reduced inter and intrahemispheric coherences in the alpha (9.5–10.5 Hz) band than those of the control group. During a 5-Hz photic stimulation, the AD patients had significantly lower intrahemispheric coherence in theta, alpha, and beta bands. Hogan et al. (2003) examined memory-related EEG power and coherence over temporal and central recording sites in patients with early AD and found that dementia subjects had reduced upper alpha coherence between the central and right temporal cortex than observed in the healthy control group. Zheng et al. (2007) investigated inter and intrahemispheric coherence during a three-level working memory task undertaken by patients with MCI. The coherence in MCI patients was significantly higher than in the controls. Their findings indicate that the alpha frequency band for coherence studies may be the characteristic band in distinguishing MCI patients from normal controls during working memory tasks. MCI patients exhibit larger interhemispheric connectivity than intrahemispheric connectivity when memory demand increases.

Coherences between prefrontal–parietal and prefrontal–occipital regions may have a role in determining the resulting activity in parietal or in occipital regions. Our groups' findings on coherences (Güntekin et al., 2008; Başar et al., 2010) are consistent with functional imaging studies in AD, showing relatively large attenuation of activations in parieto-occipital (Bradley et al., 2002; Prvulovic et al., 2002; Bentley et al., 2008) than in temporo-occipital areas. The observed hyperexcitability of primary visual areas following simple visual stimulation in AD

(Yener et al., 2009) could be partially related to several factors: (1) the decreased SE coherence (connectivity) between frontal and posterior parts of the brain; (2) the decreased frontal lobe modulation (Yener et al., 2007, 2008; Caravaglios et al., 2008, 2010); and (3) the relatively preserved sensory and motor cortical areas (Braak et al., 1993). The motor cortex hyperexcitability in AD was previously shown by Ferreri et al. (2003).

Furthermore, selectively distributed and selective coherent oscillatory activities in neural populations describe integration over the spatial axis (Başar, 1980). Consequently, integrative activity is a function of the coherences between spatial locations of the brain. These coherences vary according to the type of sensory and/or cognitive event and possibly the state of consciousness of the species (Başar, 1999, 2004). The work of Bressler and Kelso (2001) emphasized that within the coordinated large-scale cortical network, the participating sites are much more interrelated to one another than to non-network sites. These coordinated areas undergo re-entrant processing, and later re-entrant interactions will constrain the local spatial activity patterns in these areas. In this manner, re-entrant transmissions define local expression of information. As areas interact reciprocally, some areas reach a consensus through the process of large-scale relative coordination, in which those areas temporarily manifest consistent local spatial activity patterns. This mechanism also provides dynamic creation of local context in a highly adaptive manner in visual functions. Varela et al. (2001) state that the emergence of a unified cognitive moment depends on the coordination of scattered parts of functionally specialized brain regions. The mechanisms of large-scale integration enable the emergence of coherent behavior and cognition. These authors argue that the most plausible candidate is the formation of dynamic links mediated by synchrony over multiple frequency bands. Von Stein and Sarnthein (2000) propose that long-range fronto-parietal interactions during working memory retention and mental imagery evolve, instead, in the theta and alpha (4–8 Hz, 8–12 Hz) frequency ranges. This large-scale integration is performed by synchronization among neurons and neuronal assemblies evolving in different frequency ranges.

16.4. Neurotransmitters

The dysfunction of cognitive network in AD may be a result of balance disorder between neural excitation and inhibition through neurotransmitters, and disorder of long-term potentiation that strengthens or weakens the synaptic connections (Lisman and Spruston, 2005).

16.4.1. Main neurotransmitter systems and their effects on cognitive network

Acetylcholine (ACh)-containing projections from the nucleus basalis Meynert degenerates first in AD (Mesulam et al., 2004). This depletion seems to have a role in dysfunction in visuospatial system and memory-related tasks in AD. ACh promotes visual feature detection or signal-to-noise ratios in sensory processing (Hasselmo and Giacomo, 2006) and cholinergic medication can improve a normal pattern of task-dependent parietal activation in AD. Working memory tasks (Saykin et al., 2004), visual search (Hao et al., 2005), or visual attention (Balducci et al., 2003) studies indicate enhanced prefrontal cortex activity after cholinergic medication, similar to the electrophysiological findings shown by our group (Yener et al., 2007; Güntekin et al., 2008). An fMRI study in mild AD/MCI also showed a similar pattern in left prefrontal regions during attentional demands (Dannhauser et al., 2005). The diffuse innervation of cortical cholinergic neurons (Sarter et al., 2001) can lead to cholinergic modulation in both higher-level (e.g., fronto-parietal) and lower-level (e.g., visual) areas. It is possible that visual ERO deficits in AD may be related to reduction in cholinergic modulation of visual cortex and attention-related fronto-parietal cortices (Perry and Hodges, 1999).

Understanding how the cholinergic system affects visual sensory or cognitive function is important for AD. When two types of tasks (i.e., deep minus shallow visual stimulation) were given to AD patients and controls, fMRI showed that the right parietal (Hao et al., 2005), left prefrontal, and superomedial prefrontal cortices were less activated by this task effect in AD patients than in controls (Bentley et al., 2008). The extent of involvement of visual and higher order association cortex increased with greater complexity in AD. Visual tests activate both primary and secondary visual areas in dorsal stream (Förster et al., 2010). Visual dorsal stream, which involves the parietal lobe, is activated before the ventral stream, which includes the temporal lobe. The parietal lobe is activated within 30 ms after occipital activation, occurring at about 56 ms. Visual sensory areas generally continue to be active for 100–400 ms prior to motor output. The feedback processes between sensory, parietal, and prefrontal cortices take about 200 ms for an interactive process. This initial volley of sensory afference through the visual system, and involving top-down influences from parietal and frontal regions, occurs much earlier than the early ERP components (Foxe and Simpson, 2002). Using visuospatial paradigms, these regions are particularly sensitive to cholinergic modulation (Sarter et al., 2001). Acetylcholine seems to have a role in promoting visual feature detection or signal-to-noise ratios in sensory processing (Hasselmo and Giocomo, 2006) and cholinergic medication can improve a normal pattern of task-dependent parietal activation in AD.

16.4.2. Changes in AD subjects on cholinergic medication

Cortical ACh is hypothesized to modulate either the general efficacy of the cortical processing of sensory or associational information, or, more specifically, to mediate the subjects' abilities to select stimuli and associations for further processing (Sarter et al., 2005). The basal forebrain is the main source of ACh in the neocortex and Alzheimer patients show depletion of cortical ACh due to degeneration of the basal forebrain early in the course of the illness (Mesulam et al., 2004). Therefore, for almost the past 20 years, cholinergic treatment was the main

treatment option in AD. In addition, increased cholinergic input can restore hemodynamics in clinical responders (Claassen and Jansen, 2006). An early study on resting EEG showed that alpha power decreased following experimental damage to this cholinergic pathway (Holschneider et al., 1998). In addition to the basal forebrain, glutamatergic and cholinergic mechanisms within the prefrontal cortex may also regulate ACh release in other parts of the cortex such as the posterior parietal cortex (Nelson et al., 2005). The ability of prefrontal cortex to regulate transmission in more posterior cortical regions may represent a "top-down" mechanism to control attention (Sarter et al., 2005). For example, thalamocortical fibers are suppressed much less than intracortical connections by acetylcholine, thus possibly enabling the afferent input to have a relative effect in the cortex (Kimura et al., 1999). Therefore, the detrimental performance effects of an ongoing distracter are most likely diminished by increasing the cholinergic processing of sensory inputs (Sarter et al., 2005). These agents can improve the latencies of the visual P300 in AD patients (Reeves et al., 1999). Earlier functional imaging studies showed that, after administration of AChEI, clinical responders to treatment selectively displayed improvements over left cingulate and prefrontal–parietal areas (Potkin et al., 2001; Nobili et al., 2002; Vennerica et al., 2002; Mega et al., 2005).

16.5. Summary

The results of the present review permit tentative concluding remarks related to neurophysiological markers for AD patients. In defining one type of neurophysiological marker, we prefer to categorize the presented results according to their functions: (a) spontaneous EEG or resting EEG; (b) SEO responses and coherences following a simple sensory stimulus without a cognitive load; and (c) ERO responses and coherences following a cognitive stimulus (i.e., oddball paradigm). Our tentative proposal indicates that the collection of information, and especially their comparison, could provide a solid construct as "an ensemble of neurophysiologic biomarkers." Furthermore, we propose that this type of strategy will be useful for analysis of neuro-psychiatric disorders in general (see Yener and Başar, this volume).

16.5.1. Spontaneous EEG activity

An extended review of spontaneous EEG activity of AD/MCI patients is described by Vecchio et al. in this issue. The spontaneous EEG activity of AD shows characteristically increased delta and theta power in temporo-occipital regions and decreased power in beta and alpha power in parieto-occipital regions. Also, fronto-parietal coherences were abnormal in amnesic MCI, reflecting a functional disconnection among cortical regions.

16.5.2. SE oscillations

Some brain areas (sensorial and motor cortices) seem to be hyperexcitable in AD, as shown by increased theta responses over primary and secondary sensory areas (Yener et al., 2009), and increased gamma responses (Haupt et al., 2008; Van Deursen et al., 2011). The hyperexcitability of the sensory areas is indicated by the findings of Ferreri et al. (2003) and Rossini et al. (2006), indicating hyperexcitability of motor cortex in AD. These findings are in accordance with relative preservation of primary sensory and motor cortical areas in this disorder. It is highly important to note that pure sensory stimulation in AD does not display a remarkable change in frontal brain regions from that of healthy controls (Table 1 and Fig. 7).

16.5.3. ER oscillations

Contrary to results on SEOs, the cognitive paradigm (EROs) elicits: (a) attenuated delta responses over frontal and central modulating regions (Figs. 5 and 6); (b) decreased frontal phase-locking (i.e., synchronization among single sweeps) in the theta frequency range (Fig. 4); and (c) improved theta phase-locking with cholinesterase inhibitor medication (Fig. 4 and Table 1).

16.5.4. Coherences

SE coherence elicited upon simple sensory stimulation displays decreased values between only frontal lobe and primary sensory (i.e., in visual tasks, occipital) regions in the delta frequency range (Fig. 11). However, event-related coherence recorded upon a cognitive task shows decreased values between frontal and all other brain connections in the many frequency ranges, including alpha, theta, and delta (Fig. 12). It is important to note that, in higher frequency ranges (beta, gamma), no significant changes are evident in coherences. This finding implies that selective connectivity is disturbed in AD depending on the cognitive load of stimuli. Furthermore, regardless of group effect, there was great difference in coherence values between those elicited after SE and ER stimulations. The event-related coherence values (approximately 0.70) were up to double those of SE coherence (approximately 0.35) (Fig. 10). This finding implies that, upon application of a cognitive task, greater brain connectivity is reached, as expected. In addition, cholinergic agents promote improvements in alpha event-related coherences in AD subjects (Table 1, Figs. 10 and 12).

16.6. Conclusion

The most important conclusion of the present review is the following: according to Luria (1966), there are no anatomical centers for the psychological functions of the mind. Mental functions, too, are the products of complex systems, the component parts of which may be distributed throughout the structures of the brain. The task of neuroscience is therefore not to localize the "centers" but, rather, to identify the components of the various complex

264

systems that interact to generate the mental functions. Luria called this task "dynamic localization."

Mental functions, in short, are not localized in any of the component structures, but rather distributed between them. Like the mental apparatus as a whole, they are virtual entities (Solms and Turnbull, 2002). According to the present review, the understanding of whole brain function also requires the analysis of functional coherences, i.e., the increased connectivity between structures upon cognitive load, together with enhanced temporal oscillatory responses. Furthermore, in addition to Luria's view, it seems that Brodmann's areas should be extended to a more dynamic presentation, in which sensory and cognitive areas should be described as superposition of multiple primary and secondary functions.

Only in this way it may be possible to open new avenues for description of whole cortex organization. As a consequence, we propose that all information gathered from sensory or cognitive paradigms must be jointly analyzed in terms of oscillatory responses and related coherences in order to validate an electrophysiological biomarker. We tentatively assume that prefrontal areas have a modulating effect on other parts of the brain, depending on stimulation modality (i.e., sensory or cognitive). However, the modulation of the prefrontal lobe may be different on the projecting areas, depending on the cognitive load of the stimulus and on interconnected brain areas, such as primary sensory, primary motor, or heteromodal cortical areas. Among the electrophysiological parameters, the ER (or cognitive) coherences comprehend activation of a greater number of neural networks and merit special attention among the assembly of electrophysiological parameters. Therefore, ER coherence variables can be suggested as a candidate electrophysiological biomarker for diagnosis and monitoring of treatment effects in AD in the first instance. Other methods, such as phase-locking, may also provide insights into cognitive networks and their modulation by neurotransmitter changes. Oscillatory response peak-to-peak amplitudes, especially those

in delta frequencies at frontal locations, seem to be a candidate for a static (i.e., for using in diagnosis), rather than a dynamic (i.e., for understanding change over time or in response to medication) biomarker.

The results presented in this review provide evidence for the existence of separate sensory and cognitive networks that are activated either on sensory or on cognitive stimulation and show the group differences. These observations may serve to increase the physiological understanding of distributed functional networks and, in turn, the possibility of determining biomarkers for either diagnosis or monitoring of medical treatment in AD/MCI. However, it is also important to state that a greater number of subjects are needed to study either the effects of pharmacological applications or its diagnostic role on an individual basis. The standardization and harmonization of user-friendly acquisition and analysis protocols in larger cohort populations must be the main focus among researchers working on this field in order to incorporate electrophysiology as a part of the clinical criteria of AD.

Abbreviations

Aβ42 = amyloid β42 peptide
ACh = acetylcholine
AD = Alzheimer's disease
ADHD = attention deficit hyperactivity disorder
ADNI = Alzheimer's disease neuroimaging initiative
ASSR = auditory steady-state responses
BD = bipolar disorder
CSF = cerebrospinal fluid
EEG = electroencephalography
ER = event-related
ERO = event-related oscillation
fMRI = functional magnetic resonance imaging
FDG-PET = fluorodeoxyglucose positron emission tomography
MCI = mild cognitive impairment
MRI = magnetic resonance imaging

PIB-PET = Pittsburgh compound B positron emission tomography

PLF = phase-locking factor

P-tau = phospho-tau protein

SE = sensory evoked

SEO = sensory-evoked oscillation

TMS = transcranial magnetic stimulation

T-tau = total tau protein

References

Adaya-Villanueva, A., Ordaz, B., Balleza-Tapia, H., Márquez-Ramos, A. and Peña-Ortega, F. (2010) Beta-like hippocampal network activity is differentially affected by amyloid beta peptides. *Peptides*, 31: 1761–1766.

Adey, W.R., Dunlop, C.W. and Hendrix, C.E. (1960) Hippocampal slow waves: distribution and phase relationships in the course of approach learning. *Arch. Neurol. (Chic.)*, 3: 74–90.

Ahiskali, M., Green, D., Kounios, J., Clark, C.M. and Polikar, R. (2009) ERP based decision fusion for AD diagnosis across cohorts. *Proc. IEEE Eng. Med. Biol. Soc.*, 2009: 2494–2497.

Alexopoulos, P., Grimmer, T., Perneczky, R., Domes, G. and Kurz, A. (2006) Progression to dementia in clinical subtypes of mild cognitive impairment. *Dement. Geriatr. Cogn. Disord.*, 22: 27–34.

American Psychiatric Association (2000) *Diagnostic and Statistical Manual of Mental Health Disorders*. APA, Washington, DC, 980 pp.

Babiloni, C., Binetti, G., Cassetta, E., Cerboneschi, D., Dal Forno, G., Del Percio, C., Ferreri, F., Ferri, R., Lanuzza, B., Miniussi, C., Moretti, D.V., Nobili, F., Pascual-Marqui, R.D, Rodriguez, G., Romani, G.L., Salinari, S., Tecchio, F., Vitali, P., Zanetti, O., Zappasodi, F. and Rossini, P.M. (2004) Mapping distributed sources of cortical rhythms in mild Alzheimer's disease. a multicenter EEG study. *Neuroimage*, 22: 57–67.

Babiloni, C., Cassetta, E., Chiovenda, P., Del Percio, C., Ercolani, M., Moretti, D.V., Moffa, F., Pasqualetti, P., Pizzella, V., Romani, G.L., Tecchio, F., Zappasodi, F. and Rossini, P.M. (2005) Alpha rhythms in mild dements during visual delayed choice reaction time tasks: a MEG study. *Brain Res. Bull.*, 65: 457–470.

Babiloni, C., Binetti, G., Cassetta, E., Dal Forno, G., Del Percio, C., Ferreri, F., Ferri, F., Frisoni, F., Hirata, K., Lanuzza, B., Miniussi, C., Moretti, D.V., Nobili, F., Rodriguez, G., Romani, G.L., Salinari, S. and Rossini, P.M. (2006a) Sources of cortical rhythms change as a function of cognitive impairment in pathological aging: a multicenter study. *Clin. Neurophysiol.*, 117: 252–268.

Babiloni, C., Cassetta, E., Dal Forno, G., Del Percio, C., Ferreri, F., Ferri, R., Lanuzza, B., Miniussi, C., Moretti, D.V., Nobili, F., Pascual-Marqui, R.D., Rodriguez, G., Luca Romani, G., Salinari, S., Zanetti, O.

and Rossini, P.M. (2006b) Donepezil effects on sources of cortical rhythms in mild Alzheimer's disease: responders vs. non-responders. *Neuroimage*, 31: 1650–1665.

Babiloni, C., Frisoni, G., Steriade, M., Bresciani, L., Binetti, G., Del Percio, C., Geroldi, C., Miniussi, C., Nobili, F., Rodriguez, G., Zappasodi, F., Carfagna, T. and Rossini, P.M. (2006c) Frontal white matter volume and delta EEG sources negatively correlate in awake subjects with mild cognitive impairment and Alzheimer's disease. *Clin. Neurophysiol.*, 117: 1113–1129.

Babiloni, C., Frisoni, G.B., Pievani, M., Vecchio, F., Lizio, R., Buttiglione, M., Geroldi, C., Fracassi, C., Eusebi, F., Ferri, R. and Rossini, P.M. (2009a) Hippocampal volume and cortical sources of EEG alpha rhythms in mild cognitive impairment and Alzheimer disease. *Neuroimage*, 44: 123–135.

Babiloni, C., Pievani, M., Vecchio, F., Geroldi, C., Eusebi, F., Fracassi, C., Fletcher, E., De Carli, C., Boccardi, M., Rossini, P.M. and Frisoni, G.B. (2009b) White-matter lesions along the cholinergic tracts are related to cortical sources of EEG rhythms in amnesic mild cognitive impairment. *Hum. Brain Mapp.*, 30: 1431–1443.

Babiloni, C., Visser, P.J., Frisoni, G., De Deyn, P.P., Bresciani, L., Jelic, V., Nagels, G., Rodriguez, G., Rossini, P.M., Vecchio, F., Colombo, D., Verhey, F., Wahlund, L.O. and Nobili, F. (2010) Cortical sources of resting EEG rhythms in mild cognitive impairment and subjective memory complaint. *Neurobiol. Aging*, 31: 1787–1798.

Balducci, C., Nurra, M., Pietropoli, A., Samanin, R. and Carli, M. (2003) Reversal of visual attention dysfunction after AMPA lesions of the nucleus basalis magnocellularis (NBM) by the cholinesterase inhibitor donepezil and by a 5-HT1A receptor antagonist WAY 100635. *Psychopharmacology (Berl.)*, 167: 28–36.

Başar, E. (1980) *EEG-Brain Dynamics. Relation between EEG and Brain Evoked Potentials*. Elsevier, Amsterdam, pp. 1–411.

Başar, E. (1992) Brain natural frequencies are causal factors for resonances and induced rhythms. In: E. Başar and T. Bullock (Eds.), *Induced Rhythms in the Brain*. Birkhäuser, Boston, MA, pp. 425–457.

Başar, E. (1999) *Brain Function and Oscillations II. Integrative Brain Function. Neurophysiology and Cognitive Processes*. Springer, Berlin, pp. 1–476.

Başar, E. (2004) *Memory and Brain Dynamics. Oscillations Integrating Attention, Perception, Learning, and Memory*. CRC Press, Boca Raton, FL, pp. 1–261.

Başar, E. and Güntekin, B. (2008) A review of brain oscillations in cognitive disorders and the role of neurotransmitters. *Brain Res.*, 1235: 172–193.

Başar, E. and Stampfer, H.G. (1985) Important associations among EEG-dynamics, event-related potentials, short-term memory and learning. *Int. J. Neurosci.*, 26: 161–180.

Başar, E., Başar-Eroğlu, C., Rosen, B. and Schütt, A. (1984) A new approach to endogenous event-related potentials in man: relation between EEG and P300 wave. *Int. J. Neurosci.*, 24: 1–21.

Başar, E., Schürmann, M., Başar-Eroğlu, C. and Karakaş, S. (1997) Alpha oscillations in brain functioning: an integrative theory. *Int. J. Psychophysiol.*, 26: 5–29.

Başar, E., Özgören, M. and Karakaş, S. (2001) A brain theory based on neural assemblies and superbinding. In: H. Reuter, P. Schwab, D. Kleiber and G. Gniech (Eds.), *Wahrnehmen und Erkennen*. PABST Science Publishers, Lengerich, pp. 11–24.

Başar, E., Güntekin, B., Tülay, E. and Yener, G.G. (2010) Evoked and event related coherence of Alzheimer patients manifest differentiation of sensory-cognitive networks. *Brain Res.*, 1357: 79–90.

Başar-Eroğlu, C. and Başar, E. (1991) A compound P300–40 Hz response of the cat hippocampus. *Int. J. Neurosci.*, 60: 227–237.

Başar-Eroğlu, C., Başar, E., Demiralp, T. and Schürmann, M. (1992) P300-response: possible psychophysiological correlates in delta and theta frequency channels. *Int. J. Psychophysiol.*, 13: 161–179.

Başar-Eroğlu, C., Demiralp, T., Schürmann, M. and Başar, E. (2001) Topological distribution of oddball 'P300' responses. *Int. J. Psychophysiol.*, 39: 213–220.

Bennys, K., Portet, F., Touchon, J. and Rondouin, G. (2007) Diagnostic value of event-related evoked potentials N200 and P300 subcomponents in early diagnosis of Alzheimer's disease and mild cognitive impairment. *J. Clin. Neurophysiol.*, 24: 405–412.

Bentley, P., Driver, J. and Dolan, R.J. (2008) Cholinesterase inhibition modulates visual and attentional brain responses in Alzheimer's disease and health. *Brain*, 131: 409–424.

Besthorn, C., Zerfass, R., Geiger-Kabisch, C., Sattel, H., Daniel, S., Schreiter-Gasser, U. and Förstl, H. (1997) Discrimination of Alzheimer's disease and normal aging by EEG data. *Electroencephalogr. Clin. Neurophysiol.*, 103: 241–248.

Bhattacharya, B.S., Coyle, D. and Maguire, L.P. (2011) Alpha and theta rhythm abnormality in Alzheimer's disease: a study using a computational model. *Adv. Exp. Med. Biol.*, 718: 57–73.

Blennow, K., Zetterberg, H., Minthon, L., Lannfelt, L., Strid, S., Annas, P., Basun, H. and Andreasen, N. (2007) Longitudinal stability of CSF biomarkers in Alzheimer's disease. *Neurosci. Lett.*, 419: 18–22.

Blennow, K., Hampel, H., Weiner, M. and Zetterberg, H. (2010) Cerebrospinal fluid and plasma biomarkers in Alzheimer disease. *Nat. Rev. Neurol.*, 6: 131–144.

Bobes, M.A., García, Y.F., Lopera, F., Quiroz, Y.T., Galán, L., Vega, M., Trujillo, N., Valdes-Sosa, M. and Valdes-Sosa, P. (2010) ERP generator anomalies in presymptomatic carriers of the Alzheimer's disease E280A PS-1 mutation. *Hum. Brain Mapp.*, 31: 247–265.

Bonanni, L., Franciotti, R., Onofrj, V., Anzellotti, F., Mancino, E., Monaco, D., Gambi, F., Manzoli, L., Thomas, A. and Onofrj, M. (2010) Revisiting P300 cognitive studies for dementia diagnosis: early dementia with Lewy bodies (DLB) and Alzheimer disease (AD). *Neurophysiol. Clin.*, 40: 255–265.

Braak, H., Braak, E. and Bohl, J. (1993) Staging of Alzheimer-related cortical destruction. *Eur. Neurol.*, 33: 403–408.

Bradley, K.M., O'Sullivan, V.T. and Soper, N.D. (2002) Cerebral perfusion SPECT correlated with Braak pathological stage in Alzheimer's disease. *Brain*, 125: 1772–1781.

Bressler, S.L. and Kelso, J.A. (2001) Cortical coordination dynamics and cognition. *Trends Cogn. Sci.*, 1: 26–36.

Bullock, T.H. (2006) How do brains evolve complexity? An essay. *Int. J. Psychophysiol.*, 60: 106–109.

Bullock, T.H. and Başar, E. (1988) Comparison of ongoing compound field potentials in the brain of invertebrates and vertebrates. *Brain Res. Rev.*, 13: 57–75.

Bullock, T.H., McClune, M.C., Achimowicz, J.Z., Iragui-Madoz, V.J., Duckrow, R.B. and Spencer, S.S. (1995) EEG coherence has structure in the millimeter domain: subdural and hippocampal recordings from epileptic patients. *Electroencephalogr. Clin. Neurophysiol.*, 95: 161–177.

Bullock, T.H., McClune, M.C. and Enright, J.T. (2003) Are the electroencephalograms mainly rhythmic? Assessment of periodicity in wide-band time series. *Neuroscience*, 121: 233–252.

Buscema, M., Grossi, E., Capriotti, M., Babiloni, C. and Rossini, P. (2010) The I.F.A.S.T. model allows the prediction of conversion to Alzheimer disease in patients with mild cognitive impairment with high degree of accuracy. *Curr. Alzh. Res.*, 7: 173–187.

Caravaglios, G., Costanzo, E., Palermo, F. and Muscoso, E.G. (2008) Decreased amplitude of auditory event-related delta responses in Alzheimer's disease. *Int. J. Psychophysiol.*, 70: 23–32.

Caravaglios, G., Castro, G., Costanzo, E., Di Maria, G., Mancuso, D. and Muscoso, E. (2010) Theta power responses in mild Alzheimer's disease during an auditory oddball paradigm: lack of theta enhancement during stimulus processing. *J. Neural Transm.*, 117: 1195–1208.

Chapman, R.M., Nowlis, G.H., McCrary, J.W., Chapman, J.A., Sandoval, T.C., Guillily, M.D., Gardner, M.N. and Reilly, L.A. (2007) Brain event-related potentials: diagnosing early-stage Alzheimer's disease. *Neurobiol. Aging*, 28: 194–201.

Chapman, R.M., McCrary, J.W., Gardner, M.N., Sandoval, T.C., Guillily, M.D., Reilly, L.A. and DeGrush, E. (2011) Brain ERP components predict which individuals progress to Alzheimer's disease and which do not. *Neurobiol. Aging*, 32: 1742–1755.

Chen, K., Ayutyanont, N., Langbaum, J.B., Fleisher, A.S., Reschke, C., Lee, W., Liu, X., Bandy, D., Alexander, G.E., Thompson, P.M., Shaw, L., Trojanowski, J.Q., Jack, C.R., Jr., Landau, S.M., Foster, N.L., Harvey, D.J., Weiner, M.W., Koeppe, R.A., Jagust, W.J., Reiman, E.M. and Alzheimer's Disease Neuroimaging Initiative (2011) Characterizing Alzheimer's disease using a hypometabolic convergence index. *Neuroimage*, 56: 52–60.

Cichocki, A., Shishkin, S.L. and Musha, T. (2005) EEG filtering based on blind source separation (BSS) for early detection of Alzheimer's disease. *Clin. Neurophysiol.*, 116: 729–737.

Claassen, J.A. and Jansen, R.W. (2006) Cholinergically mediated augmentation of cerebral disease and related cognitive disorders: the cholinergic-vascular hypothesis. *J. Gerontol. Biol. Sci. Med. Sci.*, 61: 267–271.

Coben, L.A., Danziger, W. and Storandt, M. (1985) A longitudinal EEG study of mild senile dementia of Alzheimer type: changes at 1 year and at 2.5 years. *Electroencephalogr. Clin. Neurophysiol.*, 61: 101–112.

Consensus report of the Working Group on: Molecular and Biochemical Markers of Alzheimer's Disease (1998) The Ronald and Nancy Reagan Research Institute of the Alzheimer's Association and the National Institute on Aging Working Group. *Neurobiol. Aging*, 19(2), 109–116.

Cummins, T.A.D., Broughton, M. and Finnigan, S. (2008) Theta oscillations are affected by mild cognitive impairment (amnestic domain) and cognitive load. *Int. J. Psychophysiol.*, 70: 75–81.

Dannhauser, T.M., Walker, Z., Stevens, T., Lee, L., Seal, M. and Shergill, S.S. (2005) The functional anatomy of divided attention in amnestic mild cognitive impairment. *Brain*, 128: 1418–1427.

Dauwels, J., Vialatte, F. and Cichocki, A. (2010a) Diagnosis of Alzheimer's disease from EEG signals, where are we standing? *Curr. Alzh. Res.*, 7: 487–505.

Dauwels, J., Vialatte, F., Musha, T. and Cichocki, A.A. (2010b) Comparative study of synchrony measures for the early diagnosis of Alzheimer's disease based on EEG. *Neuroimage*, 49: 668–693.

De Carli, C., Frisoni, G.B., Clark, C.M., Harvey, D., Grundman, M., Petersen, R.C., Thal, L.J., Jin, S., Jack, C.R., Jr., Scheltens, P. and Alzheimer's Disease Cooperative Study Group (2007) Qualitative estimates of medial temporal atrophy as a predictor of progression from mild cognitive impairment to dementia. *Arch. Neurol. (Chic.)*, 64: 108–115.

Deiber, M.P., Missonnier, P., Bertrand, O., Gold, G., Fazio-Costa, L., Ibañez, V. and Giannakopoulos, P. (2007) Distinction between perceptual and attentional processing in working memory tasks, a study of phase-locked and induced oscillatory brain dynamics. *J. Cogn. Neurosci.*, 19(1): 158–172.

Deiber, M.P., Ibañez, V., Missonnier, P., Herrmann, F., Fazio-Costa, L., Gold, G. and Giannakopoulos, P. (2009) Abnormal-induced theta activity supports early directed-attention network deficits in progressive MCI. *Neurobiol. Aging*, 30: 1444–1452.

Delatour, B., Blanchard, V., Pradier, L. and Duyckaerts, C. (2004) Alzheimer pathology disorganizes cortico-cortical circuitry, direct evidence from a transgenic animal model. *Neurobiol. Dis.*, 16: 41–47.

Demiralp, T. and Ademoğlu, A. (2001) Decomposition of event-related brain potentials into multiple functional components using wavelet transform. *Clin. Electroencephalogr.*, 32: 122–138.

Demiralp, T., Başar-Eroglu, C., Rahn, E. and Başar, E. (1994) Event-related theta rhythms in cat hippocampus and prefrontal cortex during an omitted stimulus paradigm. *Int. J. Psychophysiol.*, 18: 35–48.

Demiralp, T., Ademoğlu, A., Schürmann, M., Başar-Eroğlu, C. and Başar, E. (1999) Detection of P300 waves in single trials by the wavelet transform (WT). *Brain Lang.*, 66: 108–128.

De Waal, H., Stam, C.J., Blankenstein, M.A., Pijnenburg, Y.A., Scheltens, P. and Van der Flier, W.M. (2011) EEG abnormalities in early and late onset Alzheimer's disease, understanding heterogeneity. *J. Neurol. Neurosurg. Psychiatry*, 82: 67–71.

Dierks, T., Jelic, V., Pascual-Marqui, R.D., Wahlund, L., Julin, P., Linden, D.E., Maurer, K., Winblad, B. and Nordberg, A. (2000) Spatial pattern of cerebral glucose metabolism (PET) correlates with localization of intracerebral EEG generators in Alzheimer's disease. *Clin. Neurophysiol.*, 111: 1817–1824.

Duara, R., Loewenstein, D.A., Potter, E., Appel, J., Greig, M.T., Urs, R., Shen, Q., Raj, A., Small, B., Barker, W., Schofield, E., Wu, Y. and Potter, H. (2008) Medial temporal lobe atrophy on MRI scans and the diagnosis of Alzheimer disease. *Neurology*, 71: 1986–1992.

Dubois, B., Feldman, H.H., Jacova, C., Dekosky, S.T., Barberger-Gateau, P., Cummings, J., Delacourte, A., Galasko, D., Gauthier, S., Jicha, G., Meguro, K., O'Brien, J., Pasquier, F., Robert, P., Rossor, M., Salloway, S., Stern, Y., Visser, P.J. and Scheltens, P. (2007) Research criteria for the diagnosis of Alzheimer's disease, revising the NINCDS-ADRDA criteria. *Lancet Neurol.*, 6: 734–746.

Ertekin-Taner, N., Allen, M., Fadale, D., Scanlin, L., Younkin, L., Petersen, R.C. and Graff-Radford, N. (2004) Genetic variants in a haplotype block spanning IDE are significantly associated with plasma Aβ42 levels and risk for Alzheimer disease. *Hum. Mutat.*, 23: 334–342.

Ertekin-Taner, N., Ronald, J., Feuk, L., Prince, J., Tucker, M., Younkin, L., Hella, M., Jain, S., Hackett, A., Scanlin, L., Kelly, J., Kihiko-Ehman, M., Neltner, M., Hersh, L., Kindy, M., Markesbery, W., Hutton, M., Andrade, M., Petersen, R.C., Graff-Radford, N., Estus, S., Brookes, A.J. and Younkin, S.G. (2005) Elevated amyloid β protein (Aβ42) and late onset Alzheimer's disease are associated with single nucleotide polymorphisms in the urokinase-type plasminogen activator gene. *Hum. Mol. Genet.*, 14: 447–460.

Fernandez, R., Kavcic, V. and Duffy, C.J. (2007) Neurophysiologic analyses of low- and high-level visual processing in Alzheimer disease. *Neurology*, 68: 2066–2076.

Ferreri, F., Pauri, F., Pasqualetti, P., Fini, R., Dal Forno, G. and Rossini, P.M. (2003) Motor cortex excitability in Alzheimer's disease. A transcranial magnetic stimulation study. *Ann. Neurol.*, 53: 102–108.

Ferri, C.P., Prince, M., Brayne, C., Brodaty, H., Fratiglioni, L., Ganguli, M., Hall, K., Hasegawa, K., Hendrie, H., Huang, Y., Jorm, A., Mathers, C., Menezes, P.R., Rimmer, E. and Scazufca, M. (2005) Alzheimer's disease. International global prevalence of dementia, a Delphi consensus study. *Lancet*, 366: 2112–2117.

Förster, S., Teipel, S., Zach, C., Rominger, A., Cumming, P., Fougere, C., Yakushev, I., Haslbeck, M., Hampel, H., Bartenstein, P. and Bürger, K. (2010) FDG-PET mapping the brain substrates of visuo-constructive processing in Alzheimer's disease. *J. Psychiatr. Res.*, 44: 462–469.

Foxe, J.J. and Simpson, G.V. (2002) Flow of activation from V1 to frontal cortex in humans. A framework for defining "early" visual processing. *Exp. Brain Res.*, 142: 139–150.

Fuster, J.M. (1990) Prefrontal cortex and the bridging of temporal gaps in the perception–action cycle. *Ann. N Y Acad. Sci.*, 608: 318–329.

Gardner, W.A. (1992) Unifying view of coherence in signal processing. *Signal. Process.*, 29: 113–140.

Golob, E.J., Ringman, J.M., Irimajiri, R., Bright, S., Schaffer, B., Medina, L.D. and Starr, A. (2009) Cortical event-related potentials in preclinical familial Alzheimer disease. *Neurology*, 73: 1649–1655.

Grady, C.L., Furey, M.L., Pietrini, P., Horwitz, B. and Rapoport, S.I. (2001) Altered brain functional connectivity and impaired short-term memory in Alzheimer's disease. *Brain*, 124: 739–756.

Grunwald, M., Busse, F., Hensel, A., Riedel-Heller, S., Kruggel, F., Arendt, T., Wolf, H. and Gertz, H.J. (2002) Theta-power differences in patients with mild cognitive impairment under rest condition and during haptic tasks. *Alzhimer. Dis. Assoc. Disord.*, 16: 40–48.

Güntekin, B. and Başar, E. (2010) A new interpretation of P300 responses upon analysis of coherences. *Cogn. Neurodyn.*, 4: 107–118.

Güntekin, B., Saatçi, E. and Yener, G. (2008) Decrease of evoked delta, theta and alpha coherence in Alzheimer patients during a visual oddball paradigm. *Brain Res.*, 1235: 109–116.

Halgren, E., Boujon, C., Clarke, J., Wang, C. and Chauvel, P. (2002) Rapid distributed fronto-parieto-occipital processing stages during working memory in humans. *Cereb. Cortex*, 12: 710–728.

Hao, J., Li, K., Li, K., Zhang, D., Wang, W., Yang, Y., Yan, B., Shan, B. and Zhou, X. (2005) Visual attention deficits in Alzheimer's disease, an fMRI study. *Neurosci. Lett.*, 385: 18–23.

Hardy, J. and Selkoe, D.J. (2002) The amyloid hypothesis of Alzheimer's disease, progress and problems on the road to therapeutics. *Science*, 297: 353–356.

Hasselmo, M.E. and Giocomo, L.M. (2006) Cholinergic modulation of cortical function. *J. Mol. Neurosci.*, 30: 133–136.

Haupt, M., González-Hernández, J.A. and Scherbaum, W.A. (2008) Regions with different evoked frequency band responses during early-stage visual processing distinguish mild Alzheimer dementia from mild cognitive impairment and normal aging. *Neurosci. Lett.*, 442: 273–278.

Heister, D., Brewer, J.B., Magda, S., Blennow, K. and McEvoy, L.K. (2011) Alzheimer's disease neuroimaging initiative predicting MCI outcome with clinically available MRI and CSF biomarkers. *Neurology*, 77: 1619–1628.

Helkala, E.L., Koivisto, K., Hänninen, T., Vanhanen, M., Kervinen, K., Kuusisto, J., Mykkänen, L., Kesäniemi, Y.A., Laakso, M. and Riekkinen, S.P. (1996) Memory functions in human subjects with different apolipoprotein E phenotypes during a 3-year population-based follow-up study. *Neurosci. Lett.*, 204: 177–180.

Herholz, K. (2010) Cerebral glucose metabolism in preclinical and prodromal Alzheimer's disease. *Exp. Rev. Neurother.*, 10: 1667–1673.

Herrmann, C.S. and Demiralp, T. (2005) Human EEG gamma oscillations in neuropsychiatric disorders. *Clin. Neurophysiol.*, 116: 2719–2733.

Hillyard, S.A. and Kutas, M. (1983) Electrophysiology of cognitive processing. *Annu. Rev. Psychol.*, 34: 33–61.

Hogan, M.J., Swanwick, G.R., Kaiser, J., Rowan, M. and Lawlor, B. (2003) Memory-related EEG power and coherence reductions in mild Alzheimer's disease. *Int. J. Psychophysiol.*, 49: 147–163.

Holschneider, D.P., Leuchter, A.F., Scremin, O.U., Treiman, D.M. and Walton, N.Y. (1998) Effects of cholinergic deafferentation and NGF on brain electrical coherence. *Brain Res. Bull.*, 45: 531–541.

Huang, C., Wahlund, L., Dierks, T., Julin, P., Winblad, B. and Jelic, V. (2000) Discrimination of Alzheimer's disease and mild cognitive impairment by equivalent EEG sources, a cross-sectional and longitudinal study. *Clin. Neurophysiol.*, 111: 1961–1967.

Hyman, B.T., Gomez-Isla, T., Rebeck, G.W., Briggs, M., Chung, H., West, H., Greenberg, S., Mui, S., Nichols, S., Wallace, R. and Growdon, J.H. (1996) Epidemiological, clinical, and neuropathological study of apolipoprotein E genotype in Alzheimer's disease Apolipoprotein E genotyping in Alzheimer's disease. *Ann. N Y Acad. Sci.*, 802: 1–5.

Jack, C.R., Jr., Shiung, M.M., Weigand, S.D., O'Brien, P.C., Gunter, J.L., Boeve, B.F., Boeve, B.F., Knopman, D.S., Smith, G.E., Ivnik, R.J., Tangalos, E.G. and Petersen, R.C. (2005) Brain atrophy rates predict subsequent clinical conversion in normal elderly and amnestic MCI. *Neurology*, 65: 1227–1231.

Jack, C.R., Jr., Barkhof, F., Bernstein, M.A., Cantillon, M., Cole, P.E., DeCarli, C., Dubois, B., Duchesne, S., Fox, N.C., Frisoni, G.B., Hampel, H., Hill, D.L., Johnson, K., Mangin, J.F., Scheltens, P., Schwarz, A.J., Sperling, R., Suhy, J., Thompson, P.M., Weiner, M. and Foster, N.L. (2011a) Steps to standardization and validation of hippocampal volumetry as a biomarker in clinical trials and diagnostic criterion for Alzheimer's disease. *Alzh. Dement.*, 7: 474–485.

Jack, C.R., Jr., Vemuri, P., Wiste, H.J., Weigand, S.D., Aisen, P.S., Trojanowski, J.Q., Shaw, L.M., Bernstein, M.A., Petersen, R.C., Weiner, M.W., Knopman, D.S. and Alzheimer's Disease Neuroimaging Initiative (2011b) Evidence for ordering of Alzheimer disease biomarkers. *Arch. Neurol. (Chic.)*, 68(12): 1526–1535.

Jackson, C.E. and Snyder, P.J. (2008) Electroencephalography and event related potentials as biomarkers of mild cognitive impairment and mild Alzheimer disease. *Alzh. Dement.*, 4: 137–143.

Jagust, W., Reed, B., Mungas, D., Ellis, W. and De Carli, C. (2007) What does fluorodeoxyglucose PET imaging add to a clinical diagnosis of dementia? *Neurology*, 69: 871–877.

Jagust, W.J., Landau, S.M., Shaw, L.M., Trojanowski, J.Q., Koeppe, R.A., Reiman, E.M., Foster, N.L., Petersen, R.C., Weiner, M.W., Price, J.C. and Mathis, C.A. Alzheimer's Disease Neuroimaging Intiative (2009) Relationships between biomarkers in aging and dementia. *Neurology*, 73: 1193–1199.

Jelic, V. and Kowalski, J. (2009) Evidence-based evaluation of diagnostic accuracy of resting EEG in dementia and mild cognitive impairment. *Clin. Electroencephalogr. Neurosci.*, 40: 129–142.

Jelic, V., Johansson, S.E., Almkvist, O., Shigeta, M., Julin, P., Nordberg, A., Winblad, B. and Wahlund, L.O. (2000) Quantitative electroencephalography in mild cognitive impairment, longitudinal changes and possible prediction of Alzheimer's disease. *Neurobiol. Aging*, 21: 533–540.

Jeong, J. (2004) EEG dynamics in patients with Alzheimer's disease. *Clin. Neurophysiol.*, 115: 1490–1505.

Julkunen, P., Jauhiainen, A.M., Westeren-Punnonen, S., Pirinen, E., Soininen, H., Könönen, M., Pääkkönen, A., Maatta, S. and Karhu, J. (2008) Navigated TMS combined with EEG in mild cognitive impairment and Alzheimer's disease. A pilot study. *J. Neurosci. Meth.*, 172: 270–276.

Karakaş, S., Erzengin, O.U. and Başar, E. (2000) The genesis of human event-related responses explained through the theory of oscillatory neural assemblies. *Neurosci. Lett.*, 285: 45–48.

Karow, D.S., McEvoy, L.K., Fennema-Notestine, C., Hagler, D.J., Jr., Jennings, R.G., Brewer, J.B., Hoh, C.K., Dale, A.M. and Alzheimer's Disease Neuroimaging Initiative (2010) Relative capability of MR imaging and FDG PET to depict changes associated with prodromal and early Alzheimer disease. *Radiology*, 256: 932–942.

Karrasch, M., Laine, M.O., Rinne, J., Rapinoja, P., Sinerva, E. and Krause, C.M. (2006) Brain oscillatory responses to an auditory-verbal working memory task in mild cognitive impairment and Alzheimer's disease. *Int. J. Psychophysiol.*, 59: 168–178.

Keskinoğlu, P., Giray, H., Picakciefe, M., Bilgic, N. and Ucku, R. (2006) The prevalence and risk factors of dementia in the elderly population in a low socio-economic region of Izmir, Turkey. *Arch. Gerontol. Geriatr.*, 43: 93–100.

Kikuchi, M., Wada, Y. and Koshino, Y. (2002) Differences in EEG harmonic driving responses to photic stimulation between normal aging and Alzheimer's disease. *Clin. Electroencephalogr.*, 33: 86–92.

Kimura, F., Fukuda, M. and Tsumoto, T. (1999) Acetylcholine suppresses the spread of excitation in the visual cortex revealed by optical recording, possible differential effect depending on the source of input. *Eur. J. Neurosci.*, 11: 3597–3609.

Klimesch, W., Schack, B., Schabus, M., Doppelmayr, M., Gruber, W. and Sauseng, P. (2004) Phase-locked alpha and theta oscillations generate the P1–N1 complex and are related to memory performance. *Cogn. Brain Res.*, 19: 302–316.

Klimesch, W., Hanslmayr, S., Sauseng, P., Gruber, W., Brozinsky, C.J., Kroll, N.E., Yonelinas, A.P. and Doppelmayr, M. (2006) Oscillatory EEG correlates of episodic trace decay. *Cereb. Cortex*, 16: 280–290.

Knopman, D. (2001) Cerebrospinal fluid beta-amyloid and tau proteins for the diagnosis of Alzheimer disease. *Arch. Neurol. (Chic.)*, 58: 349–350.

Koivunen, J., Scheinin, N., Virta, J.R., Aalto, S., Vahlberg, T., Någren, K., Helin, S., Parkkola, R., Viitanen, M. and Rinne, J.O. (2011) Amyloid PET imaging in patients with mild cognitive impairment, a 2-year follow-up study. *Neurology*, 76: 1085–1090.

Kolev, V., Demiralp, T., Yordanova, J., Ademoğlu, A. and Isoğlu-Alkac, Ü. (1997) Time–frequency analysis reveals multiple functional components during oddball P300. *NeuroReport*, 8: 2061–2065.

Lachaux, J.P., Lutz, A., Rudrauf, D., Cosmelli, D., Quyen, M.L.V., Martinerie, J. and Varela, F. (2002) Estimating the time-course of coherence between single-trial brain signals, an introduction to wavelet coherence. *Neurophysiol. Clin.*, 32: 157–174.

Lai, C.L., Lin, R.T., Liou, L.M. and Liu, C.K. (2010) The role of event-related potentials in cognitive decline in Alzheimer's disease. *Clin. Neurophysiol.*, 121: 194–199.

Lehmann, C., Koenig, T., Jelic, V., Prichep, L., John, R.E., Wahlund, L.O., Dodge, Y. and Dierks, T. (2007) Application and comparison of classification algorithms for recognition of Alzheimer's disease in electrical brain activity (EEG). *J. Neurosci. Meth.*, 161: 342–350.

Leuchter, A.F., Newton, T.F., Cook, I.A., Walter, D.O., Rosenberg-Thompson, S. and Lachenbruch, P.A. (1992) Changes in brain functional connectivity in Alzheimer-type and multi-infarct dementia. *Brain*, 115: 1543–1561.

Lisman, J. and Spruston, N. (2005) Postsynaptic depolarization requirements for LTP and LTD, a critique of spike timing-dependent plasticity. *Nat. Neurosci.*, 8: 839–841.

Lizio, R., Vecchio, F., Frisoni, G.B., Ferri, R., Rodriguez, G. and Babiloni, C. (2011) Electroencephalographic rhythms in Alzheimer's disease. *Int. J. Alzh. Dis.*, 927573. Epub 2011 May 12.

Lopes da Silva, F.H., Vos, J.E., Mooibroek, J. and Rotterdam, A.V. (1980) Relative contributions of intra-cortical and thalamo-cortical processes in the generation of alpha rhythms, revealed by partial coherence analysis. *Electroencephalogr. Clin. Neurophysiol.*, 50: 449–456.

Luria, A.R. (1966) *Higher Cortical Functions in Man.* Basic Books, New York, 513 pp.

Mathis, C.A., Klunk, W.E., Price, J.C. and DeKosky, S.T. (2005) Imaging technology for neurodegenerative diseases, progress toward detection of specific pathologies. *Arch. Neurol. (Chic.)*, 62: 196–200.

Matthews, F.E., Chatfield, M., Brayne, C. and Medical Research Council Cognitive Function and Ageing Study (2006) An investigation of whether factors associated with short-term attrition change or persist over ten years. Data from the Medical Research Council Cognitive Function and Ageing Study (MRC CFAS). *BMC Publ. Health*, 6: 185.

Mattsson, N., Zetterberg, H., Hansson, O., Andreasen, N., Parnetti, L., Jonsson, M., Herukka, S.K., Van der Flier, W.M., Blankenstein, M.A., Ewers, M., Rich, K., Kaiser, E., Verbeek, M., Tsolaki, M., Mulugeta, E., Rosén, E., Aarsland, D., Visser, P.J., Schröder, J., Marcusson, J., De Leon, M., Hampel, H., Scheltens, P., Pirttilä, T., Wallin, A., Jönhagen, M.E., Minthon, L., Winblad, B. and Blennow, K. (2009) CSF biomarkers and incipient Alzheimer disease in patients with mild cognitive impairment. *J. Am. Med. Ass.*, 302: 385–393.

McKhann, G., Drachman, D., Folstein, M., Katzman, R., Price, D. and Stadlan, E.M. (1984) Clinical diagnosis of Alzheimer's disease. Report of the NINCDS-ADRDA Work Group under the auspices of Department of Health and Human Services Task Force on Alzheimer's Disease. *Neurology*, 34: 939–944.

McKhann, G.M., Knopman, D.S., Chertkow, H., Hyman, B.T., Jack, C.R., Jr. Kawas, C.H., Klunk, W.E., Koroshetz, W.J., Manly, J.J., Mayeux, R., Mohs, R.C., Morris, J.C.,

Rossor, M.N., Scheltens, P., Carrillo, M.C., Thies, B., Weintraub, S. and Phelps, C.H. (2011) The diagnosis of dementia due to Alzheimer's disease. Recommendations from the National Institute on Aging-Alzheimer's Association workgroups on diagnostic guidelines for Alzheimer's disease. *Alzh. Dement.*, 7: 263–269.

Mega, M.S., Dinov, I.D., Porter, V., Chow, G., Reback, E., Davoodi, P., O'Connor, S.M., Cater, M.F., Amezcua, H. and Cummings, J.L. (2005) Metabolic patterns associated with the clinical response to galantamine therapy. *Arch. Neurol. (Chic.)*, 62: 721–728.

Mesulam, M., Shaw, P., Mash, D. and Weintraub, S. (2004) Cholinergic nucleus basalis tauopathy emerges early in the aging-MCI-AD continuum. *Ann. Neurol.*, 55(6): 815–828.

Missonnier, P., Gold, G., Fazio-Costa, L., Michel, J.P., Mulligan, R., Michon, A., Ibáñez, V. and Giannakopoulos, P. (2005) Early event-related potential changes during working memory activation predict rapid decline in mild cognitive impairment. *J. Gerontol. A Biol. Sci. Med. Sci.*, 60(5): 660–666.

Missonnier, P., Gold, G., Herrmann, F.R., Fazio-Costa, L., Michel, J.P., Deiber, M.P., Michon, A. and Giannakopoulos, P. (2006a) Decreased theta event-related synchronization during working memory activation is associated with progressive mild cognitive impairment. *Dement. Geriatr. Cogn. Disord.*, 22: 250–259.

Missonnier, P., Deiber, M.P., Gold, G., Millet, P., Gex-Fabry Pun, M., Fazio-Costa, L., Giannakopoulos, P. and Ibañez, V. (2006b) Frontal theta event-related synchronization, comparison of directed attention and working memory load effects. *J. Neural Transm.*, 113: 1477–1486.

Missonnier, P., Deiber, M.P., Gold, G., Herrmann, F.R., Millet, P., Michon, A., Fazio-Costa, L., Ibañez, V. and Giannakopoulos, P. (2007) Working memory load-related electroencephalographic parameters can differentiate progressive from stable mild cognitive impairment. *Neuroscience*, 150: 346–356.

Missonnier, P., Herrmann, F.R., Michon, A., Fazio-Costa, L., Gold, G. and Giannakopoulos, P. (2010) Early disturbances of gamma band dynamics in mild cognitive impairment. *J. Neural Transm.*, 117: 489–498.

Nelson, C.L., Sarter, M. and Bruno, J.P. (2005) Prefrontal cortical modulation of acetylcholine release in posterior parietal cortex. *Neuroscience*, 132: 347–359.

Nobili, F., Vitali, P., Canfora, M., Girtler, N., De Leo, C., Mariani, G., Pupi, A. and Rodriguez, G. (2002) Effects of long term donepezil therapy on CBF of Alzheimer's patients. *Clin. Neurophysiol.*, 113: 1241–1248.

Nunez, P.L. (1997) EEG coherence measures in medical and cognitive science, a general overview of experimental methods, computer algorithms, and accuracy. In: M. Eselt, U. Zwiener and H. Witte (Eds.), *Quantative and Topological EEG and MEG Analysis.* Universitätsverlag Druckhaus Mayer, Jena, pp. 1–427.

O'Brien, J.T., Colloby, S., Fenwick, J., Williams, E.D., Firbank, M., Burn, D., Aarsland, D. and McKeith, I.G. (2004) Dopamine transporter loss visualized with FP-CIT SPECT in the differential diagnosis of dementia with Lewy bodies. *Arch. Neurol. (Chic.)*, 61: 919–925.

Olichney, J.M., Taylor, J.R., Gatherwright, J., Salmon, D.P., Bressler, A.J., Kutas, M. and Iragui-Madoz, V.J. (2008) Patients with MCI and N400 or P600 abnormalities are at very high risk for conversion to dementia. *Neurology*, 70: 1763–1770.

Olichney, J.M., Yang, J.C., Taylor, J. and Kutas, M. (2011) Cognitive event-related potentials, biomarkers of synaptic dysfunction across the stages of Alzheimer's disease. *J. Alzh. Dis.*, 26: 215–228.

Öniz, A. and Başar, E. (2009) Prolongation of alpha oscillations in auditory oddball paradigm. *Int. J. Psychophysiol.*, 71: 235–241.

Osipova, D., Ahveninen, J., Jensen, O., Ylikoski, A. and Pekkonen, E. (2005) Altered generation of spontaneous oscillations in Alzheimer's disease. *Neuroimage*, 27: 835–841.

Osipova, D., Pekkonen, E. and Ahveninen, J. (2006) Enhanced magnetic auditory steady-state response in early Alzheimer's disease. *Clin. Neurophysiol.*, 117: 1990–1995.

Papaliagkas, V., Kimiskidis, V., Tsolaki, M. and Anogianakis, G. (2008) Usefulness of event-related potentials in the assessment of mild cognitive impairment. *BMC Neurosci.*, 9: 107.

Papaliagkas, V.T., Anogianakis, G., Tsolaki, M.N., Koliakos, G. and Kimiskidis, V.K. (2009) Progression of mild cognitive impairment to Alzheimer's disease, improved diagnostic value of the combined use of N200 latency and beta-amyloid (1–42) levels. *Dement. Geriatr. Cogn. Disord.*, 28: 30–35.

Papaliagkas, V., Tsolaki, M., Kimiskidis, V. and Anogianakis, G. (2011a) New neurophysiological marker for mild cognitive impairment progression to Alzheimer's disease. *Neurosci. Lett.*, 500: e7–e8.

Papaliagkas, V.T., Kimiskidis, V.K., Tsolaki, M.N. and Anogianakis, G. (2011b) Cognitive event-related potentials, longitudinal changes in mild cognitive impairment. *Clin. Neurophysiol.*, 122: 1322–1326.

Perry, R.J. and Hodges, J.R. (1999) Attention and executive deficits in Alzheimer's disease. A critical review. *Brain*, 122: 383–404.

Petersen, R.C., Stevens, J.C., Ganguli, M., Tangalos, E.G., Cummings, J.L. and DeKosky, S.T. (2001) Practice parameter, early detection of dementia, mild cognitive impairment (an evidence-based review). Report of the Quality Standards Subcommittee of the American Academy of Neurology. *Neurology*, 56: 1133–1142.

Polich, J. (1997) EEG and ERP assessment of normal aging. *Electroencephalogr. Clin. Neurophysiol.* 104: 244–256 (Evoked Potentials Section).

Polich, J. and Corey-Bloom, J. (2005) Alzheimer's disease and P300, review and evaluation of task and modality. *Curr. Alzh. Res.*, 2: 515–525.

Polich, J. and Herbst, K.L. (2000) P300 as a clinical assay, rationale, evaluation, and findings. *Int. J. Psychophysiol.*, 38: 3–19.

Polikar, R., Topalis, A., Green, D., Kounios, J. and Clark, C.M. (2007) Comparative multiresolution wavelet analysis of ERP spectral bands using an ensemble of classifiers approach for early diagnosis of Alzheimer's disease. *Comput. Biol. Med.*, 37: 542–558.

Polikar, R., Tilley, C., Hillis, B. and Clark, C.M. (2010) Multimodal EEG, MRI and PET data fusion for Alzheimer's disease diagnosis. *Proc. IEEE Eng. Med. Biol. Soc.*, 2010: 6058–6061.

Potkin, S.G., Anand, R., Fleming, K., Gustavo, A., Keator, D., Carreon, D., Messina, J., Wu, J.C., Hartman, R. and Fallon, J.H. (2001) Brain metabolic and clinical effects of rivastigmine in Alzheimer's disease. *Int. J. Neuropsychopharmacol.*, 4: 223–230.

Poza, J., Hornero, R., Escudero, J., Fernandez, A. and Gomez, C. (2008) Analysis of spontaneous MEG activity in Alzheimer's disease using time-frequency parameters. *Proc. IEEE Eng. Med. Biol. Soc.*, 2008: 5712–5715.

Price, J.L. and Morris, J.C. (1999) Tangles and plaques in nondemented aging and "preclinical" Alzheimer's disease. *Ann. Neurol.*, 45: 358–368.

Prvulovic, D., Hubl, D., Sack, A.T., Melillo, L., Maurer, K., Frölich, L., Lanfermann, H., Zanella, F.E., Goebel, R., Linden, D.E.J. and Dierks, T. (2002) Functional imaging of visuospatial processing in Alzheimer's disease. *Neuroimage*, 17: 1403–1414.

Quigley, H., Colloby, S.J. and O'Brien, J.T. (2011) PET imaging of brain amyloid in dementia, a review. *Int. J. Geriatr. Psychiatry*, 26: 991–999.

Quiroz, Y.T., Ally, B.A., Celone, K., McKeever, J., Ruiz-Rizzo, A.L., Lopera, F., Stern, C.E. and Budson, A.E. (2011) Event-related potential markers of brain changes in preclinical familial Alzheimer disease. *Neurology*, 77: 469–475.

Rabinovici, G.D. and Miller, B.L. (2010) Frontotemporal lobar degeneration, epidemiology, pathophysiology, diagnosis and management. *CNS Drugs*, 24: 375–398.

Rappelsberger, P., Pockberger, H. and Petsche, H. (1982) The contribution of the cortical layers to the generation of the EEG: field potential and current source density analyses in the rabbit's visual cortex. *Electroencephalogr. Clin. Neurophysiol.*, 53(3): 254–269.

Rasquin, S.M., Lodder, J., Visser, P.J., Lousberg, R. and Verhey, F.R. (2005) Predictive accuracy of MCI subtypes for Alzheimer's disease and vascular dementia in subjects with mild cognitive impairment, a 2-year follow-up study. *Dement. Geriatr. Cogn. Disord.*, 19: 113–119.

Ray, S., Britschgi, M., Herbert, C., Takeda-Uchimura, Y., Boxer, A., Blennow, K., Friedman, L.F., Galasko, D.R., Jutel, M., Karydas, A., Kaye, J.A., Leszek, J., Miller, B.L., Minthon, L., Quinn, J.F., Rabinovici, G.D., Robinson, W.H., Sabbagh, M.N., So, Y.T., Sparks, D.L., Tabaton, M., Tinklenberg, J., Yesavage, J.A., Tibshirani, R. and Wyss-Coray, T. (2007) Classification and prediction of clinical Alzheimer's diagnosis based on plasma signaling proteins. *Nat. Med.*, 13: 1359–1362.

Reeves, R.R., Frederick, D.O., Struve, A., Patrick, G., Booker, J.G. and Nave, D.W. (1999) The effects of donepezil on the P300 auditory and visual cognitive evoked potentials of patients with Alzheimer's disease. *Am. J. Geriatr. Psychiatry*, 7: 349–352.

Reitz, C. and Mayeux, R. (2009) Endophenotypes in normal brain morphology and Alzheimer's disease, a review. *Neuroscience*, 164: 174–190.

Rektor, I., Bareš, M., Kaňovský, P., Brázdil, M., Klajblová, I., Streitová, H., Rektorová, I., Sochůrková, D., Kubová, D., Kuba, R. and Daniel, P. (2004) Cognitive potentials in the basal ganglia–frontocortical circuits. An intracerebral recording study. *Exp. Brain Res.*, 158: 289–301.

Rogaeva, E. (2007) The neuronal sortilin-related receptor SORL1 is genetically associated with Alzheimer disease. *Nat. Genet.*, 39: 168–177.

Rossini, P.M., Del Percio, C., Pasqualetti, P., Cassetta, E., Binetti, G., Dal Forno, G., Ferreri, F., Frisoni, G., Chiovenda, P., Miniussi, C., Parisi, L., Tombini, M., Vecchio, F. and Babiloni, C. (2006) Conversion from mild cognitive impairment to Alzheimer's disease is predicted by sources and coherence of brain electroencephalography rhythms. *Neuroscience*, 143: 793–803.

Rossini, P.M., Rossi, S., Babiloni, C. and Polich, J. (2007) Clinical neurophysiology of aging brain, from normal aging to neurodegeneration. *Prog. Neurobiol.*, 83: 375–400.

Sarter, M., Givens, B. and Bruno, J.P. (2001) The cognitive neuroscience of sustained attention, where top-down meets bottom-up. *Brain Res. Rev.*, 35: 146–160.

Sarter, M., Hasselmo, M.E., Bruno, J.P. and Givens, B. (2005) Unraveling the attentional functions of cortical cholinergic inputs, interactions between signal-driven and cognitive modulation of signal detection. *Brain Res. Rev.*, 48: 98–111.

Sauseng, P., Klimesch, W., Doppelmayr, M., Pecherstorfer, T., Freunberger, R. and Hanslmayr, S. (2005) EEG alpha synchronization and functional coupling during top-down processing in a working memory task. *Hum. Brain Mapp.*, 26: 148–155.

Saykin, A.J., Wishart, H.A. and Rabin, L.A. (2004) Cholinergic enhancement of frontal lobe activity in mild cognitive impairment. *Brain*, 127: 1574–1583.

Schürmann, M., Nikouline, V.V., Soljanlahti, S., Ollikainen, M., Başar, E. and Risto, J. (2001) EEG responses to combined somatosensory and transcranial magnetic stimulation. *Clin. Neurophysiol.*, 112: 19–24.

Shaw, L.M., Vanderstichele, H., Knapik-Czajka, M., Clark, C.M., Aisen, P.S., Petersen, R.C., Blennow, K., Soares, H., Simon, A., Lewczuk, P., Dean, R., Siemers, E., Potter, W., Lee, V.M.Y. and Trojanowski, J.Q. (2009) Cerebrospinal fluid biomarker signature in Alzheimer's disease neuroimaging initiative subjects. *Ann. Neurol.*, 110: 403–413.

Smits, L.L., Liedorp, M., Koene, T., Roos-Reuling, I.E., Lemstra, A.W., Scheltens, P., Stam, C.J. and Van der Flier, W.M. (2011) EEG abnormalities are associated with different cognitive profiles in Alzheimer's disease. *Dement. Geriatr. Cogn. Disord.*, 31: 1–6.

Soares, H.D., Chen, Y., Sabbagh, M., Rohrer, A., Schrijvers, E. and Breteler, M. (2009) Identifying early markers of Alzheimer's disease using quantitative multiplex proteomic immunoassay panels. Biomarkers in brain disease. *Ann. N Y Acad. Sci.*, 1180: 56–67.

Soininen, H., Partanen, J., Laulumaa, V., Pääkkönen, A., Helkala, E.L. and Riekkinen, P.J. (1991) Serial EEG in Alzheimer's disease, 3 year follow-up and clinical outcome. *Electroencephalogr. Clin. Neurophysiol.*, 79: 342–348.

Solms, M. and Turnbull, O. (2002) *The Brain and the Inner World. An Introduction to the Neuroscience of Subjective Experience.* Other Press/Karnac Books, New York, 342 pp.

Spencer, K.M. and Polich, J. (1999) Poststimulus EEG spectral analysis and P300, attention, task, and probability. *Psychophysiology*, 36: 220–232.

Sperling, R.A., Aisen, P.S., Beckett, L.A., Bennett, D.A., Craft, S., Fagan, A.M., Iwatsubo, T., Jack, C.R., Jr., Kaye, J., Montine, T.J., Park, D.C., Reiman, E.M., Rowe, C.C., Siemers, E., Stern, Y., Yaffe, K., Carrillo, M.C., Thies, B., Morrison-Bogorad, M., Wagster, M.V. and Phelps, C.H. (2011) Toward defining the preclinical stages of Alzheimer's disease. Recommendations from the National Institute on Aging-Alzheimer's Association workgroups on diagnostic guidelines for Alzheimer's disease. *Alzh. Dement.*, 7: 280–292.

Stampfer, H.G. and Başar, E. (1985) Does frequency analysis lead to better understanding of human event related potentials. *Int. J. Neurosci.*, 26: 181–196.

Stephen, J.M., Montano, R., Donahue, C.H., Adair, J.C., Knoefel, J., Qualis, C., Hart, B., Ranken, D. and Aine, C.J. (2010) Somatosensory responses in normal aging, mild cognitive impairment, and Alzheimer's disease. *J. Neural Transm.*, 117: 217–225.

Tallon-Baudry, C. and Bertrand, O. (1999) Oscillatory gamma activity in humans and its role in object representation. *Trends Cogn. Sci.*, 3: 151–162.

Uhlhaas, P.J. and Singer, W. (2006) Neural synchrony in brain review disorders, relevance for cognitive dysfunctions and pathophysiology. *Neuron*, 52: 155–168.

Van der Hiele, K., Vein, A.A., Reijntjes, R.H.A.M., Westendorp, R.G.J., Bollen, E.L.E.M., Van Buchem, M.A., Van Dijk, J.G. and Middelkoop, H.A.M. (2007) EEG correlates in the spectrum of cognitive decline. *Clin. Neurophysiol.*, 118: 1931–1939.

Van Deursen, J.A., Vuurman, E.F., Verhey, F.R., Van Kranen-Mastenbroek, V.H. and Riedel, W.J. (2008) Increased EEG gamma band activity in Alzheimer's disease and mild cognitive impairment. *J. Neural Transm.*, 115: 1301–1311.

Van Deursen, J.A., Vuurman, E.F., Van Kranen-Mastenbroek, V.H., Verhey, F.R. and Riedel, W.J. (2011) 40-Hz steady state response in Alzheimer's disease and mild cognitive impairment. *Neurobiol. Aging*, 32: 24–30.

Varela, F., Lachaux, J.P., Rodriguez, E. and Martinerie, J. (2001) The brainweb, phase synchronization and large-scale integration. *Nat. Rev. Neurosci.*, 2: 229–232.

Vennerica, A., Shanks, M.F., Staff, R.T., Pestell, S.J., Forbes, K.E., Gemmell, H.G. and Murray, A.D. (2002) Cerebral blood flow and cognitive responses to rivastigmine treatment in Alzheimer's disease. *NeuroReport*, 13: 83–87.

Villemagne, V.L., Pike, K.E., Darby, D., Maruff, P., Savage, G., Ng, S., Ackermann, U., Cowie, T.F., Currie, J., Chan, S.G., Jones, G., Tochon-Danguy, H., O'Keefe, G., Masters, C.L. and Rowe, C.C. (2008) Aβ deposits in older non-demented individuals with cognitive decline are indicative of preclinical Alzheimer's disease. *Neuropsychologia*, 46: 1688–1697.

Visser, P.J., Verhey, F., Knol, D.L., Scheltens, P., Wahlund, L.O., Freund-Levi, Y., Tsolaki, M., Minthon, L., Wallin, A.K., Hampel, H., Bürger, K., Pirttila, T., Soininen, H., Rikkert, M.O., Verbeek, M.M., Spiru, L. and Blennow, K. (2009) Prevalence and prognostic value of CSF markers of Alzheimer's disease pathology in patients with subjective cognitive impairment or mild cognitive impairment in the DESCRIPA study, a prospective cohort study. *Lancet Neurol.*, 8: 619–627.

Vitali, P., Maccagnano, E., Caverzasi, E., Henry, R.G., Haman, A., Torres-Chae, C., Johnson, D.Y., Miller, B.L. and Geschwind, M.D. (2011) Diffusion-weighted MRI hyperintensity patterns differentiate CJD from other rapid dementias. *Neurology*, 76: 1711–1719.

Von Stein, A. and Sarnthein, J. (2000) Different frequencies for different scales of cortical integration, from local gamma to long distance alpha-theta synchronization. *Int. J. Psychophysiol.*, 38: 301–313.

Waldemar, G., Dubois, B., Emre, M., Georges, J., McKeith, I.G., Rossor, M., Scheltens, P., Tariska, P. and Winblad, B. (2007) EFNS recommendations for the diagnosis and management of Alzheimer's disease and other disorders associated with dementia, EFNS guideline. *Eur. J. Neurol.*, 14: 1–26.

Walhovd, K.B., Fjell, A.M., Brewer, J., McEvoy, L.K., Fennema-Notestine, C., Hagler, D.J., Jr., Jennings, R.G., Karow, D., Dale, A.M. and Alzheimer's Disease Neuroimaging Initiative (2010) Combining MR imaging, positron-emission tomography, and CSF biomarkers in the diagnosis and prognosis of Alzheimer disease. *Am. J. Neuroradiol.*, 3: 347–354.

Wimo, A., Jonsson, L. and Winblad, B. (2006) An estimate of the worldwide prevalence and direct costs of dementia in 2003. *Dement. Geriatr. Cogn. Disord.*, 21: 175–181.

Wright, C.F., Hall, A., Matthews, F.E. and Brayne, C. (2009) Biomarkers, dementia, and public health. *Ann. N Y Acad. Sci.*, 1180: 11–19.

Yener, G.G. and Başar, E. (2010) Sensory evoked and event related oscillations in Alzheimer's disease, a short review. *Cogn. Neurodyn.*, 4: 263–274.

Yener, G.G., Leuchter, A.F., Jenden, D., Read, S.L., Cummings, J.L. and Miller, B.L. (1996) Quantitative EEG in frontotemporal dementia. *Clin. Electroencephalogr.*, 27: 61–68.

Yener, G., Güntekin, B., Öniz, A. and Başar, E. (2007) Increased frontal phase-locking of event related theta oscillations in Alzheimer patients treated with acetylcholine-esterase inhibitors. *Int. J. Psychophysiol.*, 64: 46–52.

Yener, G.G., Güntekin, B. and Başar, E. (2008) Event-related delta oscillatory responses of Alzheimer patients. *Eur. J. Neurol.*, 15: 540–547.

Yener, G.G., Güntekin, B., Tülay, E. and Başar, E. (2009) A comparative analysis of sensory visual evoked oscillations with visual cognitive event related oscillations in Alzheimer's disease. *Neurosci. Lett.*, 462: 193–197.

Yener, G., Rosen, H. and Papatriantafyllou, J. (2010) The frontotemporal degeneration. *Am. Acad. Neurol. Contin. Lifelong Learn. Neurol.*, 16: 191–211.

Yener, G.G., Güntekin, B. and Başar, E. (2011) Evoked and event related oscillations in Alzheimer's disease and a preliminary report on mild cognitive impairment. In: *Brain Oscillations in Cognitive Impairment and Neurotransmitters Conference/Workshop, Istanbul, 29 April–01 May 2011.* Abstract Book, pp. 15–16.

Yener, G.G., Güntekin, B., Orken, D.N., Tülay, E., Forta, H. and Başar, E. (2012) Auditory delta event-related oscillatory responses are decreased in Alzheimer's disease. *Behav. Neurol.*, 25: 3–11.

Yordanova, J. and Kolev, V. (1998) A single-sweep analysis of the theta frequency band during an auditory oddball task. *Psychophysiology*, 35: 116–126.

Yordanova, J., Devrim, M., Kolev, V., Ademoğlu, A. and Demiralp, T. (2000) Multiple time-frequency components account for the complex functional reactivity of P300. *NeuroReport*, 11: 1097–1103.

Zervakis, M., Michalopoulos, K., Iordanidou, V. and Sakkalis, V. (2011) Intertrial coherence and causal interaction among independent EEG components. *J. Neurosci. Meth.*, 197: 302–314.

Zhang, D., Wang, Y., Zhou, L., Yuan, H., Shen, D. and Alzheimer's Disease Neuroimaging Initiative (2011) Multimodal classification of Alzheimer's disease and mild cognitive impairment. *Neuroimage*, 55: 856–867.

Zheng, L.L., Jiang, Z.Y. and Yu, E.Y. (2007) Alpha spectral power and coherence in the patients with mild cognitive impairment during a three-level working memory task. *J. Zhejiang Univ. Sci. B*, 8: 584–592.

Zheng-yan, J. (2005) Abnormal cortical functional connections in Alzheimer's disease, analysis of inter- and intrahemispheric EEG coherence. *J. Zhejiang Univ. Sci. B*, 6: 259–264.

Application of Brain Oscillations in Neuropsychiatric Diseases
(Supplements to Clinical Neurophysiology, Vol. 62)
Editors: E. Başar, C. Başar-Eroğlu, A. Özerdem, P.M. Rossini, G.G. Yener

Chapter 17

Resting state brain oscillations and symptom profiles in attention deficit/hyperactivity disorder

Robert J. Barry* and Adam R. Clarke

Brain & Behaviour Research Institute and School of Psychology, University of Wollongong, Wollongong, NSW 2522, Australia

ABSTRACT

Our perspective on resting-state electroencephalogram (EEG) is that it provides a window into the substrate of cognitive and perceptual processing, reflecting the dynamic potential of the brain's current functional state. In an extended research program into the electrophysiology of attention deficit/hyperactivity disorder (AD/HD), we have examined resting-state EEG power and coherence, and event-related potentials (ERPs), in children, adolescents, and adults with the disorder. We sought initially to identify consistent AD/HD anomalies in these measures, relative to normal control subjects, and then to understand how these differences related to existing models of AD/HD. An emergent strand in this program has been to clarify the EEG correlates of "arousal" and to understand the role of arousal dysfunction as a core anomaly in AD/HD. To date, findings in this strand serve to rule out a commonly held dictum in the AD/HD field: that elevated theta/beta ratio is an indicator of hypo-arousal. In turn, this requires further work to elucidate the ratio's functional significance in the disorder. Our brain dynamics studies relating prestimulus EEG amplitude and phase states to ERP outcomes are expected to help in this regard, but we are still at a relatively early stage, currently examining these relationships in control children, in order to better understand normal aspects of brain dynamics before turning to children with AD/HD. This range of studies provides a framework for our recent work relating resting-state EEG anomalies, in individuals with AD/HD, to their symptom profile. This has had promising results, indicating links between increased inattention scores and reduced resting EEG gamma power. With resting-state EEG coherence, reduced left lateralized coherences across several bands have correlated negatively with inattention scores, while reduced frontal interhemispheric coherence has been correlated negatively with hyperactivity/impulsivity scores. Such linkages appear to provide encouraging leads for future EEG research in AD/HD.

KEYWORDS

EEG power; EEG coherence; Event-related potential; Symptom; Attention deficit/hyperactivity disorder

17.1. Introduction

Our laboratory has had a long-term major interest in electroencephalogram (EEG) and its development,

focused particularly on attention deficit/hyperactivity disorder (AD/HD). This program of research has largely used measures of absolute and relative power in the four traditional bands (delta, theta, alpha, and beta) and coherence measures exploring regional linkages. The work has recently been extended into the gamma band in several studies. Over the years, we have included studies of the relationships between EEG power measures and electrodermal activity, exploring the energetics

Correspondence to: Dr. R.J. Barry, Brain & Behaviour Research Institute and School of Psychology, University of Wollongong, Northfields Avenue, Wollongong, NSW 2522, Australia.
Tel.: +61 2 4221 4421; Fax: +61 2 4221 4421;
E-mail: robert_barry@uow.edu.au

dimension in studies of *arousal* versus *activation*. This appears to be very useful in helping us to understand the nature of EEG anomalies in AD/HD. In addition to this emphasis on spontaneous oscillations, we have also studied event-related potentials (ERPs) for many years, in a range of populations, and currently have a major interest in the brain dynamics involved in ERP generation. Within the AD/HD field, we are now working to relate the EEG/ERP anomalies already established to the behavioral symptoms characterizing the disorder.

Because of the limited space available, it is not possible to place each of the studies sketched here in the wider literature that originally provided its context. That context is critically discussed within the original studies cited and should be consulted by the interested reader.

17.2. Anomalous oscillations in AD/HD

17.2.1. Eyes-closed EEG power in children with AD/HD

We have published detailed historical reviews of EEG in AD/HD in Barry et al. (2003a), and a detailed overview of data from approximately 50 of our own studies of this syndrome was presented in Barry and Clarke (2009). Graphical presentations of eyes-closed resting EEG data, as shown in Fig. 1, allow identification of similarities and differences between typically developing children and those with AD/HD. The most common DSM-IV types of AD/HD are the inattentive and combined groups, with the former showing developmentally inappropriate levels of inattention, and the latter showing developmentally inappropriate levels of both inattention and hyperactivity. EEG profiles from both these types are illustrated.

With absolute power, the top panel in Fig. 1 shows that the major markers of AD/HD are elevated delta and theta; there is also evidence of less extreme reductions in alpha and beta power. The topographies of all bands in both AD/HD types are broadly similar to the control

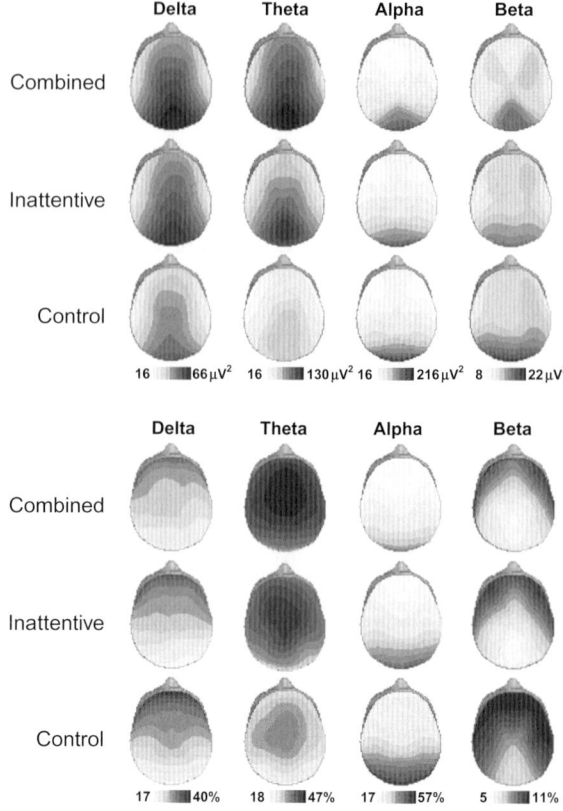

Fig. 1. Topographic head maps showing absolute (top panel) and relative power (bottom panel) for children with both types of AD/HD versus typically developing controls.

group, although there are some commonly reported topographic differences. With relative power (Fig. 1, lower panel), the major markers of AD/HD in both types are globally elevated theta, with globally reduced alpha and beta power. In general, it can be seen that EEG profiles of children with the inattentive type are less aberrant than those of children with the combined type of AD/HD.

The best general marker of AD/HD is the theta/beta ratio, where the elevated theta and reduced beta are synergistically combined into a single marker. Indeed, Monastra's group (e.g., Monastra et al., 1999, 2001) has consistently reported elevated theta/beta ratio in large samples of children and adolescents with AD/HD, with high classification accuracy, and proposed the use of the theta/beta ratio recorded at the vertex as a stand-alone diagnostic test for AD/HD.

This picture of EEG power in AD/HD is complicated by developmental changes in the EEG patterning occurring with age. In broad terms, with increasing age in normal children, slow wave EEG activity decreases and fast wave activity increases. Changes occur faster in the posterior than anterior regions (Gasser et al., 1988a,b; Clarke et al., 2001a). The rates of change in EEG patterns also differ with gender, with girls appearing to develop more mature EEG power patterns later than boys (Clarke et al., 2001a). Our research has indicated that similar developmental patterns occur in children with AD/HD and that many of the differences described above are maintained relative to age-matched control children, although the EEG differences between the DSM types decrease with age (Clarke et al., 2001b).

The EEG profile of children with AD/HD is also complicated by the great range of comorbidities commonly associated with the disorder. We have reported that those with AD/HD and comorbid learning disabilities are distinguishable by their more aberrant EEG profiles, particularly with the addition of increased left posterior relative delta, and a reduction in posterior relative alpha, associated with the learning disability (Clarke et al., 2002b). In contrast, further work has suggested that there is little impact on the AD/HD EEG profile that can be associated with the behavioral anomalies of oppositional defiant disorder or conduct disorder, and we have suggested that much of the symptomatology associated with this comorbidity is learned rather than of neurological origin (e.g., Clarke et al., 2002a). Learning disabilities and behavioral problems are the two most common comorbid disorders found with AD/HD, but anxiety and depression, as well as other childhood disorders, add to the clinical complexity. Overall, this range of possible comorbidities obscures the clinical picture of AD/HD and the EEG power profile obtained at the individual level.

17.2.2. EEG-based models of AD/HD

In order to understand AD/HD, we must attempt to understand the causes of the EEG anomalies described above. Comparison of the AD/HD EEG profile with typical developmental data has been taken to suggest the existence of developmental deviations, or maturational delay, in AD/HD. This model sees the major EEG differences between children with AD/HD and age-matched controls — increased slow wave and decreased fast wave activity — as reflecting an immaturity of brain development. In relation to this model, the first reported EEG study of child, adolescent, and adult AD/HD patients was that of Bresnahan et al. (1999). In this study, we examined patient and control EEGs in eyes-open resting baseline conditions. The eyes-open paradigm introduces EEG changes that are addressed later, but one of the important findings in this study was that elevated slow wave activity (particularly absolute and relative theta) persisted from childhood, through adolescence, to adulthood in AD/HD. This was confirmed in subsequent studies of specificity (Bresnahan and Barry, 2002), and good responders to stimulant medication (Bresnahan et al., 2006) in adults. Hobbs et al. (2007) broadly confirmed these data in adolescent males in an eyes-closed condition. Thus, elevated slow wave activity is an enduring characteristic of AD/HD, occurring in children, adolescents, and adults. Such data strongly suggest that AD/HD cannot be solely a maturational problem. Even if some atypical development is present in children with the disorder, it cannot be core to the symptoms remaining in adulthood.

Another influential EEG-based model of AD/HD sees the increased slow wave and decreased fast wave activity, described above, as reflecting CNS hypo-arousal and suggests that this causes the inattention and hyperactivity symptoms of the disorder (Satterfield and Cantwell, 1974). This model provides an account of the paradoxical effect of small doses of stimulants in AD/HD: they normalize arousal levels and temporarily reduce behavior problems. This model emerged following

Lubar's (1991) hypothetical linkage of resting EEG frequency increases during activation (Jasper et al., 1938) with reports of reduced skin conductance level (SCL), and hence CNS hypo-arousal, in AD/HD (Satterfield and Dawson, 1971). The hypothesis that children with AD/HD are chronically under-aroused, as reflected in their reduced beta and increased theta, was supported by Mann et al. (1992), and the AD/HD elevated theta/beta ratio was taken to represent hypo-arousal. The hypo-arousal model has had a continuing impact on EEG interpretation in AD/HD, but a long-standing problem is that the link between low SCL (reflecting CNS under-arousal) and elevated theta and reduced beta was not specifically validated. Although SCL has had a long tradition as an index of CNS arousal (e.g., Raskin, 1973; Raine et al., 1990; Barry and Sokolov, 1993), it was not directly established that the theta/beta ratio measures arousal.

17.2.3. Arousal effects in EEG power

From our autonomic work, we had defined arousal, following Pribram and McGuiness (1975, 1992), as the current energetic state of the organism, and supported the use of SCL as its measure (e.g., Barry and Sokolov, 1993). Our consistent position has been that arousal differences should be apparent as global EEG effects across the scalp, in contrast to topographic differences that can be related to effects in specific focal/regional brain processing. In that context, we began our exploration of arousal in the EEG with a study of normal boys. Barry et al. (2004a) recorded simultaneous EEG and SCL in an eyes-closed resting state in 24 control children. A median split of the group on SCL showed that a high CNS arousal group (mean SCL = 14.2 microSiemens, µS) had a global (across-scalp) reduction in alpha power, with no global differences in relative theta or beta, compared to a low arousal group (mean SCL = 4.7 µS). These EEG data are displayed in Fig. 2. There was no

significant difference in the theta/beta ratio between these groups, contradicting the concept of the theta/beta ratio as an indicator of cortical hypo-arousal, at least in typically developing children.

We then examined arousal changes in studies using caffeine as a stimulant (Barry et al., 2005, 2008). For example, Barry et al. (2005) examined the effects of 250 mg caffeine in a placebo-controlled double-blind study with 18 adults. At 30 min after ingestion, caffeine led to significantly increased SCL and globally reduced alpha power (see Fig. 3) relative to placebo; other effects were topographic. We saw these data as confirmation that the major impact of caffeine was increased arousal. This suggested that caffeine could be used to manipulate arousal without the confounding effects associated with manipulations of task difficulty, commonly used to explore the arousal dimension. We subsequently found similar effects with 80 mg caffeine in children (Barry et al., 2009c).

In further work exploring the inverse link between SCL and alpha, Barry et al. (2007) compared eyes-closed and eyes-open resting conditions in young adults. Opening the eyes produced an increase in arousal, as defined by an increase in SCL, and a global decrease in alpha power. Changes in the other EEG bands were topographically focal (reduced lateral frontal delta and posterior theta, and decreased posterior/increased frontal beta), as shown in Fig. 4. These focal changes were considered as indicating regional activation involved in processing the visual input in the eyes-open condition. These data have been confirmed subsequently in typically developing children (Barry et al., 2009b). Based on these studies, we propose that arousal can be measured by SCL and global mean alpha power. These two measures are negatively correlated in both adults and children; thus an increase in arousal is indicated by a joint increase in SCL and decrease in mean alpha power. Barry et al. (2011b) reported the additive effects of these two manipulations (opening the eyes and caffeine)

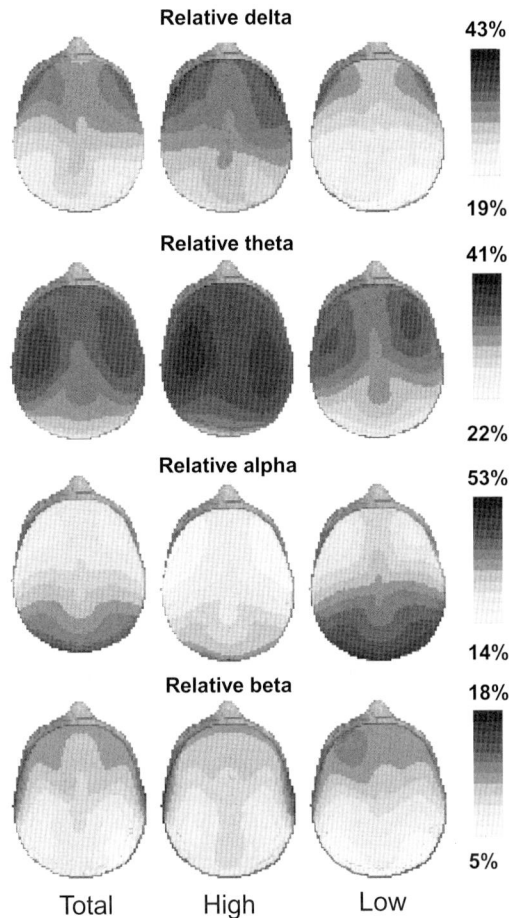

Fig. 2. Topographic head maps showing relative power in the four traditional EEG bands for a group of control children (total), and when subdivided into groups with high and low arousal levels (based on SCL). There is a group difference in global alpha, with lower levels in the high arousal group.

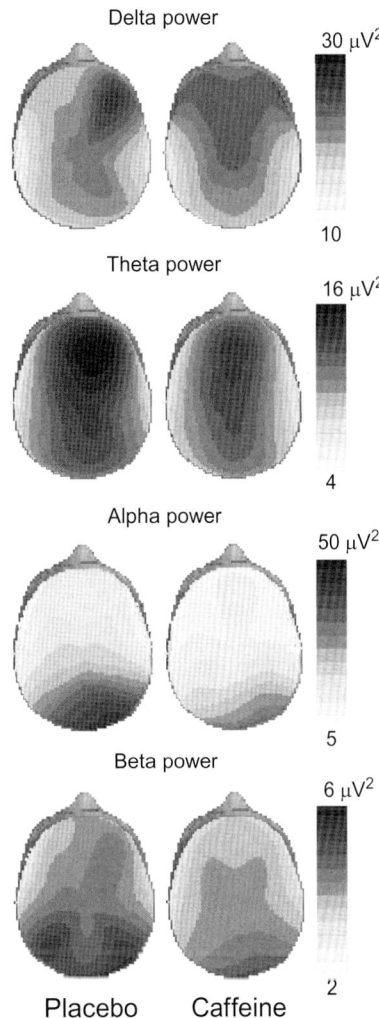

Fig. 3. Caffeine changes in absolute power are shown in the four traditional EEG bands for young adults. There is a global reduction in alpha with caffeine.

on both SCL and EEG alpha power. Importantly, this confirmed the stability of our arousal conceptualization, and its measure in terms of inverse changes in SCL and mean alpha power.

In this context, we recently examined EEG and SCL in boys with AD/HD, in comparison with age-matched controls (Barry et al., 2009d). We confirmed that the AD/HD group showed both reduced SCL and an elevated theta/beta ratio compared to controls, as shown in Fig. 5 (top panel). These results are compatible with the bulk of the AD/HD literature. Mean alpha level was also lower in the AD/HD group than controls (bottom panel). There was no correlation between the theta/beta ratio and SCL, ruling it out as an arousal index. However, alpha activity and SCL were similarly (negatively) correlated in both the control and AD/HD groups, reinforcing their joint use as indices of arousal. Interestingly, while this inverse relationship would lead us to expect

280

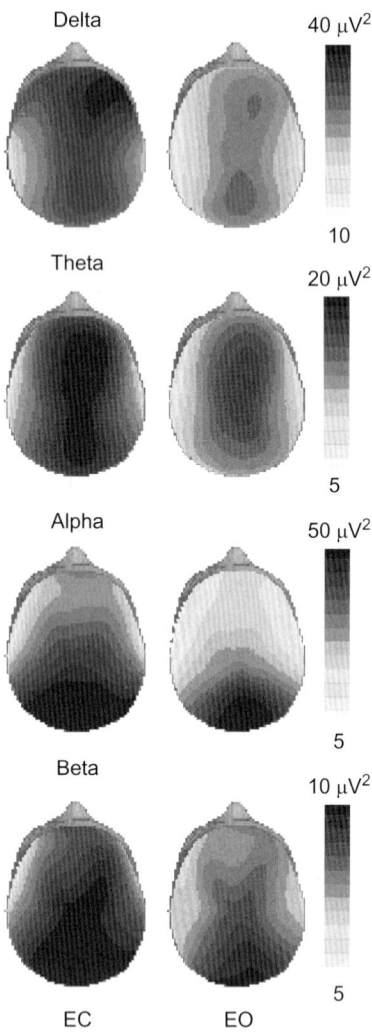

Fig. 4. Topographic head maps showing absolute power in the four traditional EEG bands for counterbalanced eyes-open and eyes-closed conditions in young adults. There is a global reduction in alpha in the eyes-open condition.

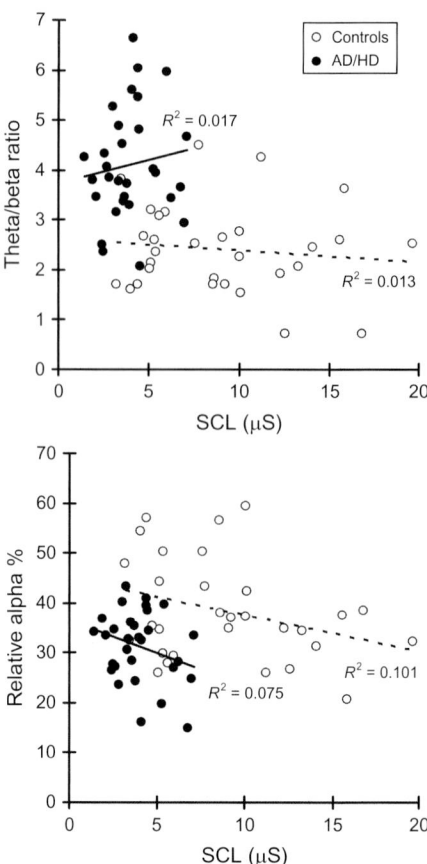

Fig. 5. Theta/beta (top panel) and relative alpha (bottom panel) as functions of SCL. Each point represents the data for one child. The top panel shows elevated theta/beta ratio and lower SCL in AD/HD; there is no significant relation between the two measures in either group. The bottom panel shows reduced alpha and lower SCL in AD/HD; these two measures are significantly correlated (negatively) in each group.

enhanced alpha associated with the hypo-aroused AD/HD children, the converse was found. This means that AD/HD in this study was associated with a reduction in alpha activity in addition to hypo-arousal — two deficits involving the one EEG measure.

This series of studies has confirmed that AD/HD patients are hypo-aroused, compared with age-matched controls, and has ruled out the theta/beta ratio as an EEG marker of arousal. Hence, the meaning of the elevated theta activity and reduced beta activity commonly reported in AD/HD, and the combined theta/beta ratio, must be reconsidered. That is, we have excluded both the developmental delay and arousal interpretations of the major EEG marker of AD/HD, and this signature now requires definitive clarification.

281

17.2.4. EEG coherence in AD/HD

Cognition and behavior depend on the integrated activity of different brain regions, and hence we have studied the EEG coupling between regions. The coherence of the EEG activity between two electrodes reflects time-locked EEG activity, within a particular frequency range, in different brain regions (Shaw, 1981). Importantly, coherence measures are independent of EEG power levels, providing a different set of information than that usually considered in relation to EEG power. Our first AD/HD coherence study (Barry et al., 2002) confirmed marked deviations in collaborative activity between different brain regions in age- and gender-matched groups of 8–12-year-old children. Children with AD/HD had elevated intrahemispheric coherences at shorter interelectrode distances in the theta band, and reduced lateral differences in the theta and alpha bands. At longer interelectrode distances, they had lower intrahemispheric alpha coherences than controls. We interpreted such differences following Thatcher et al.'s (1986) developmental model of coherences at different interelectrode distances. They proposed that short-range coherences increase with normal development, while long-range coherences decrease. Our results thus provided evidence for reduced cortical differentiation and specialization in AD/HD, particularly in the neural circuits involving theta and alpha. With interhemispheric electrode pairs, children with AD/HD had frontal coherences elevated in the delta and theta bands and reduced in the alpha band. Temporal coherence was reduced in alpha, and central/parietal/occipital coherence was enhanced in theta. We have related such differences to dysfunctional circuitry within specific brain regions and frequency bands in AD/HD. Subsequently we have investigated coherence in a range of normal and atypical samples, exploring age, gender, and AD/HD-type differences. Clarke et al. (2008) found that adults with AD/HD displayed reduced hemispheric differences in the delta band, and lower alpha coherences at short

interelectrode differences, compared with age- and gender-matched controls. This suggests that coherence anomalies remain in adults with the disorder, but that these have changed from the childhood profile with increasing age. An updated general model of our understanding of coherence anomalies in AD/HD children, based on Barry et al. (2011a), is shown in Fig. 6, indicating a wide range of regional connectivity anomalies in this disorder.

17.2.5. Event-related potentials in AD/HD

There are currently two dominant models of ERP generation. The *evoked* model considers the ERP as stimulus-locked electrical activity evoked by the stimulus processing, and adding to the ongoing EEG (Jervis et al., 1983; Lopes da Silva, 1999). The *phase-reset* model does not call on evoked activity — rather, stimulus processing is proposed to reset the ongoing EEG phase, resulting in activity at particular frequencies becoming phase-locked (Başar, 1980; Brandt et al., 1991; Makeig et al., 2002). These are not mutually exclusive processes — e.g., Barry (2009) provided evidence

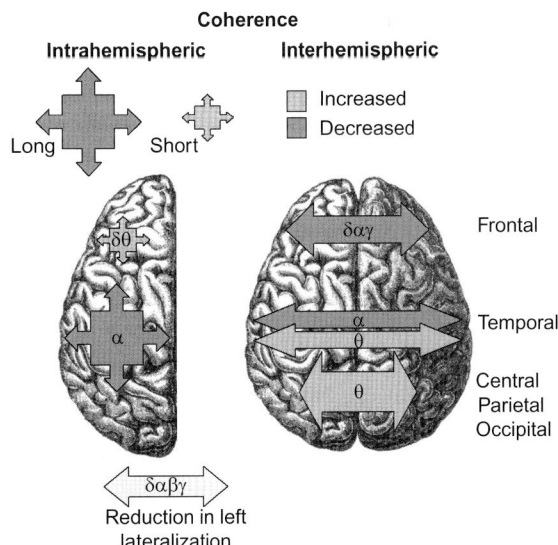

Fig. 6. A model of coherence anomalies in children with AD/HD.

282

that both evoked activity and phase locking of ongoing EEG activity contributed substantially to the different ERP components in a Go/NoGo paradigm. A major research stream in our laboratory has sought to understand the dynamics of the phase-resetting mechanism in paradigms with a fixed interstimulus interval — reviewed in Chapter 3 in this volume. For example, we have reported substantial effects of the alpha phase at stimulus onset on P3 in the auditory oddball task (Barry et al., 2004b). In a different line of research, we have also demonstrated substantial effects of prestimulus alpha power on the P3 (Barry et al., 2000). Given the alpha anomalies reported in this syndrome (described above), pursuit of such links in AD/HD should be fruitful. Our brain dynamics studies to date are still at a relatively early stage, currently examining these relationships in control children, in order to better understand normal aspects of brain dynamics before turning to children with AD/HD. We have established that the preferential phase-occurrence phenomenon with fixed interstimulus interval does occur reliably in children, and we are pressing forward with both this research strand and a new project exploring prestimulus EEG amplitude effects upon the subsequent ERPs in a Go/NoGo task.

For our present purposes in relation to raising awareness of processing anomalies in AD/HD, it is sufficient to note that our brain dynamics work argues that the ongoing spontaneous EEG is prepotent in determining the ERP correlates of stimulus processing. If this is accepted, the EEG anomalies in AD/HD described above would lead us to expect substantive ERP anomalies marking atypical stimulus processing in this disorder. Such anomalies are readily apparent in the extensive ERP–AD/HD literature (see Barry et al., 2003b, for a historic review, and Barry and Clarke, 2009, for a recent review of our own work).

For example, ERPs from children and adolescents in response to targets in an auditory oddball task (see Fig. 7) suggest that, compared with age- and gender-matched controls, there are signs of

impaired processing in many ERP components. The most commonly reported of these anomalies is reduced P3 amplitudes, clearly evident here. Note, however, that these data suggest that atypical processing is apparent even in the early N1, and it has not been adequately established to what extent the P3 differences arise from such earlier processing anomalies. These data also indicate that the ERP anomalies apparent in patients with the inattentive type of AD/HD are reduced compared with those in patients with the combined type. This type difference echoes findings in the EEG literature (e.g., see Fig. 1).

As another example, ERPs across the scalp in adults with and without AD/HD, in response to auditory targets in an intermodal auditory-visual oddball task, are shown in Fig. 8. Anomalies are apparent in the clinical group across the time span of the ERP, from the reduced N1 to the reduced P3.

These two examples illustrate ERP correlates of processing anomalies in children, adolescents, and adults with AD/HD, indicating widespread impairments in this disorder across the lifespan. Our current working hypothesis is that the anomalously elevated theta/beta ratio, the major EEG marker of AD/HD, reflects cortical processing deficiencies responsible for anomalous cognitive processing in the disorder and underpins these ERP markers.

17.2.6. Summary

From the material presented above, it can be seen that AD/HD is characterized by anomalies in resting EEG oscillations, whether these are measured in terms of absolute or relative power. Compared with age- and gender-matched controls, these differences are generally global in the theta and beta bands, with topographic differences less consistently reported in other bands. Alpha differences are not always reported, but this may be the result of competition between a hypo-arousal-related *increase*, and a different anomaly of alpha *reduction*,

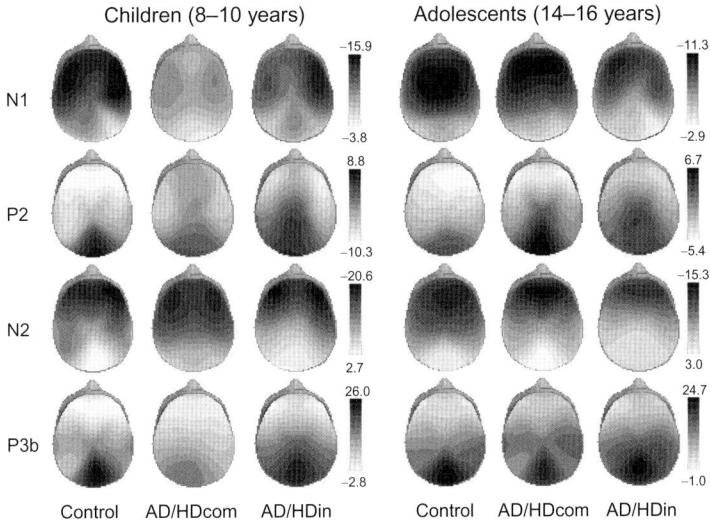

Fig. 7. ERP component topography in children and adolescents in response to targets in an auditory oddball task. Impaired responses in all components are apparent in AD/HD; anomalies are greater for those with the combined type (AD/HDcom) than the inattentive type (AD/HDin).

producing different net outcomes in different samples. Spontaneous gamma has not been widely studied in this disorder, but some recent results indicate global reduction in resting gamma power in AD/HD (Barry et al., 2009a, 2010). Age, gender, DSM type, and comorbidities all complicate these EEG profiles of AD/HD. There are also anomalies in regional connectivity, as indicated above using EEG coherence analysis. Finally, and not unexpectedly after consideration of these anomalies in spontaneous oscillations, consistent and substantial ERP anomalies are reported in a range of paradigms.

17.3. Anomalies in resting oscillations and symptoms of AD/HD

After many years of exploring these anomalies, the field is now turning its efforts to the relationships between these complex brain anomalies and the defining characteristics of AD/HD patients — their symptom profiles. Some general aspects of these have long been reported, such as developmental changes over the lifespan and the differences

between the DSM types of the disorder. In relation to the first of these, the balance of AD/HD symptoms changes over the lifespan: in particular, hyperactivity reduces with age. Bresnahan et al. (1999) reported that elevated slow wave activity persisted from childhood, through adolescence, to adulthood in AD/HD, but the reduced beta prominent in childhood disappeared with age. This parallel with the reduction in hyperactivity suggests an important EEG–behavior link. In relation to the second of these, in contrast, many of the electrophysiological data presented above suggest that the anomalies associated with the combined type of AD/HD are more severe than those from the inattentive type, rather than being qualitatively different. From this perspective, more symptoms have been thought to be simply reflected in more extensive EEG anomalies, rather than in different anomalies (Clarke et al., 1998). However, such interpretations are at least partly attributable to an earlier simplistic assessment of the disorder in "either/or" terms, rather than in terms of detailed symptom severity ratings. Increased use of

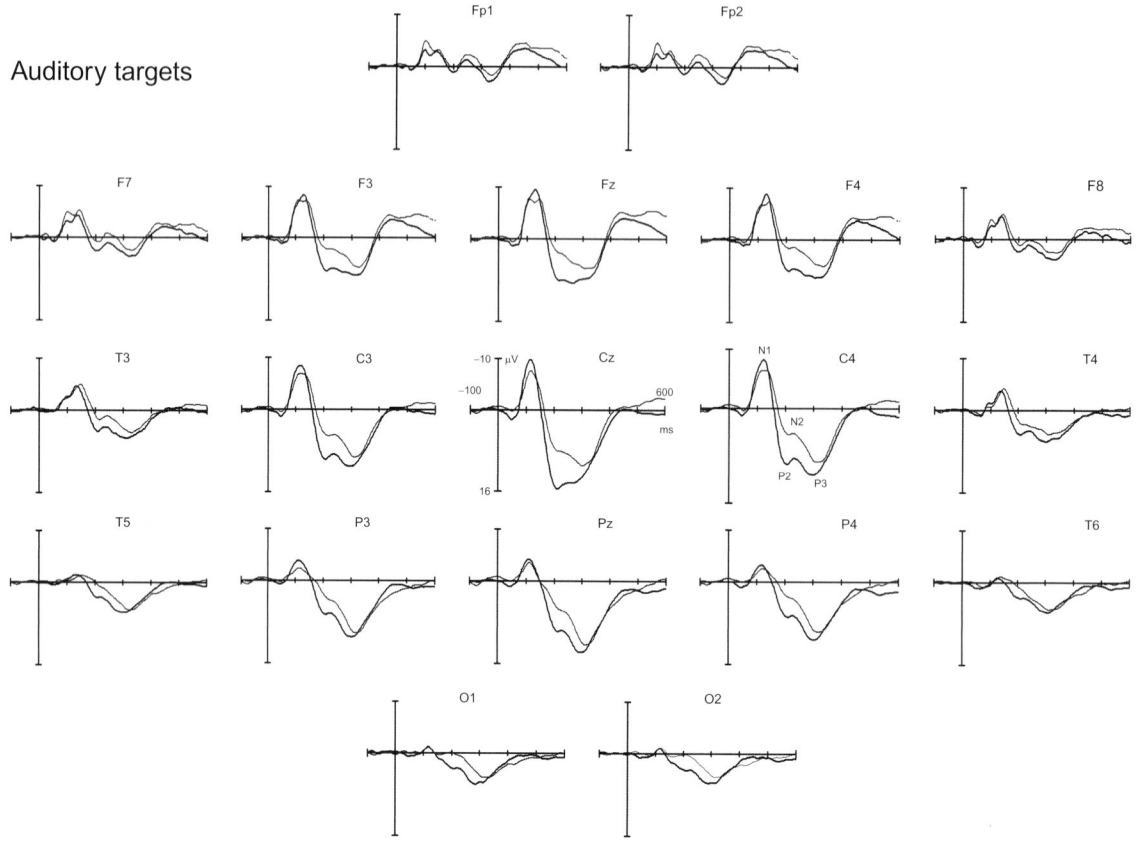

Fig. 8. ERPs to auditory targets in an intermodal auditory-visual oddball task. Heavy line represents control adults; light line represents AD/HD. Anomalies are apparent in the AD/HD group for all components.

symptom rating scales is ushering in a new focus on the detailed examination of EEG anomalies in relation to specific symptom profiles. The following sections briefly sketch a few more recent studies from our laboratory with this changing focus.

17.3.1. Three resting EEG power examples

The electrophysiological studies described above considered the clinical groups as being homogeneous, but this overlooks substantial variability between subjects. As a first example, despite reduced beta being consistently reported as a group marker of AD/HD, a number of years ago we found that some 20% of subjects with AD/HD of the combined type had elevated levels of beta activity

(Clarke et al., 1998). Case notes indicated that these children were more moody and prone to temper tantrums than the typical child with AD/HD. A similar enhanced beta group had been reported by Chabot and Serfontein (1996), and we confirmed such a group in a larger combined type study (Clarke et al., 2001c). However, we have failed to find the excess beta group in a study of boys with the inattentive type (Clarke et al., 2002c), or in a study of females with AD/HD (Clarke et al., 2003).

A second example comes from a recent cluster study of 155 boys with AD/HD, which included scores on the Conners' (Parent) rating scale, the Child Behavior Checklist, the Depression and Anxiety Youth Scale, and the Developmental Behavior Checklist (Clarke et al., 2011). We found four EEG-defined clusters in this study. Cluster 1

(23%) was a high beta group, with symptoms of increased delinquent behavior with reduced signs of guilt and reduced inattention, self-harming/ suicidal ideation, strange ideas, and physical problems. Clearly this overlaps with and clarifies the symptomatology of the high-beta group described in our first example in this section. Cluster 2 (36%) had elevated total power and theta and reduced alpha and beta. This group showed fewer problems across most scales than other groups and can be considered as representing the typical profile of boys with AD/HD. Cluster 3 (25%) had elevated slow wave activity and reduced alpha. These children showed more impulsivity, inattention, and bad language. Cluster 4 (17%) had reduced delta and increased hyperactivity and ritualistic behaviors. Interpretation of clusters 3 and 4 are beyond the scope of the present chapter, but are clearly of interest to the understanding of EEG profiles in AD/HD.

A recent gamma study of EEG in AD/HD (Barry et al., 2010) provides a third example. It found that inattention scores on the Conners DSM scale correlated positively with theta (which is increased in AD/HD) and negatively with gamma (which is reduced in AD/HD). Hyperactivity–impulsivity scores on the Conners scale correlated positively with the theta/beta ratio, which is increased in AD/HD. That is, in this study, the major AD/HD symptoms of inattention and hyperactivity–impulsivity were positively correlated with the extent of specific EEG anomalies associated with AD/HD. Such a direct link between symptoms and EEG anomalies provides an incentive for future targeted EEG studies in this syndrome.

17.3.2. An EEG coherence example

In the context of the model of EEG coherence in AD/HD presented in Fig. 6, Barry et al. (2011a) found that smaller left lateralized coherences in AD/HD correlated negatively with Conners' Innattentive and Total scores. This was true for coherences in the delta, alpha, beta, and gamma bands. Smaller frontal interhemispheric coherences in AD/HD in the alpha band correlated negatively with Conners' Hyperactive–Impulsive scores. We consider that the negative values obtained for these correlations suggest compensatory brain function for these coherence anomalies, perhaps reducing the impact of brain anomalies in left frontal regions. Such novel findings are very exciting, suggesting new insights into brain plasticity in this disorder. Obviously, such innovative studies are in need of stringent replication in future work.

17.4. Conclusions and future directions

It has not been the purpose of this chapter to evaluate the significance of the contributions mentioned above, but rather to provide a brief overview of this narrow slice of research exploring the importance of brain oscillations in the understanding of AD/HD. That work has occurred amidst a huge explosion in the range of methodologies in neuroscience and related fields researching AD/HD, but consideration of the place of this work in the wider context is not possible here.

To this end, the chapter has briefly outlined a wide range of evidence showing the existence of anomalous EEG oscillations in AD/HD. We have shown the impact of these anomalous oscillations in the resting-state EEG, in coherence measuring the coupling between regions of interest, and in the ERPs marking stimulus processing and subsequent cognitive elaboration in this disorder. We consider that all these flow from the underlying anomalies in spontaneous EEG oscillations and their patterning. The importance of these findings is highlighted by recent EEG/symptom linkage studies, suggesting that there is a close relation between specific EEG deficits and specific symptoms in this disorder. We are pursuing such linkages as the current major AD/HD focus in our laboratory and expect that this will reward us with significant insights into the etiology and expression of AD/HD across the age span.

286

Acknowledgments

This research was funded by grants from the Australian Research Council Discovery funding scheme (Project Numbers DP0558989 and DP0665531).

References

Barry, R.J. (2009) Evoked activity and EEG phase-resetting in the genesis of auditory Go/NoGo ERPs. *Biol. Psychol.*, 80: 292–299.

Barry, R.J. and Clarke, A.R. (2009) Spontaneous EEG oscillations in children, adolescents, and adults: typical development, and pathological aspects in relation to AD/HD. *J. Psychophyiol.*, 23: 157–173.

Barry, R.J. and Sokolov, E.N. (1993) Habituation of phasic and tonic components of the orienting reflex. *Int. J. Psychophysiol.*, 15: 39–42.

Barry, R.J., Kirkaikul, S. and Hodder, D. (2000) EEG alpha activity and the ERP to target stimuli in an auditory oddball paradigm. *Int. J. Psychophysiol.*, 39: 39–50.

Barry, R.J., Clarke, A.R., McCarthy, R. and Selikowitz, M. (2002) EEG coherence in attention-deficit/hyperactivity disorder: a comparative study of two DSM-IV types. *Clin. Neurophysiol.*, 113: 579–585.

Barry, R.J., Clarke, A.R. and Johnstone, S.J. (2003a) A review of electrophysiology in attention-deficit/hyperactivity disorder. I. Qualitative and quantitative electroencephalography. *Clin. Neurophysiol.*, 114: 171–183.

Barry, R.J., Johnstone, S.J. and Clarke, A.R. (2003b) A review of electrophysiology in attention-deficit/hyperactivity disorder. II. Event-related potentials. *Clin. Neurophysiol.*, 114: 184–198.

Barry, R.J., Clarke, A.R., McCarthy, R., Selikowitz, M., Rushby, J.A. and Ploskova, E. (2004a) EEG differences in children as a function of resting-state arousal level. *Clin. Neurophysiol.*, 115: 402–408.

Barry, R.J., Rushby, J.A., Johnstone, S.J., Clarke, A.R., Croft, R.J. and Lawrence, C. (2004b) Event-related potentials in the auditory oddball as a function of EEG alpha phase at stimulus onset. *Clin. Neurophysiol.*, 115: 2593–2601.

Barry, R.J., Rushby, J.A., Wallace, M.J., Clarke, A.R., Johnstone, S.J. and Zlojutro, I. (2005) Caffeine effects on resting-state arousal. *Clin. Neurophysiol.*, 116: 2693–2700.

Barry, R.J., Clarke, A.R., Johnstone, S.J., Magee, C.A. and Rushby, J.A. (2007) EEG differences between eyes-closed and eyes-open resting conditions. *Clin. Neurophysiol.*, 118: 2765–2773.

Barry, R.J., Clarke, A.R., Johnstone, S.J. and Rushby, J.A. (2008) Timing of caffeine's impact on autonomic and central nervous system measures: clarification of arousal effects. *Biol. Psychol.*, 7: 304–316.

Barry, R.J., Clarke, A.R., Hajos, M., McCarthy, R., Selikowitz, M. and Bruggemann, J.M. (2009a) Acute atomoxetine effects on the EEG of children with attention-deficit/hyperactivity disorder. *Neuropharmacology*, 57: 702–707.

Barry, R.J., Clarke, A.R., Johnstone, S.J. and Brown, C.R. (2009b) EEG differences in children between eyes-closed and eyes-open resting conditions. *Clin. Neurophysiol.*, 120: 1806–1811.

Barry, R.J., Clarke, A.R., Johnstone, S.J., Brown, C.R., Bruggemann, J.M. and Van Rijbroek, I. (2009c) Caffeine effects on resting-state arousal in children. *Int. J. Psychophysiol.*, 73: 355–361.

Barry, R.J., Clarke, A.R., Johnstone, S.J., McCarthy, R. and Selikowitz, M. (2009d) Electroencephalogram θ/β ratio and arousal in AD/HD: evidence of independent processes. *Biol. Psychiatry*, 66: 398–401.

Barry, R.J., Clarke, A.R., Hajos, M., McCarthy, R., Selikowitz, M. and Dupuy, F. (2010) Resting-state EEG gamma activity in children with attention-deficit/hyperactivity disorder. *Clin. Neurophysiol.*, 121: 1871–1877.

Barry, R.J., Clarke, A.R., Hajos, M., Dupuy, F.E., McCarthy, R. and Selikowitz, M. (2011a) EEG coherence and symptom profiles of children with attention-deficit/hyperactivity disorder. *Clin. Neurophysiol.*, 122: 1327–1332.

Barry, R.J., Clarke, A.R. and Johnstone, S.J. (2011b) Caffeine and opening the eyes have additive effects on resting arousal measures. *Clin. Neurophysiol.*, 122: 2010–2015.

Başar, E. (1980) *EEG Brain Dynamics: Relation between EEG and Brain Evoked Potentials.* Elsevier, Amsterdam.

Brandt, M.E., Jansen, B.H. and Carbonari, J.P. (1991) Pre-stimulus spectral EEG patterns and the visual evoked response. *Electroencephalogr. Clin. Neurophysiol.*, 80: 16–20.

Bresnahan, S.M. and Barry, R.J. (2002) Specificity of quantitative EEG analysis in adults with attention deficit hyperactivity disorder. *Psychiatr. Res.*, 112: 133–144.

Bresnahan, S.M., Anderson, J.W. and Barry, R.J. (1999) Age-related changes in quantitative EEG in attention-deficit/hyperactivity disorder. *Biol. Psychol.*, 46: 1690–1697.

Bresnahan, S.M., Barry, R.J., Clarke, A.R. and Johnstone, S.J. (2006) Quantitative EEG analysis in dexamphetamine-responsive adults with attention deficit/hyperactivity disorder. *Psychiatr. Res.*, 141: 151–159.

Chabot, R.J. and Serfontein, G. (1996) Quantitative electroencephalographic profiles of children with attention deficit disorder. *Biol. Psychol.*, 40: 951–963.

Clarke, A.R., Barry, R.J., McCarthy, R. and Selikowitz, M. (1998) EEG analysis in attention deficit/hyperactivity disorder: a comparative study of two subtypes. *Psychiatr. Res.*, 81: 19–29.

Clarke, A.R., Barry, R.J., McCarthy, R. and Selikowitz, M. (2001a) Age and sex effects in the EEG: development of the normal child. *Clin. Neurophysiol.*, 112: 806–814.

Clarke, A.R., Barry, R.J., McCarthy, R. and Selikowitz, M. (2001b) Age and sex effects in the EEG: differences in two subtypes of attention-deficit/hyperactivity disorder. *Clin. Neurophysiol.*, 112: 815–826.

Clarke, A.R., Barry, R.J., McCarthy, R. and Selikowitz, M. (2001c) EEG-defined subtypes of children with attention-deficit/hyperactivity disorder. *Clin. Neurophysiol.*, 112: 2098–2105.

Clarke, A.R., Barry, R.J., McCarthy, R. and Selikowitz, M. (2002a) Children with attention-deficit/hyperactivity disorder and comorbid oppositional defiant disorder: an EEG analysis. *Psychiatr. Res.*, 111: 181–190.

Clarke, A.R., Barry, R.J., McCarthy, R. and Selikowitz, M. (2002b) EEG analysis of children with attention-deficit/

hyperactivity disorder and comorbid reading disabilities. *J. Learn. Disabil.*, 35: 276–285.

Clarke, A.R., Barry, R.J., McCarthy, R., Selikowitz, M. and Brown, C.R. (2002c) EEG evidence for a new conceptualisation of attention deficit hyperactivity disorder. *Clin. Neurophysiol.*, 113: 1036–1044.

Clarke, A.R., Barry, R.J., McCarthy, R., Selikowitz, M., Clarke, D. and Croft, R.J. (2003) EEG activity in girls with attention-deficit/hyperactivity disorder. *Clin. Neurophysiol.*, 114: 319–328.

Clarke, A.R., Barry, R.J., Heaven, P.C.L., McCarthy, R., Selikowitz, M. and Byrne, M. (2008) EEG coherence in adults with attention-deficit/hyperactivity disorder. *Int. J. Psychophysiol.*, 67: 35–40.

Clarke, A.R., Barry, R.J., Dupuy, F.E., Heckel, L.D., McCarthy, R. and Selikowitz, M. (2011) Behavioural differences between EEG-defined subgroups of children with attention-deficit/hyperactivity disorder. *Clin. Neurophysiol.*, 122: 1333–1341.

Gasser, T., Jennen-Steinmetz, C., Sroka, L., Verleger, R. and Mocks, J. (1988a) Development of the EEG of school age children and adolescents. II. Topography. *Electroencephalogr. Clin. Neurophysiol.*, 69: 100–109.

Gasser, T., Verleger, R., Bacher, P. and Sroka, L. (1988b) Development of the EEG of school age children and adolescents. I. Analysis of band power. *Electroencephalogr. Clin. Neurophysiol.*, 69: 91–99.

Hobbs, M.J., Clarke, A.R., Barry, R.J., McCarthy, R. and Selikowitz, M. (2007) EEG abnormalities in adolescent males with AD/HD. *Clin. Neurophysiol.*, 118: 363–371.

Jasper, H., Solomon, P. and Bradley, C. (1938) Electroencephalographic analyses of behavior problem children. *Am. J. Psychiatry*, 95: 641–658.

Jervis, B.W., Nichols, M.J., Johnson, T.E., Allen, E. and Hudson, N.R. (1983) A fundamental investigation of the composition of auditory evoked potentials. *IEEE Trans. Biomed. Eng.*, 30: 43–50.

Lopes da Silva, F.H. (1999) Event-related potentials: methodology and quantification. In: E. Niedermeyer and F.H. Lopes da Silva (Eds.), *Electroencephalography: Basic Principles, Clinical Applications, and Related Fields*. Williams and Wilkins, Baltimore, MD.

Lubar, J. (1991) Discourse on the development of EEG diagnostic and biofeedback for attention-deficit/hyperactivity disorder. *Biofeedb. Self Regul.*, 16: 201–225.

Makeig, S., Westerfield, M., Jung, T.P., Enghoff, S., Townsend, J., Courchesne, E. and Sejnowski, T.J. (2002) Dynamic brain sources of visual evoked responses. *Science*, 295: 690–694.

Mann, C., Lubar, J.H., Zimmerman, A., Miller, C. and Munchen, R. (1992) Quantitative analysis of EEG in boys with attention deficit hyperactivity disorder: controlled study with clinical implications. *Pediatr. Neurol.*, 8: 30–36.

Monastra, V.J., Lubar, J.F., Linden, M.K., Van Deusen, P., Green, G., Wing, W., Phillips, A. and Nick, F.T. (1999) Assessing attention deficit hyperactivity disorder via quantitative electroencephalography: an initial validation study. *Neuropsychology*, 13: 424–433.

Monastra, V.J., Lubar, J.F. and Linden, M.K. (2001) The development of a quantitative electroencephalographic scanning process for attention deficit/hyperactivity disorder: reliability and validity studies. *Neuropsychology*, 15: 136–144.

Pribram, K.H. and McGuiness, D. (1975) Arousal, activation and effort in the control of attention. *Psychol. Rev.*, 2: 116–149.

Pribram, K.H. and McGuiness, D. (1992) Attention and para-attentional processing: event-related brain potentials as tests of a model. In: D. Friedman and G.E. Bruder (Eds.), *Psychophysiology and Experimental Psychopathology: A Tribute to Samuel Sutton. Annals of the New York Academy of Sciences*, vol. 658. New York Academy of Sciences, New York, pp. 65–92.

Raine, A., Venables, P.H. and Williams, M. (1990) Relationships between central and autonomic measures of arousal at age 15 years and criminality at age 24 years. *Arch. Gen. Psychiatry*, 152: 1595–1600.

Raskin, D.C. (1973) Attention and arousal. In: W.F. Prokasy and D.C. Raskin (Eds.), *Electrodermal Activity in Psychological Research*. Academic Press, New York, pp. 125–155.

Satterfield, J.H. and Cantwell, D.P. (1974) CNS function and response to methylphenidate in hyperactive children. *Psychopharmacol. Bull.*, 10: 36–38.

Satterfield, J.H. and Dawson, M.E. (1971) Electrodermal correlates of hyperactivity in children. *Psychophysiology*, 8: 191–197.

Shaw, J. (1981) An introduction to the coherence function and its use in the EEG signal analysis. *J. Med. Eng. Technol.*, 5: 279–288.

Thatcher, R., Krause, P. and Hrybyk, M. (1986) Cortico-cortical associations and EEG coherence: a two-compartmental model. *Electroencephalogr. Clin. Neurophysiol.*, 64: 123–143.

Application of Brain Oscillations in Neuropsychiatric Diseases
(Supplements to Clinical Neurophysiology, Vol. 62)
Editors: E. Başar, C. Başar-Eroğlu, A. Özerdem, P.M. Rossini, G.G. Yener
© 2013 Elsevier B.V. All rights reserved

Chapter 18

Event-related oscillations reflect functional asymmetry in children with attention deficit/hyperactivity disorder

Juliana Yordanova[a,*], Vasil Kolev[a], and Aribert Rothenberger[b]

[a]*Institute of Neurobiology, Bulgarian Academy of Sciences, Acad. G. Bonchev Str., Bl. 23, 1113 Sofia, Bulgaria*
[b]*Child and Adolescent Psychiatry, University of Göttingen, D-37075 Göttingen, Germany*

ABSTRACT

Previous studies have found that event-related theta and gamma oscillations elicited in an auditory selective attention task are deviant in children with attention deficit/hyperactivity disorder (ADHD). It has been suggested that these deviations are associated with deficient motor inhibition in ADHD, which may lead to increased excitability of not only the motor generation networks but also the networks involved in sensory and cognitive processing of the stimulus requiring motor response.

Within this suggestion, the present study used the same experimental database to compare the motor cortical activation of healthy controls and children with ADHD during the performance of the auditory selective attention task. Electroencephalography mu (8–12 Hz) activity at C3 and C4 electrodes was used as a measure of motor cortical activation. Mu power was analyzed for four stimulus conditions of the task (attended target, unattended target, attended nontarget, and unattended nontarget). It was found that motor cortical activation as reflected by mu power suppression was not overall greater in ADHD than healthy children. However, stimuli that possessed only partial target features and did not require motor responding (unattended target and attended nontarget) produced a significant reduction of mu activity in ADHD patients. These results suggest that motor cortical excitability is not generally increased in ADHD children. Rather, the co-existence of conflict features in complex stimuli induces task-irrelevant motor activation in these children. The deficient inhibition of motor cortical networks contralateral to the response may therefore be responsible for the functional asymmetry in stimulus processing in ADHD.

KEYWORDS

Attention deficit/hyperactivity disorder; Selective attention; Event-related oscillation; Motor activation; Functional asymmetry

18.1. The concept of event-related oscillations

Neuroelectric oscillations provide important tools to study brain functions. In addition to spontane-

Correspondence to: Dr. Juliana Yordanova, Ph.D., Institute of Neurobiology, Bulgarian Academy of Sciences, Acad. G. Bonchev Str., Bl. 23, 1113 Sofia, Bulgaria.
Tel./fax: +359-2-979-37-49;
E-mail: jyord@bio.bas.bg

ous electroencephalographic (EEG) activity, event-related oscillations (EROs) have been introduced to explore the neurophysiologic mechanisms of information processing (Başar, 1980, 1998). There are several conceptual and methodological advantages of EEG oscillations that help reveal new specific aspects of neural dynamics (e.g., Yordanova et al., 2009). First, within the concept of neuroelectric oscillations, signals from unitary frequency-specific systems produce both the spontaneous and stimulus-related EEG activity, and frequency-specific EROs originate from the reorganization of the spontaneous (ongoing) EEG activity from the same frequency range (Başar, 1998). Second, the functional involvement of a system can be assessed by its ability to reorganize neural networks and synchronize them in space and time during active information processing (Başar et al., 2001; Yordanova and Kolev, 2008). The important consequences of the ERO concept are (1) the understanding of distributed neural systems which are defined by frequency specificity and subserve neural coding and connectivity, (2) the introduction of new approaches to explore functionality by analysis of event-related reorganization (spatial and temporal synchronization and power changes), and (3) the possibility to explore the neurobiological status of an oscillatory system (normal or pathological) reflected by spontaneous EEG oscillations independently of functional competence reflected by EROs (Yordanova and Kolev, 1996, 1998, 2008; Başar et al., 1997).

18.2. Spontaneous EEG oscillations in ADHD

Recently, the application of EROs to brain functions in psychopathological conditions has gained increased attention (Herrmann and Demiralp, 2005; Ford et al., 2007; Rossini et al., 2007; Başar and Güntekin, 2008; Rothenberger, 2009). Among other cognitive disturbances, attention deficit/hyperactivity disorder (ADHD) is one of the most intensively studied syndromes in child psychiatry because of its prevalence and great social impact (Rothenberger, 1990; Swanson et al., 1998; Tannock, 1998). Yet, pathophysiological mechanisms leading to the ADHD core symptoms of inattention, impulsivity, and hyperactivity remain to be clarified (Swanson et al., 1998; Sergeant, 2000; Yordanova et al., 2011). In addition to neuroanatomical, pharmacological' and genetic research, studies of the neuroelectric substrate of cognitive functioning have provided important clues to ADHD-related dysfunctions (Swanson et al., 1998). Both earlier (e.g., Dykman et al., 1982; Matoušek et al., 1984; Woerner et al., 1987; Matsuura et al., 1993) and more recent research of spontaneous EEG activity (Clarke et al., 1998, 2001; Lazzaro et al., 1998, 1999) have demonstrated that, typically, children with ADHD have elevated levels of absolute delta and theta power and decreased levels of absolute beta and gamma power compared to controls. For relative power measures, an enhancement of delta and theta activities and reduction of alpha, beta' and gamma activities are often found in children with ADHD (review Barry et al., 2003a, 2010; Monastra, 2008). These differences in the patterns of the spontaneous EEG power along with measures of EEG coherence have differentiated not only ADHD co-morbidity with other child psychiatric disorders such as tic disorder, autism, reading disability, oppositional defiant disorder, etc. (Rothenberger, 1982; Barry et al., 2007, 2009; Clarke et al., 2011) but also ADHD sub-types based on DSM diagnostic criteria (Clarke et al., 2001). Thus, spontaneous neuroelectric patterns have provided convincing evidence for deviations in the neurobiological development of neural networks in ADHD. Much less is known, however, about the functional reactivity and competence of neural oscillatory networks involved in sensory and cognitive information processing in ADHD.

18.3. EROs in ADHD: auditory selective attention

Event-related potentials (ERPs) have been used extensively as a standard tool to study neurophysiologic mechanisms of stimulus information processing in ADHD (Barry et al., 2003b; Banaschewski and Brandeis, 2007; Albrecht et al., 2008). Just a few previous reports have addressed, however, the issue of EROs and their associations with information processing networks in ADHD (Heinrich et al., 2001; Yordanova et al., 2001, 2006; Lenz et al., 2008, 2010).

In our previous studies (Yordanova et al., 2001, 2006), EROs in ADHD were analyzed based on the concept of the reorganization of oscillatory EEG activity (Başar, 1980, 1998). In these studies, an auditory selective attention task was used, where two tones differing in frequency (target and nontarget) were presented either on the right or on the left. There were two conditions, in which the side of stimulus appearance had to be attended to as requiring a motor response to one of the stimulus types (target, see also Appendix). Equal numbers of each stimulus type were presented to the left and right ear. In the first condition, subjects were instructed to press a button in response to the targets presented to the right, while in the second condition, the attended targets were presented to the left. Thus, there were four signal types in each series: target–attended (T–A), target–nonattended (T–NA), nontarget–attended (NT–A), and nontarget–nonattended (NT–NA). A total of 28 children (14 children with ADHD and 14 healthy controls matched for age, IQ, and gender) were studied (details of group characteristics are presented in the Appendix). EEG responses in the theta and gamma frequency ranges for each stimulus type were recorded and analyzed at left, midline, and right electrodes over frontal, central, and parietal cortical regions (for details, see Yordanova et al., 2001, 2006). The statistical analysis was designed to address two major questions: (1) Do EROs from the theta and gamma ranges provide biological markers of ADHD? (2) Do EROs from theta and gamma ranges reveal differences between healthy children and children with ADHD in information processing during auditory selective attention? Specifically, the functional reactivity of theta and gamma oscillations to two cognitive variables, spatial attention and target features discrimination, was compared between the groups.

18.3.1. Event-related theta oscillations

Fig. 1 presents event-related theta oscillations in average ERPs in two groups of children (control and ADHD) in an auditory selective attention task. The figure demonstrates that in the theta (3–7.5 Hz) frequency range, two responses emerged with different latencies. The first, termed early theta response (ETR), was observed in the first 0–200 ms after stimulus at anterior (bilateral fronto-central and midline frontal) locations. The ETR was most prominent for T–A ERPs but was also observed for other stimulus types. A second theta response from approximately the same frequency band (3–7.5 Hz) emerged at fronto-central electrodes between 200 and 450 ms after stimulus (late theta response, LTR). The LTR was not generated after attended targets. It was especially enhanced after nonattended nontargets (NT–NA) and was much less evident after T–NA and NT–A stimulus types.

The study of Yordanova et al. (2006) yielded several major results about ADHD psychopathology. First, as demonstrated in the figure, the two theta responses, early and late, were generated in children with ADHD, similar to controls. Second, the LTR was substantially elevated in children with ADHD symptoms, irrespective of whether these symptoms were behaviorally expressed in a single nosology, or in combination with tic disorder symptoms. Since the LTR was specifically associated with hyperactivity scores, it presented a biological marker of hyperactivity in children (for details, see Yordanova et al., 2006). Importantly, the LTR was determined by ongoing theta activity in the spontaneous EEG that was also enhanced in ADHD and thus reflected a modulation of biologically altered theta networks during irrelevant information processing in ADHD. Third, while the ETR did not manifest an overall difference between the groups, it revealed a specific variation in the mechanisms of spatial attention in children with ADHD. The ETR in controls was larger for attended than unattended stimuli at

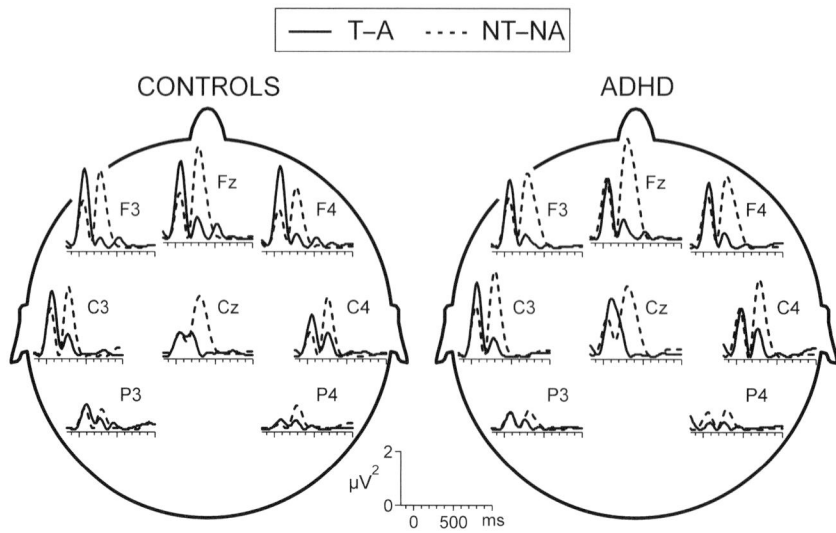

Fig. 1. Grand average time–frequency components in the theta frequency range (wavelet scale 3–7.5 Hz of event-related theta power) for two stimulus conditions (T–A, target–attend and NT–NA, nontarget–nonattend) in two groups, controls and ADHD. For clarity of illustration power envelopes are shown. The impression that the theta response starts before stimulus is due to envelope presentation. Note that theta responses of two stimulus types (T–A and NT–NA) are shown, whereas the description of statistical results in the text refers to effects from all four stimulus types. (After Yordanova et al., 2006, with modifications.)

electrodes contralateral to the side of attention, whereas in ADHD children, the ETR to attended stimuli was larger at left hemisphere electrodes, irrespective of whether the attended channel was on the right or on the left.

18.3.2. Event-related gamma oscillations

Fig. 2 demonstrates event-related gamma oscillations of average ERPs in the same groups of children in the same conditions. In the average ERPs of both control and ADHD children, the gamma band response (GBR) was generated within 0–120 ms after stimulus and was maximal at frontal and minimal at parietal locations (Yordanova et al., 2001). No significant main between-group differences were found. However, the most intriguing result was that GBRs to right-side stimuli were significantly larger in ADHD relative to control children, independently of whether stimuli

were targets or nontargets, and whether the attended channel was on the right or on the left. Notably, as also shown in Fig. 2, the increase of GBR to the right-side stimuli in ADHD was more pronounced at left-hemisphere electrodes. Analyses of the phase locking of GBR also showed that a significant increase of the phase synchronization in ADHD versus controls was observed for right-side stimuli over the left hemisphere. The differences between the two groups were significant at left parietal and central locations (for details, see Yordanova et al., 2001).

18.4. Objectives of the current study

According to these results, both early theta and gamma EROs in ADHD displayed variations in functional reactivity at the left-hemisphere electrodes as compared to healthy controls. These observations have been suggested to reflect an effect of left-hemisphere disinhibition related to

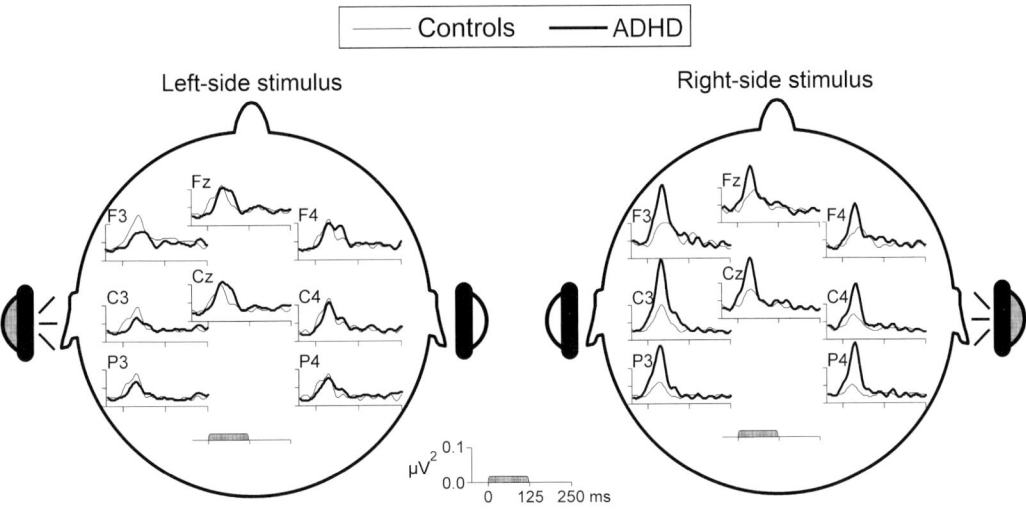

Fig. 2.   Grand average of gamma band power (envelopes shown) of control and ADHD children for left- and right-side auditory stimuli in selective attention task. The increase of GBR to the right-side stimuli in ADHD is clearly observed. (After Yordanova et al., 2001, with modifications.)

the requirement to produce motor responses with the right hand (see Appendix). It was proposed that a transient overactivation of left motor cortical regions occurring in relation to motor response production could not be dynamically controlled in ADHD, which affected the functioning of internal attention networks as reflected by theta oscillations and external attention networks as reflected by gamma oscillations.

Here, we tested this hypothesis by analyzing the activation of motor cortical regions in the same groups of subjects performing the auditory selective attention task. As a relevant parameter, the power of 8–12 Hz EEG activity was used. It has been previously demonstrated that the EEG frequency from the 8–12 Hz band corresponds to the mu rhythm in children and adolescents from 6 to 18 years of age (Bender et al., 2005). Also, these authors have observed that the power of 8–12 Hz activity is reduced over motor regions contralateral to the response in the foreperiod of a warned reaction time task, thus indicating that the reduction in 8–12 Hz power in children reflects a motor cortical activation. Therefore, the power of 8–12 Hz activity was analyzed here for left

and right motor cortical electrodes (C3 and C4) in a time window during task processing where no active stimulus or response generation processes were implicated. This was a period starting late after stimulus occurrence (later than the response time for T–A stimuli) and preceding next stimulus appearance (see Appendix for methodological details). This epoch was chosen to minimize effects related to active stimulus processing in terms of sensory, cognitive, and motor evaluation. It was expected that a response-related overactivation of the motor cortical regions in ADHD would be associated with a suppression of 8–12 Hz mu activity at the left motor cortex (contralateral to the response), which would be especially pronounced after T–A stimuli as a specific reflection of the motor dysinhibition deficit.

There are other accounts that may explain the left- versus right-hemispheric differences in oscillatory responses between the two groups. Previous studies have consistently shown laterality deviations in ADHD (Roessner et al., 2004). At the behavioral level, ADHD children have manifested deficits in re-orienting attention, particularly for targets in the left visual field (Bellgrove et al., 2008, 2009). This left-sided inattention (spatial rightward bias) has been found for both externally and internally guided responses (Bellgrove et al., 2009) and has been extended to the movement domain (Johnson et al., 2010) and to spontaneous EEG alpha rightward asymmetry (Hale et al., 2010). With regard to possible laterality effects on neurobiological alpha networks in ADHD, 8–12 Hz power in the spontaneous EEG was also analyzed in the present study and compared between the groups (see Appendix).

18.5. Motor cortical activation during auditory selective attention in ADHD

To reflect the effects of task variables (attended channel and stimulus type) on the activation of motor cortical regions, the power of 8–12 Hz mu EEG activity was subjected to a statistical analysis similar to the one used in the previous studies where EROs from the theta and gamma frequency bands were explored. There was one between-subjects variable group (controls vs. ADHD) and four within-subjects variables, attended channel (attended vs. unattended), stimulus type (target vs. nontarget), side of stimulation (right vs. left), and lead (C3 vs. C4).

No significant effect of the group factor was found, indicating no overall difference in the activation state of motor regions between the groups. As demonstrated in Fig. 3, mu activity was significantly smaller following a stimulus in the attended channel relative to the unattended channel (attended channel, F $(1/26) = 15.3$, $p < 0.001$), and following stimulus with target characteristics relative to nontarget characteristics (stimulus type, F $(1/26) = 14.2$, $p < 0.001$). However, as expected, these effects were produced by the attended targets (Fig. 3), only after which the mu activity was significantly reduced (attended channel $\times$ stimulus type, F $(1/26) = 10.8$, $p = 0.003$), indicating a prolonged overactivation of the motor cortical regions after motor response

generation. Importantly, this expected pattern was only observed in healthy control children but not in ADHD children (attended channel $\times$ stimulus type $\times$ group, F $(1/26) = 4.5$, $p = 0.04$; Fig. 3). In controls (attended channel $\times$ stimulus type, F $(1/13) = 16.3$, $p < 0.001$), mu activity was reduced for T–A, but it did not differ among stimulus types that did not require a motor cortical activation (NT–A, T–NA, and NT–NA). In ADHD children, not only the T–A stimulus but also the NT–A and the T–NA stimuli produced a reduction of mu EEG activity, while the NT–NA type was less effective (attended channel $\times$ stimulus type, F $(1/13) = 0.66$, $p = 0.4$). These results demonstrate that motor cortical activation as reflected by mu suppression is sustained in healthy children only when the stimulus has been processed as a response generation stimulus. In contrast, ADHD children manifest a prolonged motor cortical activation not only in relation to response generation, but even when partial target characteristics are identified.

Another major question of the present analysis was if the left motor cortical regions would demonstrate a higher state of activation in children with ADHD relative to controls. No main effect of lead (C3 vs. C4) or a significant lead $\times$ group interaction was found. There was, however, a significant lead $\times$ group $\times$ attended channel interaction (F $(1/26) = 4.9$, $p = 0.035$). Fig. 4 demonstrates (graphically and in difference time–frequency plots) that in contrast to controls, children with ADHD reduced the mu activity more strongly at C3 than C4 following a stimulus in the attended channel. No such laterality effect existed for stimuli in the unattended channel in any of the groups (Fig. 4).

To control for the topographic specificity of these effects, the same analyses were performed for frontal and parietal electrodes. Attended channel $\times$ stimulus type $\times$ group interaction was significant for frontal ($F (1/26) = 6.14$, $p = 0.02$) but not for parietal sites ($F (1/26) = 0.4$, $p > 0.5$) In none of these analyses, was the lead $\times$ group $\times$ attended channel interaction significant (F $(1/26) < 0.9$, $p > 0.3$).

295

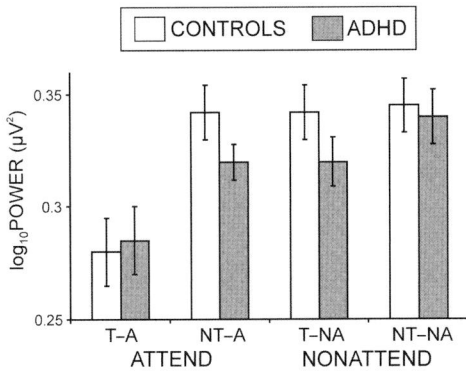

Fig. 3. The effect of stimulus type on alpha band total power in selective attention task in attend and nonattend conditions for control and ADHD groups. T–A, target–attend; NT–A, nontarget–attend; T–NA, target–nonattend; NT–NA, nontarget–nonattend. It is demonstrated that in controls, alpha activity did not differ among stimulus types that did not require a motor cortical activation (NT–A, T–NA, and NT–NA), whereas in ADHD children not only the T–A stimulus but also the NT–A and the T–NA stimuli produced a reduction of event-related alpha (mu) activity.

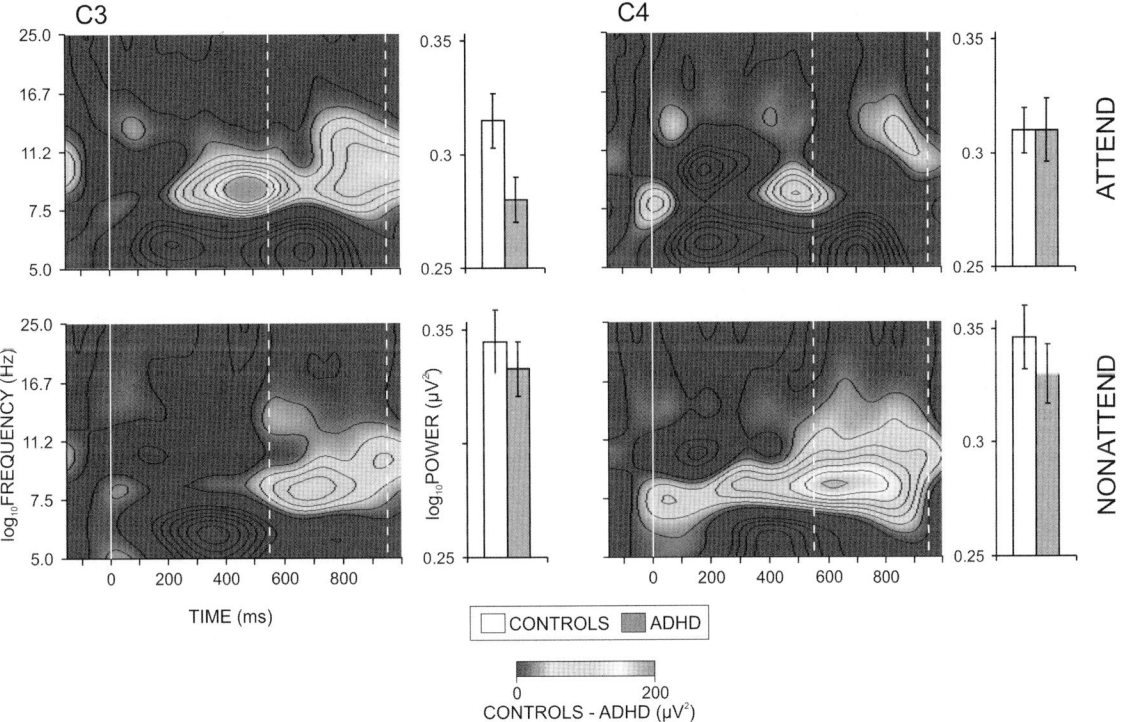

Fig. 4. The effect of electrode position (C3, C4) on alpha band total power in selective attention task in attend and nonattend conditions for control and ADHD groups. Difference time–frequency plots show the grand average total power of ADHD children subtracted from the grand average total power of controls for attended (upper row) and nonattended (lower row) stimuli at C3 and C4. Positive values in the analyzed epoch (marked with white dash lines) indicate controls > ADHD. Bar graphs present group mean values. It is demonstrated that in contrast to controls, children with ADHD reduced alpha (mu) activity more strongly at C3 than C4 following a stimulus in the attended channel. (For color figures, please refer to the color figures in last section of the book.)

The power of the spontaneous 8–12 Hz activity (Appendix) was analyzed at nine electrodes (left, midline, and right for frontal, central, and parietal areas). After being log10 transformed, power values were subjected to a group × lead analysis of variance with repeated measures. No significant main effect of group or group × lead interaction was found ($p > 0.3$). For the two groups, 8–12 Hz activity in the spontaneous EEG was maximal parietally and minimal frontally (lead, $F (1/26) = 39.1$, $p < 0.001$).

18.6. Discussion and conclusions

The present study tested if previously found deviations in the functional reactivity of event-related theta and gamma oscillations in children with ADHD are associated with overactivation of motor cortical regions during an auditory selective attention task. The major suggestion has been that deficient motor inhibition in ADHD would increase the excitability of not only motor generation networks but also networks involved in sensory and cognitive evaluation of motor-related stimuli (Yordanova et al., 2001, 2006).

Analyses of 8–12 Hz power at motor cortical regions demonstrated that in the two groups, mu activity was markedly reduced during and following response generation after target-attended stimuli. This observation confirms the validity of the analysis parameter (Bender et al., 2005) and indicates that motor generation produces comparable levels of activation of the motor cortices in healthy subjects and children with ADHD. A second observation was that the activation of motor cortical regions as reflected by mu power suppression was not overall greater in ADHD than healthy children, nor was there a general sustained overactivation of the left motor cortex (contralateral to response) in ADHD as compared to controls. Together, these results imply that it may not be an unspecific increase in motor cortical excitability that affects the reactivity of sensorimotor or

cognitive–motor networks during stimulus information processing in ADHD.

Instead, the present results demonstrate that mu activity was specifically reduced in ADHD after stimuli that did not require motor response by possessing only partial target features. These were attended nontargets sharing the spatial characteristics and unattended targets sharing the physical characteristics of the motor-related targets. Since no greater mu reduction was obvious in ADHD for either attended targets or unattended nontargets, the presence of conflict Go and NoGo features in complex stimuli appears efficient to trigger motor cortical activation in ADHD. As indicated by control analyses, processing of simultaneous Go and NoGo features of an auditory stimulus also is accompanied by increased cortical activation of frontal cortical regions in ADHD patients, pointing to an abnormal involvement of a larger anteriorly distributed network possibly regulating conflict processing (Ullsperger and Von Cramon, 2001; Albrecht et al., 2008). Analysis of the spontaneous 8–12 Hz EEG verifies that these effects may not be due to between-group differences in the background oscillatory activity.

Further, when the Go feature was based on internally focused spatial attention, the suppression of mu activity in ADHD was greater at the left motor regions reflecting an overactivation of motor-related networks in the hemisphere contralateral to the responding hand. Hence, increased activity of the reacting motor cortex is a plausible source of modulation of theta and gamma responses in children with ADHD (Yordanova et al., 2001, 2006). However, as the present results suggest, such a motor cortical overactivation is produced by a deficient functional control by spatial attention networks rather than unspecific enhancement of motor neuron excitability. This notion is consistent with previous laterality studies of ADHD demonstrating increased right-hemisphere contribution and left-hemisphere deficits during early stage or basic forms of lateralized information processing (Hale et al., 2005,

2006, 2010). It is also consistent with models for ADHD according to which right-hemisphere fronto-parietal attention networks subserving attention re-orienting and bilateral spatial attention networks are deficient in ADHD (Epstein et al., 1997; Nigg et al., 1997; Bellgrove et al., 2009; Chan et al., 2009), as well as models according to which processing strategies during active cognition in ADHD are determined by visual/spatial and motoric neural systems (Fassbender and Schweitzer, 2006).

It is notable that at the behavioral level, no laterality performance deficits were detected for ADHD children. As reported in Yordanova et al. (2001), reaction time and error rate did not differentiate healthy children and ADHD patients depending on the side of attention. Thus, event-related theta, alpha, and gamma oscillations help reveal covert alterations in sensory, cognitive, and motor processing in children with ADHD, which can be associated with abnormal modulation of motor cortical activation by attention control systems.

18.7. Appendix

18.7.1. Task procedure

In each of the two recording conditions, a total of 240 auditory stimuli were used. Two stimulus types were presented randomly to the left and right ear via headphones. The stimuli were nontarget (1000 Hz, $n = 144$, $p = 0.6$) and target (1500 Hz, $n = 96$, $p = 0.4$) tones with a duration of 120 ms, rise/fall time of 10 ms, and intensity of 85 dB sound pressure level. Interstimulus intervals varied randomly from 1150 to 1550 ms. Equal numbers of each stimulus type were presented to the left and right ear. In the first condition, subjects were instructed to press a button in response to the targets presented to the right, while in the second condition, the attended targets were the higher tones presented to the left. Thus, there were four signal types in each series: target–attended (T–A, $n = 48$), target–nonattended (T–A, $n = 48$), nontarget–attended (NT–A, $n = 72$), and nontarget–nonattended (NT–NA, $n = 72$).

18.7.2. Subjects

Within the framework of a multilevel longitudinal study on central nervous regulatory mechanisms and child psychiatric disorders, a total of 28 subjects participated in the experiment. They belonged to two groups (healthy controls vs. ADHD patients, $n = 14$ each), matched for gender, age, and full-scale IQ. Psychopathological characteristics of the two groups are presented in Table A1.

The entire study received prior approval by the local ethical review board. Informed consent was obtained from the parents of each investigated subject. Subjects were totally unmedicated, or drug-free for at least 4 weeks prior to the experiment. Healthy controls were devoid of child psychiatric disorders and gross neurological or other organic disorders. Patients, most of them outpatients, fulfilled the DSM-III-R criteria (American Psychiatric Association, 1987) for ADHD (314.01). Detailed information on psychopathology and level of social functioning according to the Children's Global Assessment Scale (CGAS; Shaffer et al., 1983) was gathered by clinical investigation (including a structured parent interview, several questionnaires, and neuropsychological testing) and pooled to yield solidly based diagnoses by board certified child psychiatrists. For all children, the Child Behavior Checklist (CBCL; Achenbach and Edelbrock, 1983) was used as a screening instrument for child psychiatric symptoms based on parents' reports. The level of hyperactivity was assessed by the 10-item Conners parent questionnaire (Goyette et al., 1978). In addition, the Matching Familiar Figures Test (MFFT; Kagan and Kogan, 1970) was administered to assess cognitive impulse control, which is often a great problem in hyperkinetic children, while the child version of the Leyton Obsessional Inventory (Berg et al., 1986) was used to evaluate

TABLE A1

PSYCHOLOGICAL CHARACTERISTICS OF CHILDREN ACCORDING TO CLINICAL GROUP (MEAN VALUES)

	Group		Controls vs. ADHD
	Controls ($n = 14$)	ADHD ($n = 14$)	
Age (months)			
Mean	137.2	138.2	—
S.D.	21.2	23.4	
SES (low = 1... high = 5)	3.0	3.0	—
IQ (full-scale)			
Mean	105.8	99.4	—
S.D.	10.8	10.8	
Conners (10 items)			
Mean	3.4	19.9	***
S.D.	3.0	3.3	
CBCL t values			
Total	49.4	69.9	***
Externalizing	50.8	74.1	***
Internalizing	49.5	66.6	***
Severity of psychopathology (0–4)	0.2	3.4	***
MFFT			
Time (s)	238.6	148.8	*
Errors	3.0	9.0	***
Leyton			
Total ("yes" answers)	14.0	19.9	*
Resistance	11.4	19.0	*
Interference	11.3	25.9	**
CGAS (0–100)	87.1	46.1	***

— not significant, * $p < 0.05$, ** $p < 0.01$, *** $p < 0.001$.
Significance levels are given for two-tailed Mann–Whitney U tests.
ADHD, attention deficit hyperactivity disorder; SES, socioeconomic status; CBCL, Child Behavior Checklist; MFFT, Matching Familiar Figures Test; CGAS, Children's Global Assessment Scale.

obsessive–compulsive behavior, since such symptoms frequently accompany ADHD (Moll et al., 2000; see also Table A1). All subjects were right-handed, except for two children from each group.

18.7.3. Data recording

EEG activity was recorded via Nihon Kohden Ag/AgCl cup electrodes (impedance kept below 3 kΩ) fixed to the scalp at F3, Fz, F4, C3, Cz, C4, P3, and P4 locations according to the International 10/20 system and referred to the two mastoid electrodes, which were connected via a 10 kΩ resistor (voltage divider, cf., Nunez, 1981, pp. 191–193). Spontaneous EEG was registered also at Oz. Vertical and horizontal electro-oculograms (EOGs) were simultaneously recorded from electrodes above and below the right eye and at the outer canthi. Reaction time data were collected as behavioral measures.

The EEG and EOG signals were amplified and filtered with cutoff frequencies of 0.03 and 120 Hz for EEG channels, and 0.03 and 70 Hz for EOG channels. Analysis epochs of 150 ms before and 1000 ms after stimulus onset were sampled with a frequency of 500 Hz. Epochs contaminated with ocular or muscle artifacts were rejected, with only traces lower than 200 μV peak-to-peak being accepted. Next, slight horizontal and vertical eye movements preserved in the accepted trials were corrected by means of a linear regression method for EOG correction (Dumais-Huber and Rothenberger, 1992).

18.7.4. Data analysis

18.7.4.1. Spontaneous alpha band EEG activity

The spontaneous alpha activity was evaluated for artifact-free EEG epochs of 20 s recorded while the subjects were relaxing with closed eyes. The 20-s epochs were divided into 10 time windows of 2 s duration each. Each 2-s epoch was transformed to the frequency domain by means of Fast Fourier Transform (FFT). Afterward, averaging in the frequency domain was performed to increase statistical validity of frequency-domain measures. Alpha power was measured as the mean value in the frequency range of 8.1–12.1 Hz for each subject and electrode. Power values were log10-transformed to normalize the distributions.

18.7.4.2. Time–frequency analysis of event-related alpha activity

To analyze alpha power changes to the four stimulus types, time–frequency (TF) decomposition of single sweeps was performed. TF analysis was done by means of a continuous wavelet transform (CWT; Mallat, 1999) with Morlet wavelets as basis functions. Here, the TF energy was analyzed using a modification of a method described in, for example, Tallon-Baudry et al. (1997). Complex Morlet wavelets w can be generated in the time domain for different frequencies, f, according to the equation:

$$w(t,f) = A\exp\left(-t^2/2\sigma_t^2\right)\exp(2i\pi ft)$$

where t is time, $A = \left(\sigma_t\sqrt{\pi}\right)^{-1/2}$, σ_t is the wavelet duration, and $i = \sqrt{-1}$. For analysis, a ratio of $f_0/\sigma_f = 5$ was used, where f_0 is the central frequency and σ_f is the width of the Gaussian shape in the frequency domain. The analysis was performed in the frequency range 5–25 Hz with a central frequency at 0.5 Hz intervals. For different f_0, time and frequency resolutions can be calculated as $2\sigma_t$ and $2\sigma_f$, respectively, where σ_t and σ_f are related by the equation $\sigma_t = 1/(2\pi\sigma_f)$. For example, for $f_0 = 10$ Hz, $2\sigma_t = 160$ ms and $2\sigma_f = 4$ Hz.

For each trial, the time-varying power was calculated, which was obtained by squaring the absolute value of the convolution of the signal with the complex wavelet. For 8–12 Hz range, frequency-relevant TF power was extracted with central frequency $f_0 = 10.08$ Hz. The mean TF power was measured within the time window 550–950 ms after stimulus presentation. A time window of 150 ms prior to the stimulus was used to estimate background activity. The mean of this baseline epoch was subtracted from the TF power measures at each time point of the analysis epoch. For statistical analysis, TF power was log10-transformed to normalize the distributions.

References

Achenbach, T. and Edelbrock, C. (1983) *Manual for the Child Behavior Checklist and Revised Child Behavior Profile*. Department of Psychiatry, University of Vermont, Burlington, VT.

Albrecht, B., Brandeis, D., Uebel, H., Heinrich, H., Mueller, U.C., Hasselhorn, M., Steinhausen, H.C., Rothenberger, A. and Banaschewski, T. (2008) Action monitoring in boys with attention-deficit/hyperactivity disorder, their nonaffected siblings, and normal control subjects: evidence for an endophenotype. *Biol. Psychiatry*, 64: 615–625.

American Psychiatric Association (1987) *Diagnostic and Statistical Manual DSM-III-R*, 3rd Rev. Edn. American Psychiatric Association, Washington, DC.

Banaschewski, T. and Brandeis, D. (2007) Annotation: what electrical brain activity tells us about brain function that other techniques cannot tell us — a child psychiatric perspective. *J. Child Psychol. Psychiatry*, 48: 415–435.

Barry, R.J., Clarke, A.R. and Johnstone, S.J. (2003a) A review of electrophysiology in attention-deficit/hyperactivity disorder. I. Qualitative and quantitative electroencephalography. *Clin. Neurophysiol.*, 114: 171–183.

Barry, R.J., Johnstone, S.J. and Clarke, A.R. (2003b) A review of electrophysiology in attention-deficit/hyperactivity disorder. II. Event-related potentials. *Clin. Neurophysiol.*, 114: 184–198.

Barry, R.J., Clarke, A.R., McCarthy, R. and Selikowitz, M. (2007) EEG coherence in children with attention-deficit/hyperactivity disorder and comorbid oppositional defiant disorder. *Clin. Neurophysiol.*, 118: 356–362.

Barry, R.J., Clarke, A.R., McCarthy, R. and Selikowitz, M. (2009) EEG coherence in children with attention-deficit/hyperactivity disorder and comorbid reading disabilities. *Int. J. Psychophysiol.*, 71: 205–210.

Barry, R.J., Clarke, A.R., Hajos, M., McCarthy, R., Selikowitz, M. and Dupuy, F.E. (2010) Resting-state EEG gamma activity in children with attention-deficit/hyperactivity disorder. *Clin. Neurophysiol.*, 121: 1871–1877.

Başar, E. (1980) *EEG Brain Dynamics. Relation between EEG and Brain Evoked Potentials.* Elsevier, Amsterdam.

Başar, E. (1998) *Brain Oscillations: Principles and Approaches. Brain Function and Oscillations,* Vol. 1. Springer, Berlin.

Başar, E. and Güntekin, B. (2008) A review of brain oscillations in cognitive disorders and the role of neurotransmitters. *Brain Res.*, 1235: 172–193.

Başar, E., Yordanova, J., Kolev, V. and Başar-Eroğlu, C. (1997) Is the alpha rhythm a control parameter for brain responses? *Biol. Cybern.*, 76: 471–480.

Başar, E., Schürmann, M. and Sakowitz, O. (2001) The selectively distributed theta system: functions. *Int. J. Psychophysiol.*, 39: 197–212.

Bellgrove, M.A., Barry, E., Johnson, K.A., Cox, M., Dáibhis, A., Daly, M., Hawi, Z., Lambert, D., Fitzgerald, M., McNicholas, F., Robertson, I.H., Gill, M. and Kirley, A. (2008) Spatial attentional bias as a marker of genetic risk, symptom severity, and stimulant response in ADHD. *Neuropsychopharmacology*, 33: 2536–2545.

Bellgrove, M.A., Johnson, K.A., Barry, E., Mulligan, A., Hawi, Z., Gill, M., Robertson, I. and Chambers, C.D. (2009) Dopaminergic haplotype as a predictor of spatial inattention in children with attention-deficit/hyperactivity disorder. *Arch. Gen. Psychiatry*, 66: 1135–1142.

Bender, S., Weisbrod, M., Bornfleth, H., Resch, F. and Oelkers-Ax, R. (2005) How do children prepare to react? Imaging maturation of motor preparation and stimulus anticipation by late contingent negative variation. *Neuroimage*, 27: 737–752.

Berg, C., Rapoport, J. and Flament, M. (1986) The Leyton obsessional inventory — child version. *J. Am. Acad. Child Adolesc. Psychol.*, 25: 84–91.

Chan, E., Mattingley, J.B., Huang-Pollock, C., English, T., Hester, R., Vance, A. and Bellgrove, M.A. (2009) Abnormal spatial asymmetry of selective attention in ADHD. *J. Child Psychol. Psychiatry*, 50: 1064–1072.

Clarke, A.R., Barry, R.J., McCarthy, R. and Selikowitz, M. (1998) EEG analysis in attention-deficit/hyperactivity disorder: a comparative study of two subtypes. *Psychiatry Res.*, 81: 19–29.

Clarke, A.R., Barry, R.J., McCarthy, R. and Selikowitz, M. (2001) Electroencephalogram differences in two subtypes of attention-deficit/hyperactivity disorder. *Psychophysiology*, 38: 212–221.

Clarke, A.R., Barry, R.J., Irving, A.M., McCarthy, R. and Selikowitz, M. (2011) Children with attention-deficit/hyperactivity disorder and autistic features: EEG evidence for comorbid disorders. *Psychiatry Res.*, 185: 225–231.

Dumais-Huber, C. and Rothenberger, A. (1992) Psychophysiological correlates of orienting, anticipation, and contingency changes in children with psychiatric disorders. *J. Psychophysiol.*, 6: 225–239.

Dykman, R., Holcomb, P., Oglesby, D. and Ackerman, P. (1982) Electrocortical frequencies in hyperactive, learning-disabled, mixed, and normal children. *Biol. Psychiatry*, 17: 675–685.

Epstein, J.N., Conners, C.K., Erhardt, D., March, J.S. and Swanson, J.M. (1997) Asymmetrical hemispheric control of visual-spatial attention in adults with attention deficit hyperactivity disorder. *Neuropsychology*, 11: 467–473.

Fassbender, C. and Schweitzer, J.B. (2006) Is there evidence for neural compensation in attention deficit hyperactivity disorder? A review of the functional neuroimaging literature. *Clin. Psychol. Rev.*, 26: 445–465.

Ford, J.M., Krystal, J.H. and Mathalon, D.H. (2007) Neural synchrony in schizophrenia: from networks to new treatments. *Schizophr. Bull.*, 33: 848–852.

Goyette, C.H., Conners, C.K. and Ulrich, R.F. (1978) Normative data on revised Conners parent and teacher rating scales. *J. Abnorm. Child Psychol.*, 6: 221–236.

Hale, T.S., McCracken, J.T., McGough, J.J., Smalley, S.L., Phillips, J.M. and Zaidel, E. (2005) Impaired linguistic processing and atypical brain laterality in adults with ADHD. *Clin. Neurosci. Res.*, 5: 255–263.

Hale, T.S., Zaidel, E., McGough, J.J., Phillips, J.M. and McCracken, J.T. (2006) Atypical brain laterality in adults with ADHD during dichotic listening for emotional intonation and words. *Neuropsychologia*, 44: 896–904.

Hale, T.S., Smalley, S.L., Dang, J., Hanada, G., Macion, J., McCracken, J.T., McGough, J.J. and Loo, S.K. (2010) ADHD familial loading and abnormal EEG alpha asymmetry in children with ADHD. *J. Psychiatr. Res.*, 44: 605–615.

Heinrich, H., Moll, G.H., Dickhaus, H., Kolev, V., Yordanova, J. and Rothenberger, A. (2001) Time-on-task analysis using wavelet networks in an event-related potential study on attention-deficit hyperactivity disorder. *Clin. Neurophysiol.*, 112: 1280–1287.

Herrmann, C.S. and Demiralp, T. (2005) Human EEG gamma oscillations in neuropsychiatric disorders. *Clin. Neurophysiol.*, 116: 2719–2733.

Johnson, K.A., Dáibhis, A., Tobin, C.T., Acheson, R., Watchorn, A., Mulligan, A., Barry, E., Bradshaw, J.L., Gill, M. and Robertson, I.H. (2010) Right-sided spatial difficulties in ADHD demonstrated in continuous movement control. *Neuropsychologia*, 48: 1255–1264.

Kagan, J. and Kogan, N. (1970) Individual variation in cognitive processes. In: P.H. Mussen (Ed.), *Carmichael's Manual* of Child Psychology, 3rd Edn. Wiley, New York, pp. 273–365.

Lazzaro, I., Gordon, E., Whitmont, S., Plahn, M., Li, W., Clarke, S., Dosen, A. and Meares, R. (1998) Quantified EEG activity in adolescent attention deficit hyperactivity disorder. Clin. Electroencephalogr., 29: 37–42.

Lazzaro, I., Gordon, E., Li, W., Lim, C., Plahn, M., Whitmont, S., Clarke, S., Barry, R., Dosen, A. and Meares, R. (1999) Simultaneous EEG and EDA measures in adolescent attention deficit hyperactivity disorder. Int. J. Psychophysiol., 34: 123–134.

Lenz, D., Krauel, K., Schadow, J., Baving, L., Duzel, E. and Herrmann, C.S. (2008) Enhanced gamma-band activity in ADHD patients lacks correlation with memory performance found in healthy children. Brain Res., 1235: 117–132.

Lenz, D., Krauel, K., Flechtner, H.H., Schadow, J., Hinrichs, H. and Herrmann, C.S. (2010) Altered evoked gamma-band responses reveal impaired early visual processing in ADHD children. Neuropsychologia, 48: 1985–1993.

Mallat, S. (1999) A Wavelet Tour of Signal Processing (2nd Edn.). Academic Press, San Diego.

Matoušek, M., Rasmussen, P. and Gilberg, C. (1984) EEG frequency analysis in children with so-called minimal brain dysfunction and related disorders. Adv. Biol. Psychiatry, 15: 102–108.

Matsuura, M., Okubo, Y., Toru, M., Kojima, T., He, Y., Hou, Y., Shen, Y. and Lee, C. (1993) A cross-national EEG study of children with emotional and behavioural problems: a WHO collaborative study in the Western Pacific region. Biol. Psychiatry, 34: 52–58.

Moll, G.H., Eysenbach, K., Woerner, W., Banaschewski, T., Schmidt, M.H. and Rothenberger, A. (2000) Quantitative and qualitative aspects of obsessive–compulsive behaviour in children with attention-deficit hyperactivity disorder compared with tic disorder. Acta Psychiatr. Scand., 101: 389–394.

Monastra, V.J. (2008) Quantitative electroencephalography and attention-deficit/hyperactivity disorder: implications for clinical practice. Curr. Psychiatry Rep., 10: 432–438.

Nigg, J.T., Swanson, J.M. and Hinshaw, S.P. (1997) Covert visual spatial attention in boys with attention deficit hyperactivity disorder: lateral effects, methylphenidate response and results for parents. Neuropsychologia, 35: 165–176.

Nunez, P.L. (1981) Electric Fields of the Brain: The Neurophysics of EEG. Oxford University Press, New York, pp. 191–193.

Roessner, V., Banaschewski, T., Uebel, H., Becker, A. and Rothenberger, A. (2004) Neuronal network models of ADHD — lateralization with respect to interhemispheric connectivity reconsidered. Eur. Child Adolesc. Psychiatry, 13: 71–79.

Rossini, P.M., Rossi, S., Babiloni, C. and Polich, J. (2007) Clinical neurophysiology of aging brain: from normal aging to neurodegeneration. Prog. Neurobiol., 83: 375–400.

Rothenberger, A. (Ed.) (1982) Event-related Potentials in Children. Elsevier Biomedical Press, Amsterdam.

Rothenberger, A. (Ed.) (1990) The Role of the Frontal Lobes in Child Psychiatric Disorders. Springer, Berlin.

Rothenberger, A. (2009) Brain oscillations forever — neurophysiology in future research of child psychiatric problems. J. Child Psychol. Psychiatry, 50: 79–86.

Sergeant, J. (2000) The cognitive-energetic model: an empirical approach to attention-deficit hyperactivity disorder. Neurosci. Biobehav. Rev., 24: 7–12.

Shaffer, D., Gould, M.S., Brasic, J., Ambrosini, P., Fisher, P., Bird, H. and Aluwahlia, S. (1983) A children's global assessment scale (CGAS). Arch. Gen. Psychiatry, 40: 1228–1231.

Swanson, J., Castellanos, F.X., Murias, M., La Hoste, G. and Kennedy, J. (1998) Cognitive neuroscience of attention deficit hyperactivity disorder and hyperkinetic disorder. Curr. Opin. Neurobiol., 8: 263–271.

Tallon-Baudry, C., Bertrand, O., Delpuech, C. and Permier, J. (1997) Oscillatory gamma-band (30–70 Hz) activity induced by a visual search task in humans. J. Neurosci., 17: 722–734.

Tannock, R. (1998) Attention deficit hyperactivity disorder: advances in cognitive, neurobiological, and genetic research. J. Child Psychol. Psychiatry, 39: 65–99.

Ullsperger, M. and Von Cramon, D.Y. (2001) Subprocesses of performance monitoring: a dissociation of error processing and response competition revealed by event-related fMRI and ERPs. Neuroimage, 14: 1387–1401.

Woerner, W., Rothenberger, A. and Lahnert, B. (1987) Test–retest reliability of spectral parameters of the resting EEG in a field sample: a 5 year follow-up in schoolchildren with and without psychiatric disturbances. Electroencephalogr. Clin. Neurophysiol. Suppl., 40: 629–632.

Yordanova, J. and Kolev, V. (1996) Brain theta response predicts P300 latency in children. NeuroReport, 8: 277–280.

Yordanova, J. and Kolev, V. (1998) A single-sweep analysis of the theta frequency band during an auditory oddball task. Psychophysiology, 35: 116–126.

Yordanova, J. and Kolev, V. (2008) Event-related brain oscillations in normal development. In: L.A. Schmidt and S.J. Segalowitz (Eds.), Developmental Psychophysiology. Theory, Systems, and Methods. Cambridge University Press, New York, pp. 15–68.

Yordanova, J., Banaschewski, T., Kolev, V., Woerner, W. and Rothenberger, A. (2001) Abnormal early stages of task stimulus processing in children with attention-deficit hyperactivity disorder — evidence from event-related gamma oscillations. Clin. Neurophysiol., 112: 1096–1108.

Yordanova, J., Heinrich, H., Kolev, V. and Rothenberger, A. (2006) Increased event-related theta activity as a psychophysiological marker of comorbidity in children with tics and attention-deficit/hyperactivity disorders. Neuroimage, 32: 940–955.

Yordanova, J., Kolev, V. and Rothenberger, A. (2009) Functional neuroelectric oscillations along the lifespan. J. Psychophysiol., 23: 153–156.

Yordanova, J., Albrecht, B., Uebel, H., Kirov, R., Banaschewski, T., Rothenberger, A. and Kolev, V. (2011) Independent oscillatory patterns determine performance fluctuations in children with attention deficit/hyperactivity disorder. Brain, 134: 1740–1750.

Application of Brain Oscillations in Neuropsychiatric Diseases
(Supplements to Clinical Neurophysiology, Vol. 62)
Editors: E. Başar, C. Başar-Eroğlu, A. Özerdem, P.M. Rossini, G.G. Yener
© 2013 Elsevier B.V. All rights reserved

Chapter 19

Review of delta, theta, alpha, beta, and gamma response oscillations in neuropsychiatric disorders

Erol Başar* and Bahar Güntekin

Brain Dynamics, Cognition and Complex Systems Research Center, Istanbul Kultur University, Istanbul 34156, Turkey

ABSTRACT

Method and concepts of brain oscillations pervade the neuroscience literature, especially in cognitive processes. Electrophysiological changes in patients with cognitive impairment will provide fundamental knowledge, not only for clinical studies but also, in turn, for understanding cognitive processes in healthy subjects. This review includes description of brain oscillations in schizophrenia, bipolar disorder, mild cognitive impairment, Alzheimer's disease, and attention deficit hyperactivity disorder. The reviewed publications include several methodological approaches: analysis of spontaneous electroencephalogram (EEG) spectra, evoked oscillations, event-related oscillations, and coherences both in spontaneous EEG and event-related oscillations. The review clearly shows that, in cognitive impairment, fundamental changes are observed in all diseases under study. Accordingly, oscillations can most probably be used as biomarkers in clinical studies. The conclusions of this review include several remarks indicating the nature of brain oscillations, their application to cognitive processes, and the usefulness of recording brain oscillations in memory loss, attention deficit, and learning.

KEYWORDS

Electroencephalogram; Event-related potential; Evoked oscillation; Event-related oscillations; Delta; Theta; Alpha; Beta; Gamma; Neuropsychiatric disorder; Schizophrenia; Alzheimer's disease; Mild cognitive impairment; Bipolar disorder; Attention deficit hyperactivity disorder; EEG coherence; Oddball paradigm; Go/No-Go paradigm; N-Back task; Steady-state response; Auditory; Visual; Transcranial magnetic stimulation

19.1. Introduction

Neuroscience has provided us some astonishing breakthroughs, from non-invasive imaging of the human brain to uncovering the molecular mechanisms of some complex processes and disease states. Nevertheless, what makes the brain so special and fundamentally different from all other living tissue is its organized action in time. This temporal domain is where the importance of research on neural oscillators is indispensable in human and animal brains (Başar-Eroğlu et al., 1991; Schürmann et al., 1995, 2000; Demiralp et al., 2001; Başar, 2006, 2010; Buszáki, 2006).

As presented by O'Donnell et al., Vecchio et al., and Yener and Başar (2013, all in this volume), biomarkers are proposed for diagnosis in cognitive

---

*Correspondence to: Prof. Dr. Erol Başar, Director, Istanbul Kultur University, Brain Dynamics, Cognition and Complex Systems Research Center, Istanbul 34156, Turkey.
Tel.: +90 212 498 43 92; Fax: +90 212 498 45 46;
E-mail: e.basar@iku.edu.tr

impairment. A preparative review was published in 2008 (Başar and Güntekin, 2008), during the intervening 4 years, the number of reports has increased considerably. However, reviews are written only on schizophrenia and mostly centered on the gamma window; the present review therefore aims to fill this gap.

In the coming sections, we will discuss results related to schizophrenia (SZ), Alzheimer's disease (AD), mild cognitive impairment (MCI), bipolar disorders (BD), and attention deficit hyperactivity disorder (ADHD). At the end of the review a conceptual conclusion and synopsis will be presented.

19.2. Schizophrenia

After the first review of brain oscillations in cognitive impairment by Başar and Güntekin (2008), an increasing number of publications appeared in this field. Therefore, in this review we emphasize the new results on schizophrenia. On the other hand, this volume includes two reviews on AD (Spontaneous activity, Vecchio et al., 2013, this volume; Event-related oscillations, Yener and Başar, 2013, this volume).

We have encountered around 10 reviews of evoked/event-related oscillations in schizophrenia patients (Lee et al., 2003a; Herrmann and Demiralp, 2005; Schnitzler and Gross, 2005; Başar and Güntekin, 2008; Uhlhaas et al., 2008; Brenner et al., 2009; Uhlhaas and Singer, 2010; Haenschel and Linden, 2011; Luck et al., 2011; Sun et al., 2011). In these reviews, the authors mostly reviewed research on gamma response oscillations in schizophrenia. The present review differs in that it tries to be more comprehensive, covering all frequencies, and is not restricted to steady-state paradigms. Table 1 provides a chronological overview of studies of schizophrenia patients in different frequency bands (delta, theta, alpha, beta, and gamma) upon application of different stimuli. The text is divided into four sections, reviewing the results of oscillatory dynamics in schizophrenia in different paradigms. In order to present the reviewed studies from two different perspectives,

the table is organized by frequency bands, whereas the text is organized according to paradigms.

The preliminary aim of the present paper was not to review abnormalities in spontaneous electroencephalogram (EEG) of schizophrenic subjects (the reader is referred to Boutros et al., 2008). Instead, the present review aims to review studies on evoked or event-related oscillations. The literature includes several paradigms used to differentiate between healthy subjects and schizophrenic patients by means of evoked/event-related oscillations. These paradigms can be summarized as follows: auditory/visual steady-state stimuli; somatosensory/auditory/visual sensory stimuli; TMS stimuli; and working memory (WM) paradigms such as oddball, Go/No-go, N-back, etc. The following section reviews and discusses the results of studies reported in the literature.

19.2.1. Steady-state auditory/visual evoked oscillations in schizophrenia patients

19.2.1.1. Auditory steady-state evoked oscillations in schizophrenia patients

Several paradigms are used in research of evoked/event-related oscillations in schizophrenia. One of the most commonly used paradigms is auditory/visual steady-state paradigm (Brenner et al., 2009). Most of the auditory steady-state studies used 40-Hz auditory tones. In auditory steady-state studies, schizophrenia patients showed reduced power in 40-Hz responses to 40-Hz auditory tones. Furthermore, schizophrenia patients showed reduction in phase-locking factor (PLF) across trials for 40-Hz response to 40-Hz auditory tones (Kwon et al., 1999; Brenner et al., 2003; Light et al., 2006; Spencer et al., 2008b, 2009; Teale et al., 2008; Vierling-Claassen et al., 2008; Wilson et al., 2008; Krishnan et al., 2009; Maharajh et al., 2010; Hamm et al., 2011; Mülert et al., 2011).

Kwon et al. (1999) demonstrated that schizophrenia patients had selectively reduced averaged evoked EEG power in response to 40-Hz auditory stimulation, but normal power responses to 20- and 30-Hz stimulation. Brenner et al. (2003)

TABLE 1

THE RESULTS OF STUDIES IN SCHIZOPHRENIA PATIENTS IN DIFFERENT FREQUENCY BANDS (DELTA, THETA, ALPHA, BETA, AND GAMMA) UPON APPLICATION OF DIFFERENT PARADIGMS

Schizophrenia	Modality and paradigms	Methods	Results
Delta			
Ergen et al., 2008	Visual oddball paradigm	Evoked power (WT)	Evoked delta activity and P3 amplitude to target stimuli were both reduced significantly in patients with schizophrenia, whereas no such difference was observed for total delta activity
Ford et al., 2008	Auditory oddball	Phase-locking	Reduced delta synchrony in patients
Bates et al., 2009	Go/No-Go	ERS/ERD	Reduced delta activity for task-relevant events in schizophrenia
Doege et al., 2010b	Go/No-Go	Evoked power (WT)	Compared with controls, patients showed reduced evoked delta for correct reject trials
Theta			
Schmiedt et al., 2005	Cognitive and working memory demand	EROs amplitude	Reduced late theta response in all tasks
Ford et al., 2008	Auditory oddball	Phase-locking	Reduced theta synchrony in patients
Pachou et al., 2008	N-back task	Evoked power	Compared with controls, patients showed reduced theta activity at frontal electrode sites
Bates et al., 2009	Go/No-Go	ERS/ERD	Reduced theta activity for task-relevant events in schizophrenia
Haenschel et al., 2009	Working memory task	Evoked and induced power	In controls, evoked activity in theta, alpha, and beta band activity during encoding predicted the number of successfully encoded items. Patients showed reduced evoked activity in these frequency bands
Doege et al., 2010a	Auditory oddball	Phase-locking	SZ patients displayed reduced phase-locked delta and theta responses in comparison to healthy subjects
Doege et al., 2010b	Go/No-Go	Evoked power (WT)	Compared with controls, patients displayed less evoked theta for correct hit trials; and less evoked delta and theta for correct reject trials
Riečanský et al., 2010	Steady-state gamma frequency (40 Hz) photic stimulation	Evoked power; phase-locking	Lower phase-locking in theta (4–8 Hz) frequency over the anterior cortex
Alpha			
Rice et al., 1989; Jin et al., 1990, 1995, 1997, 2000; Wada et al., 1995	Periodic photic stimuli, visual steady state	Evoked power	Schizophrenia patients exhibited reduced power in the alpha frequency range compared to healthy controls

Continued

TABLE 1

THE RESULTS OF STUDIES IN SCHIZOPHRENIA PATIENTS IN DIFFERENT FREQUENCY BANDS (DELTA, THETA, ALPHA, BETA, AND GAMMA) UPON APPLICATION OF DIFFERENT PARADIGMS — CONT'D

Schizophrenia	Modality and paradigms	Methods	Results
Bachman et al., 2008	Match to sample task	ERD/ERS	Schizophrenia patients and their co-twins showed a greater increase in ERS magnitude with increasing memory loads, relative to controls
Başar-Eroğlu et al., 2008	Visual oddball	Evoked power and phase-locking	Neither amplitude enhancement after stimulus onset nor intertrial coherence was generally reduced in patients. Healthy controls elicited maximum early alpha and late theta response over occipital electrode sites, while the maximum response in patients was shifted to anterior electrode locations
Brockhaus-Dumke et al., 2008	Auditory paired-click paradigm	Phase-locking analyses, single-trial amplitudes	Phase-locking of the alpha frequency band was significantly reduced in patients
Başar-Eroğlu et al., 2009	Auditory continuous performance task	Peak-to-peak amplitudes of averaged and single-trial data	Amplitudes from patients were reduced at F_z and C_z locations only for the early time window (0–250 ms) upon non-target stimuli
Ramos-Loyo et al., 2009	Three oddball paradigm tasks (face and facial expression)	Peak-to-peak amplitudes of averaged data, root mean square (RMS)	Grand-averaged alpha oscillations demonstrated higher RMS values in the occipital leads in schizophrenia compared to controls and the opposite over frontal regions
Haenschel et al., 2010	Delayed discrimination task	Phase-locking	Alpha phase-locking increased with working memory (WM) load in both SZ and control subjects. Alpha phase locking was generally reduced in SZ compared to healthy controls
White et al., 2010	Vibrotactile somatosensory task	EEG-fMRI evoked power	In healthy individuals, the strongest component was dominated by alpha oscillations, and was associated with activity in somatosensory regions, the insula, anterior cingulate cortex. In schizophrenia, the strongest component had low alpha power and activity was limited mainly to somatosensory regions
Koh et al., 2011	Auditory oddball	MEG evoked power and inter-trial coherence	SZ patients showed diminished alpha ERD compared with control subjects, alpha inter-trial phase coherence was lower in the SZ patients than ultra-high-risk subjects, and lower in ultra-high-risk subjects than normal control subjects

TABLE 1

THE RESULTS OF STUDIES IN SCHIZOPHRENIA PATIENTS IN DIFFERENT FREQUENCY BANDS (DELTA, THETA, ALPHA, BETA, AND GAMMA) UPON APPLICATION OF DIFFERENT PARADIGMS — CONT'D

Schizophrenia	Modality and paradigms	Methods	Results
Beta			
Spencer et al., 2003	Gestalt stimuli	Phase-locking and phase coherence	Absence of posterior component of 20- to 26-Hz band response in SZ patients. Interhemispheric coherence decreased in patients
Krishnan et al., 2005	Visual steady state	Evoked power	Subjects showed reduced signal power compared to healthy control subjects at higher frequencies (above 17 Hz), but not at 4 and 8 Hz at occipital regions
Uhlhaas et al., 2006	Gestalt stimuli	Phase-locking	Reduced phase synchrony in the beta band (20–30 Hz) in Gestalt perception among schizophrenia patients compared to healthy controls
Pachou et al., 2008	N-back task	Evoked power	Reduced beta band activity in patients, compared to controls, at frontal electrode sites
Barr et al., 2010	N-back task	Evoked power	Reduced frontal β activity at all WM loads was also observed in patients with SZ compared to healthy subjects
Riečanský et al., 2010	Steady-state gamma frequency (40 Hz) photic stimulation	Evoked power; phase-locking	Lower phase-locking in beta (13–24 Hz) frequency over the anterior cortex
Arnfred et al., 2011	Proprioceptive stimulus consisted of an abrupt increase of weight on a hand-held load	Evoked power (WT)	Contralateral evoked beta (latency 90 ms, frequency 21 Hz) oscillations were attenuated in the patient group
Gamma			
Kwon et al., 1999	Auditory steady state	Evoked power	Schizophrenia patients had selectively reduced averaged evoked-EEG power in response to 40-Hz auditory stimulation
Haig et al., 2000	Auditory oddball	Amplitude of EROs	For targets: reduced gamma response at left hemisphere and frontal side; increased gamma response in right hemisphere and parieto-occipital sides. For non-targets: widespread reduction in gamma response
Lee et al., 2001	Auditory oddball	Evoked power	Schizophrenia patients had reduced early evoked gamma amplitude compared to healthy subjects
Brenner et al., 2003	Auditory steady state	Evoked power	SZ patients exhibited lower power in response to steady-state auditory

Continued

308

TABLE 1

THE RESULTS OF STUDIES IN SCHIZOPHRENIA PATIENTS IN DIFFERENT FREQUENCY BANDS
(DELTA, THETA, ALPHA, BETA, AND GAMMA) UPON APPLICATION OF DIFFERENT
PARADIGMS — CONT'D

Schizophrenia	Modality and paradigms	Methods	Results
			stimuli compared to non-psychiatric subjects
Green et al., 2003	Visual masking task	Evoked power	Event-related gamma activity concurrent with backward masking reflected increased gamma activity in healthy subjects but not for SZ patients
Lee et al., 2003b	Auditory oddball	Phase-locking	SZ patients had decreased frontal (gamma-1: − 150 to 150 ms; gamma-2: 200–550 ms), and left hemisphere (gamma-1) synchrony. Increased posterior synchrony (gamma-2: 200–550 ms)
Gallinat et al., 2004	Auditory oddball	Evoked power (WT)	In response to standard stimuli, early evoked gamma-band responses (20–100 ms) did not show significant group differences. Schizophrenic patients showed reduced evoked gamma-band responses in a late latency range (220–350 ms), particularly after target stimuli
Hong et al., 2004	Auditory steady state	Evoked power	Patients, as a group, did not significantly differ from controls; patients taking new generation antipsychotics had significantly enhanced 40-Hz synchronization compared to patients taking conventional antipsychotics
Slewa-Younan et al., 2004	Auditory oddball	Phase-locking	Chronic schizophrenia subjects showed lower gamma phase synchrony compared to healthy subjects. This reduction was most apparent in chronic female patients
Spencer et al., 2004	Gestalt stimuli	Evoked power (WT)	Negative symptoms correlated with decreased gamma responses, whereas a significant increase in gamma amplitudes was observed during positive symptoms such as hallucinations
Johannesen et al., 2005	Auditory click	Evoked power	Reduced gamma power in the response following the first auditory click
Wynn et al., 2005	Backward masking task	Evoked power	Patients showed overall lower gamma activity
Symond et al., 2005	Auditory oddball	Phase-locking	Schizophrenia patients showed decreased magnitude and delayed latency for global gamma-1 (0–150 ms) synchrony in relation to healthy comparison subjects

TABLE 1

THE RESULTS OF STUDIES IN SCHIZOPHRENIA PATIENTS IN DIFFERENT FREQUENCY BANDS
(DELTA, THETA, ALPHA, BETA, AND GAMMA) UPON APPLICATION OF DIFFERENT
PARADIGMS — CONT'D

Schizophrenia	Modality and paradigms	Methods	Results
			By contrast, there were no group differences in gamma-2 (200–550 ms) synchrony
Cho et al., 2006	Stimulus–response compatibility task	Evoked power	Controls, but not patients, showed increased induced gamma band activity for the incongruent condition
Light et al., 2006	Auditory steady state	Evoked power and phase-locking	Reduced evoked power and phase-synchronization in response to 30–40 Hz stimulation
Başar-Eroğlu et al., 2007	N-back task	ERO amplitude	High-amplitude gamma oscillations remained constant in patients, regardless of task difficulty
Bucci et al., 2007	Auditory	Gamma power event-related coherence	Induced gamma power and event-related coherence was observed in patients with non-deficit schizophrenia, but not in those with deficit schizophrenia
Ferrarelli et al., 2008	Participants underwent 3–5 TMS/high-density EEG sessions at various TMS doses	Amplitude, synchronization, and source localization	Relative to healthy controls, schizophrenia patients had a marked decrease in evoked gamma oscillations that occurred within the first 100 ms after TMS, particularly in a cluster of electrodes located in a fronto-central region
Flynn et al., (2008)	Auditory oddball	Phase-locking	In first-episode patients, gamma-phase synchrony was generally increased during auditory oddball task processing, especially over left centro-temporal sites in 800 ms poststimulus time window
Pachou et al., 2008	N-back task	Evoked power	Compared to controls, patients showed reduced activity at temporal sites in the gamma band
Roach and Mathalon, 2008	Auditory oddball	phase-locking	The results showed prominent gamma band phase-locking at frontal electrodes between 20 and 60 ms following tone onset in healthy controls that was significantly reduced in patients with schizophrenia
Spencer et al., 2008a	Visual and auditory oddball tasks. Standard stimuli were analyzed	Evoked power and phase-locking (WT)	Visual evoked gamma oscillation phase-locking at occipital electrodes was reduced in SZ compared with HC. In contrast, auditory evoked gamma oscillation phase-locking and evoked power did not differ between groups

Continued

310

TABLE 1

THE RESULTS OF STUDIES IN SCHIZOPHRENIA PATIENTS IN DIFFERENT FREQUENCY BANDS (DELTA, THETA, ALPHA, BETA, AND GAMMA) UPON APPLICATION OF DIFFERENT PARADIGMS — CONT'D

Schizophrenia	Modality and paradigms	Methods	Results
Spencer et al., 2008b	20, 30, and 40 Hz binaural click trains	Evoked power; phase-locking (WT)	At 40-Hz stimulation, SZ patients had significantly reduced phase-locking compared with healthy controls. Evoked power at 40 Hz was also reduced in patients compared with HC. At 30- Hz stimulation, phase-locking and evoked power were reduced in patient groups
Teale et al., 2008	Steady-state auditory tones	MEG phase-locking; mean evoked and induced amplitude	Schizophrenic subjects showed reduced phase-locking in both hemispheres. For the pure tone stimulus, only the left hemisphere PLFs in the transient window were reduced. In contrast, subjects with schizophrenia exhibited higher induced 40 Hz power in response to both stimulus types, consistent with the reduced PLF findings
Vierling-Claassen et al., 2008	Steady-state auditory tones	Evoked power	Reduced 40-Hz, but increased 20-Hz response in SZ patients compared to healthy controls
Haenschel et al., 2009	Working memory task	Evoked and induced power	During the late maintenance period, patients showed an increase in induced gamma band amplitude in response to WM load 2 and failed to sustain induced gamma band activity for the highest WM load
Krishnan et al., 2009	Steady-state auditory tones from 5 to 50 Hz	Evoked power; phase-locking factor	Patients with SZ showed broad-band reductions in both PLF and MP. Induced gamma (around 40 Hz) response to unmodulated tone stimuli was also reduced in SZ
Spencer et al., 2009	Steady-state auditory tones (40 Hz)	Evoked power; phase-locking (WT)	Phase-locking factor (PLF) and evoked power were reduced in SZ at fronto-central electrodes. Left hemisphere source PLF in SZ was positively correlated with auditory hallucination symptoms, and was modulated by delta phase
Barr et al., 2010	N-back task	Evoked power	SZ patients showed increased evoked frontal gamma oscillatory activity that was most pronounced in the 3-back compared to healthy subjects
Leicht et al., 2010	Auditory reaction task	Evoked power (WT)	Patients with schizophrenia showed a significant reduction of power

TABLE 1

THE RESULTS OF STUDIES IN SCHIZOPHRENIA PATIENTS IN DIFFERENT FREQUENCY BANDS
(DELTA, THETA, ALPHA, BETA, AND GAMMA) UPON APPLICATION OF DIFFERENT
PARADIGMS — CONT'D

Schizophrenia	Modality and paradigms	Methods	Results
			and phase-locking of the early auditory evoked GBR
Oribe et al., 2010	Speech sounds and pure tones	MEG evoked power (WT)	SZ subjects showed delayed evoked oscillations and phase-locking to speech sounds specifically in the left hemisphere
Maharajh et al., 2010	Steady-state auditory tones (40 Hz)	MEG, source localization, spatial and temporal filtering	Results indicated reduced phase-synchronization of the ASSR and the stimulus reference signal in SZ patients compared to control subjects, in addition to reduced inter-hemispheric phase synchronization between contralateral and ipsilateral hemispheric responses in SZ patients
White et al., 2010	Vibrotactile somatosensory task	EEG-fMRI evoked power	In the healthy group, but not the patients, significant correlation was observed between the strongest component and evoked gamma power
Başar-Eroğlu et al., 2011	Auditory sensory and auditory oddball	Evoked power (WT)	At the single-trial level, auditory stimuli elicited higher gamma responses at both anterior and occipital sites in patients with schizophrenia compared to controls. In patients with schizophrenia, target detection compared to passive listening to stimuli was related to increased single-trial gamma power at frontal sites
Hall et al., 2011	Auditory oddball	Evoked power	Reduced event-related gamma power during an auditory oddball task in schizophrenia patients and their unaffected identical twins
Hamm et al., 2011	Steady-state auditory tones	MEG inter-trial phase coherence	Schizophrenia patients had reduced gamma response to 40-Hz stimuli in right hemisphere. SZ showed normal beta range ASSRs (20 Hz) but reduced gamma range entrainment bilaterally at the harmonic (40 Hz)
Lenz et al., 2011	Auditory oddball	Evoked power (WT)	Schizophrenic patients presented decreased gamma power in both deviant and target stimuli compared to healthy participants
Mülert et al., 2011	Steady-state auditory tones	SLoreta	The major finding was reduced phase synchronization in schizophrenia only

Continued

312

TABLE 1

THE RESULTS OF STUDIES IN SCHIZOPHRENIA PATIENTS IN DIFFERENT FREQUENCY BANDS (DELTA, THETA, ALPHA, BETA, AND GAMMA) UPON APPLICATION OF DIFFERENT PARADIGMS — CONT'D

Schizophrenia	Modality and paradigms	Methods	Results
			between the left and right primary auditory cortex. A positive correlation between auditory hallucination symptom scores and interhemispheric phase synchronization was present only for primary auditory cortices
Sharma et al., 2011	Choice–reaction task	Event-related coherence	Reduced event-related coherence in SZ patients during time intervals (0–250 ms poststimulus)

The results are reviewed in chronological order.
ASSR = auditory steady-state response; ERD = event-related desynchronization; ERS = event-related synchronization; MEG = magnetoencephalography; MP = mean power; PLF = phase-locking factor; SZ = schizophrenia; WM = working memory; TMS = transcranial magnetic stimulation; WT = wavelet transform.

subsequently analyzed auditory steady-state responses (ASSRs) in a combined group of 21 subjects with schizophrenia or schizoaffective disorder, 11 subjects with schizotypal personality disorder, and 22 non-psychiatric comparison subjects. The authors reported that the schizophrenia and schizoaffective disorder groups exhibited decreased power compared to the schizotypal personality disorder and non-psychiatric comparison groups. Accordingly, the authors concluded that deficit may reflect less efficient local neural synchronization to external stimuli in the sensory cortex or in thalamic-sensory oscillations.

Light et al. (2006) analyzed schizophrenia patients ($n = 100$) and non-psychiatric subjects ($n = 80$) undergoing auditory steady-state event-related potential testing. They also found that patients had reductions in both evoked power and phase synchronization in response to 30- and 40-Hz stimulation, but a normal response to 20-Hz stimulation. Light et al. (2006) concluded that schizophrenia patients have frequency-specific deficits in the generation and maintenance of coherent gamma-range oscillations, reflecting a fundamental degradation of the basic integrated neural network activity.

Spencer et al. (2008b) included 16 first-episode schizophrenia patients, 16 first-episode affective disorder patients (13 with BD), and 33 healthy control subjects. The study used 20-, 30-, and 40-Hz binaural click trains as stimuli and analyzed ASSR phase-locking and evoked power. It was reported that, at 40-Hz stimulation, schizophrenia patients and affective disorder patients had significantly reduced phase-locking compared with healthy control subjects. This deficit was more pronounced over the left hemisphere in schizophrenia patients. Evoked power at 40 Hz was also reduced in the patients compared with healthy controls. At 30-Hz stimulation, phase-locking and evoked power were reduced in both patient groups. The 20-Hz ASSR did not differ between groups, but phase-locking and evoked power of the 40-Hz harmonic of the 20 Hz ASSR were reduced in both schizophrenia patients and affective disorder patients. Phase-locking of this 40-Hz harmonic was correlated with total positive symptoms in schizophrenia patients.

Spencer et al. (2009) further analyzed 40-Hz ASSRs in schizophrenia patients. These authors examined whether the 40-Hz auditory ASSR generated in the left primary auditory cortex was positively correlated with auditory hallucination symptoms in schizophrenia. They reported that left hemisphere source PLF in schizophrenia was positively correlated with auditory hallucination symptoms and was modulated by delta phase.

Accordingly, the results of Spencer et al. (2008b, 2009) and of other groups (Teale et al., 2008; Oribe et al., 2010) suggest that the reduction in 40-Hz auditory steady-state evoked power of schizophrenia subjects may be more pronounced for the left hemisphere generators. Oribe et al. (2010) reported that schizophrenia subjects showed delayed evoked neural oscillations and phase-locking to speech sounds, specifically in the left hemisphere.

Krishnan et al. (2009) obtained steady-state event-related oscillations to amplitude modulated tones from 5 to 50 Hz (5 Hz steps) in subjects with schizophrenia (SZ) and healthy control subjects. These authors used time–frequency spectral analysis to differentiate EEG activity synchronized in phase across trials using PLF and mean power. These authors reported that schizophrenia patients showed broad-band reductions in both PLF and mean power. In addition, control subjects showed a more pronounced increase in PLF with increases in power compared to SZ subjects. Accordingly, these authors concluded that reduction of the PLF along with reduced mean power may reflect abnormalities in the auditory cortical circuits, such as a reduction in pyramidal cell volume, spine density, and alterations in GABAergic neurons.

Studies analyzing steady-state responses indicate reduction of gamma response oscillations not only in EEG but also in MEG. Teale et al. (2008) analyzed magnetoencephalographic (MEG) recordings to estimate the phase and amplitude behavior

of sources in primary auditory cortex in both hemispheres of schizophrenic and comparison subjects. These authors evaluated both ipsi- and contralateral cases using a driving (40-Hz modulated, 1-kHz carrier) and a non-driving (1-kHz tone) stimulus. Schizophrenic subjects showed reduced PLF and evoked source strength for contralateral generators responding to the driving stimulus in both hemispheres. For the pure tone stimulus, only the left hemisphere PLFs in the transient window were reduced. In contrast, subjects with schizophrenia exhibited higher induced 40-Hz power in response to both stimulus types, consistent with the reduced PLF findings.

Maharajh et al. (2010) used whole head MEG to detect ASSR from both hemispheres in SZ patients and control counterparts. The results indicated reduced phase synchronization of the ASSR and the stimulus reference signal in SZ patients compared to control subjects, in addition to reduced interhemispheric phase synchronization between contralateral and ipsilateral hemispheric responses in SZ patients. In a recent paper, Hamm et al. (2011) demonstrated that schizophrenia patients had reduced MEG gamma response to 40-Hz stimuli in the right hemisphere. Furthermore, SZ showed normal beta range ASSRs (20 Hz) but reduced gamma range entrainment bilaterally at the harmonic (40 Hz). Wilson et al. (2008) had also reported that gamma power was significantly weaker and peaked later in adolescents with psychosis relative to their normally developing peers. However, it should be noted that not all the patients in their study were schizophrenia patients. The authors used a mixed subject group with psychosis (three patients diagnosed with schizoaffective disorder, three with bipolar I disorder, and four schizophrenia patients).

Although most studies on auditory steady state stimuli indicated reduced gamma responses, Hong et al. (2004) reported some contradictory results. These authors tested a group of first-degree relatives of schizophrenic probands with schizophrenia spectrum personality symptoms,

314

and a group of schizophrenic patients, to examine whether individuals with increased tendency towards schizophrenia have reduced gamma synchronization. These authors reported that relatives with schizophrenic spectrum personality symptoms had reduced power at 40-Hz synchronization compared to normal controls. Previous findings of reduced steady-state gamma band synchronization in schizophrenic patients were not directly replicated in their study. Patients as a group did not significantly differ from controls, but patients taking new generation antipsychotics had significantly enhanced 40-Hz synchronization compared to patients taking conventional antipsychotics.

19.2.1.2. Visual steady-state evoked oscillations in schizophrenia patients

To our knowledge, the first study of visual steady-state responses in schizophrenia patients was conducted by Rice et al. (1989). These authors reported that subjects with schizophrenia exhibited reduced power in the alpha frequency range upon application of periodic photic stimuli. The results of Rice et al. (1989) were subsequently supported by those of Jin et al. (1990, 1995, 1997) and Wada et al. (1995). Jin et al. (1995) showed that visual steady-state response reduction in schizophrenia occurred at higher alpha frequencies (12.5 Hz) and not at lower alpha frequencies (9.375 Hz). Further, these authors reported that group differences were primarily located in the mid-frontal, central, and parietal areas. Temporal and lateral frontal lobe alpha remained the same in the two groups. Jin et al. (2000) later showed that schizophrenia subjects showed reduced power at 10, 11, and 12 Hz in all regions except centro-temporal regions when evaluating the harmonics in the alpha frequency range.

Clementz et al. (2008) presented a visual target detection task and reported that, for both schizophrenia and healthy subjects, attending to specific parts of the attended image enhanced brain activity related to attended bars and reduced activity evoked by unattended bars.

Krishnan et al. (2005) evaluated the visual steady-state response for seven different frequencies of stimulation (4, 8, 17, 20, 23, 30, and 40 Hz) using a sinusoidally modulated high-luminance stimulus. These authors found that schizophrenia subjects showed reduced signal power compared to healthy control subjects at higher frequencies (above 17 Hz), but not at 4 and 8 Hz in the occipital region.

Riečanský et al. (2010) analyzed phase-locking of neural responses in schizophrenia upon application of steady-state gamma frequency (40 Hz) photic stimulation. Compared with healthy control subjects, patients showed higher phase-locking of early evoked activity in the gamma band (36–44 Hz) over the posterior cortex, but lower phase-locking in theta (4–8 Hz), alpha (8–13 Hz), and beta (13–24 Hz) frequencies over the anterior cortex.

Among the visual steady-state studies in schizophrenia, only Krishnan et al. (2005) and Riečanský et al. (2010) employed a frequency higher than 30 Hz. Krishnan et al. (2005) reported no significant difference between patients and healthy subjects upon application of photic driving at 40 Hz photic stimuli. However, Riečanský et al. (2010) indicated that, compared with healthy control subjects, patients showed higher phase locking of early evoked activity in the gamma band (36–44 Hz) over the posterior cortex. In their study, Riečanský et al. (2010) suggested that this difference was due to the different methodology used in these two different studies. In the study of Riečanský et al. (2010), significant group differences were observed only in a short time period following the onset of visual stimulation, whereas Krishnan et al. (2005) did not analyze the temporal dynamics of the evoked oscillations.

19.2.2. Somatosensory/auditory/visual sensory evoked oscillations in schizophrenia patients

Studies that tested early phase-locked gamma activity in response to simple visual stimuli in schizophrenia patients reported no difference (Wynn et al., 2005) or a decrease (Spencer et al., 2008a) in comparison to healthy subjects. Spencer et al. (2008a) analyzed the phase locking evoked by standard stimuli in visual and auditory oddball task in schizophrenia patients and healthy matched controls. The authors reported reduced gamma phase-locking in visual paradigm. Spencer et al. (2008a) further reported that auditory evoked gamma response was not abnormal in schizophrenia, which was consistent with the finding of Gallinat et al. (2004) that auditory evoked sensory gamma response did not differ between healthy individuals and unmedicated, mainly first-episode schizophrenia subjects. These two studies suggested that auditory sensory evoked gamma response is generally not affected in schizophrenia. Başar-Eroğlu et al. (2011) investigated gamma oscillations during auditory sensory processing and reported that averaged gamma response did not differ between schizophrenia and healthy controls. However, at the single-trial level, auditory stimuli elicited higher gamma responses at both anterior and occipital sites in patients with schizophrenia compared to controls.

Başar Eroğlu et al. (2008) used a simple visual evoked potential and a visual oddball paradigm to investigate discrepancies in various frequency components in patients with schizophrenia. They found that patients showed higher alpha post-stimulus amplitude enhancement and phase coupling than healthy controls in the early time windows for all conditions (VEPs, non-target, and target) at fronto-central sites, whereas the healthy group only showed this effect over occipital locations.

White et al. (2010) analyzed evoked alpha and gamma power in schizophrenia patients upon application of a vibrotactile somatosensory task. The authors reported that, in schizophrenia patients, the strongest component had low alpha power and activity was limited mainly to somatosensory regions.

Arnfred et al. (2011) analyzed proprioceptive beta and gamma responses in schizophrenia patients and healthy controls. They demonstrated that, when hand posture was disturbed by increased load, the schizophrenia patients demonstrated generally attenuated amplitude of contralateral high frequency (18–45 Hz) activity in the 40- to 120-ms latency range. On the other hand, frontal beta activity in the 100- to 150-ms time period and lower frequency range (14–24 Hz) did not differ across any of the groups.

According to the results discussed above, it seems that visual oscillatory deficits might be a general phenomenon in schizophrenia independent of task and stimulus type, as concluded by Spencer et al. (2008a). On the other hand, it should also be noted that there are few studies analyzing pure sensory stimulation. The results of Gallinat et al. (2004) and Spencer et al. (2008a) used standard stimuli in an oddball task to investigate sensory networks. However, standard stimuli in an oddball task could have required cognitive functions. Further research is needed with pure visual and auditory sensory stimuli to reach more robust conclusions.

19.2.3. The applications of transcranial magnetic stimulation–EEG combination in schizophrenia research

Transcranial magnetic stimulation (TMS) studies in patients with schizophrenia (Daskalakis et al., 2002; Fitzgerald et al., 2002, 2003) demonstrated deficits in cortical inhibition in the motor cortex. There is evidence that repetitive transcranial magnetic stimulation (rTMS) is an efficient method in the treatment of negative symptoms of schizophrenia (Cohen et al., 1999; D'Alfonso et al., 2002; Hoffman et al., 2003; Jandl et al., 2005; Jin et al., 2006; Fitzgerald et al., 2008; Schneider et al., 2008; Freitas et al., 2009; Přikryl, 2011).

Studies comparing schizophrenia patients with healthy controls upon application of a combined TMS–EEG method were begun very recently. Jin et al. (2006) hypothesized that frontal lobe rTMS with individualized stimulus rate at subjects' peak alpha EEG frequency (8–13 Hz) would be most effective as a treatment (αTMS). These authors reported that individualized αTMS demonstrated a significantly larger therapeutic effect than the other three conditions (3 Hz, 20 Hz, sham stimulus). Furthermore, these clinical improvements were found to be correlated with increases in frontal alpha amplitude following αTMS. Accordingly, Jin et al. (2006) concluded that their results affirm that the resonant features of alpha frequency EEG play an important role in the pathophysiology of schizophrenia.

Ferrarelli et al. (2008) stimulated the premotor cortex in schizophrenia patients and healthy comparison subjects and analyzed the TMS-evoked EEG activity. These authors reported delayed and reduced amplitude and synchronization of gamma oscillations in schizophrenia patients within the first 100 ms, especially in a fronto-central region.

Farzan et al. (2010) analyzed the TMS-evoked EEG activity in schizophrenia patients compared to bipolar disordered patients and healthy subjects. The authors stimulated the dorsolateral prefrontal cortex (DLPFC) of all subjects groups. It was demonstrated that the inhibition of gamma oscillations was significantly reduced in DLPFC of schizophrenia patients compared to bipolar disordered patients and healthy subjects. Furthermore, there were no differences in inhibition of other oscillatory frequencies in the DLPFC or in the motor cortex between groups.

Barr et al. (2011) analyzed the effect of 20-Hz rTMS on gamma oscillatory activity elicited during the N-back task in schizophrenia patients and healthy controls. The authors performed their experiment over 2 testing days. On the first day, subjects performed the N-back test while their EEG was recorded. One week later, the authors administered rTMS over the DLPFC; 20 min after the rTMS administration, EEG was recorded upon application of N-back task. Consistent with their previous findings (Barr et al., 2009), the authors reported that patients with schizophrenia elicited excessive frontal gamma and reduced frontal beta oscillatory activity compared to healthy subjects prior to rTMS. Following rTMS, excessive frontal gamma oscillatory activity in schizophrenia patients was significantly reduced. Furthermore, rTMS reduced delta activity in patients only (Barr et al., 2011).

These studies seem to be important for future research on combinations of TMS–EEG methods. Important clues may exist within EEG research on schizophrenia. The reduction of different EEG frequencies may help to identify better treatment strategies in the TMS research. In future, studies of individualized gamma TMS could also provide important improvements in treatment.

19.2.4. Evoked/event-related oscillations upon application of WM paradigms in schizophrenia patients

19.2.4.1. Application of oddball paradigm

Haig et al. (2000) examined gamma response amplitudes upon application of auditory oddball stimuli in medicated schizophrenics and healthy controls. Significant differences were observed between groups in the amplitude of the second poststimulus peak in gamma activity in targets. The results indicated amplitude reduction of gamma response oscillations in schizophrenia patients compared to healthy controls over the left hemisphere in frontal sites and an increase in the right hemisphere and parieto-occipital sites. There were no significant between-group differences in the first gamma peak, which occurred around stimulus onset.

The results of Gallinat et al. (2004) were in good accordance with Haig et al. (2000). These authors found that, in response to standard stimuli, early evoked gamma band responses (GBRs) (20–100 ms) did not show significant between-group differences. However, schizophrenic patients showed reduced evoked GBRs in a late latency range (220–350 ms), particularly after target stimuli. This deficit occurred over the right frontal scalp regions.

Slewa-Younan et al. (2004) reported that chronic schizophrenia subjects showed lower late gamma phase synchrony compared to healthy subjects during auditory oddball task processing. This reduction was most apparent in female patients. Furthermore, analysis of early gamma phase synchrony indicated that chronic schizophrenia subjects showed lower early gamma phase synchrony compared to healthy subjects over the left hemisphere. First-episode female patients showed a faster latency of early gamma activity when compared to first-episode male patients. This study showed the importance of testing for gender-based differences in subject responses. Gender differences in evoked oscillations exist even in simple visual sensory stimulation in healthy subjects, as reported previously by Güntekin and Başar (2007a). Gender difference in evoked oscillations was also shown in different modalities (Güntekin and Başar, 2007b; Jaušovec and Jaušovec, 2009a,b, 2010). Comparing chronic SZ patients versus first-episode SZ patients also may provide important findings. Furthermore, several studies demonstrated the importance of including two time periods in the analysis of gamma band (early gamma, late gamma) (Haig et al., 2000; Lee et al., 2001; Gallinat et al., 2004; Slewa-Younan et al., 2004; Symond et al., 2005; Başar-Eroğlu et al., 2009; Lenz et al., 2011).

Symond et al. (2005) used a conventional auditory oddball paradigm to study 40 first-episode schizophrenia patients and 40 age- and sex-matched healthy controls. The authors then examined the magnitude and latency of both early (gamma-1: −150 to 150 ms post stimulus) and late (gamma-2: 200 to 550 ms post stimulus) synchrony with multiple analysis of variance. First-episode schizophrenia patients showed a decreased magnitude and delayed latency for global gamma-1 synchrony in relation to the healthy comparison subjects. In contrast, there were no group differences in gamma-2 synchrony.

Reinhart et al. (2011) investigated the relation between prestimulus gamma band activity, reaction times and P300 amplitude upon application of an auditory oddball paradigm. The authors reported that, in healthy controls, the single-trial prestimulus gamma power was positively correlated with reaction times. Furthermore, in healthy controls, average P300 amplitude was positively correlated with average, prestimulus gamma power; however, in schizophrenia patients, neither reaction times nor P300 amplitude were related to prestimulus gamma power. Accordingly, the authors concluded that their results suggested a breakdown in the preparatory brain state in schizophrenia patients.

Başar-Eroğlu et al. (2011) investigated evoked gamma oscillations upon application of auditory oddball paradigm. These authors found that, in patients with schizophrenia, the target detection compared to passive listening to stimuli was related to increased single-trial gamma power at frontal sites. Furthermore, averaged gamma response did not differ between schizophrenia and healthy controls. Accordingly, the authors emphasized the importance of considering single-trial gamma response analysis.

Ford et al. (2008) showed that P300 amplitude and delta and theta synchrony were reduced in schizophrenia patients upon application of auditory oddball paradigm. Delta power and synchrony were better distinguished between groups than the P300 amplitude. In healthy controls, but not in the patient group, gamma synchrony predicted P300 amplitude.

Roach and Mathalon (2008) compared the degree of phase-locking of the GBR in 22 healthy controls and 21 medicated patients with schizophrenia upon application of auditory oddball task. The results showed prominent gamma band phase-locking at frontal electrodes between 20 and 60 ms following tone onset in healthy controls that was significantly reduced in patients with schizophrenia. Flynn et al. (2008) reported that, in first-episode patients, gamma phase synchrony was generally increased during auditory oddball task processing, especially over left centro-temporal sites in the 800-ms post-stimulus time window. On the other hand, Hall et al. (2011)

reported that schizophrenia patients and their unaffected identical co-twins exhibited significantly reduced EAGBR power compared with control subjects upon application of auditory oddball paradigm. Lenz et al. (2011) investigated evoked gamma oscillations upon application of passive auditory oddball paradigm in three different patient groups (schizophrenia, mood disorder, personality disorders) and in healthy participants. Their results showed that only schizophrenic patients presented decreased amplitude in both deviant and target stimuli compared to healthy participants, whereas no significant differences were observed between healthy participants and the other psychiatric groups.

Ergen et al. (2008) investigated delta response oscillations in schizophrenic and matched healthy control subjects upon the application of visual oddball tasks. The authors analyzed the evoked (phase-locked) and total (phase-locked and non-phase-locked) delta responses. Evoked delta activity and P3 amplitude to target stimuli were both reduced significantly in patients with schizophrenia, whereas no such difference was obtained for the total delta activity. The authors concluded that the significant reduction of the evoked delta response and the absence of such a difference in the total delta response of schizophrenia patients indicated that the delta band response is weakly phase-locked to stimulus in schizophrenia. Furthermore, this result suggests that the reduced P3 amplitudes in the averaged ERPs of schizophrenia patients result from a temporal jitter in the activation of neural circuits engaged in P3 generation (Ergen et al., 2008). On the other hand, increased delta and theta oscillatory activity in spontaneous EEG and MEG were reported by Begic et al. (2000) and Fehr et al. (2001, 2003) in schizophrenia patients compared to healthy controls.

Başar-Eroğlu et al. (2008) analyzed theta and alpha response oscillations in schizophrenia patients upon application of visual oddball paradigm. Neither the amplitude enhancement after stimulus onset nor the intertribal coherence were generally reduced in patients. However, healthy controls elicited their maximum early alpha and late theta response over occipital electrode sites, while the maximum response in patients was shifted to anterior electrode positions. The authors further commented that their results imply that not only temporal, but also regional coordination dysfunctions appear to be of importance even under simple tasks conditions, such as VEPs and non-target processing.

Ramos-Loyo et al. (2009) evaluated event-related oscillations during emotional recognition of happiness and fear compared to facial identity recognition in schizophrenic patients versus healthy controls. Subjects performed three oddball paradigm tasks, evaluating face identity recognition and facial emotional recognition of happiness and fear. The authors analyzed the event-related theta and alpha oscillations for each task and reported that theta oscillations showed significantly lower RMS values in schizophrenia patients between 250- and 500-ms poststimuli in frontal and central regions.

19.2.4.2. Application of Go/No-Go, N-back task, Gestalt stimuli

Although most of the studies on evoked/event-related oscillations in schizophrenia research on WM were performed upon application of oddball paradigms, there are also some studies that used other memory paradigms. The results of these studies are described in the following paragraphs.

Bates et al. (2009) examined event-related evoked and induced delta and theta activity in 17 people with schizophrenia and 17 healthy controls in two Go/No-Go task variants. Their results revealed that SZ patients exhibited less evoked and induced delta and theta responses. Doege et al. (2010a,b) also examined evoked delta and theta oscillations in schizophrenia patients and healthy controls in a Go/No-Go task. In accordance with the results of Bates et al. (2009), these authors reported that, compared with controls, patients displayed less evoked theta for correct hit trials and less evoked delta and theta for correct reject trials.

Schmiedt et al. (2005) focused on event-related changes in poststimulus theta oscillatory activity during three N-back task levels in healthy controls and schizophrenia patients. The results showed significant WM load and rule switching-related increases of poststimulus theta amplitude at fronto-central locations in controls. In patients with schizophrenia, there were generally reduced late theta responses in all tasks and at all locations.

Cho et al. (2006) analyzed evoked gamma response upon application of stimulus–response compatibility task. Their results showed that controls, but not patients, showed increased induced gamma band activity for the incongruent condition, which correlated with performance. Başar-Eroğlu et al. (2007) investigated the modulation of event-related gamma responses in tasks varying the WM load in schizophrenia patients and healthy controls. Gamma amplitude values were obtained for a simple choice–reaction task, a low WM demand task, and a high WM demand task. A gradual increase in gamma amplitudes after stimulus onset was associated with an increase in WM load in controls. In contrast, high amplitude gamma oscillations remained constant in patients, regardless of task difficulty.

Consistent with Başar-Eroğlu et al. (2007), Barr et al. (2010) reported that SZ patients generated increased evoked frontal gamma oscillatory activity that was most pronounced in the 3-back compared to healthy subjects. The authors also reported a reduction in beta oscillatory activity in schizophrenia patients. In contrast, Pachou et al. (2008) reported reduced gamma activity in patients, as compared to controls, at temporal electrode sites upon application of the N-back task. Furthermore, these authors reported reduced activity in both theta and beta bands in patients, as compared to controls, at frontal electrode sites. Haenschel et al. (2009) demonstrated that patients show reduced evoked theta, alpha, and beta oscillatory activity during WM encoding upon presentation of a delayed discrimination task that

probes load effects in visual WM. In a recent study, Heanschel et al. (2010) reported that both patients and healthy controls demonstrated an increase in alpha phase-locking with WM load. However, they also reported that patients differed from control subjects, in that they showed generally reduced levels of alpha phase-locking over frontal and occipital electrode sites. On the contrary, Bachman et al. (2008) demonstrated that schizophrenia patients and their co-twins were found to display a larger increase in event-related synchronization (ERS) magnitude with increasing memory loads, relative to controls. Recently, Koh et al. (2011) reported that schizophrenia patients showed diminished alpha event-related desynchronization (ERD) compared with control subjects in an MEG study upon application of auditory oddball paradigm. Furthermore, these authors also showed that alpha inter-trial phase coherence was lower in the schizophrenia patients than the ultra-high-risk subjects, and lower in the ultra-high-risk subjects than the normal control subjects. Abnormal delta and alpha oscillatory responses in SZ patients, compared to healthy controls, were also reported by Ince et al. (2009). Future research is needed to clarify the contradictory results on evoked/event-related alpha responses in WM paradigms.

Spencer et al. (2003) used measures of phase-locking and phase coherence in the EEG to examine the synchronization of neural circuits in schizophrenia patients upon presentation of Gestalt stimuli. Compared with matched control subjects, schizophrenia patients demonstrated an absence of the posterior component of the early visual GBR to Gestalt stimuli. Furthermore, the authors found that the healthy subject group had more coherence increases than the SZ group, particularly in the 20 to 26 Hz frequency range. In accordance with Spencer et al. (2003), Uhlhaas et al. (2006) reported reduced phase synchrony in the beta band (20–30 Hz), in Gestalt perception in schizophrenia patients compared to healthy controls. Green et al. (2003) demonstrated that event-related gamma activity concurrent with backward masking reflected increased gamma activity in healthy subjects but not for SZ patients.

Minzenberg et al. (2010) recorded EEGs of 53 first-episode schizophrenia patients (21 without antipsychotic medication treatment) and 29 healthy control subjects during the performance of a preparatory cognitive control task. Theta power was not impaired in the full patient group nor in the unmedicated patient subgroup. Furthermore, impaired cognitive control-related gamma cortical oscillatory activity was present at the first psychotic episode in schizophrenia and was independent of medication status.

In addition to these studies, which used measures of power, PLF, coherence analysis, etc., there are also measures of functional connectivity in neural networks obtained by graph theory (Micheloyannis et al., 2006; De Vico Fallani et al., 2010). Earlier studies have also documented abnormalities in measures of gamma band power in mental arithmetic task during spontaneous EEG recording in schizophrenia patients compared to healthy controls (Kissler et al., 2000).

Bucci et al. (2007) investigated evoked and induced 40-Hz gamma power as well as frontal–parietal and frontal–temporal event-related coherence in patients with deficit and non-deficit schizophrenia and in matched healthy controls. In patients, correlations between gamma oscillations and psychopathological dimensions were also investigated. A reduction of both induced gamma power and event-related coherence was observed in patients with non-deficit schizophrenia, but not in those with deficit schizophrenia.

It is also important to note that, in schizophrenic patients, negative symptoms correlate with a decrease in gamma responses, whereas a significant increase in gamma amplitudes is observed during positive symptoms such as hallucinations (Baldeweg et al., 1998; Lee et al., 2003b; Ropohl et al., 2004; Spencer et al., 2004, 2008b, 2009; Herrmann and Demiralp, 2005). Mülert et al. (2011) demonstrated positive correlation between auditory hallucination symptom scores and interhemispheric phase synchronization only

for primary auditory cortices, but not for secondary auditory cortices.

19.2.5. General remarks and summary of evoked/event-related studies of schizophrenia

(1) Event-related delta response to WM stimuli (auditory–visual oddball, Go/No-Go) was significantly reduced in patients with schizophrenia compared to healthy subjects (Ergen et al., 2008; Ford et al., 2008; Bates et al., 2009; Doege et al., 2010b; Table 1 and Fig. 1).

(2) Similar to delta, event-related theta response to WM stimuli (auditory–visual oddball, Go/No-Go, N-back task) was also significantly reduced in patients with schizophrenia when compared to healthy subjects (Schmiedt et al., 2005; Ford et al., 2008; Pachou et al., 2008; Haenschel et al., 2009; Doege et al., 2010a). Furthermore, evoked theta response was reduced in visual steady-state responses in schizophrenia patients when compared with healthy controls (see Table 1 and Fig. 1 for details).

(3) Most studies on auditory steady-state evoked gamma responses showed reduced gamma response oscillations in schizophrenia patients compared to healthy controls. To our knowledge, there is only one study in which previous findings of reduced steady-state gamma band synchronization in schizophrenic patients were not directly replicated (Hong et al., 2004). Hong et al. (2004) reported that patients, as a group, did not significantly differ from controls, but patients taking new generation antipsychotics had significantly enhanced 40-Hz synchronization compared to patients taking conventional antipsychotics (see Table 1 and Fig. 1 for details).

(4) Studies on visual steady-state evoked alpha responses indicated reduced alpha response in patients with schizophrenia when compared to healthy subjects. The few studies that analyzed visual evoked gamma steady-state responses (Rice et al., 1989; Jin et al., 1990,

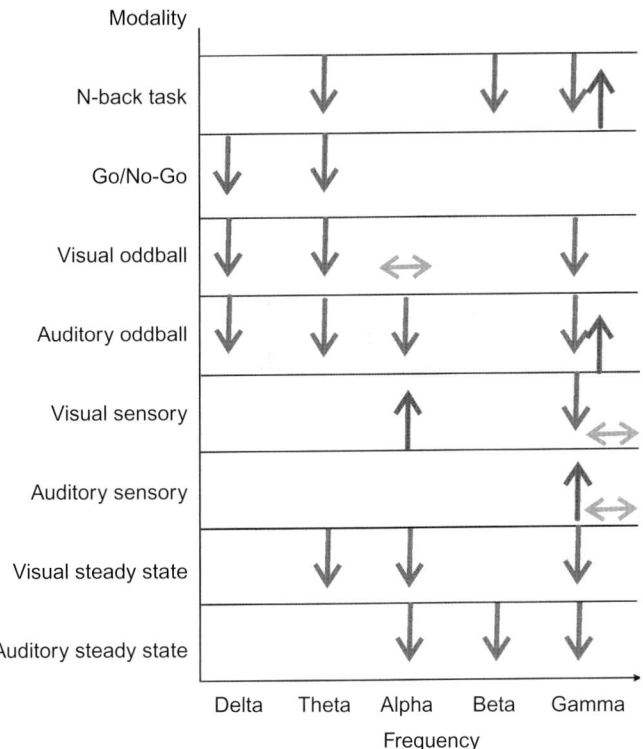

Fig. 1. Summary of evoked/event-related studies in schizophrenia upon application of several paradigms. The summary is based on the results described in Table 1. The "↓" and "↑"signs indicate that the evoked/event-related oscillation is decreased or increased, respectively, in SZ patients for a given paradigm compared to healthy controls. The "↔" sign describes that there is no difference between SZ patients and healthy controls in a given paradigm. (For color figures, please refer to the color figures in last section of the book.)

1995, 1997, 2000; Wada et al., 1995; Krishnan et al., 2005) reported no significant difference between patients and healthy subjects upon application of photic driving at 40-Hz photic stimuli. On the other hand, Riečanský et al. (2010) indicated that, compared with healthy control subjects, patients showed higher phase-locking of early evoked activity in the gamma band (36–44 Hz) over the posterior cortex. Further research is needed for clarification of results on visual steady-state gamma responses.

(5) Spontaneous alpha activity and visual steady-state alpha responses were reported to be reduced in schizophrenia patients compared to healthy controls (Itil et al., 1972, 1974; Iacono, 1982; Rice et al., 1989; Jin et al., 1990, 1995, 1997, 2000; Miyauchi et al., 1990;

Sponheim et al., 1994, 2000; Wada et al., 1995; Alfimova and Uvarova, 2008). However, the results for evoked/event-related alpha responses show contradictory results in WM paradigms. Başar-Eroğlu et al. (2008) reported that neither the amplitude enhancement after stimulus onset nor the inter-trial coherence was generally reduced in patients upon application of a visual oddball paradigm. Later in a different paradigm, Başar-Eroğlu et al. (2009) showed that amplitudes from patients were reduced at Fz and Cz locations only for the early time window (0–250 ms) upon non-target stimuli of auditory continuous performance task. Consistent with the results of Başar-Eroğlu et al. (2009), Koh et al. (2011) reported that the alpha inter-trial phase coherence was lower in schizophrenia patients than in ultra-high-risk subjects, and lower in ultra-high-risk subjects than in normal control subjects upon application of an auditory oddball paradigm. Haenschel et al. (2010) demonstrated that alpha phase-locking was generally reduced in SZ compared to healthy controls upon delayed discrimination task.

(6) Spencer et al. (2003) and Uhlhaas et al. (2006) reported reduced phase synchrony in the beta band in Gestalt perception in schizophrenia patients compared to healthy controls. In healthy controls, beta oscillations were reported to be increased in identification of angry face expression (Güntekin and Başar, 2007c). Beta oscillations seem to have important roles in face recognition and face expression recognition paradigms as well as in other emotional paradigms (IAPS, Güntekin and Başar, 2010b). In future studies, the differences in beta oscillations between schizophrenia subjects and healthy controls in emotional paradigms should also be studied. Evoked/event-related beta responses were also reduced in WM paradigms and auditory steady-state stimuli (Pachou et al., 2008).

(7) In auditory oddball paradigms, previous authors mostly evaluated event-related gamma responses in two different time windows (early and late time window). Some studies showed that early evoked GBRs did not show significant group differences. However, schizophrenic patients showed reduced evoked GBRs in late latency range stimuli (Haig et al., 2000; Gallinat et al., 2004). On the other hand, other studies (Lee et al., 2001; Slewa-Younan et al., 2004; Symond et al., 2005; Lenz et al., 2011) reported that schizophrenia subjects showed lower early gamma phase synchrony compared to healthy subjects. Some studies reported increased gamma response in schizophrenic subjects compared to healthy controls upon application of an auditory paradigm. Başar-Eroğlu et al. (2011) reported that passive listening to stimuli was related to increased single-trial gamma

power at frontal sites. Flynn et al. (2008) reported that, in first-episode patients, gamma phase synchrony was generally increased during auditory oddball task processing, especially over left centro-temporal sites in the 800-ms poststimulus time window. Further research is needed to make robust conclusions on gamma response in auditory oddball paradigm in schizophrenia.

(8) Accordingly, the results by Spencer et al. (2008b, 2009) and other groups (Teale et al., 2008; Oribe et al., 2010) suggest that the reduction in the 40-Hz auditory steady-state evoked power of schizophrenia subjects may be more pronounced for the left hemisphere generators.

(9) The results of the above studies showed that there could be differences between schizophrenia subgroups; therefore, future studies should compare first-episode versus chronic schizophrenia, schizophrenia with positive symptoms versus schizophrenia with negative symptoms, and also medicated versus unmedicated schizophrenia patients to provide clearer results. Furthermore, the effects of gender on event-related oscillations in healthy subjects were observed by Güntekin and Başar (2007a,b), and Jaušovec and Jaušovec (2009a,b, 2010). There are also gender effects on evoked oscillations in schizophrenia patients, as reported by Slewa-Younan et al. (2004). The effects of gender on evoked oscillations in schizophrenia patients should also be analyzed in future studies.

19.3. Bipolar disorder

In terms of EEG in BD, most previous studies analyzed spontaneous EEG or ERP components upon stimulation using different paradigms. However, there are few studies of evoked/event-related oscillation in BD patients compared with the number of studies in schizophrenia. The main aim of the present report was not to review spontaneous EEG or ERP studies in BD; instead, we aimed to review and discuss evoked/event-related oscillation studies of BD (for spontaneous EEG and

ERP in BD, please see the reviews of Degabriele and Lagopoulos (2009) and Onitsuka et al. (2013, this volume)).

Although we did not aim to review spontaneous EEG and ERP research in BD, some important points should be noted before reviewing evoked/event-related oscillations in BD patients. The literature includes several previous investigations of spontaneous EEG, ERP, and spontaneous MEG in bipolar patients (Cook et al., 1986; Dewan et al., 1988; Small et al., 1989, 1998; Gerez and Tello, 1992; Kano et al., 1992; Clementz et al., 1994; Koles et al., 1994; Souza et al., 1995; Schulz et al., 2000; El-Badri et al., 2001; Ikeda et al., 2002; Başar et al., 2012). These studies found generalized slowing, increased delta and theta power. Furthermore, some studies found significant differences in alpha asymmetry in bipolar individuals (Kano et al., 1992; Allen et al., 1993). In comparison with non-bipolar individuals, BD patients showed greater left frontal cortical activation in preparation for the hard/win trials (Harmon-Jones et al., 2008). The degree of resting state long-range synchrony was reduced in manic patients compared to healthy controls in all frequency bands (Bhattacharya, 2001). On the other hand, El-Badri et al. (2001) demonstrated higher power in all frequency bands in bipolar patients compared to healthy subjects. In an MEG study, Chen et al. (2008) reported increased delta synchronization and decreased beta synchronization in the frontal regions of bipolar patients. Clementz et al. (1994) investigated alpha activity (analyzed only C_3, C_z, C_4 electrodes) in a group of bipolar psychosis patients, schizophrenia patients, and their first-degree relatives. EEG data obtained from patients and their first-degree relatives showed that patients with schizophrenia and BD had reduced alpha in comparison to healthy subjects. In a recent study, Başar et al. (2012) analyzed spontaneous alpha activity and evoked alpha response upon presentation of visual sensory stimuli in drug-free euthymic bipolar patients. This study showed that spontaneous EEG alpha power was significantly higher in healthy subjects than euthymic

patients for all electrodes and in both eyes-open and eyes-closed recording sessions.

Furthermore, the most significant differences between groups were found during eyes-closed recording session in occipital electrodes. Visual evoked sensory alpha power of healthy subjects was also significantly higher than visual evoked alpha power of euthymic patients (Başar et al., 2012). Clementz et al. (1994) included a mixed patient group in their study and the bipolar patient group was not all in a euthymic stage and was not all drug-free. In contrast, the patient group in Başar et al. (2012) provides the strongest advantages, making the study unique in the literature. The results of Başar et al. (2012) indicated a reduction in alpha activity in the range of 70% within a group of euthymic patients, compared with healthy controls. This was not observed in earlier studies and can even be considered a breakdown of alpha activity and visual alpha response.

Several studies analyzed P50, N100, and P300 components of ERP in BD compared with healthy controls. Several studies (Olincy and Martin, 2005; Schulze et al., 2007; Sánchez-Morla et al., 2008) reported reduced P50 response in BD patients. Other authors demonstrated that N100 amplitude did not differ between BD patients and healthy controls (O'Donnell et al., 2004b; Force et al., 2008; Fridberg et al., 2009). O'Donnell et al. (2004b) and Schulze et al. (2008) demonstrated that P300 response was delayed in BD patients. Salisbury et al. (1999) reported reduced P300 amplitude in BD patients compared to healthy controls. Controversially, some studies reported that the amplitude of P300 response did not differ between groups (O'Donnell et al., 2004b; Schulze et al., 2008).

19.3.1. Auditory steady-state evoked oscillations in BD patients

The studies analyzing evoked/event-related oscillations in BD used different paradigms: auditory steady-state paradigm (O'Donnell et al., 2004a; Spencer et al., 2008b; Rass et al., 2010), dual-click paradigm (Hall et al., 2011), auditory oddball paradigm (Hall et al., 2011), visual sensory paradigm (Özerdem et al., 2011), visual oddball paradigm (Özerdem et al., 2008, 2010, 2011), and facial expression paradigm (Lee et al., 2010).

O'Donnell et al. (2004a) reported that patients in the manic or mixed state showed reduced power in 20-, 30-, 40-, and 50-Hz activity during click entrainment paradigm. Spencer et al. (2008b) reported reduced phase-locking and reduced evoked power at 30- and 40-Hz stimulation as well as at 40-Hz harmonic of the 20-Hz ASSRs in first-episode affective disorder patients (13 out of the 16 subjects were BD patients) compared to healthy controls. Consistent with O'Donnell et al. (2004a), Spencer et al. (2008b), and Rass et al. (2010) reported reduced auditory steady-state gamma responses in BD patients in a larger sample size (68 BD patients). Furthermore, these authors showed that unmedicated patients showed gamma range phase-locking values comparable to those of control participants. The 40-Hz response was also larger in unmedicated compared to medicated patients (Rass et al., 2010). Reite et al. (2009) demonstrated that BD patients failed to demonstrate normal laterality of steady-state gamma responses in primary auditory cortex.

19.3.2. Evoked/event-related oscillations upon application of WM paradigms in BD patients

To our knowledge, event-related oscillation studies in BD patients upon cognitive load begun with the studies of Özerdem et al. (2008), who reported decreased alpha response but increased beta response to visual target stimuli in manic BD patients compared to healthy controls. Furthermore, the results showed that abnormally increased beta response in BD patients was reduced after valproate monotherapy.

Özerdem et al. (2010) analyzed event-related coherence in response to visual oddball paradigm in a group of medication-free manic BD patients in comparison to healthy controls. The coherence to the target stimuli at the right fronto-temporal location was significantly reduced in BD patients compared to controls. In a subsequent study, Özerdem et al. (2011) analyzed evoked/event-related coherence in response to visual sensory stimuli and visual oddball paradigm in a group of drug-free euthymic patients with BD in comparison to healthy controls. The patients showed bilaterally reduced long-distance event-related gamma-coherence between frontal and temporal as well as frontal and temporo-parietal regions compared to healthy controls. However, no significant sensory evoked coherence reduction was recorded in the patient group compared to the healthy controls. The authors concluded that the occurrence of a large coherence decrease only under cognitive load, but not in response to simple sensory stimuli, was a major finding with regard to cognitive dysfunction across all states of BD (Özerdem et al., 2011). Hall et al. (2011) analyzed gamma response oscillations in BD patients, unaffected relatives of BD patients, and healthy controls upon application of an auditory oddball paradigm and dual-click paradigm. They reported that, although BD patients showed smaller gamma response power to both standard and target stimuli compared to control subjects, these differences were not statistically significant (Hall et al., 2011). On the other hand, upon application of dual-click paradigm, BD patients showed significantly reduced gamma response power. Hall et al. (2011) concluded that evoked gamma response in oddball paradigm did not emerge as an endophenotype for psychotic BD patients.

Lee et al. (2010) investigated the event-related MEG signals in healthy subjects, patients with BD, and patients with major depressive disorder upon application of facial expression stimuli. These authors reported that, compared with healthy controls, BD patients and major depressive disorder patients had decreased gamma response in the frontal and parietal regions. Furthermore, these authors stated that BD patients had increased alpha–beta activities in the bilateral temporal and occipital regions in comparison to healthy controls. Güntekin and Başar (2007c) showed that presentation of angry facial expression stimuli elicited higher occipital alpha and higher frontal beta response in comparison to presentation of happy and neutral facial expression stimuli in healthy subjects. In a recent study, Güntekin and Başar (2010b) demonstrated that, in healthy subjects, unpleasant pictures elicited higher beta response in comparison to pleasant and neutral emotional stimuli. Accordingly, it seems that alpha and beta oscillations are involved in emotional processes. In future, analysis of evoked/event-related oscillations upon application of different emotional paradigms in BD patients could provide important clues to understanding the emotional processes in BD.

Oribe et al. (2010) analyzed evoked oscillations to speech sound in BD patients, schizophrenia patients, and healthy controls. These authors reported that BD patients exhibited higher 20- to 45-Hz evoked oscillations in response to speech sounds compared to healthy subjects and schizophrenia subjects. On the other hand, no significant differences were observed in the response to pure tones among the three groups (Oribe et al., 2010).

Similar to research on schizophrenia, studies of evoked/event-related oscillations in BD patients mainly analyzed gamma response oscillations. The studies analyzing auditory steady-state evoked gamma response showed that BD patients had reduced gamma response upon presentation of auditory steady-state stimuli (O'Donnell et al., 2004a; Spencer et al., 2008b; Rass et al., 2010). These results are very similar to those reported for schizophrenia, in which the schizophrenia patients showed decreased gamma response upon presentation of auditory steady-state stimuli. Auditory steady-state stimuli seem not to be an ideal stimulus in the search for identical differences in evoked/event-related oscillations between schizophrenia and BD patients. The decrease in gamma response oscillations in auditory state stimuli could be a general phenomenon in both psychiatric illnesses. On the other hand, in an auditory oddball paradigm, the gamma response did not reduce in bipolar patients in comparison to healthy subjects (Hall et al., 2011). Although there were no differences in local gamma synchrony between BD patients and healthy controls, there were differences in long-range connections. Özerdem et al. (2010, 2011) showed that BD patients showed reduced long distance event-related gamma coherence upon application of a visual oddball paradigm. Hall et al. (2011) used an auditory oddball paradigm, whereas Özerdem et al. (2010, 2011) used a visual paradigm. Accordingly, in future, analysis of local gamma synchrony in visual oddball paradigm and analysis of long distance gamma coherence in an auditory paradigm are needed. The results of these analyses could clarify the conclusion on gamma response oscillation in BD patients upon cognitive loads (Table 2).

19.4. Mild cognitive impairment and AD

Several spontaneous EEG and MEG studies have shown that AD patients had reduced posterior alpha rhythms when compared to healthy controls and/or amnesic MCI subjects. On the other hand, AD patients had increased delta and theta rhythms when compared to healthy controls and/or amnesic MCI subjects. (Dierks et al., 1993, 2000; Huang et al., 2000; Jelic et al., 2000; Ponomareva et al., 2003; Jeong, 2004; Babiloni et al., 2006). For a review of spontaneous EEG and/or ERP, see Adamis et al. (2005), Rossini et al. (2007), Jackson and Synder (2008), Babiloni et al. (2011), Lizio et al. (2011); and Vecchio et al. (2013); for evoked/event-related oscillations, see Başar and Güntekin (2008), Dauwels et al. (2010), and Yener and Başar (2010).

In recent years, our group published several analyses of evoked/event-related oscillations in AD upon application of sensory and/or cognitive paradigms. Yener et al. (2007) analyzed the phase-locking of theta oscillations upon application of a visual oddball paradigm and reported that an untreated AD group had lower phase-locking in

326

visual event-related theta oscillations than that of controls over the left frontal region. However, the treated AD group showed phase-locking in the theta frequency range, which did not differ from the control group. Polikar et al. (2007) reported decreased delta response (P_z) in AD patients compared to healthy controls upon presentation of auditory oddball paradigm. Consistent with Polikar et al. (2007), Caravaglios et al. (2008) reported decreased single-trial delta response in AD patients compared to healthy controls in F_z, C_z, and P_z electrode sites. In a visual oddball paradigm, Yener et al. (2008) reported that Alzheimer subjects (both treated and untreated groups) had decreased central (C_3, C_z) delta responses in comparison to healthy controls. Furthermore, the

TABLE 2

THE RESULTS OF STUDIES IN BIPOLAR DISORDER PATIENTS IN DIFFERENT FREQUENCY BANDS (ALPHA, BETA, AND GAMMA) UPON APPLICATION OF DIFFERENT PARADIGMS

Bipolar disorder	Modality and paradigms	State of BD	Methods	Results
Alpha, beta, gamma				
O'Donnell et al., 2004a	Auditory steady state	Manic or mixed state	Evoked power	Reduced power in 20-, 30-, 40-, 50-Hz activity in BD patients
Spencer et al., 2008b	Auditory steady state	First-episode affective disorder patients	Phase locking, evoked power	Reduced phase-locking and reduced evoked power at 30- and 40-Hz stimulation as well as at 40-Hz harmonic of the 20-Hz ASSRs
Özerdem et al., 2008	Visual oddball paradigm	Manic BD	Filtered event-related response	Decreased alpha response but increased beta response to visual target stimuli in BD patients. Increased beta response was normalized after valproate monotherapy
Reite et al., 2009	Auditory steady state	Mixed group of medicated and unmedicated euthymic BD	Filtered event-related response	BD patients failed to demonstrate normal laterality of steady-state gamma responses in primary auditory cortex
Rass et al., 2010	Auditory steady state	Mixed group of medicated and unmedicated euthymic and acute BD	Mean trial power, phase locking	BD patients had reduced gamma response Unmedicated patients showed gamma range phase-locking values comparable to those of control participants. Forty hertz was larger in unmedicated compared to medicated patients

TABLE 2

THE RESULTS OF STUDIES IN BIPOLAR DISORDER PATIENTS IN DIFFERENT FREQUENCY BANDS
(ALPHA, BETA, AND GAMMA) UPON APPLICATION OF DIFFERENT PARADIGMS — CONT'D

Bipolar disorder	Modality and paradigms	State of BD	Methods	Results
Özerdem et al., 2010	Visual oddball paradigm	Manic BD	Event-related coherence	The event-related gamma coherence to the target stimuli at the right fronto-temporal location was significantly reduced in BD
Lee et al., 2010	Facial expression paradigm	Medicated euthymic BD	Evoked power	BD patients had decreased gamma response in the frontal and parietal regions. BD patients had increased alpha–beta activities in the bilateral temporal and occipital regions
Hall et al., 2011	Auditory oddball, dual-click paradigm	Mixed group of medicated and unmedicated euthymic and depression BD	Evoked power	BD patients showed significantly reduced gamma response power in response to dual-click paradigm
Özerdem et al., 2011	Visual oddball paradigm	Drug-free euthymic BD	Evoked/event-related coherence	BD patients showed bilaterally reduced long-distance event-related gamma coherence between frontal and temporal as well as frontal and temporo-parietal regions. No significant sensory evoked coherence reduction was recorded between groups
Oribe et al., 2010	Speech sounds	Medicated euthymic BD	MEG phase-locking, evoked power	BD patients exhibited higher 20–45 Hz in response to speech sounds compared to healthy subjects and schizophrenia subjects. No significant differences were observed in the response to pure tones among the three groups
Başar et al., 2012	Sensory visual	Drug-free euthymic BD	Evoked power	BD patients had reduced evoked alpha response

The results are reviewed in chronological order.

authors reported that cholinesterase inhibitors did not have effect on delta oscillatory responses. Significant between-groups differences were revealed at the level of single sweep amplitude at the three midline sites (F_z, C_z, P_z), during target tone processing. Yener et al. (2009) compared visual sensory evoked oscillatory responses of subjects with AD to those of healthy elderly controls elicited by simple light stimuli. The visual evoked oscillatory responses in AD subjects without cholinergic treatment showed significant differences from both controls and AD subjects treated with a cholinesterase inhibitor. Higher theta oscillatory responses in untreated AD subjects were seen on the electrode locations over bi-parietal and right occipital regions after simple light stimuli with less, if any, cognitive load. These changes were restricted to the theta frequency range only and were related to location, frequency bands, and drug effects.

Güntekin et al. (2008) investigated event-related coherence of patients with AD using a visual oddball paradigm. The authors demonstrated that the control group showed higher evoked coherence in the delta, theta, and alpha bands in the left fronto-parietal electrode pairs versus the untreated AD group. The control group showed higher values of evoked coherence in the left fronto-parietal electrode pair in the theta frequency band and higher values of evoked coherence in the right fronto-parietal electrode pair in the delta band when compared to the treated AD group. With a larger patient group, Başar et al. (2010) reported that the healthy control group showed significantly higher values of event-related coherence in delta, theta, and alpha bands in comparison to the de novo and medicated AD groups ($p < 0.01$ for the delta, theta, and alpha) upon application of a target stimuli. In contrast, almost no changes in event-related coherences were observed in beta and gamma frequency bands. Furthermore, no differences were recorded between healthy and AD groups upon application of simple light stimuli. Besides this, coherence values upon application of target stimuli were higher than sensory evoked coherence in all groups and in all frequency bands ($p < 0.01$). Based on the findings of this study, Güntekin and Başar (2010a) subsequently analyzed the evoked/event-related coherences in young healthy subjects upon application of auditory paradigm. In this study, the authors reported that the coherence values to target responses were higher than the non-target and simple auditory response coherence. This difference was significant for the delta coherence for both hemispheres and for theta coherences over the left hemisphere. The results presented in these studies provide evidence for the existence of separate sensory and cognitive networks that are activated either on sensory or cognitive stimulation. Furthermore, the cognitive networks of AD patients were highly impaired, whereas sensory networks activated by sensory stimulation were not impaired in AD patients (Başar et al., 2010).

Karrasch et al. (2006) analyzed ERD and ERS in elderly controls, MCI patients, and mild probable AD patients upon stimulation of an auditory–verbal Sternberg memory task. The authors demonstrated that the elderly control group had significant EEG synchronization in the 3- to 6-Hz and 12- to 14-Hz frequency bands during encoding of the memory set. Although the responses in the 10- to 20-Hz frequencies were characterized by ERS in the control group, the responses were characterized by ERD in the MCI group.

Missonnier et al. (2006) conducted a longitudinal study that analyzed ERS in MCI patients upon application of N-back WM task. They recorded EEG of 24 MCI subjects. On follow-up, 13 MCI subjects showed progressive MCI and 11 MCI subjects remained stable. Their results showed that progressive MCI subjects demonstrated lower theta synchronization in comparison to stable MCI subjects. In a longitudinal study, Deiber et al. (2009) analyzed ERS in MCI patients upon application of the N-back task. There was no significant effect of group or task on global theta activity; however, there were group differences

329

in induced theta activity. The results demonstrated that an early decrease in induced theta amplitude occurred in progressive MCI cases; in contrast, induced theta amplitude in stable MCI cases did not differ from elderly controls.

Cummins et al. (2008) analyzed event-related theta oscillations in MCI patients and elderly healthy controls during the performance of a modified Sternberg word recognition task. Their results demonstrated that MCI subjects exhibited lower recognition interval power than controls at F_3 and C_3 electrodes. Retention interval theta power was also lower in the MCI subjects in comparison to healthy subjects; however, differences during retention were observed at parietal and temporal electrodes.

Babiloni et al. (2005) recorded MEG of AD patients, vascular dementia patients, young and elderly healthy controls upon application of a visual-delayed choice–reaction time task. These authors analyzed event-related alpha desynchronization and reported that the alpha ERD peak had a greater amplitude in the demented patients than in the normal subjects.

Caravaglios et al. (2010) analyzed single-trial theta power responses in two time windows (0–250 ms; 250–500 ms) and then compared the results to prestimulus theta power during both target tone and standard tone processing in AD patients and in elderly healthy controls. AD patients had an increased prestimulus theta power and had no significant poststimulus theta power increase upon both target and non-target stimulus processing. On the other hand, healthy elderly controls had an enhancement of both early and late theta responses relative to the prestimulus baseline only during target tone processing.

Haupt et al. (2008) applied cLORETA to see topological differences between AD patients and healthy controls. They identified topographic differences that differentiate healthy elderly, MCI, and mild AD subjects during early visual processing. Zervakis et al. (2011) analyzed event-related inter-trial coherence in mild probable AD patients and elderly controls upon stimulation of

an auditory oddball paradigm. The authors reported that the theta band in AD patients is reflected in slightly more energy than in controls. The authors further indicated that non-phase-locked late alpha activity is non-existent in AD patients. On the other hand, their study early observed alpha activity only in some AD subjects, which appeared as phase-locked activity. The authors commented that the increased theta in AD patients could be due to drug effects, since all the AD patients included in their study were treated with ACh-esterase inhibitors. Yener et al. (2007) showed that cholinergic treatment modulates theta synchrony and the treated AD group had better synchronization and positive response to medication at left frontal site.

Lou et al. (2011) applied the methods of spatial complexity, field strength, and frequency of field changes to analyze event-related oscillations of vascular dementia patients and healthy controls. Vascular dementia patients showed a significantly higher spatial complexity value in the delta and theta frequency bands. Furthermore, vascular dementia patients had a lower field strength value and a higher field change value in the delta frequency band compared with normal controls.

Missonnier et al. (2010) performed gamma band analysis in MCI patients during the N-back task. Recordings were performed at baseline and at a 1-year follow-up. These authors reported that progressive cognitive decline cases displayed significantly lower average changes in gamma values than the patients remained stable both in detection and 2-back tasks.

Osipova et al. (2006) analyzed 40-Hz auditory steady-state responses in AD patients. These authors demonstrated that the amplitude of the auditory 40-Hz steady-state responses was significantly increased in AD compared to controls. Recently, Van Deursen et al. (2011) reported results consistent with Osipova et al. (2006). A study by Van Deursen et al. (2011) showed a significant increase of 40-Hz SSR power in the AD group compared to MCI and controls. The results by Osipova et al. (2006), Yener et al. (2009), and

Van Deursen et al. (2011) showed that sensory evoked oscillations were higher in AD subjects upon application of sensory stimuli. This could be due to the lack of frontal inhibition on sensory cortical areas in AD patients. As Yener and Başar (2010) discussed in their paper, decreased inhibition of cortical auditory/visual sensory processing, possibly due to decreased prefrontal activity, may lead to increased sensory evoked cortical responses in AD.

Other groups also studied evoked and/or event-related coherence in AD patients upon application of simple stimuli or cognitive stimuli. Hogan et al. (2003) examined memory-related EEG power and coherence over temporal and central recording sites in patients with early AD and normal controls. While the behavioral performance of very mild AD patients did not differ significantly from that of normal controls, the AD patients had reduced upper alpha coherence between the central and right temporal cortex compared with controls. Zheng-yan (2005) stated that, during photic stimulation, inter- and intra-hemispheric EEG coherences of AD patients showed lower values in the alpha (9.5–10.5 Hz) band than those of the control group.

The above-mentioned studies showed that delta responses in AD patients were decreased in comparison to healthy controls upon presentation of cognitive stimuli (Yener et al., 2008). Event-related theta responses were also decreased in AD patients in comparison to healthy controls upon application of several cognitive paradigms (Missonnier et al., 2006; Cummins et al., 2008; Deiber et al., 2009). Yener et al. (2007) demonstrated that untreated AD patients did not have synchronous theta activity in comparison to treated AD patients and healthy controls. Caravaglios et al. (2010) showed that AD patients had increased prestimulus theta power and had no significant post-stimulus theta power increase upon both target and non-target stimulus processing. Several publications reported increased phase-locking of theta oscillatory responses upon presentation of cognitive

load in P300 target paradigm (Başar- Eroğlu et al., 1992; Demiralp et al., 1994; Klimesch et al., 2004). Accordingly, decreased theta responses in AD patients seem to reflect cognitive deficits seen in this group of patients. Decrease in event-related delta and theta coherence (Güntekin et al., 2008; Başar et al., 2010), upon application of cognitive paradigms, showed that not only local connections but also impaired long-range connections could also be represented in brain oscillations.

19.5. Attention deficit hyperactivity disorder

ADHD patients had increased absolute and/or relative delta and theta power, and decreased absolute and/or relative beta and gamma power in comparison to age-matched healthy controls (Dykman et al., 1982; Matoušek et al., 1984; Woerner et al., 1987; Matsuura et al., 1993; Clarke et al., 1998, 2001; Lazzaro et al., 1998, 1999; Barry et al., 2003a,b, 2010; Monastra, 2008). Since the theta activity is increased and beta activity is reduced in ADHD patients, the theta/beta ratio is one of the most important components of abnormal EEG in ADHD patients (see Barry et al., 2003a; Barry and Clarke, 2013, this volume for a review of spontaneous EEG in ADHD patients).

There are few papers analyzing event-related oscillations of ADHD patients. Yordanova et al. (2001) analyzed children with ADHD disorder in auditory task and found larger and more strongly phase-locked GBR than controls only in response to right-side stimuli, irrespective of whether these were the attended or the ignored stimuli. Based on their findings, they concluded that association between auditory GBR and motor task stimulus in children suggests that phase-locked gamma oscillations may reflect processes of sensorimotor integration. Lenz et al. (2008) analyzed EEG of ADHD patients during the encoding phase of a visual memory paradigm. Analysis of evoked GBRs during stimulus encoding revealed a strong task-related enhancement for ADHD patients in parieto-occipital areas. Furthermore, these authors stated that this augmentation was not associated with recognition performance, whereas healthy subjects exhibited a strong positive correlation between evoked gamma activity during stimulus encoding and subsequent recognition performance. The authors commented that ADHD patients had non-specific increased evoked gamma response, but they did not benefit from this increase (Lenz et al., 2008). Later, the same group (Lenz et al., 2010) analyzed evoked gamma response of ADHD patients and healthy controls during application of forced-choice–reaction task. The results showed that only healthy participants showed significantly enhanced evoked gamma response following known items compared to responses evoked by unknown, new pictures. In contrast, ADHD patients failed to show such early differentiation between known and unknown items, as they evoked similar gamma responses in both conditions (Lenz et al., 2010). These three studies indicated impairment in the GBR in ADHD patients compared to controls. In the studies by Yordanova et al. (2001) and Lenz et al. (2008), ADHD patients showed enhanced gamma response in comparison to healthy controls. However, Lenz et al. (2010) showed that GBR was not necessarily enhanced upon presentation of forced-choice–reaction task. As Lenz et al. (2010) concluded, different results in evoked gamma response of ADHD patients may be related to task demands or stimulus complexity.

Yordanova et al. (2006) analyzed early (0–200 ms) and late (200–450 ms) theta responses of ADHD patients and healthy controls upon application of auditory selective attention task. These authors showed that early theta response did not differ between groups. On the other hand, late theta responses were larger in ADHD patients compared to controls. Furthermore, late theta responses in ADHD patients were associated with hyperactivity scores. On the other hand, Groom et al. (2010) investigated evoked theta power and inter-trial phase coherence in ADHD patients and healthy controls upon application of Go/No-Go task. The results of their study revealed that ADHD patients had reduced late theta power and reduced early and late theta inter-trial coherence values. Decrease in theta response in cognitive paradigms was also reported in schizophrenia (Schmiedt et al., 2005; Ford et al., 2008), AD, and MCI (Missonnier et al., 2006; Yener et al., 2007; Cummins et al., 2008; Deiber et al., 2009; Caravaglios et al., 2010). Accordingly, the decrease in theta response seems to be a common phenomenon in different pathologies.

19.6. Concluding remarks

In this manuscript, we have reviewed oscillatory dynamic changes in different pathologies. Some common parameters show impairment in different pathologies (such as decrease in delta response upon cognitive load). On the other hand, there are also some distinct parameters between pathologies. It is difficult to compare different pathologies, since the reviewed studies were performed by different groups and applied different methods and paradigms. Although some groups have compared SZ patients and BP patients, this is made more difficult by the use of different drug therapies in these pathologies. Below, we discuss the common and distinct parameters of evoked/event-related oscillations seen in schizophrenia, BD, Alzheimer, MCI, and ADHD. (Please see Section 19.5 for more detailed concluding remarks for evoked/event-related oscillation studies of schizophrenia patients.)

After reviewing the reports cited in this manuscript, it becomes obvious that the results upon analysis of pathology (cognitive disorders, diseases) and the changes upon medication (which influence the transmitter release) strongly influence the understanding of the cognitive processes. In turn, the establishment of a new framework of cognitive processes is to be expected. Such a framework may include the following features:

(1) Various pathologies cause significant and differentiated changes in the oscillatory dynamics of patients.

    (a) One of the common parameters seen in different pathologies was the decrease in delta activity upon cognitive load. Delta response oscillations were decreased in SZ (Ergen et al., 2008; Ford et al., 2008; Bates et al., 2009; Doege et al., 2010b) and in Alzheimer patients (Yener et al., 2008) upon cognitive load. New studies analyzing event-related delta response in ADHD and bipolar patients are needed to further investigate potential differences between these pathologies.

    (b) Decreased theta responses were also reported in different pathologies upon cognitive load. SZ patients (Schmiedt et al., 2005; Ford et al., 2008; Pachou et al., 2008; Haenschel et al., 2009; Doege et al., 2010a), Alzheimer patients (Missonnier et al., 2006; Yener et al., 2007; Cummins et al., 2008; Deiber et al., 2009; Caravaglios et al., 2010), ADHD patients (Groom et al., 2010), and BP patients (Atagün et al., 2011) had reduced theta responses upon cognitive load.

    (c) Decreased auditory steady-state gamma responses were reported in SZ (Kwon et al., 1999; Brenner et al., 2003; Light et al., 2006; Spencer et al., 2008b, 2009; Teale et al., 2008; Vierling-Claassen et al., 2008; Wilson et al., 2008; Krishnan et al., 2009; Maharajh et al., 2010; Hamm et al., 2011; Mülert et al., 2011) and BP patients (O'Donnell et al., 2004a; Spencer et al., 2008a,b; Rass et al., 2010). On the other hand, increased auditory steady-state gamma responses were reported in AD patients (Osipova et al., 2006; Van Deursen et al., 2011).

    (d) Drug effect on evoked/event-related oscillations. ACh-esterase inhibitors have positive effects on theta phase synchrony (Yener et al., 2007). Özerdem et al. (2008) showed that abnormally increased beta response in BD patients was reduced after valproate monotherapy. The difficulty of including drug-free patients in studies means that it is not possible to compare the drug effects on the evoked/event-related oscillations in different pathologies.

    (e) Although this manuscript reviews evoked/event-related oscillations in different pathologies we have also mentioned some studies of spontaneous EEG research, when relevant. Decreased spontaneous alpha oscillations were reported in SZ, Alzheimer, and BP patients. However, analyzing and comparing the power of spontaneous alpha activity in different pathologies in the same laboratory circumstances could help to identify differences in the alpha activity of these patient groups. One of the important methods in spontaneous EEG research could be the ratio analysis of different oscillations. Since theta activity is increased and beta activity is reduced in ADHD patients, theta/beta ratio is one of the important components of abnormal EEG in ADHD patients (see Barry et al., 2003a). Moretti et al. (2009) indicated that theta/gamma ratio of relative power at peak frequency is significantly associated with memory decline in MCI patients. This method could also be applied to different pathologies in which one frequency is decreased while another is increased.

(2) Medication (modulation of transmitters) can partly reduce the electrophysiological manifestation caused by cognitive impairment of patients. Additionally, medication helps to reduce pathological deformation of electrical signals.

(3) Not just oscillations in a unique frequency window, but also multiple oscillations need to be jointly analyzed for the description of pathological cases. For example, see results

in AD, schizophrenia, and BD (Özerdem et al., Vecchio et al., and Yener and Başar, 2013, in this volume). The release of transmitters also selectively influences brain oscillations (see the first and second gamma and theta windows).

(4) In addition to the analysis of amplitudes of oscillatory responses, a coherence analysis is highly recommended. The latter analysis method helps in the understanding of the *selective connectivity* or the *decrease in connectivity* between distant locations. Sharma et al. (2011) describe the differential connectivity deficit.

(5) With regard to EEG coherence and phase delays: multiple frequency windows in coherence function should be analyzed in order to determine a more accurate picture of the pathology.

(6) The analysis of the *"superposition of oscillations"* is also an extremely relevant tool for the description of oscillatory responses in cognitive processes, both in healthy subjects and those with cognitive disorders.

(7) To obtain a true picture of the oscillation processes in pathology, the frequency analysis has to be performed separately in medicated and non-medicated patients. As the studies of Yener et al. (2008) and Özerdem et al. (2008) show, it is essential to perform analyses separately before and after medication.

(8) According to Bowden (2008), therapy using multiple pharmacological products (polypharmacy) is useful. The selectivity of the oscillatory response can assist in achieving optimal use of medication following the analysis of brain oscillations.

(9) The ambiguity of gamma responses can be better understood using adequate input modalities and also early and late time windows. Accordingly, it is proposed that a standard assessment methodology should be developed for this purpose.

(10) The alpha and beta frequency windows have been neglected in most studies of schizophrenia. As demonstrated by the results of Fehr et al. (2001), Başar-Eroğlu et al. (2008), Ford et al. (2008), and Özerdem et al. (2008), it is obvious that all frequency windows need to be analyzed in all cognitive disorders.

(11) The link between genetics, brain oscillations and transmitters is better understood from the work of Begleiter and Porjesz (2006). This "genetics–brain oscillation concept" will, potentially, form one of the most important areas of research in neuropathology, as this short review shows.

Acknowledgments

The authors are thankful to Elif Tülay and Melis Diktaş for arranging the reference list and overall error finding throughout.

References

Adamis, D., Sahu, S. and Treloar, A. (2005) The utility of EEG in dementia: a clinical perspective. *Int. J. Geriatr. Psychiatry*, 20: 1038–1045.

Alfimova, M.V. and Uvarova, L.G. (2008) Changes in EEG spectral power on perception of neutral and emotional words in patients with schizophrenia, their relatives, and healthy subjects from the general population. *Neurosci. Behav. Physiol.*, 38: 533–540.

Allen, J.J.B., Iacono, W.G., Depue, R.A. and Arbisi, P. (1993) Regional electroencephalographic asymmetries in bipolar seasonal affective disorder before and after exposure to bright light. *Biol. Psychiatry*, 33: 642–646.

Arnfred, S.M., Mørup, M., Thalbitzer, J., Jansson, L. and Parnas, J. (2011) Attenuation of beta and gamma oscillations in schizophrenia spectrum patients following hand posture perturbation. *Psychiatry Res.*, 185(1–2): 215–224.

Atagün, İ., Özerdem, A., Güntekin, B. and Başar, E. (2011) Evoked and event related theta oscillations are decreased in drug-free euthymic bipolar patients. In: *Society of Biological Psychiatry 66th Annual Meeting*, 12–14 May 2011, Hyatt Regency, San Francisco, CA, p. 97S.

Babiloni, C., Cassetta, E., Chiovenda, P., Del Percio, C., Ercolani, M., Moretti, D.V., Moffa, F., Pasqualetti, P., Pizzella, V., Romani, G.L., Tecchio, F., Zappasodi, F. and Rossini, P.M. (2005) Alpha rhythms in mild dements during visual delayed choice reaction time tasks: a MEG study. *Brain Res. Bull.*, 65(6): 457–470.

Babiloni, C., Binetti, G. and Cassetta, E. (2006) Sources of cortical rhythms change as a function of cognitive impairment in pathological aging: a multicenter study. *Clin. Neurophysiol.*, 117(2): 252–268.

Babiloni, C., Vecchio, F., Lizio, R., Ferri, R., Rodriguez, G., Marzano, N., Frisoni, G.B. and Rossini, P.M. (2011) Resting state cortical rhythms in mild cognitive impairment and Alzheimer's disease: electroencephalographic evidence. *J. Alzheimer's Dis.*, 26: 201–214.

Bachman, P., Kim, J., Yee, C.M., Therman, S., Manninen, M., Lönnqvist, J., Kaprio, J., Huttunen, M.O., Näätänen, R. and Cannon, T.D. (2008) Abnormally high EEG alpha synchrony during working memory maintenance in twins discordant for schizophrenia. *Schizophr. Res.*, 103(1–3): 293–297.

Baldeweg, T., Spence, S., Hirsch, S.R. and Gruzelier, J. (1998) Gamma-band electroencephalographic oscillations in a patient with somatic hallucinations. *Lancet*, 352(9128): 620–621.

Barr, M.S., Farzan, F., Rusjan, P.M., Chen, R. and Fitzgerald, P.B. (2009) Potentiation of gamma oscillatory activity through repetitive transcranial magnetic stimulation of the dorsolateral prefrontal cortex. *Neuropsychopharmacology*, 34: 2359–2367.

Barr, M.S., Farzan, F., Tran, L.C., Chen, R., Fitzgerald, P.B. and Daskalakis, Z.J. (2010) Evidence for excessive frontal evoked gamma oscillatory activity in schizophrenia during working memory. *Schizophr. Res.*, 121(1–3): 146–152.

Barr, M.S., Farzan, F., Arenovich, T., Chen, R., Fitzgerald, P.B. and Daskalakis, Z.J. (2011) The effect of repetitive transcranial magnetic stimulation on gamma oscillatory activity in schizophrenia. *PLoS One*, 6(7): e22627.

Barry, R.J. and Clarke, A.R. (2013) Resting state brain oscillations and symptom profiles in AD/HD. In: E. Başar, C. Başar-Eroğlu, A. Özerdem, P.M. Rossini and G.G. Yener (Eds.), *Application of Brain Oscillations in Neuropsychiatric Diseases. Supplements to Clinical Neurophsyiology*, Vol. 62. Elsevier, Amsterdam, Ch. 17.

Barry, R.J., Clarke, A.R. and Johnstone, S.J. (2003a) A review of electrophysiology in attention-deficit/hyperactivity disorder. I. Qualitative and quantitative electroencephalography. *Clin. Neurophysiol.*, 114: 171–183.

Barry, R.J., Johnstone, S.J. and Clarke, A.R. (2003b) A review of electrophysiology in attention-deficit/hyperactivity disorder. II. Event-related potentials. *Clin. Neurophysiol.*, 114: 184–198.

Barry, R.J., Clarke, A.R., Hajos, M., McCarthy, R., Selikowitz, M. and Dupuy, F. (2010) Resting-state EEG gamma activity in children with attention-deficit/hyperactivity disorder. *Clin. Neurophysiol.*, 121: 1871–1877.

Başar, E. (2006) The theory of the whole-brain work. *Int. J. Psychophysiol.*, 60: 133–138.

Başar, E. (2010) *Brain–Body–Mind in the Nebulous Cartesian System: A Holistic Approach by Oscillations.* Springer, Berlin.

Başar, E. and Güntekin, B. (2008) A review of brain oscillations in cognitive disorders and the role of neurotransmitters. *Brain Res.*, 1235: 172–193.

Başar, E., Güntekin, B., Tülay, E. and Yener, G.G. (2010) Evoked and event related coherence of Alzheimer patients manifest differentiation of sensory-cognitive networks. *Brain Res.*, 1357: 79–90.

Başar, E., Güntekin, B., Atagün, İ., Turp, B., Tülay, E. and Özerdem, A. (2012) Brain's alpha activity is highly reduced in euthymic bipolar disorder patients. *Cogn. Neurodyn.*, 6: 11–20.

Başar-Eroğlu, C., Başar, E. and Schmielau, F. (1991) P300 in freely moving cats with intracranial electrodes. *Int. J. Neurosci.*, 60: 215–226.

Başar-Eroğlu, C., Başar, E., Demiralp, T. and Schürmann, M. (1992) P300 response: possible psychophysiological correlates in delta and theta frequency channels. *Int. J. Psychophysiol.*, 13: 161–179.

Başar-Eroğlu, C., Brand, A., Hildebrandt, H., Kedzior, K.K., Mathes, B. and Schmiedt-Fehr, C. (2007) Working memory related gamma oscillations in schizophrenia patients. *Int. J. Psychophysiol.*, 64: 39–45.

Başar-Eroğlu, C., Schmiedt-Fehr, C., Marbach, S., Brand, A. and Mathes, B. (2008) Altered oscillatory alpha and theta networks in schizophrenia. *Brain Res.*, 1235: 143–152.

Başar-Eroğlu, C., Schmiedt-Fehr, C., Mathes, B., Zimmermann, J. and Brand, A. (2009) Are oscillatory brain responses generally reduced in schizophrenia during long sustained attentional processing? *Int. J. Psychophysiol.*, 71(1): 75–83.

Başar-Eroğlu, C., Mathes, B., Brand, A. and Schmiedt-Fehr, C. (2011) Occipital gamma response to auditory stimulation in patients with schizophrenia. *Int. J. Psychophysiol.*, 79(1): 3–8.

Bates, A.T., Kiehl, K.A., Laurens, K.R. and Liddle, P.F. (2009) Low-frequency EEG oscillations associated with information processing in schizophrenia. *Schizophr. Res.*, 115(2–3): 222–230.

Begic, D., Hotujac, L. and Begic, N.J. (2000) Quantitative EEG in F-positive and F-negative schizophrenia. *Acta Psychiatr. Scand.*, 101: 307–311.

Begleiter, H. and Porjesz, B. (2006) Genetics of human brain oscillations. *Int. J. Psychophysiol.*, 60: 162–171.

Bhattacharya, J. (2001) Reduced degree of long-range phase synchrony in pathological human brain. *Acta Neurobiol. Exp.*, 61: 309–318.

Boutros, N.N., Arfken, C., Galderisi, S., Warrick, J., Pratt, G. and Iacono, W. (2008) The status of spectral EEG abnormality as a diagnostic test for schizophrenia. *Schizophr. Res.*, 99 (1–3): 225–237.

Bowden, C.L. (2008) Bipolar pathophysiology and development of improved treatments. *Brain Res.*, 1235: 92–97.

Brenner, C.A., Sporns, O., Lysaker, P.H. and O'Donnell, B.F. (2003) EEG synchronization to modulated auditory tones in schizophrenia, schizoaffective disorder, and schizotypal personality disorder. *Am. J. Psychiatry*, 160 (12): 2238–2240.

Brenner, C.A., Krishnan, G., Vohs, J.L., Ahn, W.Y., Hetrick, W.P., Morzorati, S.L. and O'Donnell, B.F. (2009) Steady-state responses: electrophysiological assessment of sensory function in schizophrenia. *Schizophr. Bull.*, 35: 1065–1077.

Brockhaus-Dumke, A., Mueller, R., Faigle, U. and Klosterkoetter, J. (2008) Sensory gating revisited: relation between brain oscillations and auditory evoked potentials in schizophrenia. *Schizophr. Res.*, 99(1–3): 238–249.

Bucci, P., Mucci, A., Merlotti, E., Volpe, U. and Galderisi, S. (2007) Induced gamma activity and event-related coherence in schizophrenia. *Clin. EEG Neurosci.*, 38: 96–104.

Buszáki, G. (2006) *Rhythms of the Brain.* Oxford University Press, New York.

Caravaglios, G., Costanzo, E., Palermo, F. and Muscoso, E.G. (2008) Decreased amplitude of auditory event-related delta responses in Alzheimer's disease. *Int. J. Psychophysiol.*, 70 (1): 23–32.

Caravaglios, G., Castro, G., Costanzo, E., Di Maria, G., Mancuso, D. and Muscoso, E.G. (2010) Theta power responses in mild Alzheimer's disease during an auditory oddball paradigm: lack of theta enhancement during stimulus processing. *J. Neural Transm.*, 117(10): 1195–1208.

Chen, S.S., Tu, P.C., Su, T.P., Hsieh, J.C., Lin, Y.C. and Chen, L.F. (2008) Impaired frontal synchronization of spontaneous magnetoencephalographic activity in patients with bipolar disorder. *Neurosci. Lett.*, 445: 174–178.

Cho, R.Y., Konecky, R.O. and Carter, C.S. (2006) Impairments in frontal cortical gamma synchrony and cognitive control in schizophrenia. *Proc. Natl. Acad. Sci. USA*, 103: 19878–19883.

Clarke, A.R., Barry, R.J., McCarthy, R. and Selikowitz, M. (1998) EEG analysis in attention deficit/hyperactivity disorder: a comparative study of two subtypes. *Psychiatry Res.*, 81: 19–29.

Clarke, A.R., Barry, R.J., McCarthy, R. and Selikowitz, M. (2001) EEG-defined subtypes of children with attention-deficit/ hyperactivity disorder. *Clin. Neurophysiol.*, 112: 2098–2105.

Clementz, B.A., Sponheim, S.R. and Iacono, W.G. (1994) Resting EEG in first-episode schizophrenia patients, bipolar psychosis patients and their first degree relatives. *Psychophysiology*, 31: 486–494.

Clementz, B.A., Wang, J. and Keil, A. (2008) Normal electrocortical facilitation but abnormal target identification during visual sustained attention in schizophrenia. *J. Neurosci.*, 28 (50): 13411–13418.

Cohen, E., Bernardo, M. and Masana, J. (1999) Repetitive transcranial magnetic stimulation in the treatment of chronic negative schizophrenia: a pilot study. *J. Neurol. Neurosurg. Psychiatry*, 67: 129–130.

Cook, E.W., Hodes, R.L. and Lang, P.J. (1986) Preparedness and phobia: effects of stimulus content on human visceral conditioning. *J. Abnorm. Psychol.*, 95: 195–207.

Cummins, T.D., Broughton, M. and Finnigan, S. (2008) Theta oscillations are affected by amnestic mild cognitive impairment and cognitive load. *Int. J. Psychophysiol.*, 70(1): 75–81.

D'Alfonso, A.A.L., Aleman, A. and Kessels, R.P.C. (2002) Transcranial magnetic stimulation of left auditory cortex in patients with schizophrenia: effects on hallucinations and neurocognition. *J. Neuropsychiatry Clin. Neurosci.*, 14(1): 77–79.

Daskalakis, Z.J., Christensen, B.K., Chen, R., Fitzgerald, P.B., Zipursky, R.B. and Kapur, S. (2002) Evidence for impaired cortical inhibition in schizophrenia using transcranial magnetic stimulation. *Arch. Gen. Psychiatry*, 59: 347–354.

Dauwels, J., Vialatte, F., Musha, T. and Cichocki, A. (2010) A comparative study of synchrony measures for the early diagnosis of Alzheimer's disease based on EEG. *Neuroimage*, 49 (1): 668–693.

Degabriele, R. and Lagopoulos, J. (2009) A review of EEG and ERP studies in bipolar disorder. *Acta Neuropsychiatr.*, 21: 58–66.

Deiber, M.P., Ibañez, V., Missonnier, P., Herrmann, F., Fazio-Costa, L., Gold, G. and Giannakopoulos, P. (2009) Abnormal-induced theta activity supports early directed-attention network deficits in progressive MCI. *Neurobiol. Aging*, 30(9): 1444–1452.

Demiralp, T., Başar-Eroğlu, C., Rahn, E. and Başar, E. (1994) Event-related theta rhythms in cat hippocampus and prefrontal cortex during an omitted stimulus paradigm. *Int. J. Psychophysiol.*, 18(1): 35–48.

Demiralp, T., Ademoğlu, A., Istefanopulos, Y., Başar-Eroğlu, C. and Başar, E. (2001) Wavelet analysis of oddball P300. *Int. J. Psychophysiol.*, 39(2–3): 221–227.

De Vico Fallani, F., Maglione, A., Babiloni, F., Mattia, D., Astolfi, L., Vecchiato, G., De Rinaldis, A., Salinari, S., Pachou, E. and Micheloyannis, S. (2010) Cortical network analysis in patients affected by schizophrenia. *Brain Topogr.*, 23(2): 214–220.

Dewan, M.J., Haldipur, C.V., Boucher, M.F., Ramachandran, T. and Major, L.F. (1988) Bipolar affective disorder. II. EEG, neuropsychological, and clinical correlates of CT abnormality. *Acta Psychiatr.*, 77: 677–682.

Dierks, T., Frölich, R., Ihl, L. and Maurer, K. (1993) Dementia of the Alzheimer type: effects on the spontaneous EEG described by dipole sources. *Psychiatry Res.*, 50(3): 151–162.

Dierks, T., Jelic, V., Pascual-Marqui, R.D., Wahlund, L., Julin, P., Linden, D.E., Maurer, K., Winblad, B. and Nordberg, A. (2000) Spatial pattern of cerebral glucose metabolism (PET) correlates with localization of intracerebral EEG-generators in Alzheimer's disease. *Clin. Neurophysiol.*, 111: 1817–1824.

Doege, K., Jansen, M., Mallikarjun, P., Liddle, E.B. and Liddle, P.F. (2010a) How much does phase resetting contribute to event-related EEG abnormalities in schizophrenia? *Neurosci. Lett.*, 481(1): 1–5.

Doege, K., Kumar, M., Bates, A.T., Das, D., Boks, M.P. and Liddle, P.F. (2010b) Time and frequency domain event-related electrical activity associated with response control in schizophrenia. *Clin. Neurophysiol.*, 121(10): 1760–1771.

Dykman, R., Holcomb, P., Oglesby, D. and Ackerman, P. (1982) Electrocortical frequencies in hyperactive, learning-disabled, mixed, and normal children. *Biol. Psychiatry*, 17: 675–685.

El-Badri, S.M., Ashton, C.H., Moore, P.B., Mursh, V.R. and Ferrier, I.N. (2001) Electrophysiological and cognitive function in young euthymic patients with bipolar affective disorder. *Bipolar Disord.*, 3: 79–87.

Ergen, M., Marbach, S., Brand, A., Başar-Eroğlu, C. and Demiralp, T. (2008) P3 and delta band responses in visual oddball paradigm in schizophrenia. *Neurosci. Lett.*, 440(3): 304–308.

Farzan, F., Barr, M.S., Levinson, A.J., Chen, R. and Wong, W. (2010) Evidence for gamma inhibition deficits in the dorsolateral prefrontal cortex of patients with schizophrenia. *Brain*, 133: 1505–1514.

Fehr, T., Kissler, J., Moratti, S., Wienbruch, C., Rockstroh, B. and Elbert, T. (2001) Source distribution of neuromagnetic slow waves and MEG delta activity in schizophrenic patients. *Biol. Psychiatry*, 50: 108–116.

Fehr, T., Kissler, J., Wienbruch, C., Moratti, S., Elbert, T., Watzl, H. and Rockstroh, B. (2003) Source distribution of neuromagnetic slow-wave activity in schizophrenic patients: effects of activation. *Schizophr. Res.*, 63: 63–71.

336

Ferrarelli, F., Massimini, M., Peterson, M.J., Riedner, B.A., Lazar, M. and Murphy, M.J. (2008) Reduced evoked gamma oscillations in the frontal cortex in schizophrenia patients: a TMS/EEG study. *Am. J. Psychiatry*, 165: 996–1005.

Fitzgerald, P.B., Brown, T.L., Daskalakis, Z.J. and Kulkarni, J. (2002) A transcranial magnetic stimulation study of inhibitory deficits in the motor cortex in patients with schizophrenia. *Psychiatry Res.*, 114: 11–22.

Fitzgerald, P.B., Brown, T.L., Marston, N.A., Oxley, T.J., De Castella, A. and Daskalakis, Z.J. (2003) A transcranial magnetic stimulation study of abnormal cortical inhibition in schizophrenia. *Psychiatry Res.*, 118: 197–207.

Fitzgerald, P.B., Herring, S., Hoy, K., McQueen, S., Segrave, R., Kulkarni, J. and Daskalakis, Z.J. (2008) A study of the effectiveness of bilateral transcranial magnetic stimulation in the treatment of the negative symptoms of schizophrenia. *Brain Stimul.*, 1(1): 27–32.

Flynn, G., Alexander, D., Harris, A., Whitford, T., Wong, W., Galletly, C., Silverstein, S., Gordon, E. and Williams, L.M. (2008) Increased absolute magnitude of gamma synchrony in first-episode psychosis. *Schizophr. Res.*, 105(1–3): 262–271.

Force, R.B., Venables, N.C. and Sponheim, S.R. (2008) An auditory processing abnormality specific to liability for schizophrenia. *Schizophr. Res.*, 103: 298–310.

Ford, J.M., Roach, B.J., Hoffman, R.S. and Mathalon, D.H. (2008) The dependence of P300 amplitude on gamma synchrony breaks down in schizophrenia. *Brain Res.*, 1235: 133–142.

Freitas, C., Fregni, F. and Pascual-Leone, A. (2009) Meta-analysis of the effects of repetitive transcranial magnetic stimulation (rTMS) on negative and positive symptoms in schizophrenia. *Schizophr. Res.*, 108(1–3): 11–24.

Fridberg, D.J., Hetrick, W.P., Brenner, C.A., Shekhar, A., Steffen, A.N., Malloy, F.W. and O'Donnell B.F. (2009) Relationships between auditory event-related potentials and mood state, medication, and comorbid psychiatric illness in patients with bipolar disorder. *Bipolar Disord.*, 11: 857–866.

Gallinat, J., Winterer, G., Herrmann, C.S. and Senkowski, D. (2004) Reduced oscillatory gamma band responses in unmedicated schizophrenic patients indicate impaired frontal network processing. *Clin. Neurophysiol.*, 115: 1863–1874.

Gerez, M. and Tello, A. (1992) Clinical significance of focal topographic changes in the electroencephalogram (EEG) and evoked potentials (EP) of psychiatric patients. *Brain Topogr.*, 5: 3–10.

Green, M.F., Mintz, J., Salveson, D., Nuechterlein, K.H., Breitmeyer, B., Light, G.A. and Braff, D.L. (2003) Visual masking as a probe for abnormal gamma range activity in schizophrenia. *Biol. Psychiatry*, 53(12): 1113–1119.

Groom, M.J., Cahill, J.D., Bates, A.T., Jackson, G.M., Calton, T.G., Liddle, P.F. and Hollis, C. (2010) Electrophysiological indices of abnormal error-processing in adolescents with attention deficit hyperactivity disorder (ADHD). *J. Child Psychol. Psychiatry*, 51(1): 66–76.

Güntekin, B. and Başar, E. (2007a) Gender differences influence brain's beta oscillatory responses in recognition of facial expressions. *Neurosci. Lett.*, 424(2): 94–99.

Güntekin, B. and Başar, E. (2007b) Brain oscillations are highly influenced by gender differences. *Int. J. Psychophysiol.*, 65 (3): 294–299.

Güntekin, B. and Başar, E. (2007c) Emotional face expressions are differentiated with brain oscillations. *Int. J. Psychophysiol.*, 64: 91–100.

Güntekin, B. and Başar, E. (2010a) A new interpretation of P300 responses upon analysis of coherences. *Cogn. Neurodyn.*, 4(2): 107–118.

Güntekin, B. and Başar, E. (2010b) Event-related beta oscillations are affected by emotional eliciting stimuli. *Neurosci. Lett.*, 483: 173–178.

Güntekin, B., Saatçi, E. and Yener, G. (2008) Decrease of evoked delta, theta and alpha coherence in Alzheimer patients during a visual oddball paradigm. *Brain Res.*, 1235: 109–116.

Haenschel, C. and Linden, D. (2011) Exploring intermediate phenotypes with EEG: working memory dysfunction in schizophrenia. *Behav. Brain Res.*, 216(2): 481–495.

Haenschel, C., Bittner, R.A., Waltz, J., Haertling, F., Wibral, M., Singer, W., Linden, D.E. and Rodriguez, E. (2009) Cortical oscillatory activity is critical for working memory as revealed by deficits in early-onset schizophrenia. *J. Neurosci.*, 29(30): 9481–9489.

Haenschel, C., Linden, D.E., Bittner, R.A., Singer, W. and Hanslmayr, S. (2010) Alpha phase locking predicts residual working memory performance in schizophrenia. *Biol. Psychiatry*, 68(7): 595–598.

Haig, A.R., Gordon, E., Pascalis, V.D., Meares, R.A., Bahramali, H. and Harris, A. (2000) Gamma activity in schizophrenia: evidence of impaired network binding? *Clin. Neurophysiol.*, 111(8): 1461–1468.

Hall, M.H., Taylor, G., Sham, P., Schulze, K., Rijsdijk, F., Picchioni, M., Toulopoulou, T., Ettinger, U., Bramon, E., Murray, R.M. and Salisbury, D.F. (2011) The early auditory gamma-band response is heritable and a putative endophenotype of schizophrenia. *Schizophr. Bull.*, 37: 778–787.

Hamm, J.P., Gilmore, C.S., Picchetti, N.A., Sponheim, S.R. and Clementz, B.A. (2011) Abnormalities of neuronal oscillations and temporal integration to low- and high-frequency auditory stimulation in schizophrenia. *Biol. Psychiatry*, 69: 989–996.

Harmon-Jones, E., Abramson, L.Y., Nusslock, R., Sigelman, J.D., Urosevic, S., Turonie, L.D., Alloy, L.B. and Fearn, M. (2008) Effect of bipolar disorder on left frontal cortical responses to goals differing in valence and task difficulty. *Biol. Psychiatry*, 63: 693–698.

Haupt, M., González-Hernández, J.A. and Scherbaum, W.A. (2008) Regions with different evoked frequency band responses during early stage visual processing distinguish mild Alzheimer dementia from mild cognitive impairment and normal aging. *Neurosci. Lett.*, 442(3): 273–278.

Herrmann, C.S. and Demiralp, T. (2005) Human EEG gamma oscillations in neuropsychiatric disorders. *Clin. Neurophysiol.*, 116: 2719–2733.

Hoffman, R.E., Hawkins, K.A. and Gueorguieva, R. (2003) Transcranial magnetic stimulation of left temporoparietal cortex and medication-resistant auditory hallucinations. *Arch. Gen. Psychiatry*, 60: 49–56.

Hogan, M.J., Swanwick, G.R., Kaiser, J., Rowan, M. and Lawlor, B. (2003) Memory-related EEG power and coherence reductions in mild Alzheimer's disease. *Int. J. Psychophysiol.*, 49: 147–163.

Hong, L.E., Summerfelt, A., McMahon, R., Adami, H., Francis, G., Elliott, A., Buchanan, R.W. and Thaker, G.K. (2004) Evoked gamma band synchronization and the liability for schizophrenia. *Schizophr. Res.*, 70: 293–302.

Huang, C., Wahlund, L.O., Dierks, T., Julin, P., Winblad, B. and Jelic, V. (2000) Discrimination of Alzheimer's disease and mild cognitive impairment by equivalent EEG sources: a cross-sectional and longitudinal study. *Clin. Neurophysiol.*, 111: 1961–1967.

Iacono, W.G. (1982) Bilateral electrodemal habituation-dishabituation and resting EEG in remitted schizophrenics. *J. Nerv. Ment. Dis.*, 170: 91–101.

Ikeda, A., Kato, N. and Kato, T. (2002) Possible relationship between electroencephalogram finding and lithium response in bipolar disorder. *Prog. Neuropsychopharmacol. Biol. Psychiatry*, 26: 903–907.

Ince, N.F., Pellizzer, G., Tewfik, A.H., Nelson, K., Leuthold, A., McClannahan, K. and Stéphane, M. (2009) Classification of schizophrenia with spectro-temporo-spatial MEG patterns in working memory. *Clin. Neurophysiol.*, 120(6): 1123–1134.

Itil, T.M., Saletu, B. and Davis, S. (1972) EEG findings in chronic schizophrenics based on digital computer period analysis and analog power spectra. *Biol. Psychiatry*, 5: 1–13.

Itil, T.M., Saletu, B., Davis, S. and Allen, M. (1974) Stability studies in schizophrenics and normals using computer-analyzed EEG. *Biol. Psychiatry*, 8: 321–335.

Jackson, C. and Snyder, P. (2008) Electroencephalography and event-related potentials as biomarkers of mild cognitive impairment and mild Alzheimer's disease. *Alzheimer's Dement.*, 4(1): S137–S143.

Jandl, M., Bittner, R., Sack, A., Weber, B., Günther, T., Pieschl, D., Kaschka, W.P. and Maurer, K. (2005) Changes in negative symptoms and EEG in schizophrenic patients after repetitive transcranial magnetic stimulation (rTMS): an open-label pilot study. *J. Neural Transm.*, 112(7): 955–967.

Jaušovec, N. and Jaušovec, K. (2009a) Do women see things differently than men do? *Neuroimage*, 45: 198–2007.

Jaušovec, N. and Jaušovec, K. (2009b) Gender related differences in visual and auditory processing of verbal and figural tasks. *Brain Res.*, 1: 135–145.

Jaušovec, N. and Jaušovec, K. (2010) Resting brain activity: differences between genders. *Neuropsychologia*, 48(13): 3918–3925.

Jelic, S.E., Johansson, O., Almkvist, M., Shigeta, P., Julin, A., Nordberg, B., Wahlund, W. and Wahlund, L.O. (2000) Quantitative electroencephalography in mild cognitive impairment: longitudinal changes and possible prediction of Alzheimer's disease. *Neurobiol. Aging*, 21: 533–540.

Jeong, J.S. (2004) EEG dynamics in patients with Alzheimer's disease. *Clin. Neurophysiol.*, 115: 1490–1505.

Jin, Y., Potkin, S.G., Rice, D., Sramek, J., Costa, J., Isenhart, R., Heh, C. and Sandman, C.A. (1990) Abnormal EEG responses to photic stimulation in schizophrenic patients. *Schizophr. Bull.*, 4: 627–631.

Jin, Y., Sandman, C.A., Wu, J.C., Bernat, J. and Potkin, S.G. (1995) Topographic analysis of EEG photic driving in normal and schizophrenic subjects. *Clin. Electroencephalogr.*, 26: 102–107.

Jin, Y., Potkin, S.G., Sandman, C.A. and Bunney, Jr., W.E. (1997) Electroencephalographic photic driving in patients with schizophrenia and depression. *Biol. Psychiatry*, 41: 496–499.

Jin, Y., Castellanos, A., Solis, E.R. and Potkin, S.G. (2000) EEG resonant responses in schizophrenia: a photic driving study with improved harmonic resolution. *Schizophr. Res.*, 44: 213–220.

Jin, Y., Potkin, S.G., Kemp, A.S., Huerta, S.T., Alva, G., Thai, T.M., Carreon, D. and Bunney, Jr., W.E. (2006) Therapeutic effects of individualized alpha frequency transcranial magnetic stimulation (αTMS) on the negative symptoms of schizophrenia. *Schizophr. Bull.*, 32(3): 556–561.

Johannesen, J.K., Kieffaber, P.D., O'Donnell, B.F., Shekhar, A., Evans, J.D. and Hetrick, W.P. (2005) Contributions of subtype and spectral frequency analyses to the study of P50 ERP amplitude and suppression in schizophrenia. *Schizophr. Res.*, 78: 269–284.

Kano, K., Nakamura, M., Matsuoka, T., Iida, H. and Nakajima, T. (1992) The topographical features of EEGs in patients with affective disorders. *Electroencephalogr. Clin. Neurophysiol.*, 83: 124–129.

Karrasch, M., Laine, M. and Rinne, J.O. (2006) Brain oscillatory responses to an auditory-verbal working memory task in mild cognitive impairment and Alzheimer's disease. *Int. J. Psychophysiol.*, 59(2): 168–178.

Kissler, J., Müller, M.M., Fehr, T., Rockstroh, B. and Elbert, T. (2000) MEG gamma band activity in schizophrenia patients and healthy subjects in a mental arithmetic task and at rest. *Clin. Neurophysiol.*, 111(11): 2079–2087.

Klimesch, W., Schack, B., Schabus, M., Doppelmayr, M., Gruber, W. and Sauseng, P. (2004) Phase-locked alpha and theta oscillations generate the P1–N1 complex and are related to memory performance. *Cogn. Brain Res.*, 19: 302–316.

Koh, Y., Shin, K.S., Kim, J.S., Choi, J.S., Kang, D.H., Jang, J.H., Cho, K.H, O'Donnell, B.F., Chung, C.K. and Kwon, J.S. (2011) An MEG study of alpha modulation in patients with schizophrenia and in subjects at high risk of developing psychosis. *Schizophr. Res.*, 126(1–3): 36–42.

Koles, Z.J., Lind, J.C. and Flor-Henry, P. (1994) Spatial patterns in the background EEG underlying mental disease in man. *Electroencephalogr. Clin. Neurophysiol.*, 9: 319–328.

Krishnan, G.P., Vohs, J.L., Hetrick, W.P., Carroll, C.A., Shekhar, A., Bockbrader, M.A. and O'Donnell, B.F. (2005) Steadystate visual evoked potential abnormalities in schizophrenia. *Clin. Neurophysiol.*, 116(3): 614–624.

Krishnan, G.P., Hetrick, W.P., Brenner, C.A., Shekhar, A., Steffen, A.N. and O'Donnell, B.F. (2009) Steadystate and induced auditory gamma deficits in schizophrenia. *Neuroimage*, 47(4): 1711–1719.

Kwon, J.S., O'Donnell, B.F., Wallenstein, G.V., Greene, R.W., Hirayasu, Y., Nestor, P.G., Hasselmo, M.E., Potts, G.F., Shenton, M.E. and McCarley, R.W. (1999) Gamma frequency-range abnormalities to auditory stimulation in schizophrenia. *Arch. Gen. Psychiatry*, 56(11): 1001–1005.

338

Lazzaro, I., Gordon, E., Whitmont, S., Plahn, M., Li, W., Clarke, S., Dosen, A. and Meares, R. (1998) Quantified EEG activity in adolescent attention deficit hyperactivity disorder. *Clin. Electroencephalogr.*, 29: 37–42.

Lazzaro, I., Gordon, E., Li, W., Lim, C., Plahn, M., Whitmont, S., Clarke, S., Barry, R., Dosen, A. and Meares, R. (1999) Simultaneous EEG and EDA measures in adolescent attention deficit hyperactivity disorder. *Int. J. Psychophysiol.*, 34: 123–134.

Lee, K.H., Williams, L.M., Haig, A., Goldberg, E. and Gordon, E. (2001) An integration of 40 Hz gamma and phasic arousal: novelty and routinization processing in schizophrenia. *Clin. Neurophysiol.*, 112(8): 1499–1507.

Lee, K.H., Williams, L.M., Breakspear, M. and Gordon, E. (2003a) Synchronous gamma activity: a review and contribution to an integrative neuroscience model of schizophrenia. *Brain Res. Rev.*, 41: 57–78.

Lee, K.H., Williams, L.M., Haig, A. and Gordon, E. (2003b) "Gamma (40 Hz) phase synchronicity" and symptom dimensions in schizophrenia. *Cogn. Neuropsychiatry*, 81: 57–71.

Lee, P.S., Chen, Y.S., Hsieh, J.C., Su, T.P. and Chen, L.F. (2010) Distinct neuronal oscillatory responses between patients with bipolar and unipolar disorders: a magneto-encephalographic study. *J. Affect. Disord.*, 123: 270–275.

Leicht, G., Kirsch, V., Giegling, I., Karch, S., Hantschk, I., Möller, H.J., Pogarell, O., Hegerl, U., Rujescu, D. and Mulert, C. (2010) Reduced early auditory evoked gamma-band response in patients with schizophrenia. *Biol. Psychiatry*, 67(3): 224–231.

Lenz, D., Krauel, K., Schadow, J., Baving, L., Duzel, E. and Herrmann, C.S. (2008) Enhanced gamma-band activity in ADHD patients lacks correlation with memory performance found in healthy children. *Brain Res.*, 1235: 117–132.

Lenz, D., Krauel, K., Flechtner, H.H., Schadow, J., Hinrichs, H. and Herrmann, C.S. (2010) Altered evoked gamma-band responses reveal impaired early visual processing in ADHD children. *Neuropsychologia*, 48(7): 1985–1993.

Lenz, D., Fischer, S., Schadow, J., Bogerts, B. and Herrmann, C.S. (2011) Altered evoked gamma-band responses as a neurophysiological marker of schizophrenia? *Int. J. Psychophysiol.*, 79: 25–31.

Light, G.A., Hsu, J.L., Hsieh, M.H., Meyer-Gomes, K., Sprock, J., Swerdlow, N.R. and Braff, D.L. (2006) Gamma band oscillations reveal neural network cortical coherence dysfunction in schizophrenia patients. *Biol. Psychiatry*, 60: 1231–1240.

Lizio, R., Vecchio, F., Frisoni, G.B., Ferri, R., Rodriguez, G. and Babiloni, C. (2011) Electroencephalographic rhythms in Alzheimer's disease. *Int. J. Alzheimers*, doi: 10.4061/927573.

Lou, W., Xu, J., Sheng, H. and Zhao, S. (2011) Multichannel linear descriptors analysis for event-related EEG of vascular dementia patients during visual detection task. *Clin. Neurophysiol.*, 122(11): 2151–2156.

Luck, S.J., Mathalon, D.H., O'Donnell, B.F., Hämäläinen, M.S., Spencer, K.M., Javitt, D.C. and Uhlhaas, P.J. (2011) A road map for the development and validation of event-related potential biomarkers in schizophrenia research. *Biol. Psychiatry*, 70: 28–34.

Maharajh, K., Teale, P., Rojas, D.C. and Reite, M.L. (2010) Fluctuation of gamma-band phase synchronization within the auditory cortex in schizophrenia. *Clin. Neurophysiol.*, 121(4): 542–548.

Matoušek, M., Rasmussen, P. and Gilberg, C. (1984) EEG frequency analysis in children with so-called minimal brain dysfunction and related disorders. *Adv. Biol. Psychiatry*, 15: 102–108.

Matsuura, M., Okubo, Y., Toru, M., Kojima, T., He, Y., Hou, Y., Shen, Y. and Lee, C. (1993) A cross-national EEG study of children with emotional and behavioural problems: a WHO collaborative study in the Western Pacific region. *Biol. Psychiatry*, 34: 52–58.

Micheloyannis, S., Pachou, E., Stam, C.J., Breakspear, M., Bitsios, P., Vourkas, M., Erimaki, S. and Zervakis, M. (2006) Small-world networks and disturbed functional connectivity in schizophrenia. *Schizophr. Res.*, 87: 60–66.

Minzenberg, M.J., Firl, A.J., Yoon, J.H., Gomes, G.C., Reinking, C. and Carter, C.S. (2010) Gamma oscillatory power is impaired during cognitive control independent of medication status in first-episode schizophrenia. *Neuropsychopharmacology*, 35 (13): 2590–2599.

Missonnier, P., Gold, G., Herrmann, F.R., Fazio-Costa, L., Michel, J.P., Deiber, M.P., Michon, A. and Giannakopoulos, P. (2006) Decreased theta event-related synchronization during working memory activation is associated with progressive mild cognitive impairment. *Dement. Geriatr. Cogn. Disord.*, 22(3): 250–259.

Missonnier, P., Herrmann, F.R., Michon, A., Fazio-Costa, L., Gold, G. and Giannakopoulos, P. (2010) Early disturbances of gamma band dynamics in mild cognitive impairment. *J. Neural Transm.*, 117(4): 489–498.

Miyauchi, T., Tanaka, K., Hagimoto, H., Miura, T., Kishimoto, H. and Matsushita, M. (1990) Computerised EEG in schizophrenic patients. *Biol. Psychiatry*, 28: 488–494.

Monastra, V.J. (2008) Quantitative electroencephalography and attention-deficit/hyperactivity disorder: implications for clinical practice. *Curr. Psychiatry Rep.*, 10: 432–438.

Moretti, D.V., Fracassi, C., Pievani, M., Geroldi, C., Binetti, G., Zanetti, O., Sosta, K., Rossini, P.M. and Frisoni, G.B. (2009) Increase of theta/gamma ratio is associated with memory impairment. *Clin. Neurophysiol.*, 120(2): 295–303.

Mülert, C., Kirsch, V., Pascual-Marqui, R., McCarley, R.W. and Spencer, K.M. (2011) Long-range synchrony of gamma oscillations and auditory hallucination symptoms in schizophrenia. *Int. J. Psychophysiol.*, 79(1): 55–63.

O'Donnell, B.F., Hetrick, W.P., Vohs, J.L., Krishnan, G.P., Carroll, C.A. and Shekhar, A. (2004a) Neural synchronization deficits to auditory stimulation in bipolar disorder. *NeuroReport*, 15: 1369–1372.

O'Donnell, B.F., Vohs, J.L., Hetrick, W.P., Carroll, C.A. and Shekhar, A. (2004b) Auditory event-related potential abnormalities in bipolar disorder and schizophrenia. *Int. J. Psychophysiol.*, 53: 45–55.

O'Donnell, B.F., Vohs, J.L., Krishnan, G.P., Rass, O.B.A., Hetrick, W.P. and Morzorati, S.L. (2013) The auditory steady-state response (ASSR): a translational biomarker for schizophrenia. *Suppl. Clin Neurophysiol.*, 62: Ch. 6, this volume.

Olincy, A. and Martin, L. (2005) Diminished suppression of the P50 auditory evoked potential in bipolar disorder subjects with a history of psychosis. *Am. J. Psychiatry*, 162: 43–49.

Onitsuka, T., Oribe, N.M. and Kanba, S. (2013) Neurophysiological findings in patients with bipolar disorder. *Suppl. Clin. Neurophysiol*, 62: Ch. 13, this volume.

Oribe, N., Onitsuka, T., Hirano, S., Hirano, Y., Maekawa, T., Obayashi, C., Ueno, T., Kasai, K. and Kanba, S. (2010) Differentiation between bipolar disorder and schizophrenia revealed by neural oscillation to speech sounds: an MEG study. *Bipolar Disord.*, 12(8): 804–812.

Osipova, D., Pekkonen, E. and Ahveninen, J. (2006) Enhanced magnetic auditory steady-state response in early Alzheimer's disease. *Clin. Neurophysiol.*, 117(9): 1990–1995.

Özerdem, A., Güntekin, B., Tunca, Z. and Başar, E. (2008) Brain oscillatory responses in patients with bipolar disorder manic episode before and after valproate treatment. *Brain Res.*, 1235: 98–108.

Özerdem, A., Güntekin, B., Saatçi, E., Tunca, Z. and Başar, E. (2010) Disturbance in long distance gamma coherence in bipolar disorder. *Prog. Neuropsychopharmacol. Biol. Psychiatry*, 34(6): 861–865.

Özerdem, A., Güntekin, B., Atagün, I., Turp, B. and Başar, E. (2011) Reduced long distance gamma (28–48 Hz) coherence in euthymic patients with bipolar disorder. *J. Affect. Disord.*, 132(3): 325–332.

Özerdem, A., Güntekin, B., Atagün, I. and Başar, E. (2013) Brain oscillations in bipolar disorder in search of new biomarkers. *Suppl. Clin. Neurophysiol.*, 62: Ch. 14, this volume.

Pachou, E., Vourkas, M., Simos, P., Smit, D., Stam, C.J., Vasso, T. and Micheloyannis, S. (2008) Working memory in schizophrenia: an EEG study using power spectrum and coherence analysis to estimate cortical activation and network behavior. *Brain Topogr.*, 21: 128–137.

Polikar, R., Topalis, A., Green, D., Kounios, J. and Clark, C.M. (2007) Comparative multiresolution wavelet analysis of ERP spectral bands using an ensemble of classifiers approach for early diagnosis of Alzheimer's disease. *Comput. Biol. Med.*, 37(4): 542–558.

Ponomareva, N.V., Selesneva, N.D. and Jarikov, G.A. (2003) EEG alterations in subjects at high familial risk for Alzheimer's disease. *Neuropsychobiology*, 48(3): 152–159.

Přikryl, R. (2011) Repetitive transcranial magnetic stimulation and treatment of negative symptoms of schizophrenia. *Neuroendocrinol. Lett.*, 32(2): 121–126.

Ramos-Loyo, J., González-Garrido, A.A., Sánchez-Loyo, L.M., Medina, V. and Başar-Eroğlu, C. (2009) Event-related potentials and event-related oscillations during identity and facial emotional processing in schizophrenia. *Int. J. Psychophysiol.*, 71(1): 84–90.

Rass, O., Krishnan, G., Brenner, C.A., Hetrick, W.P., Merrill, C.C., Shekhar, A. and O'Donnell, B.F. (2010) Auditory steady state response in bipolar disorder: relation to clinical state, cognitive performance, medication status, and substance disorders. *Bipolar Disord.*, 12: 793–803.

Reinhart, R.M., Mathalon, D.H., Roach, B.J. and Ford, J.M. (2011) Relationships between prestimulus gamma power and subsequent P300 and reaction time breakdown in schizophrenia. *Int. J. Psychophysiol.*, 79(1): 16–24.

Reite, M., Teale, P., Rojas, D.C., Reite, E., Asherin, R. and Hernandez, O. (2009) MEG auditory evoked fields suggest altered structural/functional asymmetry in primary but not secondary auditory cortex in bipolar disorder. *Bipolar Disord.*, 11(4): 371–381.

Rice, D.M., Potkin, S.G., Jin, Y., Isenhart, R., Heh, C.W., Sramek, J., Costa, J. and Sandman, C.A. (1989) EEG alpha photic driving abnormalities in chronic schizophrenia. *Psychiatry Res.*, 30: 313–324.

Riečanský, I., Kašpárek, T., Rehulová, J., Katina, S. and Přikryl, R. (2010) Aberrant EEG responses to gamma-frequency visual stimulation in schizophrenia. *Schizophr. Res.*, 124(1–3): 101–109.

Roach, B.J. and Mathalon, D.H. (2008) Event-related EEG time-frequency analysis: an overview of measures and an analysis of early gamma band phase locking in schizophrenia. *Schizophr. Bull.*, 34(5): 907–926.

Ropohl, A., Sperling, W., Elstner, S., Tomandl, B., Reulbach, U., Kaltenhäuser, M., Kornhuber, J. and Maihöfner, C. (2004) Cortical activity associated with auditory hallucinations. *NeuroReport*, 15(3): 523–526.

Rossini, P.M., Rossi, S., Babiloni, C. and Polich, J. (2007) Clinical neurophysiology of aging brain: from normal aging to neurodegeneration. *Prog. Neurobiol.*, 83(6): 375–400.

Salisbury, D.F., Shenton, M.E. and McCarley, R.W. (1999) P300 topography differs in schizophrenia and manic psychosis. *Biol. Psychiatry*, 45: 98–106.

Sánchez-Morla, E.M., García-Jiménez, M.A., Barabash, A., Martínez-Vizcaíno, V., Mena, J., Cabranes-Díaz, J.A., Baca-Baldomero, E. and Santos, J.L. (2008) P50 sensory gating deficit is a common marker of vulnerability to bipolar disorder and schizophrenia. *Acta Psychiatr. Scand.*, 117: 313–318.

Schmiedt, C., Brand, A., Hildebrandt, H. and Başar-Eroğlu, C. (2005) Event-related theta oscillations during working memory tasks in patients with schizophrenia and healthy controls. *Brain Res. Cogn.*, 25(3): 936–947.

Schneider, A.L., Schneider, T.L. and Stark, H. (2008) Repetitive transcranial magnetic stimulation (rTMS) as an augmentation treatment for the negative symptoms of schizophrenia: a 4-week randomized placebo controlled study. *Brain Stimul.*, 1(2): 106–111.

Schnitzler, A. and Gross, J. (2005) Normal and pathological oscillatory communication in the brain. *Nat. Rev. Neurosci.*, 6(4): 285–296.

Schulz, C., Mavrogiorgou, P., Schroter, A., Hegerl, U. and Juckel, G. (2000) Lithium-induced EEG changes in patients with affective disorders. *Neuropsychobiology*, 42: 33–37.

Schulze, K.K., Hall, M.-H., McDonald, C., Marshall, N., Walshe, M., Murray, R.M. and Bramon, E. (2007) P50 auditory evoked potential suppression in bipolar disorder patients with psychotic features and their unaffected relatives. *Biol. Psychiatry*, 62: 121–128.

Schulze, K.K., Hall, M.-H., McDonald, C., Marshall, N., Walshe, M., Murray, R.M. and Bramon, E. (2008) Auditory

P300 in patients with bipolar disorder and their unaffected relatives. *Bipolar Disord.*, 10: 377–386.

Schürmann, M., Başar-Eroğlu, C., Kolev, V. and Başar, E. (1995) A new metric for analyzing single-trial event-related potentials (ERPs) — application to human visual P300-delta response. *Neurosci. Lett.*, 197: 167–170.

Schürmann, M., Demiralp, T., Başar, E. and Başar-Eroğlu, C.B. (2000) Electroencephalogram alpha (8–15 Hz) responses to visual stimuli in cat cortex, thalamus, and hippocampus: a distributed alpha network? *Neurosci. Lett.*, 292(3): 175–178.

Sharma, A., Weisbrod, M., Kaiser, S., Markela-Lerenc, J. and Bender, S. (2011) Deficits in fronto-posterior interactions point to inefficient resource allocation in schizophrenia. *Acta Psychiatr. Scand.*, 123(2): 125–135.

Slewa-Younan, S., Gordon, E., Harris, A.W., Haig, A.R., Brown, K.J., Flor-Henry, P. and Williams, L.M. (2004) Sex differences in functional connectivity in first-episode and chronic schizophrenia patients. *Am. J. Psychiatry*, 61(9): 1595–1602.

Small, J.G., Milstein, V., Kellams, J.J., Miller, M.J., Boyko, O.B. and Small, I.F. (1989) EEG topography in psychiatric diagnosis and drug treatment. *Ann. Clin. Psychiatry*, 1: 7–17.

Small, J.G., Milstein, V., Malloy, F.W., Klapper, M.H., Golay, S.J. and Medlock, C.E. (1998) Topographic EEG studies of mania. *Clin. Electroencephalogr.*, 29: 59–66.

Souza, V.B., Muir, W.J., Walker, M.T., Glabus, M.F., Roxborough, H.M., Sharp, C.W., Dunan, J.R. and Blackwood, D.H.R. (1995) Auditory P300 event-related potentials and neuropsychological performance in schizophrenia and bipolar affective disorder. *Biol. Psychiatry*, 37: 300–310.

Spencer, K.M., Nestor, P.G., Niznikiewicz, M.A., Salisbury, D.F., Shenton, M.E. and McCarley, R.W. (2003) Abnormal neural synchrony in schizophrenia. *J. Neurosci.*, 23(19): 7407–7411.

Spencer, K.M., Nestor, P.G., Perlmutter, R., Niznikiewicz, M.A., Klump, M.C., Frumin, M., Shenton, M.E. and McCarley, R.W. (2004) Neural synchrony indexes disordered perception and cognition in schizophrenia. *Proc. Natl. Acad. Sci. USA*, 101(49): 17288–17293.

Spencer, K.M., Niznikiewicz, M.A., Shenton, M.E. and McCarley, R.W. (2008a) Sensory-evoked gamma oscillations in chronic schizophrenia. *Biol. Psychiatry*, 63(8): 744–747.

Spencer, K.M., Salisbury, D.F., Shenton, M.E. and McCarley, R.W. (2008b) Gamma-band auditory steady-state responses are impaired in first episode psychosis. *Biol. Psychiatry*, 64(5): 369–375.

Spencer, K.M., Niznikiewicz, M.A., Nestor, P.G., Shenton, M.E. and McCarley, R.W. (2009) Left auditory cortex gamma synchronization and auditory hallucination symptoms in schizophrenia. *BMC Neurosci.*, 20(10): 85.

Sponheim, S.R., Clementz, B.A., Iacono, W.G. and Beiser, M. (1994) Resting EEG in first-episode and chronic-schizophrenia. *Psychophysiology*, 31: 37–43.

Sponheim, S.R., Clementz, B.A., Iacono, W.G. and Beiser, M. (2000) Clinical and biological concomitants of resting state EEG power abnormalities in schizophrenia. *Biol. Psychiatry*, 48: 1088–1097.

Sun, Y., Farzan, F., Barr, M.S., Kirihara, K., Fitzgerald, P.B., Light, G.A. and Daskalakis, Z.J. (2011) Gamma oscillations in schizophrenia: mechanisms and clinical significance. *Brain Res.*, 1413: 98–114.

Symond, M.P., Harris, A.W., Gordon, E. and Williams, L.M. (2005) "Gamma synchrony" in first-episode schizophrenia: a disorder of temporal connectivity? *Am. J. Psychiatry*, 162 (3): 459–465.

Teale, P., Collins, D., Maharajh, K., Rojas, D.C., Kronberg, E. and Reite, M. (2008) Cortical source estimates of gamma band amplitude and phase are different in schizophrenia. *Neuroimage*, 42(4): 1481–1489.

Uhlhaas, P.J. and Singer, W. (2010) Abnormal neural oscillations and synchrony in schizophrenia. *Nat. Rev. Neurosci.*, 11(2): 100–113.

Uhlhaas, P.J., Linden, D.E.J., Singer, W., Haenschel, C., Lindner, M., Maurer, K. and Rodriguez, E. (2006) Dysfunctional long-range coordination of neural activity during Gestalt perception in schizophrenia. *J. Neurosci.*, 26(31): 8168–8175.

Uhlhaas, P.J., Haenschel, C., Nikolic, D. and Singer, W. (2008) The role of oscillations and synchrony in cortical networks and their putative relevance for the pathophysiology of schizophrenia. *Schizophr. Bull.*, 34(5): 927–943.

Van Deursen, J.A., Vuurman, E.F., Van Kranen-Mastenbroek, V.H., Verhey, F.R. and Riedel, W.J. (2011) 40-Hz steady-state response in Alzheimer's disease and mild cognitive impairment. *Neurobiol. Aging*, 32(1): 24–30.

Vecchio, F., Babiloni, C., Lizio, R., De Vico, F.F., Blinowska, K., Verrienti, G., Frisoni, G.B. and Rossini, P.M. (2013) Resting state ortical EEG rhythms in Alzheimer's disease: towards EEG markers for clinical applications. A review. *Suppl. Clin. Neurophysiol.*, 62: Ch. 15, this volume.

Vierling-Claassen, D., Siekmeier, P., Stufflebeam, S. and Kopell, N.J. (2008) Modeling GABA alterations in schizophrenia, a link between impaired inhibition and altered gamma and beta range auditory entrainment. *J. Neurophysiol.*, 99(5): 2656–2671.

Wada, Y., Takizawa, Y. and Yamaguchi, N. (1995) Abnormal photic driving responses in never-medicated schizophrenia patients. *Schizophr. Bull.*, 21: 111–115.

White, T.P., Joseph, V., O'Regan, E., Head, K.E., Francis, S.T. and Liddle, P.F. (2010) Alpha-gamma interactions are disturbed in schizophrenia: a fusion of electroencephalography and functional magnetic resonance imaging. *Clin. Neurophysiol.*, 121(9): 1427–1437.

Wilson, T.W., Hernandez, O.O., Asherin, R.M., Teale, P.D., Reite, M.L. and Rojas, D.C. (2008) Cortical gamma generators suggest abnormal auditory circuitry in early-onset psychosis. *Cereb. Cortex*, 18: 371–378.

Woerner, W., Rothenberger, A. and Lahnert, B. (1987) Test–retest reliability of spectral parameters of the resting EEG in a field sample: a 5 year follow-up in schoolchildren with and without psychiatric disturbances. *Electroenceph. Clin. Neurophysiol.*, 40: 629–632.

Wynn, J.K., Light, G.A., Breitmeyer, B., Nuechterlein, K.H. and Green, M.F. (2005) Event related gamma activity in schizophrenia patients during a visual backward-masking task. *Am. J. Psychiatry*, 162(12): 2330–2336.

Yener, G. and Başar, E. (2010) Sensory evoked and event related oscillations in Alzheimer's disease: a short review. *Cogn. Neurodyn.*, 4: 263–274.

Yener, G. and Başar, E. (2013) Biomarkers in Alzheimer's disease with a special emphasis on event-related oscillatory responses. *Suppl. Clin. Neurophysiol*, 62: Ch. 20, this volume.

Yener, G.G., Güntekin, B., Öniz, A. and Başar, E. (2007) Increased frontal phase-locking of event-related theta oscillations in Alzheimer patients treated with cholinesterase inhibitors. *Int. J. Psychophysiol.*, 64(1): 46–52.

Yener, G., Güntekin, B. and Başar, E. (2008) Event related delta oscillatory responses of Alzheimer patients. *Eur. J. Neurol.*, 15(6): 540–547.

Yener, G., Güntekin, B., Tülay, E. and Başar, E. (2009) A comparative analysis of sensory visual evoked oscillations with visual cognitive event related oscillations in Alzheimer's disease. *Neurosci. Lett.*, 462: 193–197.

Yordanova, J., Banaschewski, T., Kolev, V., Woerner, W. and Rothenberger, A. (2001) Abnormal early stages of task stimulus processing in children with attention-deficit hyperactivity disorder — evidence from event-related gamma oscillations. *Clin. Neurophysiol.*, 112: 1096–1108.

Yordanova, J., Heinrich, H., Kolev, V. and Rothenberger, A. (2006) Increased event-related theta activity as a psychophysiological marker of comorbidity in children with tics and attention-deficit/hyperactivity disorders. *Neuroimage*, 32: 940–955.

Zervakis, M., Michalopoulos, K., Iordanidou, V. and Sakkalis, V. (2011) Intertrial coherence and causal interaction among independent EEG components. *J. Neurosci. Meth.*, 197 (2): 302–314.

Zheng-yan, J. (2005) Abnormal cortical functional connections in Alzheimer's disease: analysis of inter- and intra-hemispheric EEG coherence. *J. Zhejiang Univ. Sci.*, 6B(4): 259–264.

Chapter 20

Brain oscillations as biomarkers in neuropsychiatric disorders: following an interactive panel discussion and synopsis

Görsev G. Yener[a,b,*] and Erol Başar[b]

[a]*Brain Dynamics Multidisciplinary Research Center, and Departments of Neurosciences and Neurology, Dokuz Eylül University, Izmir 35340, Turkey*
[b]*Brain Dynamics, Cognition and Complex Systems Research Center, Istanbul Kultur University, Istanbul 34156, Turkey*

ABSTRACT

This survey covers the potential use of neurophysiological changes as a biomarker in four neuropsychiatric diseases (attention deficit hyperactivity disorder (ADHD), Alzheimer's disease (AD), bipolar disorder (BD), and schizophrenia (SZ)). Great developments have been made in the search of biomarkers in these disorders, especially in AD. Nevertheless, there is a tremendous need to develop an efficient, low-cost, potentially portable, non-invasive biomarker in the diagnosis, course, or treatment of the above-mentioned disorders.

Electrophysiological methods would provide a tool that would reflect functional brain dynamic changes within milliseconds and also may be used as an ensemble of biomarkers that is greatly needed in the evaluation of cognitive changes seen in these disorders. The strategies for measuring cognitive changes include spontaneous electroencephalography (EEG), sensory evoked oscillation (SEO), and event-related oscillations (ERO). Further selective connectivity deficit in sensory or cognitive networks is reflected by coherence measurements.

Possible candidate biomarkers discussed in an interactive panel can be summarized as follows: for ADHD: (a) elevation of delta and theta, (b) diminished alpha and beta responses in spontaneous EEG; for SZ: (a) decrease of ERO gamma responses, (b) decreased ERO in all other frequency ranges, (c) invariant ERO gamma response in relation to working memory demand; for euthymic BD: (a) decreased event-related gamma coherence, (b) decreased alpha in ERO and in spontaneous EEG; for manic BD: (a) lower alpha and higher beta in ERO, (b) decreased event-related gamma coherence, (c) lower alpha and beta in ERO after valproate; and for AD: (a) decreased alpha and beta, and increased theta and delta in spontaneous EEG, (b) hyperexcitability of motor cortices as shown by transcortical magnetic stimulation, (c) hyperexcitability of visual sensory cortex as indicated by increased SEO theta responses, (d) lower delta ERO, (e) lower delta, theta, and alpha event-related coherence, (f) higher theta synchrony and higher alpha event-related coherence in cholinergically treated AD subjects.

In further research in the search for biomarkers, multimodal methods should be introduced to electrophysiology for validation purposes. Also, providing the protocols for standardization and harmonization of user-friendly acquisition or analysis methods that would be applied in larger cohort populations should be used to incorporate these electrophysiologic methods into the clinical criteria. In an extension to conventional anatomical, biochemical and brain imaging biomarkers, the use of neurophysiologic markers may lead to new applications for functional interpretations and also the possibility to monitor treatments tailored for individuals.

Correspondence to: Dr. Görsev G. Yener, M.D., Ph.D.,
Department of Neurology, Dokuz Eylül University
Medical School, Balçova, Izmir 35340, Turkey.
Tel.: +90 232 412 4050; Fax: +90 232 277 7721;
E-mail: gorsev.yener@deu.edu.tr

344

KEYWORDS

Biomarker; Brain oscillation; Alzheimer's disease; Bipolar disorder; Schizophrenia; Attention deficit hyperactivity disorder; Event-related; Alpha; Beta; Theta; Gamma; Delta

20.1. Introductory remarks

Publications on cognitive processes by means of brain oscillations have increased within the neuroscience literature in the past 20–30 years. However, there are relatively few studies related to cognitive impairment within the literature, dating only from the beginning of the last decade. Accordingly, the trend to use "biomarkers" is relatively recent.

The official US National Institutes of Health's definition of a *biomarker* is: "a *characteristic* that is objectively measured and evaluated as an *indicator* of normal biological or pathogenic processes, or pharmacologic responses to a therapeutic intervention." Biomarkers can provide an objective basis for diagnosis, treatment selection, and outcome measures (Fig. 1; Wright et al., 2009).

A conference/workshop related to brain oscillation in neuropsychiatric diseases took place in Istanbul in May 2011 as a first conference during which diseases such as Alzheimer's disease (AD), mild cognitive impairment (MCI), schizophrenia (SZ), bipolar disorders (BD), attention deficit hyperactivity disorder (ADHD) and their neurophysiologic strategy modalities were jointly referenced and discussed. The present interactive survey is mostly based on the results and closing panel discussion of this conference. It also covers part of discussions, advice or remarks of lecturers, and important hints from papers of the present Supplement 62 and also relevant knowledge from previous publications.

During the panel discussion, Claudio Babiloni gave an extended and useful synopsis of discussions, and Giovanni Frisoni gave important hints and described goals for establishing brain oscillations as biomarkers in neuropsychiatric disorders based on his experience of MRI techniques. Paolo M. Rossini stated that in the next 10 years it will be very valuable to develop a low-cost, user-friendly biomarker that can be applied widely to many neuropsychiatric disorders.

The brain does not respond in a homogenous and standard manner to stimulations. The responses are highly dependent on topology, age, states, and pathology. The spontaneous electroencephalographic oscillations, evoked oscillations, event-related oscillations (EROs) and event-related coherences are selectively distributed. Accordingly, the organizers suggested that new, reliable hypotheses and biomarkers could be pronounced only after performing or surveying a wide spectrum of measurements, as described in the following section.

20.1.1. Cardinal view on multiple analysis of brain oscillations

It is necessary to emphasize that there are important functional differences between spontaneous electroencephalography (EEG), sensory evoked oscillations (SEOs), and EROs. In the analysis of spontaneous EEG, only sporadically changes of amplitudes from hidden sources are measured. SEOs reflect the property of sensory networks activated by a sensory stimulation. Event-related (or cognitive) oscillations manifest modification of sensory and cognitive networks, both triggered by a cognitive task (Fig. 2).

An important brain mechanism underlying cognitive processes is the exchange of information between brain areas. The oscillatory analyses of isolated brain areas are important (Başar et al., 1999), but not sufficient to explain all aspects of information processing within the brain. Therefore, in addition to local changes in brain dynamics, dynamics of connectivity between different brain areas must be investigated for a description

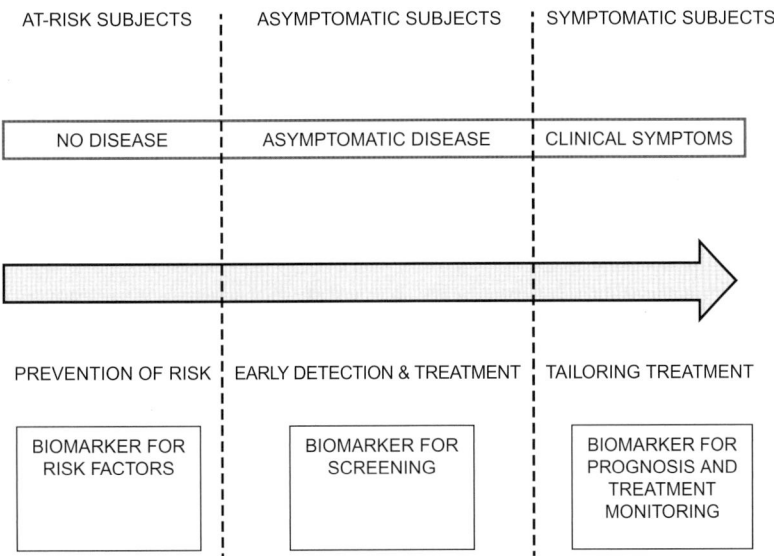

Fig. 1. Biomarkers are useful for detecting the risk factors, screening, or treatment monitoring. (Modified from Wright et al., 2009.)

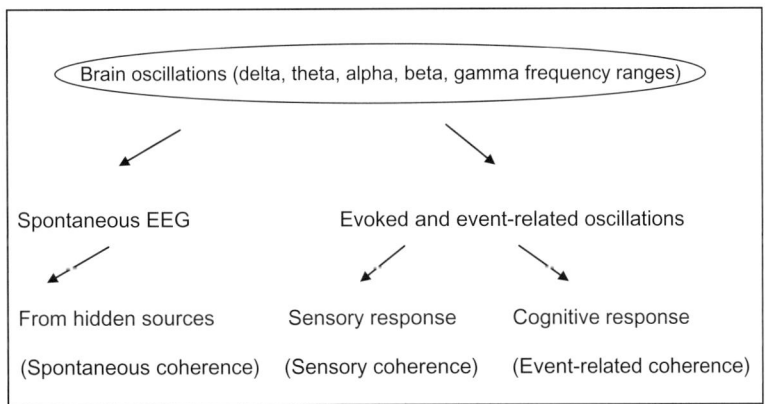

Fig. 2. A schematic presentation of differentiation in brain oscillations.

of neurophysiological mechanisms underlying cognitive deficits of neuropsychiatric diseases.

Coherence is the synchrony between neuronal activities in different parts of the brain. According to Bullock et al. (2003), increased coherence between two structures, namely A and B, can be caused by the following processes: (1) structures A and B are driven by the same generator; (2) structures A and B can mutually drive each other; (3) one of the structures, A or B, drives the other.

In resting EEG analysis, only sporadically occurring coherences from hidden sources are measured. Sensory evoked coherences reflect the degree of connectivity (links) between sensory networks activated only by a sensory stimulation. Event-related (or cognitive) coherences manifest coherent activity of sensory and cognitive networks triggered by a cognitive task. Accordingly, the cognitive response coherences comprehend activation of a greater number of neural networks that are most likely not activated or less activated in the EEG and pure sensory evoked coherences. Therefore, event-related coherences and ERO merit special attention in patients with cognitive impairment. In particular, in AD patients with strong cognitive impairment, it is relevant to analyze whether medical treatment (drug application) selectively acts upon sensory and cognitive networks manifested in topologically different places and in different frequency windows. Such an observation may serve in future to provide a deeper physiological understanding of distributed functional networks and, in turn, the possibility of determination of markers for medical treatment. Fig. 3 presents a schema for connectivity underlying sensory evoked coherence responses following simple sensory stimuli and event-related coherence responses following a cognitive task. It is not possible to define clear-cut boundaries for these neural groups that are differentiated upon application of sensory stimulation or upon cognitive stimulation. This schema indicates that there are neural populations, mostly responding to sensory signals, and other populations responding to only cognitive stimulation. Further, there is some overlap or plasticity among these networks. It is

also possible that neural groups are not separated into different structures but co-exist also in given structures. These are selectively distributed neuron clusters capable of responding to sensory/cognitive inputs. It is also expected that following sensory stimulation, cognitive neural clusters would remain silent, whereas a cognitive stimulus (i.e., target signal in oddball paradigm) would excite both sensory and cognitive neural clusters. Certainly in the case of cognitive impairment, cognitive neural clusters would be more affected, in turn, giving rise to less unclear responses. Moreover, reduced response amplitude can result from either non-responding neural units or non-phase-locked response activity.

Fig. 3 illustrates only one local area. However, isolated brain networks can explain only a limited activity. In addition to these local activities, it is important to emphasize the selective connectivity between neural elements of these networks and, more important, differential connectivity between distant areas of the brain (e.g., frontal, limbic, and parietal connections) (Fig. 4). In the case of AD, the number of neural clusters responding to cognitive stimulus is greatly reduced. Additionally, we observe a selective connectivity deficit between

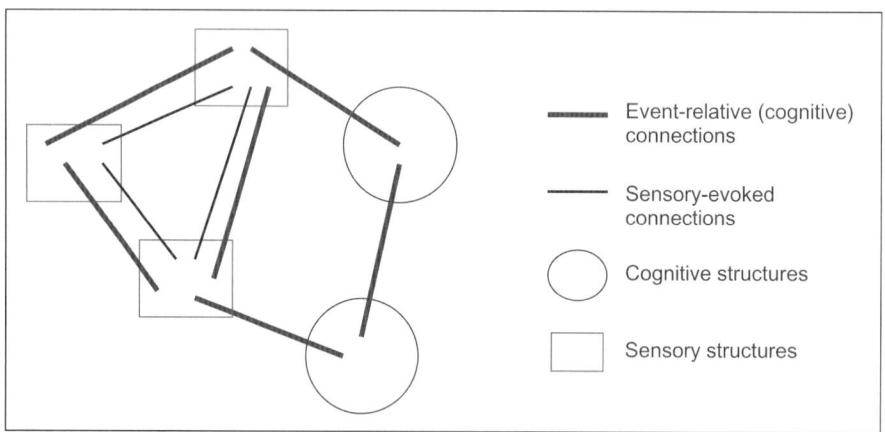

Fig. 3. Neural assemblies involved in sensory and cognitive networks. Cognitive networks (here shown by magenta lines) probably contain sensory neural elements, but also involve additional neural assemblies, as shown by magenta circles. Sensory network elements are illustrated by blue squares and connections by blue lines. It is expected that sensory signals trigger activation of sensory areas, whereas cognitive stimulation would evoke both neural groups reacting to sensory and cognitive inputs. (For color figures, please refer to the color figures in last section of the book.)

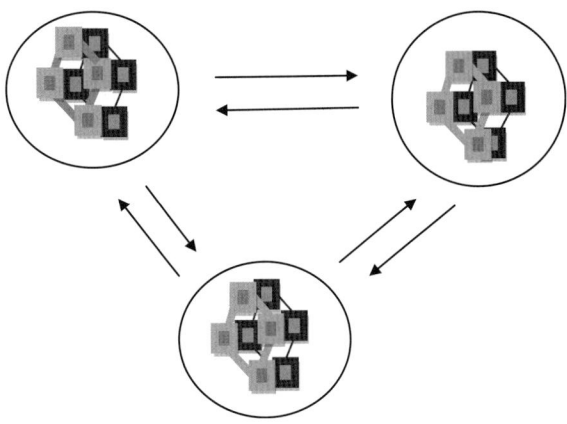

Fig. 4. Web of sensory and cognitive networks between distant neural networks. (For color figures, please refer to the color figures in last section of the book.)

distant neural networks (see Güntekin et al., 2008; Başar et al., 2010).

20.2. Interactive panel discussion, chaired by Görsev G. Yener and Erol Başar

The following section summarizes the interactive panel discussion.

Dean Salisbury stated that psychologists build models in order to understand complex behaviors. However, the model must be biologically realistic. Working with patients, neuroscientists look for abnormalities in the biological system; we therefore learn to constrain the model, based on these abnormalities. This provides a greater understanding of how our complex cognition is represented in the real brain. However, when we consider the clinical aspects in terms of potential benefits for patients, or discuss biomarkers, we need to differentiate between the larger class, which are state-dependent and may index a change or current functioning, and endophenotypes, which are trait related. In future, we aim to define complex endophenotypes using a multi-dimensional approach across the diagnostic categories; such a multivariate analysis of patterns of ERO and ERPs would allow classification of different sub-categories within neuropsychiatric disorders. That is the link

with neurotransmitter abnormalities; therefore, if we can construct multi-dimensional profiles and link them with underlying neurotransmitter abnormalities, we can develop individualized treatments.

During this interactive discussion, three main questions were discussed.

20.2.1. Question 1: After discussing the electrophysiological details of schizophrenia, AD, BDs, MCI, ADHD, etc., can we develop an ensemble of biomarkers for these disorders, and what should we be doing to translate those valuable methods into clinical practice?

Giovanni Frisoni stated that "the case of Alzheimer's disease (AD) is particularly favorable to develop neurophysiologic markers, because we have a reasonable hypothesis for the causes." Current biomarkers have various degrees of validation — a dynamic process that is ongoing. Therefore, it is possible to develop neurophysiological markers, using the already validated markers as a proof of convergent validity for diagnosis or for disease progression. Future research on neurophysiological biomarkers should therefore start from the current position, with an existing framework and biomarkers against which to validate new markers.

Markers that were discussed are for *diagnosis* — structural, metabolic, or CSF changes. However, one may also need markers to track *disease progression*, to check whether a drug is effective. Some markers may be used for diagnostic and also tracking purposes, but others may not change much over time, and so are poor markers to track disease progression (Fig. 1 and Table 1).

AD is more favorable to develop electrophysiological biomarkers. Different degrees of validation occur for these biomarkers. *Structural, metabolic,* and *CSF markers* (i.e., static) are already available for AD. Further, dynamic markers are important for tracking or progression of disease or monitoring

TABLE 1

BIOLOGICAL MARKERS USED IN ALZHEIMER'S DISEASE AND/OR MILD COGNITIVE IMPAIRMENT, AND THEIR USAGE OR ADVANTAGES

AD markers	For diagnosis	For progression	For drug effects	Non-invasiveness	Low cost
Amyloid PET	+	−	−	+	−
FDG-PET	+	+	+	+	−
CSF	+	±	−	−	−
Structural MRI	+	+	−	+	−
Electrophysiology	+	+	+	+	+

AD: Alzheimer's disease; FDG-PET: fluoro deoxy glucose positron emission tomography; CSF: cerebrospinal fluid; MRI: magnetic resonance imaging.

drug effects, since disease-modifying drugs are being widely studied in AD. In AD, Michael Weiner has launched a major project called the Alzheimer's disease neuroimaging initiative (ADNI), to follow patients with cognitive disturbances over time (every 6 months, 5 years to date), including a number of biomarkers (biological and imaging) (Weiner et al., 2012). The ADNI project has clarified much about the progression of the disease. The most obvious proposal would be to add neurophysiological markers and study how they change with time and to what extent they agree with the other markers (Karow et al., 2010; Polikar et al., 2010; Walhovd et al., 2010; Jack et al., 2011). Many years ago, the biomarker field of AD was similar to that of schizophrenia. Table 1 summarizes a few AD biomarkers.

Michael Koch commented that biomarkers could open a venue for very early therapeutic intervention, including some neuropsychiatric diseases, where the course of progression is not as rapid as in AD or Parkinson's disease. There is widespread agreement that biomarkers must be reliable not only in differentiating diseases, but also in predicting the course of the disease, thereby allowing therapeutic intervention at the presymptomatic stage.

In summary, according to G. Frisoni, M. Koch, D. Salisbury, and A. Özerdem, biomarkers can be classified based on specific functions:

(a) for diagnosis of a specific disease;
(b) for tracking the disease;
(c) for differential diagnosis;
(d) for monitoring effects of medication following therapy;
(e) for allowing therapeutic intervention at the presymptomatic stage;
(f) for detecting endophenotypes that are trait-related;
(g) studying at-risk populations to develop an early intervention;
(h) identifying subtypes.

20.2.2. Biomarkers in schizophrenia

According to Ayşegül Özerdem, in psychiatry, we need biomarkers to differentiate between disorders rather than clearly defining patients from healthy controls. This is difficult, given the diagnostic criteria we are using. However, it may help to investigate dimensions: studying schizophrenia or bipolar patients together to see how they differ over time, for example, in terms of electrophysiological parameters. Another approach for early diagnosis would be to study the at-risk population or their first-degree relatives, to track potential electrophysiological characteristics; next focus on this issue and associate it with clinical pathology; then follow up subsequent treatments (see

Onitsuka et al., this volume). According to Dan Mathalon, most of the psychiatric disorders, whose pathophysiology we still do not know well, have a neurodevelopmental basis meaning that we know that things are not normal even before the full development of the disorder is evident. Therefore, biomarkers would allow us to detect risk and to develop strategies for early intervention, because some intervention strategies may not be effective later, beyond this early window of opportunity.

Görsev G. Yener commented on these arguments as follows: "In schizophrenia or mild cognitive impairment (MCI), we may see subtle neurophysiological changes or symptoms in the early sub-clinical era. The real challenge will be developing electrophysiological methods that are inexpensive, noninvasive and user-friendly. This might help to screen wider populations and to prevent AD progression at the earliest possible stage. The epidemiological results indicate that the expansion of AD worldwide is increasing every year, and a delay of several years in the development of AD would refuse the cost."

According to G. Frisoni, there is a lack of a biomarker for the diagnosis of schizophrenia, as it is now based on the clinical criteria of the Diagnostic and Statistical Manual of Mental Disorders (DSM-IV, American Psychiatric Association, 2000). Previously, we knew very little about AD, except that there were "dementias"; this is gradually broken down into more detailed classifications, that may also be a useful approach in schizophrenia. For example a diagnostic marker to differentiate between *schizophrenia sub-types* is needed in that case.

Even though BD and schizophrenia are considered as separate neuropsychiatric entities, they share several common susceptibility genes and overlap in the confirmed linkages (Onitsuka et al., in this volume). Altered neural oscillation and synchronization can be an index of cognitive dysfunction. Studies reported larger neural oscillations and increased phase-locking in BD than healthy controls or schizophrenia. Schizophrenia subjects exhibited delayed neural oscillations and decreased phase-locking compared with healthy controls.

20.2.2. Question 2: Can we learn about cognitive impairments after application just by knowing some dynamic factors that are influenced by the disease and by looking at the disease itself; can we learn about these disorders?

Investigating the pathophysiology of neuropsychiatric diseases by means of brain oscillations can lead to an understanding of how the brain can be so disorganized that it results in this complex system of symptoms. For many researchers, this could be a more interesting topic than their potential use as biomarker as commented by Judith Ford.

The following section summarizes the analysis presented by Claudio Babiloni during the discussion on standardization, harmonization, and continuous dialogue with clinicians which is the new frontier for our field. My work and that of several others is to follow the ADNI data collection standards and to have a common language to organize and analyze the data; to link EEG oscillations in resting state in AD with respect to biomarkers, according to the most advanced standards by ADNI.

Cognitive neuroscience studies: attention and many other cognitive functions. The field now regards the cognitive functions in a refined way that focuses on sub-functions and work is ongoing to relate our EEG oscillations to this modern view of our consciousness, etc. We have a very powerful approach to capture the transmission of information within the brain at several sites according to several oscillatory codes. Translational studies to align our various EEG markers with the concept of markers in the different fields of neurological pathologies are extremely important. Further, if we are able to go beyond the limitations of EEG, like low spatial resolution, we can precisely localize the networks used for these oscillations, such as theta networks, because there are probably specific networks using specific codes or combinations of codes. So we need neuroimaging to capture, with higher spatial resolution, the cortical and subcortical networks in the brain, and studies with transition models to capture and validate oscillatory phenomena. Therefore, a multimodal approach to the study of clinical and cognitive neuroscience is crucial. An important contribution of this conference is to demonstrate the progress of several innovative multimodal studies (Rossini and Ferreri, this volume). These multimodal approaches include Professor Rossini's transcortical magnetic stimulation and EEG studies, structural connectivity studies and EEG prepulse inhibition as a model of link between brain and peripheral nervous system, and neurovegetative response to the brain as described by Başar et al. (2010).

Babiloni does not view EEG alone: the purpose of his work is not simply collecting EEG data, but is primarily to dialogue with others, providing multimodal methods including neuropsychology on AD, rather than abstract theories. This is the real core of the ongoing multi-centerwork on EEG to break into the AD frontier and research.

20.2.3. Question 3: Would it be possible to propose some common neurophysiologic grounds? What might be the methodological necessities?
Harmonized spontaneous EEG and a standardized approach to ERP and brain oscillations?

Robert Barry found that the proposal is good in principle, but very difficult to implement in practice. According to him, it is difficult to find commonalities between researchers investigating differing issues. There may be potential benefits from basic resting EEG, functional magnetic resonance imaging (fMRI). However, if one asks what might be an appropriate paradigm, these paradigms each have different efficiencies in different disorders. Therefore, there would be limited efficiency benefits from all researchers attempting to collect data on everything.

According to Dean Salisbury, we cannot simply rely on resting EEG. In psychiatry, attempts have

already been made to base diagnosis and subtyping solely on quantified EEG patterns, but the results were disappointing. Therefore, any proposed approach must be multimodal, but there are difficulties in reaching agreement. To be practical, it must be relatively inexpensive, so the use of fMRI or MRI in all cases is questionable; imaging technologies would be used in AD cases, but practical implementation must consider any method's inherent financial costs.

According to Giovanni Frisoni, the progress of the AD research resulted from the effort to organize researchers from multiple sites to generate definitive data sets. That facilitated the discovery of patterns across different imaging modalities, to the extent that these patterns are now useful for clinicians. There are other similar trends that should be encouraged: there are initiatives to conduct multi-site collection of schizophrenia data in clinically high-risk youths; as a result, large samples are rapidly being generated. This addresses a long-standing problem in our field, where the literature is dominated by studies using small samples that fail to be replicated. This problem of replication is compounded because our fields examine conditions that are inherently complex, abnormal, and heterogeneous. In the process of addressing this, we must change the process of science. It is not easy to agree on commonly applicable paradigms, but some changes are occurring, where researchers collect data that are beneficial for the wider research field. Such multi-site, large-sample studies will be necessary in order to deliver results that are of use to clinicians.

Robert Barry provided the following comments: "Listening to the presentations, it seems we are ignoring the state of the patients when they come to be assessed. Some of the differences in alpha that were presented may relate to the fact that patients may be highly anxious for a diagnosis or treatment. So some of the results we are observing are related to anxiety, not the disease itself. We should be considering universally applicable methods that would screen out some of those issues and lead to more robust results. One simple and cheap add-on might be the use of skin conductors, which showed huge differences between patients and controls in ADHD."

20.3. Open discussion

20.3.1. Summary by Claudio Babiloni

Some speakers presented an intriguing view of the brain rhythms in the resting state condition. This condition can be conceptualized as a spontaneous fluctuation in brain arousal along the time axis. This apparently simple state of the brain is very rich in information about, and the mechanisms of, neural synchronization and coordination within cortico-cortical and subcortical–cortical circuits modulating the brain arousal time by time. The speakers have shown that specific brain dynamics of the resting stage, the "default" state, express a sort of inhibition in the processing of stimuli coming from the external world and form a crucial bias in the subsequent response of the brain to external stimuli. For example, the specific phase of the brain oscillatory activity in the prestimulus period can affect the timing of the brain response to a given external stimulus, the selective involvement of the neural networks, and the relative ability of these networks to process information in order to represent events/operative states, and memories.

It has also been confirmed that brain rhythms at particular alpha frequencies (about 8–10 Hz) are related to arousal and are modulated in amplitude by caffeine. In the resting state, other brain frequencies are able to be associated with the global personality of children in the development of state; these preliminary results need to be confirmed. However, this is a positive indication that several people with different personalities and methods of processing information are characterized by particular features of the neural synchronization in the brain, together with a different functional coupling of EEG rhythms between cortical populations ("functional connectivity") as a mode to gate the transfer of signals/information across neural circuits.

Evaluation of resting state brain rhythms enlightens physiological and pathological aging and global cognitive status of the subjects. On the one hand, it has been shown that particular resting state alpha rhythms (about 8–10 Hz) are reduced in amplitude in association with brain atrophy and global cognitive status in subjects with MCI and AD. In the same vein, pathological delta rhythms (1–4 Hz) increase as a function of the disease, at least at group level. The power reduction of the alpha rhythms along the disease progression would be slowed by cholinesterase inhibitors (Donepezil) in AD patients responding to long-term therapy of 12 months, suggesting some relationship among resting state alpha rhythms, aging, and integrity of the cholinergic neuromodulation systems. Of note, intriguing analogies between AD and major depression are suggested by the finding of reduced resting state alpha rhythms in patients with depression during asymptomatic periods. On the other hand, it has been shown that, in AD patients, the power of delta rhythms is abnormal not only in the resting state, but also in response to "oddball" target stimuli as a function of the treatment with cholinesterase inhibitors (Yener et al., 2007). Impaired processing of the "oddball" target stimuli would also be related to an abnormal coupling of the EEG oscillations from delta to alpha frequencies. This is a promising neurophysiological approach to the exploration of brain function in developmental age, physiological, and pathological aging, as well as psychiatric disorders.

20.3.2. Schizophrenia

In the workgroup on schizophrenia, several speakers reviewed the state of the art in relation to the neurophysiological basis of the generation of brain gamma (<35 Hz) rhythms. A key role would be played by fine neural circuits modulated by agonists and antagonists (i.e., ketamine) of glutamate neurotransmission and NMDA receptors. Interesting original evidence has been presented in both human and animal models.

Some interesting evidence has been presented about the relationship between atrophy of the temporal lobe and abnormal EEG oscillations in oddball paradigms in schizophrenic patients, although some open issues and contrasting results suggest that the variability of the disease endophenotypes may prevent the definition of a common picture about the particular abnormalities of the brain synchronization mechanisms in schizophrenia. In this regard, the relationship between features of EEG rhythms and genotyping merits specific discussion. Some speakers have shown EEG procedures to unveil the relationships between specific endophenotypes, EEG oscillatory activity, and the progression of schizophrenia. Specifically, there would be some invariant individual features of gamma rhythms along the progression of schizophrenia from the first episode onward, and these features appear to be common to people of the same family, in terms of determining whether they depend on genetics. This is promising for a future classification of patients with different forms of the disease, possibly in relation to genetic features.

20.3.3. EEG markers in schizophrenia

Another important input from the schizophrenia workgroup was the evaluation of candidate EEG markers for schizophrenia (resting state, "oddball," etc.) in young healthy subjects who underwent to a reversible and innocuous pharmacological procedure to induce some mental states resembling positive schizophrenia symptoms. The results showed that such a procedure is not able to induce, "tout court," the typical EEG picture of schizophrenia. Only a minority of EEG markers was affected by the experimental manipulation, with only slight relationships with the subjects' mental state, in agreement with the idea that schizophrenia cannot be captured by simple pharmacological "challenge" models. However, the general methodological approach based on surrogate EEG endpoints seems to be quite promising for drug discovery in schizophrenia.

20.3.4. Hyperconnectivity

One of the most interesting findings of the schizophrenia session concerned "hyperconnectivity." One of the speakers showed that schizophrenic patients were characterized by "paradoxical" occipital EEG oscillatory responses to auditory "oddball" targets in two different experiments (Başar-Eroğlu et al., 2011). This is further evident that schizophrenia patients can display maladapted hyper-connectivity; it has been speculated that, in these patients, abnormal auditory information is distributed and triggers excitation in the occipital visual cortex, possibly producing abnormal visual imagery or visual processing. This intriguing working hypothesis will need to be tested with control experiments in schizophrenic patients to evaluate possible relationships between the "paradoxical" occipital EEG oscillatory responses to auditory "oddball" targets and structural neuroimaging indexes (i.e., tractography, diffusion tensor imaging).

20.3.5. Neurotransmitters

The symposium also addressed a new frontier for the study of EEG oscillations and neurotransmitters, namely EEG investigations of BDs. In this regard, the first preliminary results were presented on brain oscillations and major depression. ERO and coherence studies in AD also showed decreased delta and theta responses and widely diminished cortico-cortical coherences in alpha, theta, and delta ranges. Among those parameters, frontal theta phase-locking and alpha fronto-parietal coherence values were sensitive to medication effects, as reported by Yener and Başar (2010) and Güntekin et al. (2008). An intense discussion was developed about how EEG may help identify the relationship between the neural synchronization mechanisms at the basis of transfer of information between areas and mood regulation as reflected by the generation of EEG oscillations.

20.3.6. General conclusion

A general conclusion was that the EEG community must continue to inform the discussion with clinicians about the kind of evidence required to test the particular contribution of EEG oscillatory markers for early diagnosis and prognosis, individualized management, therapy monitoring, and drug discovery in psychiatric and dementia patients. Besides, understanding the brain plasticity and its underlying functional and structural components has been challenged by new neurophysiological techniques within the past 10 years as summarized by Rossini and Ferreri (this volume). There is a need for a deeper dialogue with cognitive neuroscientists using fMRI and transcranial magnetic stimulation in order to investigate the correlation between EEG oscillations and fine brain topography of hemodynamic responses and excitatory/inhibitory neurotransmitter systems. Furthermore, a deeper dialogue is necessary with cognitive psychologists involved in the fine modeling of subtypes of attention (i.e., endogenous, reflexive, exogenous, orienting, etc.) and memory (i.e., procedural, episodic, semantic), to evolve the experimental designs to be used in our EEG studies. The future role of EEG oscillations in clinical and cognitive neuroscience depends on this dialogue. The same is true for the future of clinical and cognitive neuroscience itself. Indeed, EEG oscillations are the main emerging property of the resting state and working brain. The pathway is still long but quite exciting.

After Claudio Babiloni's summary, Giovanni Frisoni stated that "as a physician, my feeling is that neuroscientists working on brain oscillations

have a great tool available, but the cross-talk with clinicians is crucial to understand how to apply this tool. For most clinicians, the neuroscience vocabulary is challenging and, previously, waveforms were difficult for physicians to interpret. The great expansion of neuroimaging within the last year allows the function to be plotted onto the anatomy, making it more recognizable for clinicians. It requires effort from all parties to use the appropriate language to communicate with each other. In AD, the great initiatives are large and multinational. This group should be expanded to mirror such approaches; if neurophysiology enters that mainstream, it could contribute enormously to the understanding of the disease and to patient treatment."

20.4. Candidate electrophysiological biomarkers for several neuropsychiatric disorders

20.4.1. Attention deficit hyperactivity disorder (ADHD)

ADHD is a condition in which a person (usually a child) has an unusually high activity level and a short attention span. People with the disorder may act impulsively and may have learning and behavioral problems. Several reports consistently reported increased gamma oscillatory responses (Perez et al., Taylor et al., Yordanova et al., all in this volume) and elevation of delta and theta along with diminished alpha and beta responses in spontaneous (resting) EEG (Monastra et al., 2001; Barry et al., 2003). One of the difficulties with ADHD is a tendency for over-diagnosis. Barry and Clarke (in this volume) suggest the theta:beta ratio as a potential biomarker for ADHD. As they state, it seems to be sensitive to medication, as improved symptoms following medication are linked to a reduction in the theta:beta ratio. An updated general model of coherence anomalies in ADHD children, based on Barry and Clarke (this volume), also indicates a wide range of regional connectivity anomalies in this disorder.

20.4.2. Schizophrenia

Schizophrenia is a psychotic disorder (or a group of disorders) marked by severely impaired thinking, emotions, and behaviors. Increased dopaminergic activity in the mesolimbic pathway of the brain is a consistent finding. The mainstay of treatment is pharmacotherapy with antipsychotic medications; these primarily work by suppressing dopamine activity.

Gamma activity induced in response to task-relevant and irrelevant auditory oddball stimuli in medicated schizophrenics showed a significant decrease in comparison to controls (Haig et al., 2000). Later other reports confirmed the reduced gamma (Wynn et al., 2005; Başar-Eroğlu et al., 2007; Spencer et al., 2008) independent of medication (Minzenberg et al., 2010), and also reduction in delta, theta, and alpha frequency bands (Başar-Eroğlu et al., 2009) in schizophrenia patients. Başar-Eroğlu et al. (2011) indicated an over-excitability of neuronal networks in schizophrenia as shown by their findings showing elevated gamma responses at both anterior and occipital sites to auditory stimuli. They also showed a less prominent anterior alpha response to simple sensory auditory input, which probably indicates less efficient processing, similar to reduced alpha responses for non-target stimuli in oddball paradigm in schizophrenia subjects (see Başar Eroğlu et al., this volume)

Herrmann and Demiralp (2005) reviewed the literature on the alterations of gamma oscillations (between 30 and 80 Hz) during the course of neuropsychiatric disorders and based on a study by Lee et al. (2003). They suggested that in schizophrenic patients, negative symptoms correlate with a decrease in gamma responses, whereas a significant increase in gamma amplitudes is observed during positive symptoms such as hallucinations.

Auditory steady-state response (ASSR) power and phase-locking to gamma range stimulation were found to be reduced in patients with schizophrenia. In a review by O'Donnell et al. (this volume), alterations of ASSRs in schizophrenia, schizotypal personality disorder, and first-degree relatives of patients with schizophrenia were reported. ASSRs are usually reduced in power or phase-locking in patients with schizophrenia following 40-Hz stimulation. Possibly, delayed phase synchronization and reduction in 40-Hz power in schizophrenia could be also considered as biomarkers.

Previously, Mathalon's and Ford's groups showed that the early evoked gamma band response to tones is poorly synchronized in schizophrenia (Roach and Mathalon, 2008), which is consistent with other reports of abnormalities in the early auditory gamma oscillatory responses in chronic schizophrenia patients (for a review, see Gandal et al., 2012). Gamma responses of young schizophrenia patients show decreased evoked power (Perez et al., this volume) and diminished phase-locking of gamma responses (Roach et al., this volume).

According to Taylor et al. (this volume), it seems likely that the early auditory gamma band responses would be reduced in schizophrenia. Roach and Mathalon (2008) suggested that wavelet parameters might play a role in the detection of group differences and reported reduced phase-locking of early auditory gamma band responses in this disorder.

The relationship between long-range fronto-posterior connectivity and local brain activity in the frontal and posterior areas is investigated by Sharma et al. (this volume). They show that abnormal functional connectivity in the fronto-posterior brain network in schizophrenia is not necessarily characterized by a global reduction of connectivity, but can either be increased (during rest) or decreased (during cognitive control), depending on the stage of the task. The sensory and frontal areas of schizophrenia patients showed reduced evoked activity and the posterior association cortex during later target evaluation and perceptual processes are more strongly reduced in schizophrenia. Fronto-posterior coherence was reduced in patients as early as 100 ms. These results indicate that connectivity disturbances may be a more fundamental deficit in schizophrenia and may manifest very early during cognitive control. This may also have an implication for the later local evoked activity, where connectivity impairments that manifested earlier could drive impairments in the later local activity.

20.4.3. Bipolar disorders

BD is not a single disorder, but a category of mood disorders defined by the presence of one or more episodes of abnormally elevated mood, clinically referred to as mania. Individuals who experience manic episodes also commonly experience depressive episodes or symptoms, or mixed episodes which present the features of both mania and depression (Bowden, 2007). The event-related oscillatory responses in various types of BDs and their response to valproate were investigated by Özerdem et al. (2008a,b, 2010). In their reports in 2008a, investigating bipolar manic and medication-free patients, they reported significantly higher occipital beta and lower occipito-frontal alpha EROs than healthy controls. After treatment with valproate, alpha ERO responses in BD patients were significantly lower. Başar et al. (2011) reported the decrease of alpha frequency band both in spontaneous EEG and sensory evoked oscillatory responses. This group concluded that alpha response is the universal operator in the brain. Increased occipital beta response in mania may be compensatory to the dysfunctional alpha operation. Its reduction after valproate may be through modulation of glutamatergic and GABAergic mechanisms. Their study on the effects of valproate euthymic and medication-free bipolar patients showed a diminished delta responses (Özerdem et al., 2008b). Later reports by the same research group have indicated decreased event-related gamma coherence both in euthymic BD (Özerdem et al., 2011) and manic BD (Özerdem et al., 2010) as another possible candidate of biomarker.

The results presented by Özerdem et al. (in this volume) and by Başar et al. (2011) suggest that the crucial decrease of alpha power, the increase of beta activity, the high reduction of long distance visual event-related gamma coherence in euthymic BD patients are candidate biomarkers in this disease.

Hall et al. (2011) examined whether or not gamma band oscillations constitute endophenotypes of BD by testing BD patients, monozygotic BD twins, unaffected relatives, and healthy subjects using the auditory oddball task. Patients with BD exhibited reduced gamma band power, whereas these changes were not observed in clinically unaffected relatives. Therefore, these responses do not appear to be an eligible criterion for endophenotypes of BD (Hall et al., 2011). Oribe et al. (2010) investigated evoked neural oscillations at 20–45 Hz and found that subjects with BD exhibited greater power in evoked neural oscillations in response to speech sounds compared to healthy subjects and schizophrenia subjects; and schizophrenia patients exhibited delayed evoked neural oscillation peak- and phase-locking to speech sounds. Their study implied that the evoked neural oscillation to speech sounds provided a useful index to distinguish BD from schizophrenia (Onitsuka et al., in this volume).

20.4.4. Alzheimer's disease

AD is the most common form of dementia, a neurological disease characterized by loss of mental ability severe enough to interfere with normal daily activities of living. In the normal aging, a reduction in total brain volume is seen; the reduction in the cortical gray matter volume in AD is more severe than in healthy controls and ranges between 8% and 9% and hippocampal loss is 8%, and olfactory/orbitofrontal cortex shows 12–15% loss. The pattern of cortical atrophy in mild AD is similar to that in prodromal AD, but the loss is more severe in the direct hippocampal pathway and sensorimotor, visual, and temporal cortices (Prestia et al., this volume). These morphometric changes are reflected in many electrophysiological measurements. In resting EEG studies (Babiloni et al., 2011; for a review, see Lizio et al., 2011), when healthy controls, MCI, and AD subjects were classified according to spectral EEG coherence and other EEG features, the successful discrimination rates of controls from mild AD were as 89–45%, from MCI to AD 92–78%, and the conversion of MCI subjects to AD 87–60%. The most sensible parameters of resting state EEG were cortical delta/theta and alpha rhythms, fronto-parietal coherence and computation of the directed transfer function that were abnormal in amnesic MCI and AD subjects (Vecchio et al., this volume).

Event-related oscillations have also shown that mild AD subjects differ from healthy controls. Polikar et al. (2007) used ERO frequency bands to classify AD and healthy controls by means of an automated program. They found oscillatory responses of 1–2 and 2–4 at P_z, and 4–8 Hz at F_z, and 2–4 Hz at C_z were the most valuable classifiers for AD subjects from healthy controls. By means of these four parameters, they reported a sensitivity rate of 77% and a specificity rate of 81%. Later studies reported a consistent decrease in fronto-central delta responses upon either visual (Yener et al., 2008) or auditory oddball stimulation (Caravaglios et al., 2008; Yener et al., 2012). Frontal theta responsiveness has been also reported, either following visual (Yener et al., 2007) or auditory oddball (Caravaglios et al., 2010) paradigm. In their study, Caravaglios et al. (2010) reported that a decreased theta responsiveness in a late time window later than poststimulus 250 ms. Diminished event-related coherence values have been reported in AD in delta, theta, and alpha ranges in fronto-parietal connections. Regarding the medication effects, the alpha event-related coherence (Güntekin et al., 2008) and theta phase-locking (Yener et al., 2007) seem to improve in AD subjects with cholinergic treatment. The most sensible ERO parameters seem to be delta and theta oscillatory responses over fronto-central regions, and fronto-parietal coherences in alpha, theta, and delta frequencies (Başar et al., 2010; Yener and Başar, Ch. 16, this volume). When electrophysiological markers are used in combination with structural MRI, SPECT, and PET markers, a comprehensive data fusion analysis may provide a more accurate analysis taking into account important variables such as validity, costs, invasiveness, and availability of the procedures in the epidemiological studies (Vecchio et al., this volume).

A chart summarizing the possible biomarkers and related neurotransmitters in mentioned neuropsychiatric disorders has been shown in Fig. 5.

20.4.5. Polymorphism

The works of Porjesz et al. (2005) and of Rangaswamy and Porjesz (2008), related to AD and a cholinergic receptor gene (CHRM2), are important, since their findings suggest the possible role of CHRM2 in the generation and modulation of evoked oscillations. Theta and delta EROs depend on the level of acetylcholine (muscarinic activation). M2 receptors inhibit presynaptic release of acetylcholine, leading to inhibition of irrelevant networks. Muscarinic receptors are particularly concentrated in the forebrain and possibly serve to maintain the effective balance of relevant/irrelevant networks, hence, directly influencing P300 generation (Frodl-Bauch et al., 1999). According to the work of the Porjesz group (Begleiter and Porjesz, 2006), the results with the CHRM2 gene and brain oscillations strongly support the role of acetylcholine in the generation of N200 (theta oscillations) and in the P300 component (delta and theta oscillations). The function of acetylcholine has been demonstrated with regard to stimulus significance (Perry et al., 1999),

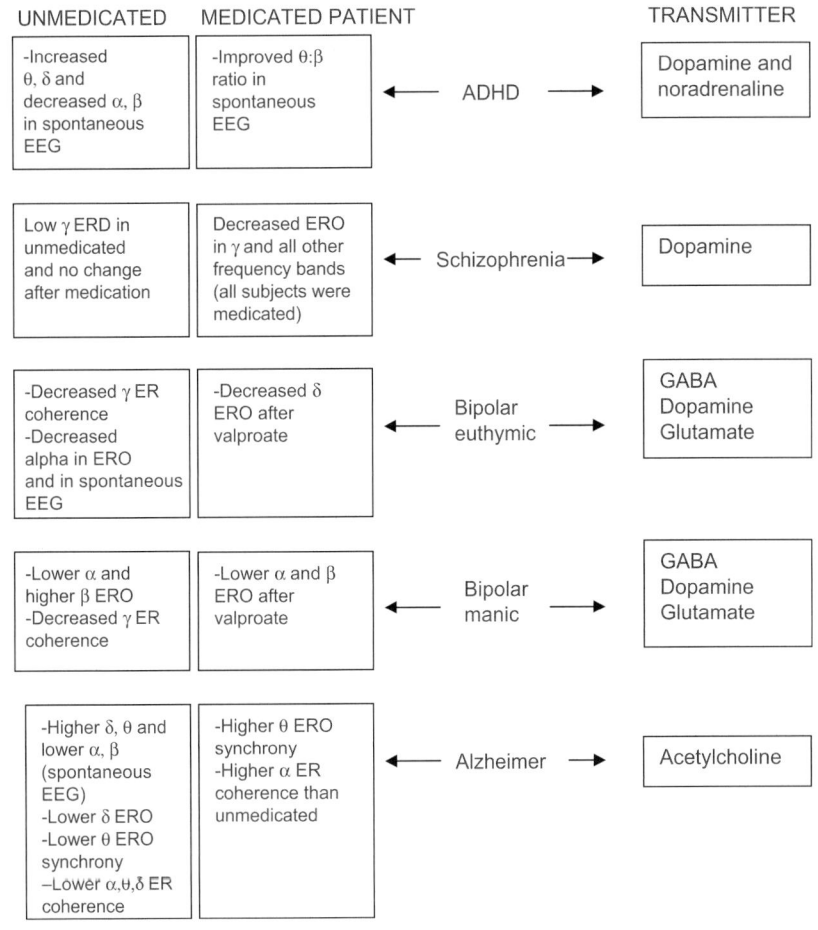

Fig. 5. The possible biomarkers and related neurotransmitters in several neuropsychiatric disorders

selective attention (Mitrofanis and Guillery, 1993), and P300 generation (Callaway et al., 1983).

Thus, genes are important for the expression of the endophenotype (brain oscillations) and help in the identification of genes that increase the propensity to develop alcohol dependence and related disorders (Begleiter and Porjesz, 2006). From the summary of the research publications of Begleiter and Porjesz and their research teams, it can be clearly stated that studies of neuroelectric endophenotypes offer a powerful strategy for identifying the genes that can create susceptibility to develop psychiatric disorders and provide novel insights into etiological factors.

20.5. Neurotransmitters and experimental studies

20.5.1. Neurotransmitters

It is important to remark that such neurotransmitter-related agents are often used as medication in certain diseases. It was long thought that a given neuron released only one kind of neurotransmitter, but today many experiments have shown that a single neuron can produce several different neurotransmitters. Below, four of the best-known transmitters that are involved in functions in both the central and the peripheral nervous systems are described; and neurotransmitters that play a role in major

358

neuropsychiatric disorders mentioned in this volume are listed in Fig. 5.

Acetylcholine is a widely distributed, excitatory neurotransmitter that triggers muscle contraction and stimulates the excretion of certain hormones. In the central nervous system, it is involved in, for example, wakefulness, attentiveness, anger, and aggression.

Norepinephrine is a neurotransmitter that is important for attentiveness, emotion, sleeping, dreaming, and learning. It is also released as a hormone into the blood, where it causes blood vessels to contract and the heart rate to increase. Norepinephrine plays a role in mood disorders such as manic depression.

Dopamine is an inhibitory neurotransmitter involved in controlling movement and posture. It also modulates mood and plays a central role in positive reinforcement and dependency. The loss of dopamine in certain parts of the brain causes the muscle rigidity typically present in Parkinson's disease.

GABA (gamma-aminobutyric acid) is an inhibitory neurotransmitter that is widely distributed in the neurons of the cortex. GABA contributes to motor control, vision, and many other cortical functions. Some drugs that increase the level of GABA in the brain are used to treat epilepsy and to calm the trembling of patients suffering from Huntington's disease. GABAergic interneurons, which are the core component of cortico-limbic circuitry, were found to be defective in the cerebral cortex of bipolar patients (Benes and Berretta, 2001). GABA spreads in neural networks involved in cognitive and emotional processing and modulates noradrenergic, dopaminergic, and serotonergic local neural circuitry (Brambilla et al., 2003). Several studies revealed low plasma (Kaiya et al., 1982; Berrettini et al., 1983) or cortical (Bhagwagar et al., 2007) GABA activity or altered genetic expression of GABA (Guidotti et al., 2000) in BD. Low GABA activity was thought to be a genetically determined trait creating a vulnerability which, with the contribution of environmental factors, can lead to the

development of either mania or depression. It is also important to note that GABAergic activity is reciprocally regulated by dopamine, hyperactivity of which also plays a role in mania (Yatham et al., 2002). Alterations in the modulation of the dopamine system may trigger the appearance of a defective GABA system (Benes and Berretta, 2001). It is important to emphasize the web of theta activity on the GABAergic and cholinergic inputs from the septum. In vivo studies suggest that the hippocampal theta rhythm depends on GABAergic and cholinergic inputs from the septum (Stewart and Fox, 1990; Brazhnik and Fox, 1997) and requires an intact hippocampal CA3 region (Wiig et al., 1994). The cholinergic inputs to the hippocampus are distributed on both the pyramidal and interneuronal cells (Frotscher and Léránth, 1985), while the GABAergic inputs selectively contact the hippocampal interneurons (Freund and Antal, 1988). Later work in vitro on septo-hippocampal cocultures showed that CA3, but not CA1, exhibited theta-like oscillations driven by septal muscarinic synaptic inputs (Fischer et al., 1999). This suggests that the hippocampus is locally capable of regulating the frequency of theta, independent of the septal inputs. Valproate was shown to augment the ability of atypical antipsychotic medications to increase dopamine (DA) and acetylcholine (ACh) efflux in the rat hippocampus and medial prefrontal cortex (Huang et al., 2006). It was also shown to lead to a significant reduction in presynaptic dopamine function in manic patients.

GABAergic interneurons and pyramidal cells were found to build and maintain complex interconnections, which lead to large-scale network oscillations, such as theta, gamma (40–100 Hz), and ultrafast (200 Hz) frequency bands (Benes and Berretta, 2001).

Glutamate is a major excitatory neurotransmitter that is associated with learning and memory and is also thought to be associated with AD, whose first symptoms include memory malfunctions. Neurons that use GABA and glutamate as neurotransmitters are used by more than 80% of the neurons in the brain and constitute the most important inhibition.

20.5.2. Animal models and neurotransmitters

The significance of 40-Hz activity in the brains of different mammals has been hypothesized by several authors (Freeman, 1975; Başar et al., 1987; Eckhorn et al., 1988; Başar-Eroğlu and Başar, 1991; Kaiser et al., 2008; Lenz et al., 2008) as an important coding channel in processing sensory and cognitive information in neural networks. These results further indicate a widely ranging function of the gamma component among the different classes of vertebrates and invertebrates. Bullock and Başar (1988), Schütt et al. (1992), and Başar et al. (1999) also examined the effect of transmitters such as acetylcholine, dopamine, noradrenalin, and serotonin on the isolated ganglia of *Helix pomatia* (snail) and showed changes in the oscillatory dynamics of these ganglia. The application of acetylcholine (ACh) induced a large increase in the theta response in the isolated visceral ganglion. Dopamine induced a crucial change in the oscillatory response, which was recorded in the gamma frequency band following the electrical stimulation in the *Helix* visceral ganglion.

According to Michael Koch (see in this volume), it seems that transmitters and animal models, and also the links between genetics, transmitters, and oscillations, will be very important in the near future. The challenge is to see whether a research group is able to combine these three factors. Koch states that animal models and endophenotypes of mental disorders are regarded as preclinical approaches for understanding the underlying mechanisms of these diseases, and in developing drug treatment strategies. A frequently used translational model of sensorimotor gating and its deficits in some neuropsychiatric disorders is prepulse inhibition (PPI) of startle. PPI is reduced in schizophrenia patients, but the exact relationship between symptoms and reduced PPI is still unclear. Recent findings suggest that the levels of PPI in humans and animals may be predictive of certain cognitive functions. Hence, this simple measure of reflex suppression may be of use for clinical research and the cannabinoid system will be one promising field of schizophrenia translational research.

20.6. Essences of the conference: advantages and efficiency of neurophysiological markers

Following the standard definition, a "biomarker" should differentiate the subject with a certain neuropsychiatric disorder from the healthy subject, track the progress of the disorder, or monitor the effects of medication. In the present report, three fundamental questions arose in relation to the principal theme of the utility of brain oscillations as biomarkers. Questions and/or remarks of conference participants are presented here in order to display knowledge related to brain oscillations in different brain diseases. Giovanni Frisoni's comments related to the nature and evolution of biomarkers in AD present important criteria for successful development of electrophysiological biomarkers in addition to structural MRI and biochemical CSF biomarkers. Claudio Babiloni's discussion presents a concise overview of the state of the art.

The advantages of electrophysiological biomarkers in comparison to other markers are as follows:

(1) These methods are non-invasive.
(2) They are inexpensive.
(3) Neurophysiological measurements enable the description of brain dynamics.
(4) These methods analyze a fast activity chain of the brain in the range of 0–500 ms.
(5) The electrophysiological measurements open the possibility to record processes of perception, attention, decision making, and working memory. In other words, it is possible to learn about dynamic brain function.

At this stage, it is vital to mention that applications of ensembles of electrophysiological recording methods and strategies are important in the search for appropriate biomarkers (Fig. 6). According to the results in the present volume, both conceptual and methodological types of strategies are needed to identify biomarkers. The conceptual strategies include (a) differentiation between evoked and EROs as they possibly reflect the activities of sensory and cognitive networks, respectively; (b) differential connectivity deficit as shown by coherence measurements; (c) changes in spontaneous EEG activity; and (d) changes under medication influence.

The present report also emphasizes the importance of the link between oscillations and neurotransmitters (Fig. 5). In this report, we also indicate the possibility that several findings described in this volume can be proposed as biomarker candidates. The search of biomarkers is certainly not limited to the results of the present issue, and the reviews of O'Donnell et al., Vecchhio et al., Yener and Başar, and Başar and Güntekin (all in this volume) indicate several other possibilities.

The present volume, Supplements to Clinical Neurophysiology, Vol. 62, and the present panel report will likely be most useful in manifesting the new strong trend to develop biomarkers related to brain oscillations in at least four

discussed neuropsychiatric diseases, namely, ADHD, AD, BD, and schizophrenia.

We hope that the results of this conference will contribute to better translational research. The most challenging topic would therefore be to develop user-friendly electrophysiological methods and a common ground that would allow discussion between clinicians, electrophysiologists, and other researchers.

Abbreviations

Aβ42 = amyloid beta 42 peptide
AD = Alzheimer's disease
ADHD = attention deficit hyperactivity disorder
ADNI = Alzheimer's disease neuroimaging initiative
ASSR = auditory steady-state responses
BACE = beta-secretase
BD = bipolar disorder
CSF = cerebrospinal fluid
EEG = electroencephalography
ERO = event-related oscillation
ERP = event-related potential
fMRI = functional magnetic resonance imaging
FDG-PET = fluoro-deoxy glucose positron emission tomography

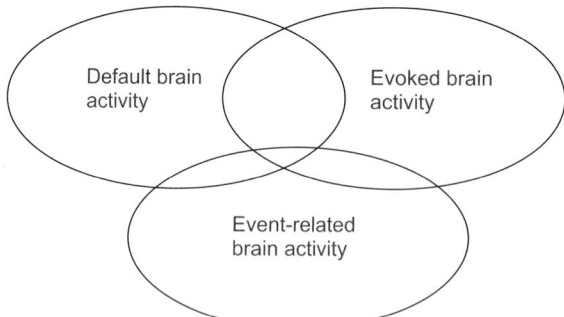

THE STRATEGIES FOR ANALYSIS OF BRAIN ACTIVITY

Fig. 6.   Analysis of brain includes combinations of default brain activity or evoked brain activity by simple sensory stimuli or event-related brain activity elicited by cognitive tasks.

HC = healthy controls
MCI = mild cognitive impairment
MRI = magnetic resonance imaging
PET = positron emission tomography
PLF = phase-locking factor
P-tau = phospho-tau protein
SZ = schizophrenia
SEO = sensory evoked oscillation
TMS = transcranial magnetic stimulation
T-tau = total tau protein

References

American Psychiatric Association (2000) *Diagnostic and Statistical Manual of Mental Health Disorders.* American Psychiatric Association, Washington, DC, 980 pp.

Babiloni, C., Vecchio, F., Lizio, R., Ferri, R., Rodriguez, G., Marzano, N., Frisoni, G.B. and Rossini, P.M. (2011) Resting state cortical rhythms in mild cognitive impairment and Alzheimer's disease: electroencephalographic evidence. *J. Alzheimers Dis.*, 26(Suppl. 3): 201–214.

Barry, R.J., Clarke, A.R. and Johnstone, S.J. (2003) A review of electrophysiology in attention deficit/hyperactivity disorder. I. Qualitative and quantitative electroencephalography. *Clin. Neurophysiol.*, 114: 171–183.

Başar, E., Rosen, B., Başar-Eroğlu, C. and Greitschus, F. (1987) The associations between 40 Hz EEG and the middle latency response of the auditory evoked potential. *Int. J. Neurosci.*, 33(1–2): 103–117.

Başar, E., Başar-Eroğlu, C., Karakaş, S. and Schürmann, M. (1999) Are cognitive processes manifested in event-related gamma, alpha, theta and delta oscillations in the EEG? *Neurosci. Lett.*, 259(3): 165–168.

Başar, E., Güntekin, B., Tülay, E. and Yener, G.G. (2010) Evoked and event related coherence of Alzheimer patients manifest differentiation of sensory-cognitive networks. *Brain Res.*, 1357: 79–90.

Başar, E., Güntekin, B., Atagün, I., Turp-Gölbaşı, B., Tülay, E. and Özerdem, A. (2011) Brain's alpha activity is highly reduced in euthymic bipolar disorder patients. *Cogn. Neurodyn.*, DOI IO 1007/s11571-011-9172-y.

Başar-Eroğlu, C. and Başar, E. (1991) A compound P300–40 Hz response of the cat hippocampus. *Int. J. Neurosci.*, 60: 227–237.

Başar-Eroğlu, C., Brand, A., Hildebrandt, H., Karolina Kedzior, K., Mathes, B. and Schmiedt, C. (2007) Working memory related gamma oscillations in schizophrenia patients. *Int. J. Psychophysiol.*, 64(1): 39–45.

Başar-Eroğlu, C., Schmiedt-Fehr, C., Mathes, B., Zimmermann, J. and Brand, A. (2009) Are oscillatory brain responses generally reduced in schizophrenia during long sustained attentional processing? *Int. J. Psychophysiol.*, 71(1): 75–83.

Başar-Eroğlu, C., Mathes, B., Brand, A. and Schmiedt-Fehr, C. (2011) Occipital gamma response to auditory stimulation in patients with schizophrenia. *Int. J. Psychophysiol.*, 79(1): 3–8.

Begleiter, H. and Porjesz, B. (2006) Genetics of human brain oscillations. *Int. J. Psychophysiol.*, 60(2): 162–171.

Benes, F.M. and Berretta, S. (2001) GABAergic interneurons: implications for understanding schizophrenia and bipolar disorder. *Neuropsychopharmacology*, 25(1): 1–27.

Berrettini, W.H., Nurnberger, J.I., Jr., Hare, T.A., Simmons-Alling, S., Gershon, E.S. and Post, R.M. (1983) Reduced plasma and CSF gamma-aminobutyric acid in affective illness: effect of lithium carbonate. *Biol. Psychiatry*, 18(2): 185–194.

Bhagwagar, Z., Wylezinska, M., Jezzard, P., Evans, J., Ashworth, F., Sule, A., Matthews, P.M. and Cowen, P.J. (2007) Reduction in occipital cortex gamma-aminobutyric acid concentrations in medication-free recovered unipolar depressed and bipolar subjects. *Biol. Psychiatry*, 61(6): 806–812.

Bowden, C.L. (2007) Spectrum of effectiveness of valproate in neuropsychiatry. *Exp. Rev. Neurother.*, 7(1): 9–16.

Brambilla, F., Biggio, G., Pisu, M.G., Bellodi, L., Perna, G., Bogdanovich-Djukic, V., Purdy, R.H. and Serra, M. (2003) Neurosteroid secretion in panic disorder. *Psychiatry Res.*, 118(2): 107–116.

Brazhnik, E.S. and Fox, S.E. (1997) Intracellular recordings from medial septal neurons during hippocampal theta rhythm. *Exp. Brain Res.*, 114(3): 442–453.

Bullock, T.H. and Başar, E. (1988) Comparison of ongoing compound field potentials in the brain of invertebrates and vertebrates. *Brain Res. Rev.*, 13: 57–75.

Bullock, T.H., McClune, M.C. and Enright, J.T. (2003) Are the electroencephalograms mainly rhythmic? Assessment of periodicity in wide-band time series. *Neuroscience*, 121: 233–252.

Callaway, E., Halliday, R. and Herning, R.I. (1983) A comparison of methods for measuring event-related potentials. *Electroencephalogr. Clin. Neurophysiol.*, 55(2): 227–232.

Caravaglios, G., Costanzo, E., Palermo, F. and Muscoso, E.G. (2008) Decreased amplitude of auditory event-related delta responses in Alzheimer's disease. *Int. J. Psychophysiol.*, 70: 23–32.

Caravaglios, G., Castro, G., Costanzo, E., Di Maria, G., Mancuso, D. and Muscoso, E. (2010) Theta power responses in mild Alzheimer's disease during an auditory oddball paradigm: lack of theta enhancement during stimulus processing. *J. Neural Transm.*, 117: 1195–1208.

Eckhorn, R., Bauer, R., Jordan, W., Brosch, M., Kruse, W., Munk, M. and Reitboeck, H. (1988) Coherent oscillations: a mechanism of feature linking in the visual cortex? Multiple electrode and correlation analyses in the cat. *Biol. Cybern.*, 60(2): 121–130.

Fischer, Y., Gähwiler, B.H. and Thompson, S.M. (1999) Activation of intrinsic hippocampal theta oscillations by acetylcholine in rat septo-hippocampal cocultures. *J. Physiol. (Lond.)*, 519(2): 405–413.

Freeman, W.J. (1975) *Mass Action in the Nervous System.* Academic Press, New York, pp. 1–507.

362

Freund, T.F. and Antal, M. (1988) GABA-containing neurons in the septum control inhibitory interneurons in the hippocampus. *Nature (Lond.)*, 336(6195): 170–173.

Frodl-Bauch, T., Bottlender, R. and Hegerl, U. (1999) Neurochemical substrates and neuroanatomical generators of the event-related P300. *Neuropsychobiology*, 40(2): 86–94.

Frotscher, M. and Léránth, C. (1985) Cholinergic innervation of the rat hippocampus as revealed by choline acetyltransferase immunocytochemistry: a combined light and electron microscopic study. *J. Comp. Neurol.*, 239(2): 237–246.

Gandal, M.J., Edgar, J.C., Klook, K. and Siegel, S.J. (2012) Gamma synchrony: towards a translational biomarker for the treatment-resistant symptoms of schizophrenia. *Neuropharmacology*, 62(3): 1504–1518.

Guidotti, A., Pesold, C. and Costa, E. (2000) New neurochemical markers for psychosis: a working hypothesis of their operation. *Neurochem. Res.*, 25(9–10): 1207–1218.

Güntekin, B., Saatçi, E. and Yener, G. (2008) Decrease of evoked delta, theta and alpha coherence in Alzheimer patients during a visual oddball paradigm. *Brain Res.*, 1235: 109–116.

Haig, A.R., Gordon, E., De Pascalis, V., Meares, R.A., Bahramali, H. and Harris, A. (2000) Gamma activity in schizophrenia: evidence of impaired network binding? *Clin. Neurophysiol.*, 111(8): 1461–1468.

Hall, M.H., Spencer, K.M., Schulze, K., McDonald, C., Kalidindi, S., Kravariti, E., Kane, F., Murray, R.M., Bramon, E., Sham, P. and Rijsdijk, F. (2011) The genetic and environmental influences of event-related gamma oscillations on bipolar disorder. *Bipolar Disord.*, 13(3): 260–271.

Herrmann, C.S. and Demiralp, T. (2005) Human EEG gamma oscillations in neuropsychiatric disorders. *Clin. Neurophysiol.*, 116: 2719–2733.

Huang, M., Li, Z., Ichikawa, J., Dai, J. and Meltzer, H.Y. (2006) Effects of divalproex and atypical antipsychotic drugs on dopamine and acetylcholine efflux in rat hippocampus and prefrontal cortex. *Brain Res.*, 1099(1): 44–55.

Jack, C.R., Jr., Vemuri, P., Wiste, H.J., Weigand, S.D., Aisen, P.S., Trojanowski, J.Q., Shaw, L.M., Bernstein, M.A., Petersen, R.C., Weiner, M.W., Knopman, D.S. and the Alzheimer's Disease Neuroimaging Initiative (2011) Evidence for ordering of Alzheimer disease biomarkers. *Arch. Neurol.*, 68(12): 1526–1535.

Kaiser, J., Heidegger, T. and Lutzenberger, W. (2008) Behavioral relevance of gamma-band activity for short-term memory-based auditory decision-making. *Eur. J. Neurosci.*, 27(12): 3322–3328.

Kaiya, H., Namba, M., Yoshida, H. and Nakamura, S. (1982) Plasma glutamate decarboxylase activity in neuropsychiatry. *Psychiatry Res.*, 6(3): 335–343.

Karow, D.S., McEvoy, L.K., Fennema-Notestine, C., Hagler, D.J., Jr., Jennings, R.G., Brewer, J.B., Hoh, C.K., Dale, A.M. and the Alzheimer's Disease Neuroimaging Initiative (2010) Relative capability of MR imaging and FDG PET to depict changes associated with prodromal and early Alzheimer disease. *Radiology*, 256: 932–942.

Lee, K.H., Williams, L.M., Breakspear, M. and Gordon, E. (2003) Synchronous gamma activity: a review and contribution to an integrative neuroscience model of schizophrenia. *Brain Res. Rev.*, 41(1): 57–78.

Lenz, D., Jeschke, M., Schadow, J., Naue, N., Ohl, F.W. and Herrmann, C.S. (2008) Human EEG very high frequency oscillations reflect the number of matches with a template in auditory short-term memory. *Brain Res.*, 1220: 81–92.

Lizio, R., Vecchio, F., Frisoni, G.B., Ferri, R., Rodriguez, G. and Babiloni, C. (2011) Electroencephalographic rhythms in Alzheimer's disease. *Int. J. Alzheimers Dis.*, 2011: 1–11. (927573. Epub 2011 May 12.)

Minzenberg, M.J., Firl, A.J., Yoon, J.H., Gomes, G.C., Reinking, C. and Carter, C.S. (2010) Gamma oscillatory power is impaired during cognitive control independent of medication status in first-episode schizophrenia. *Neuropsychopharmacology*, 35(13): 2590–2599.

Mitrofanis, J. and Guillery, R.W. (1993) New views of the thalamic reticular nucleus in the adult and the developing brain. *Trends Neurosci.*, 16(6): 240–245.

Monastra, V.J., Lubar, J.F. and Linden, M. (2001) The development of a quantitative electroencephalographic scanning process for attention deficit-hyperactivity disorder: reliability and validity studies. *Neuropsychology*, 15(1): 136–144.

Oribe, N., Onitsuka, T., Hirano, S., Hirano, Y., Maekawa, T., Obayashi, C., Ueno, T., Kasai, K. and Kanba, S. (2010) Differentiation between bipolar disorder and schizophrenia revealed by neural oscillation to speech sounds: an MEG study. *Bipolar Disord.*, 12(8): 804–812.

Özerdem, A., Güntekin, B., Tunca, Z. and Başar, E. (2008a) Brain oscillatory responses in patients with bipolar disorder manic episode before and after valproate treatment. *Brain Res.*, 1235: 98–108.

Özerdem, A., Kocaaslan, S., Tunca, Z. and Başar, E. (2008b) Event related oscillations in euthymic patients with bipolar disorder. *Neurosci. Lett.*, 444(1): 5–10.

Özerdem, A., Güntekin, B., Saatçi, E., Tunca, Z. and Başar, E. (2010) Disturbance in long distance gamma coherence in bipolar disorder. *Prog. Neuropsychopharmacol. Biol. Psychiatry*, 34(6): 861–865.

Özerdem, A., Güntekin, B., Atagün, I., Turp, B. and Başar, E. (2011) Reduced long distance gamma (28–48 Hz) coherence in euthymic patients with bipolar disorder. *J. Affect. Disord.*, 132(3): 325–332.

Perry, E., Walker, M., Grace, J. and Perry, R. (1999) Acetylcholine in mind: a neurotransmitter correlate of consciousness? *Trends Neurosci.*, 22(6): 273–280.

Polikar, R., Topalis, A., Green, D., Kounios, J. and Clark, C.M. (2007) Comparative multiresolution wavelet analysis of ERP spectral bands using an ensemble of classifiers approach for early diagnosis of Alzheimer's disease. *Comput. Biol. Med.*, 37(4): 542–558.

Polikar, R., Tilley, C., Hillis, B. and Clark, C.M. (2010) Multimodal EEG, MRI and PET data fusion for Alzheimer's disease diagnosis. *Proceedings of the IEEE Engineering in Medical and Biology Society*, 2010, pp. 6058–6061.

Porjesz, B., Rangaswamy, M., Kamarajan, C., Jones, K.A., Padmanabhapillai, A. and Begleiter, H. (2005) The utility of neurophysiological markers in the study of alcoholism. *Clin. Neurophysiol.*, 116(5): 993–1018.

Rangaswamy, M. and Porjesz, B. (2008) Uncovering genes for cognitive (dys)function and predisposition for alcoholism spectrum disorders: a review of human brain oscillations as effective endophenotypes. *Brain Res.*, 1235: 153–171.

Roach, B.J. and Mathalon, D.H. (2008) Event-related EEG time-frequency analysis: an overview of measures and an analysis of early gamma band phase locking in schizophrenia. *Schizophr. Bull.*, 34(5): 907–926.

Schütt, A., Başar, E. and Bullock, T.H. (1992) The effects of acetylcholine, dopamine and noradrenaline on the visceral ganglion of *Helix pomatia*. II. Stimulus evoked field potentials. *Comp. Biochem. Physiol. C*, 102(1): 169–176.

Spencer, K.M., Niznikiewicz, M.A., Shenton, M.E. and McCarley, R.W. (2008) Sensory-evoked gamma oscillations in chronic schizophrenia. *Biol. Psychiatry*, 63(8): 744–747.

Stewart, M. and Fox, S.E. (1990) Do septal neurons pace the hippocampal theta rhythm? *Trends Neurosci.*, 13(5): 163–168.

Walhovd, K.B., Fjell, A.M., Brewer, J., McEvoy, L.K., Fennema-Notestine, C., Hagler, D.J., Jr., Jennings, R.G., Karow, D., Dale, A.M. and Alzheimer's Disease Neuroimaging Initiative (2010) Combining MR imaging, positron-emission tomography, and CSF biomarkers in the diagnosis and prognosis of Alzheimer disease. *Am. J. Neuroradiol.*, 3: 347–354.

Weiner, M.W., Veitch, D.P., Aisen, P.S., Beckett, L.A., Cairns, N.J., Green, R.C., Harvey, D., Jack, C.R., Jagust, W., Liu, E., Morris, J.C., Petersen, R.C., Saykin, A.J., Schmidt, M.E., Shaw, L., Siuciak, J.A., Soares, H., Toga, A.W., Trojanowski, J.Q. and Alzheimer's Disease Neuroimaging Initiative (2011) The Alzheimer's disease neuroimaging initiative: a review of papers published since its inception. *Alzheimers Dement.*, 8(1, Suppl.): S1–S68. (Oct 31 (E pub ahead), PubMed PMID: 22047634.)

Wiig, K.A., Heynen, A.J. and Bilkey, D.K. (1994) Effects of kainic acid microinfusions on hippocampal type 2 RSA (theta). *Brain Res. Bull.*, 33(6): 727–732.

Wright, C.F., Hall, A., Matthews, F.E. and Brayne, C. (2009) Biomarkers, dementia, and public health. *Ann. N. Y. Acad. Sci.*, 1180: 11–19.

Wynn, J.K., Light, G.A., Breitmeyer, B., Nuechterlein, K.H. and Green, M.F. (2005) Event-related gamma activity in schizophrenia patients during a visual backward-masking task. *Am. J. Psychiatry*, 162(12): 2330–2336.

Yatham, L.N., Liddle, P.F., Lam, R.W., Shiah, I.S., Lane, C., Stoessl, A.J., Sossi, V. and Ruth, T.J. (2002) PET study of the effects of valproate on dopamine D(2) receptors in neuroleptic- and mood-stabilizer-naive patients with non-psychotic mania. *Am. J. Psychiatry*, 159(10): 1718–1723.

Yener, G. and Başar, E. (2010) Sensory evoked and event related oscillations in Alzheimer's disease, a short review. *Cogn. Neurodyn.*, 4: 263–274.

Yener, G., Güntekin, B., Öniz, A. and Başar, E. (2007) Increased frontal phase-locking of event related theta oscillations in Alzheimer patients treated with acetylcholine-esterase inhibitors. *Int. J. Psychophysiol.*, 64: 46–52.

Yener, G., Güntekin, B. and Başar, E. (2008) Event-related delta oscillatory responses of Alzheimer patients. *Eur. J. Neurol.*, 15: 540–547.

Yener, G.G., Güntekin, B., Orken, D.N., Tülay, E., Forta, H. and Başar, E. (2012) Auditory event related delta responses are decreased in Alzheimer's disease. *Behav. Neurol.*, 24: 1–9.

Subject Index

Note: Page numbers followed by "*f*" indicate figures and "*t*" indicate tables.

Color Plate

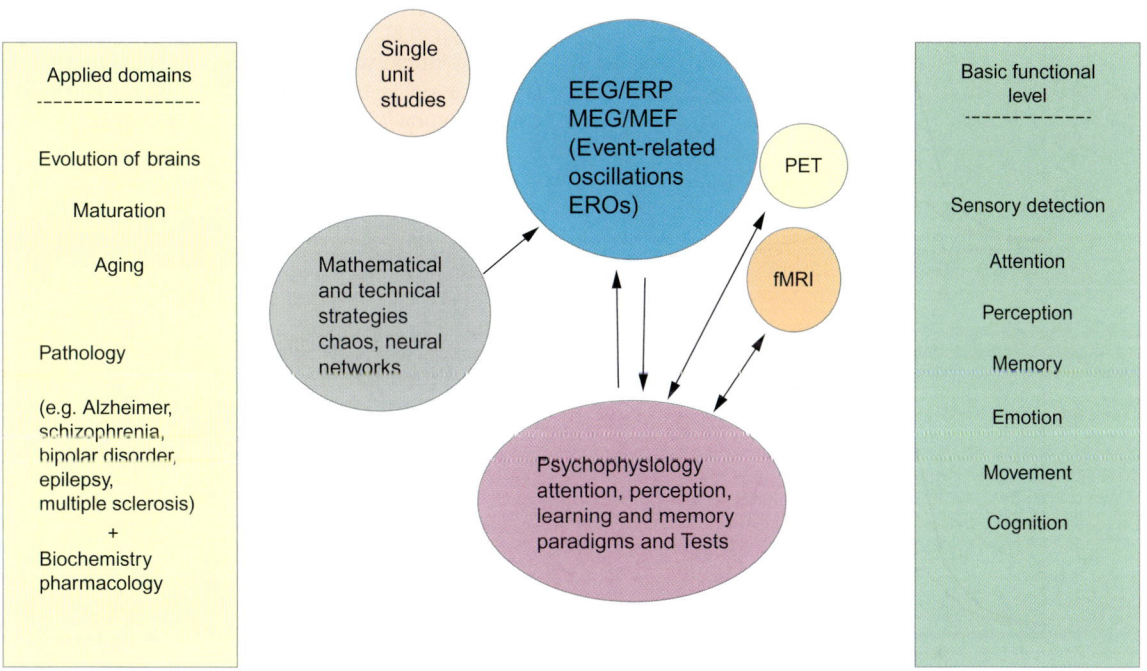

Erol Başar et al., Fig. 2.   New approaches and strategies in functional neuroscience (modified from Başar, 2004).

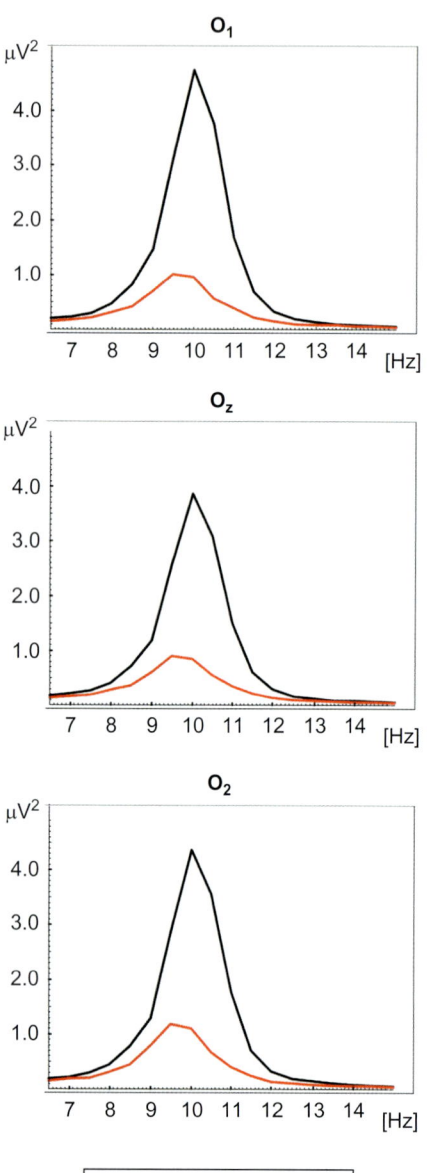

O₁

Oz

O₂

Healthy subjects
Euthymic patients

Erol Başar et al., Fig. 4. Mean eyes-closed power values for occipital electrodes (modified from Başar et al., 2012b).

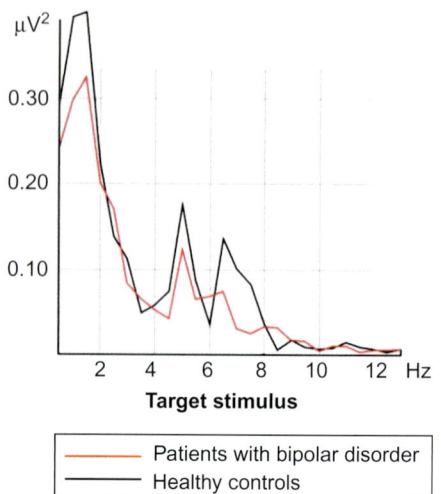

Target stimulus

Patients with bipolar disorder
Healthy controls

Erol Başar et al., Fig. 6. Grand average of power spectra of auditory event-related responses over left frontal (F₃) location in bipolar disorder subjects and healthy controls upon auditory oddball stimulation (modified from Özerdem et al., 2012, this volume).

Healthy, Alzheimer, MCI
Auditory target power spectrum
(*N*=13)

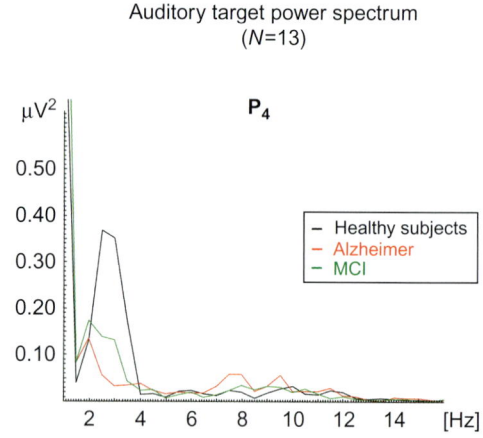

P₄

Healthy subjects
Alzheimer
MCI

Erol Başar et al., Fig. 7. Event-related spectral analysis of healthy control subjects, mild cognitive impairment (MCI), and Alzheimer's disease (AD).

Auditory event-related delta (0.5–2.2 Hz) responses (*N*=13)

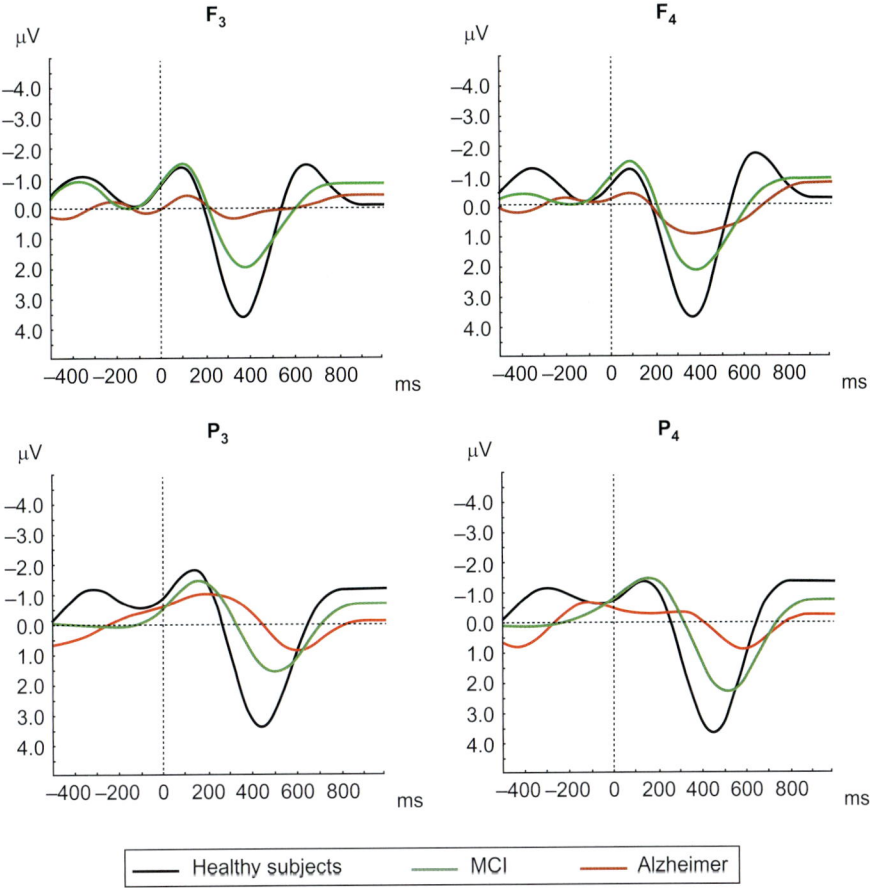

Erol Başar et al., Fig. 8. MCI and AD continuity is prominent in auditory event-related delta oscillatory activity. Results show gradually decreasing delta amplitude and increasing delta peak latency among healthy elderly subjects, MCI, and mild-stage Alzheimer subjects (MCI: mild cognitive impairment, AD: Alzheimer's disease).

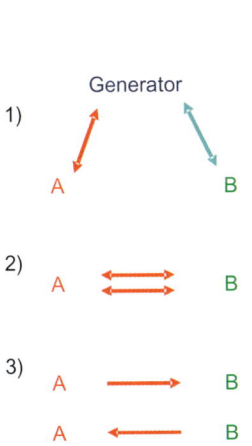

Erol Başar et al., Fig. 9. A description of possible underlying mechanism of coherence between two structures.

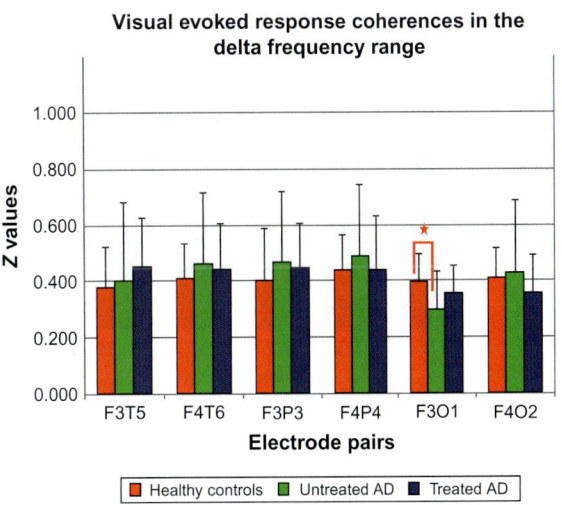

Erol Başar et al., Fig. 10. Mean *Z* values of healthy control, treated AD, and untreated AD subjects for delta frequency range upon simple light stimuli. "*" sign represents $p < 0.01$ (modified from Başar et al., 2010).

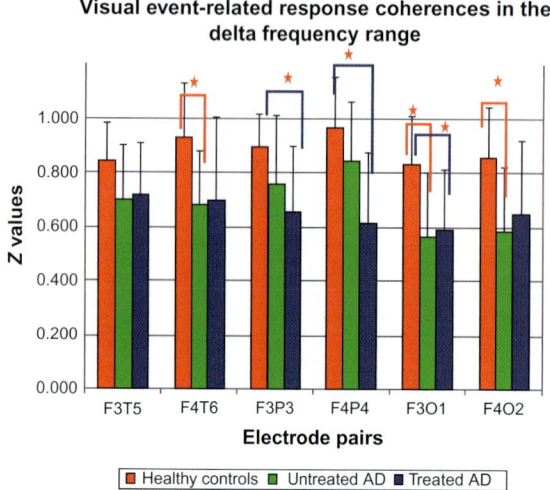

Visual event-related response coherences in the delta frequency range

Erol Başar et al., Fig. 11. Mean Z values of healthy control, treated AD, and untreated AD subjects for delta frequency range upon target stimuli. "*" sign represents $p < 0.01$ (modified from Başar et al., 2010).

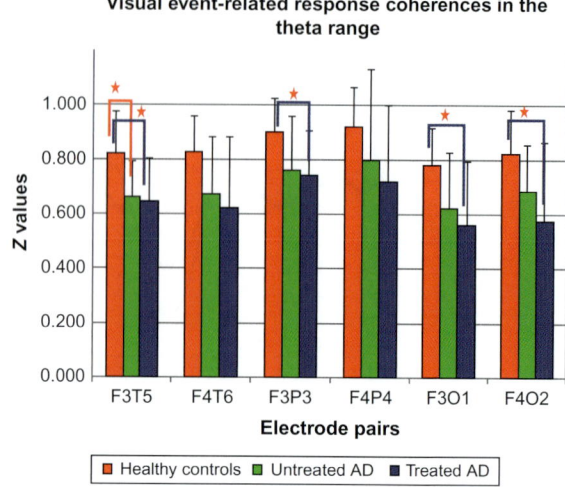

Visual event-related response coherences in the theta range

Erol Başar et al., Fig. 13. Mean Z values of healthy control, treated AD, and untreated AD subjects for theta frequency range upon target stimuli. "*" sign represents $p < 0.01$ (modified from Başar et al., 2010).

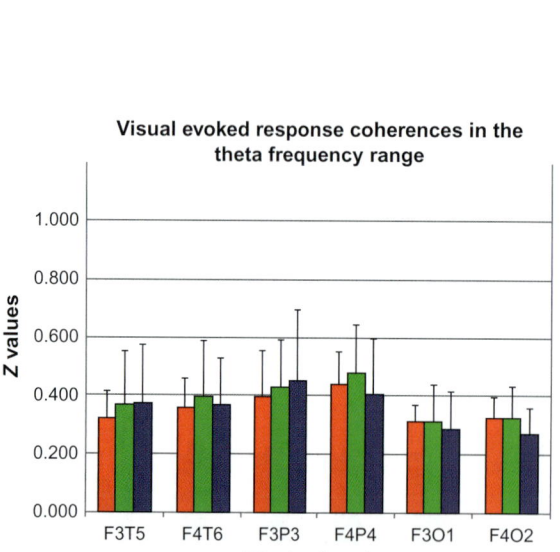

Visual evoked response coherences in the theta frequency range

Erol Başar et al., Fig. 12. Mean Z values of healthy control, treated AD, and untreated AD subjects for theta frequency range upon simple light stimuli (modified from Başar et al., 2010).

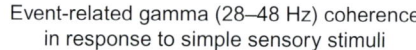
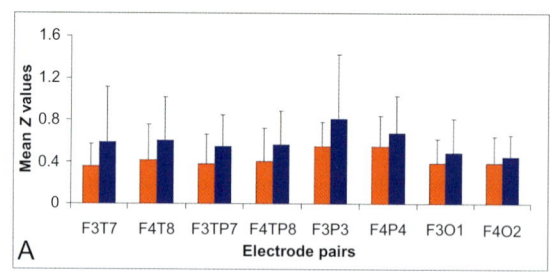
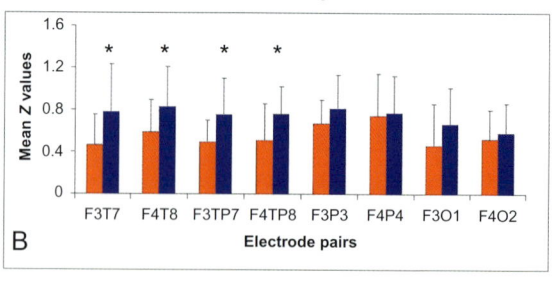

Event-related gamma (28–48 Hz) coherence in response to simple sensory stimuli

Event-related gamma (28–48 Hz) coherence in response to target stimuli

Erol Başar et al., Fig. 14. Mean Z values for sensory evoked (A) and target (B) coherence in response to visual stimuli at all electrode pairs. "*" sign represents $p < 0.05$ (modified from Özerdem et al., 2011).

Visual event-related beta responses grand averages
target
Healthy subjects

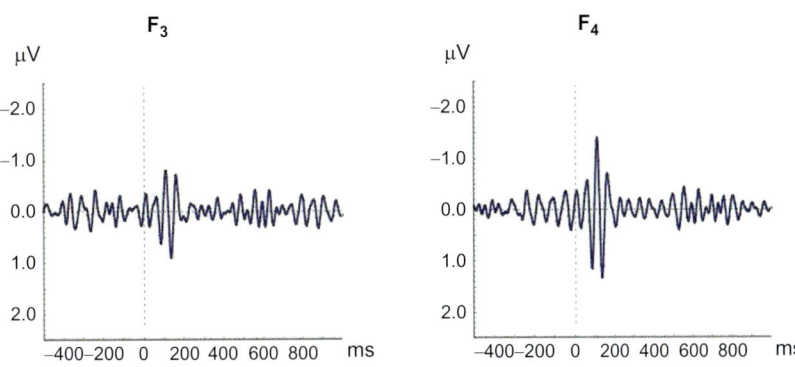

Drug-free euthymic patients

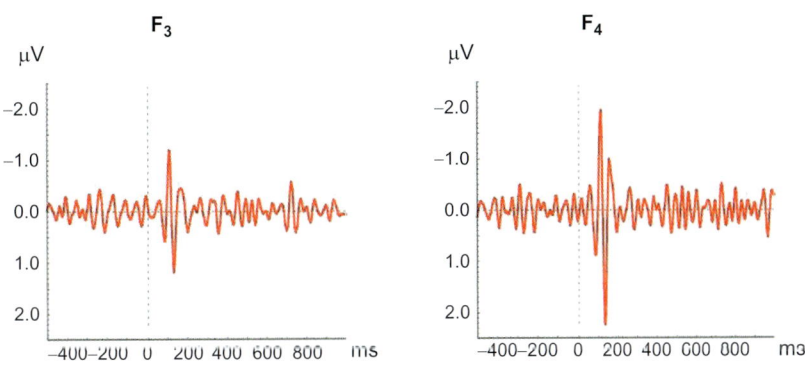

Lithium -treated euthymic patients

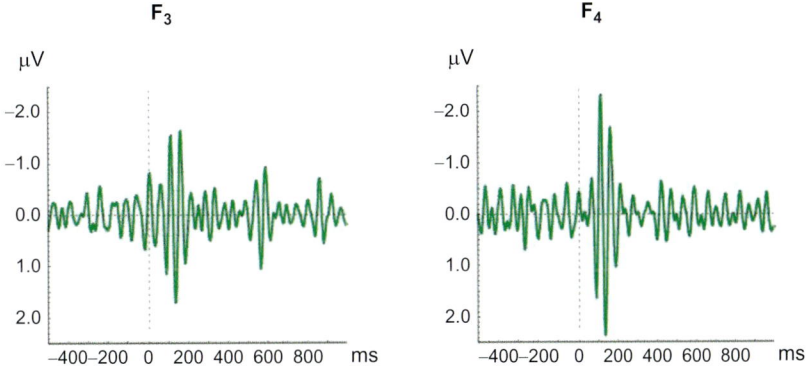

Erol Başar et al., Fig. 19.   Grand averages of event-related beta responses in left (F_3) and right (F_4) frontal electrode sites in (from top to bottom) healthy controls, euthymic drug-free patients, and in euthymic patients under lithium monotherapy (modified from Özerdem et al., 2012, this volume).

TABLE 2

OVERVIEW OF STUDIES ON ELECTROPHYSIOLOGICAL BIOMARKER CANDIDATES IN MCI OR AD

Frequency	Power spectrum			Evoked oscillations	Event-related oscillations	Phase locking	Coherence		
	Spontaneous EEG	Evoked power	Event-related power				EEG coherence	Evoked coherence	Event-related coherence
Delta	↓	↕	→ → (orange)	↕ (Yener et al., 2009, visual sensory)	→ (Yener et al., 2008, visual oddball; Yener et al., 2012, auditory oddball)		← Delta coherence in progressive MCI (Rossini et al., 2006)	↕ (Except F₃O₁ delta decrease) (Başar et al., 2010, visual oddball)	↓ (Güntekin et al., 2008, visual oddball; Başar et al., 2010)
Theta	←	←	→	← (Yener et al., 2009, visual sensory)	↕ (Yener et al., 2008, visual oddball)	↑ (orange) → (Yener et al., 2007, visual oddball)		↕ (Başar et al., 2010, visual oddball)	↓ (Güntekin et al., 2008, visual oddball; Başar et al., 2010)
Alpha	→			↕ (Yener et al., 2009, visual sensory)	↕ (Yener et al., 2008, visual oddball)		→ α1 Coherence in MCI (Babiloni et al., 2010). → α Coherence in AD (Jelic et al., 2000; Knott et al., 2000; Adler et al., 2003)	↕ (Başar et al., 2010, visual oddball)	↑ (orange) ↓ (Güntekin et al., 2008, visual oddball; Başar et al., 2010)
Beta	→			↕ (Yener et al., 2009, visual sensory)	↕ (Yener et al., 2008, visual oddball)			↕ (Başar et al., 2010, visual oddball)	↕ (Güntekin et al., 2008, visual oddball; Başar et al., 2010)
Gamma				↕→ (Yener et al., 2009, visual sensory)	↕→ (Yener et al., 2008, visual oddball)		← Gamma coherence in progressive MCI (Rossini et al., 2006)	↕→ (Başar et al., 2010, visual oddball)	↕→ (Güntekin et al., 2008, visual oddball; Başar et al., 2010)

Blue arrows represent the difference between unmedicated AD patients and healthy controls; red arrows represent the medicated AD patients. Empty cells remain to be analyzed.

TABLE 3

OVERVIEW OF STUDIES ON ELECTROPHYSIOLOGICAL BIOMARKER CANDIDATES IN BIPOLAR DISORDERS

Frequency	Power spectrum						Coherence		
	EEG	Evoked power	Event-related power	Evoked oscillations	Event-related oscillations	Phase Locking	EEG coherence	Evoked coherence	Event-related coherence
Delta									
Fast theta			↓ Atagün et al., 2011, auditory oddball						
Alpha	↓ Clementz et al., 1994; Başar et al., 2012b				↓ Özerdem et al., 2008, manic BD, visual oddball				
Beta	↑ Başar et al., 2012a				↑ Özerdem et al., 2008, manic BD visual oddball				
Gamma								↔ Özerdem et al., 2010, visual sensory	↓ Özerdem et al., 2010, visual oddball

Blue arrows represent unmedicated bipolar manic and euthymic patients. Green arrows show bipolar patients medicated with lithium. Empty cells have not yet been analyzed.

TABLE 4

OVERVIEW OF STUDIES ON ELECTROPHYSIOLOGICAL BIOMARKER CANDIDATES IN SCHIZOPHRENIA

Frequency	Power spectrum			Filtered evoked oscillations	Filtered event-related oscillations	Phase locking	Coherence		
	EEG power	Evoked power	Event-related power				EEG coherence	Evoked coherence	Event-related coherence
Delta						Ford et al., 2008; Doege et al., 2010(a)			
Theta						Ford et al. 2008; Doege et al., 2010(a)			
Alpha									Koh et al. 2011 (inter-trial phase coherence)
Beta									
Gamma	Gallinat et al., 2004; Spencer et al., 2008		Lee et al., 2001; Gallinat et al., 2004; Hall et al., 2011 / Başar-Eroğlu et al., 2011, single trail evoked power		Haig et al., 2000	Slewa-Younan et al., 2004; Symond et al. 2005 (decreased frontal, Lee et al., 2003; Roach and Mathalon, 2008) increased posterior syncrony (Lee et al., 2003)			

Hypothesized network	Cortical region	Comprised BAs
Polysynaptic hippocampal pathway	Posterior cingulate Retrosplenial cortex	23 + 31 + 26 + 29 + 30
Olfactory pathway	Prefrontal orbital cortex Subgenual cortex	11 + 25
Direct hippocampal pathway	Temporal pole Medial and inferior temporal cortex Prefrontal cortex	20 + 38 + 27 + 28 + 35 + 36 + 37 8+9+10+44+45+46+47
Sensorimotor pathway	Primary motor and somatosensory cortices	1+4+43
Visual pathway	Primary and associative visual cortices	17+18+19

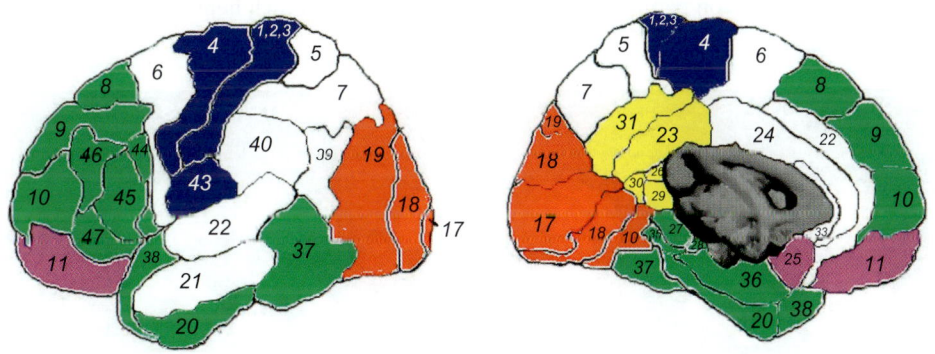

Annapaola Prestia et al., Fig. 1.   Composition of neural networks.

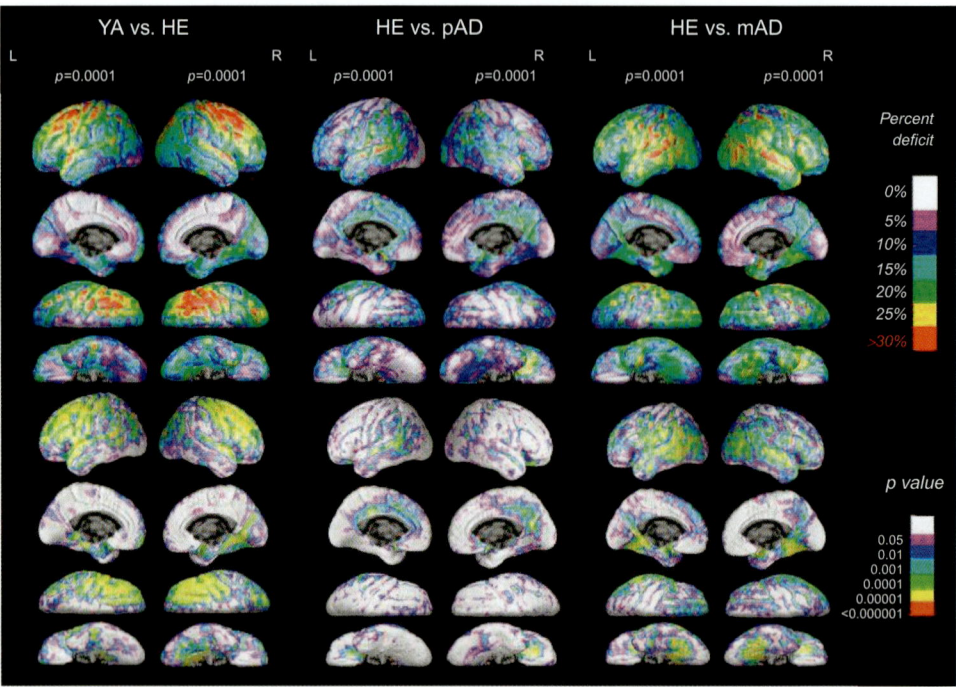

Annapaola Prestia et al., Fig. 2. Map of the differences of gray matter between study groups. Corrected set level significance on permutation test is reported on top of each hemisphere.

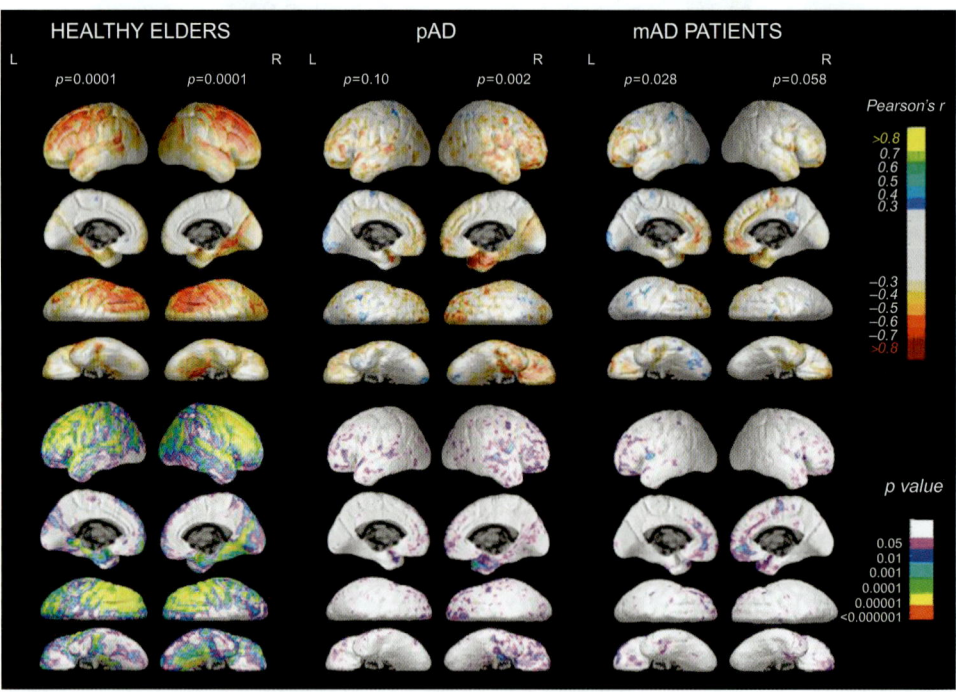

Annapaola Prestia et al., Fig. 3. Map of correlations between age and gray matter density. Corrected set level significance on permutation test is reported on top of each hemisphere.

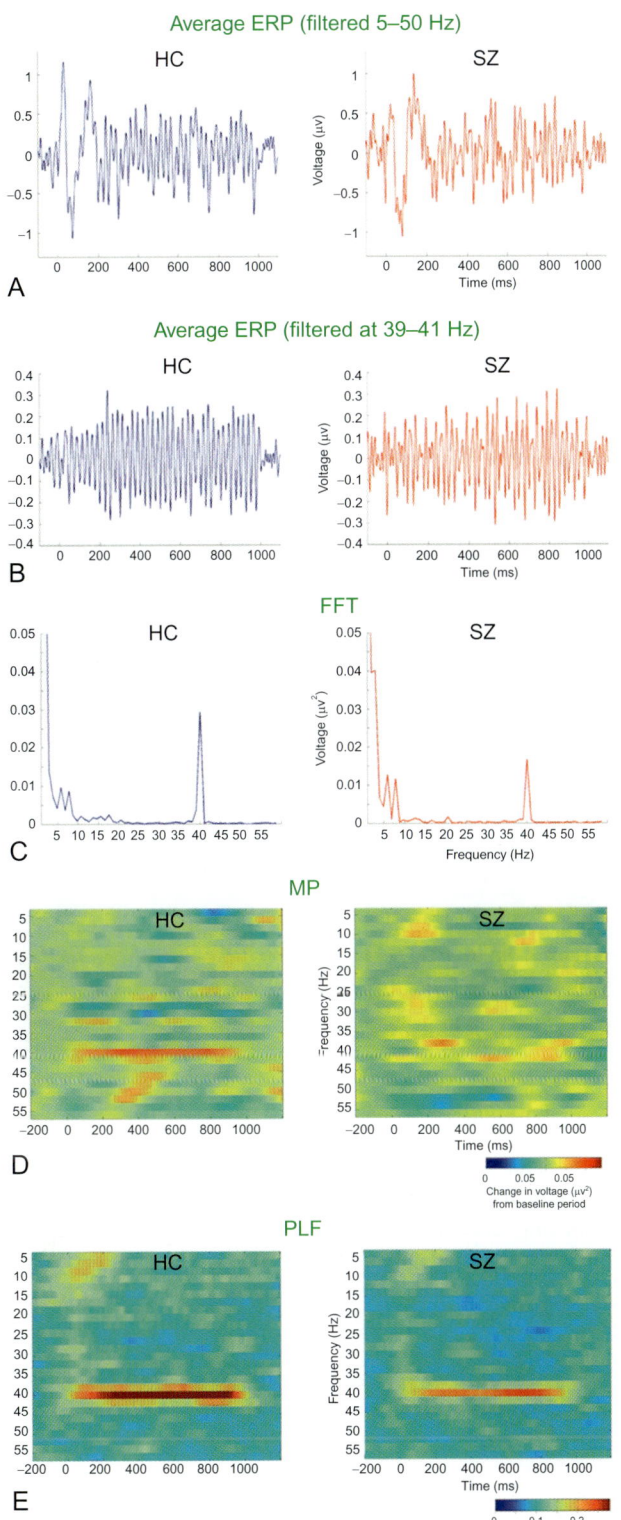

Brian F. O'Donnell et al., Fig. 1.   Auditory steady-state responses (ASSRs) to a 1-s, 40-Hz amplitude-modulated tone recorded at Cz in a healthy control group (HC; $N = 21$) and in patients with schizophrenia (SZ; $N = 21$). (A) The ERP in the time domain averaged across subjects, showing both a large onset response as well as the 40-Hz oscillation. In (B), the averaged wave form has been filtered between 39 and 41 Hz. (C) A power spectrum obtained by applying a Fast Fourier Transform on the ERPs in the two groups, showing the 40-Hz response in the HC group which is reduced in magnitude in the SZ group. (D) Mean power (MP) across the epoch which indicates the average change in power at a given frequency from the mean baseline power. The x-axis represents time in milliseconds, the y-axis represents frequency in Hertz, and the colors represent the magnitude of power. (E) The phase-locking factor (PLF) across trials. The x-axis indicates time in milliseconds, the y-axis indicates frequency, and the colors represent phase reproducibility across trials ranging from 0 (absence of synchronization) to 1 (perfect synchronization).

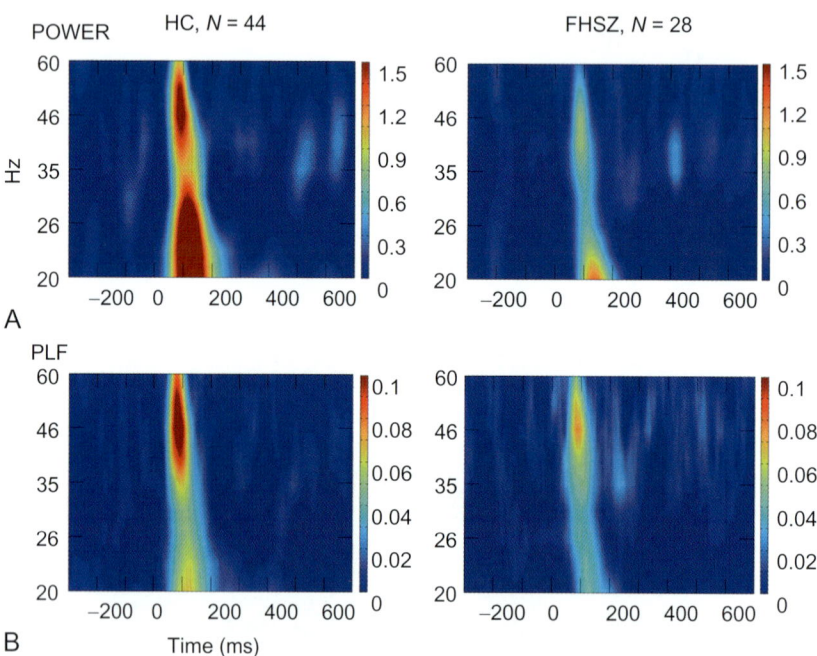

Grantley W. Taylor et al., Fig. 2.   (A) Frequency in time maps of evoked power at Cz for each group for standard stimuli. Note that patients show attenuated evoked power in that time interval relative to controls. The lower (f) activity reflects N1 and P2. (B) Phase-locking factor at Cz for each group for standard stimuli. Although maximum evoked power was observed at 46 Hz in controls, their maximum PLF was lower, closer to 40 Hz. Patients showed very little phase consistency across trials.

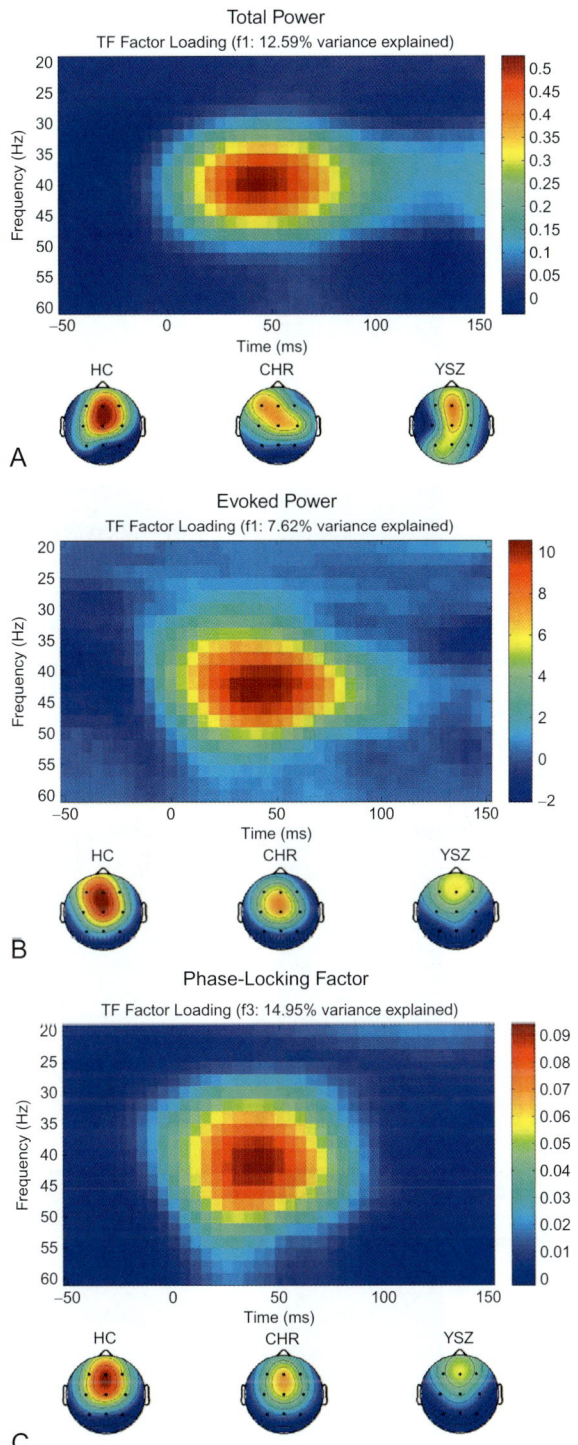

Veronica B. Perez et al., Fig. 1. GBR factor loadings. Time-frequency (TF) factor loadings are plotted from a principal component analysis (PCA) with varimax rotation for (A) total power, (B) evoked power, and (C) phase-locking factor gamma-band responses (GBR). Time (ms) is plotted on the *x*-axis; EEG frequency (Hz) is plotted on the *y*-axis. Stimulus onset occurred at 0 ms. Below each TF plot, scalp topography maps for each group (healthy control (HC), clinical high risk (CHR), and young schizophrenia (YSZ)) show a fronto-central distribution for each GBR across groups. YSZ shows reduced GBRs relative to HC. CHR is intermediate to the HC and YSZ groups. Scaling was uniform across groups. Greater total power and evoked power GBRs, and greater phase-locking consistency across trials, are shown in hot colors (red), as indicated on the color scale to the right of each TF plot.

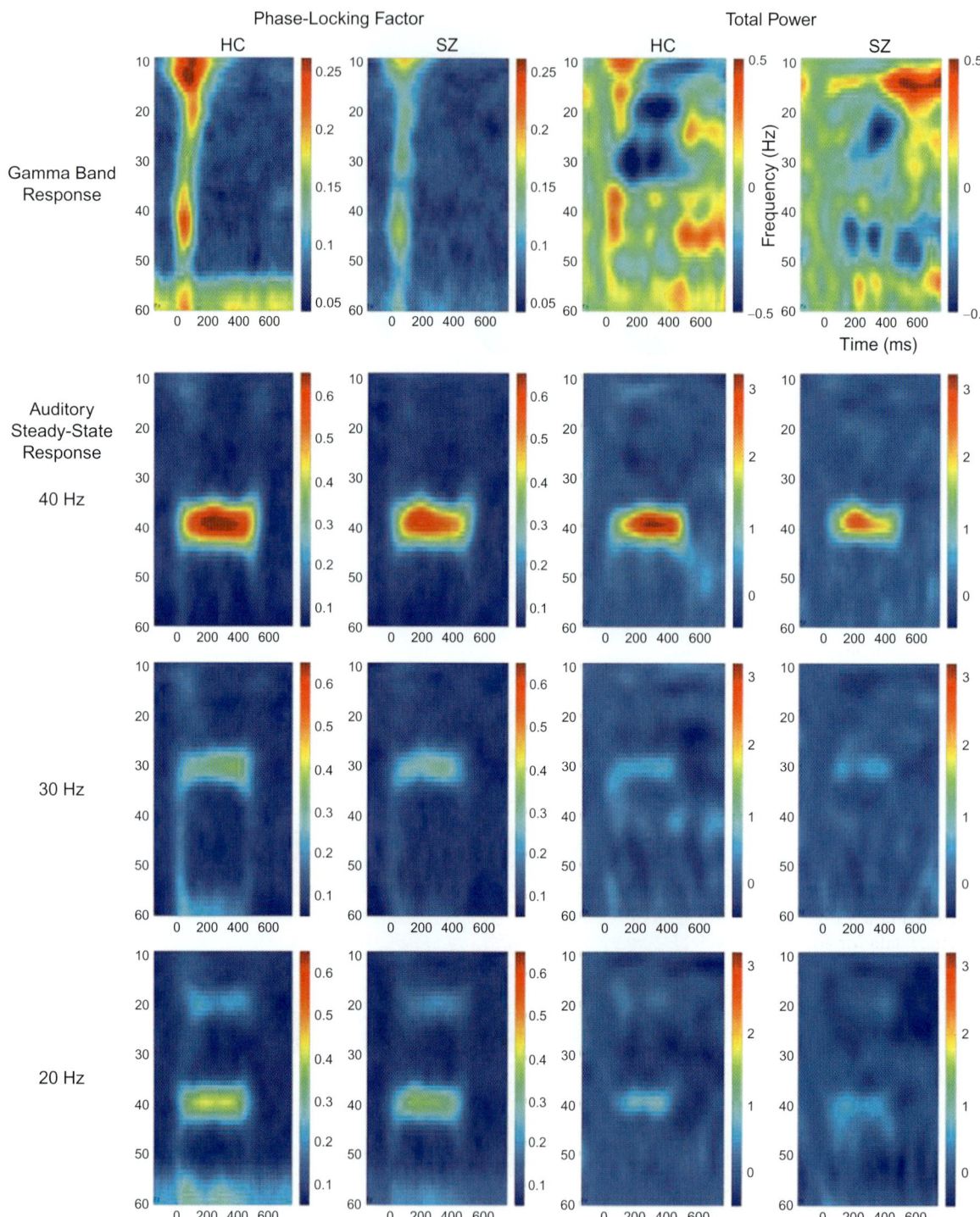

B.J. Roach et al., Fig. 1. Grand-average time-frequency maps from 25 healthy controls (HC) and 28 schizophrenia patients (SZ) are plotted with frequencies on the *y*-axis and time on the *x*-axis. Gamma-band responses are plotted on the top row while auditory steady-state responses for 40, 30, and 20 Hz driving conditions are shown on the second, third, and fourth rows, respectively. Dark red colors indicate little phase variance across trials in the first two columns, whereas dark blue colors indicate equally distributed phase variance across trials. In the third and fourth columns, total power data are plotted in decibel (dB) units, with dark red and blue showing magnitude increases or decreases relative to a 100 ms baseline.

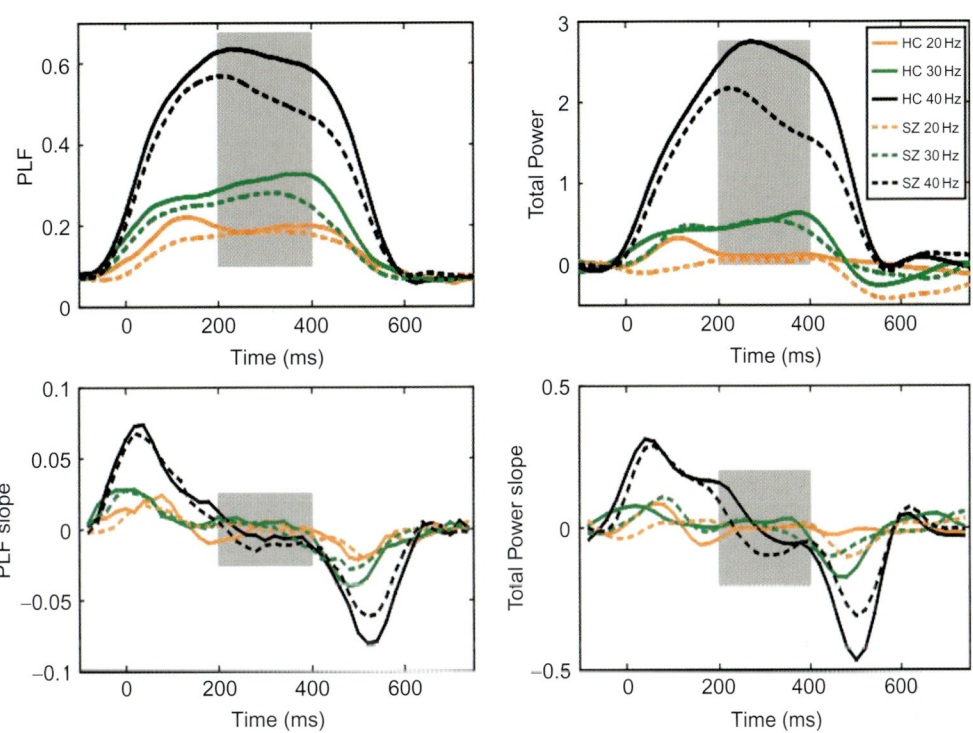

B.J. Roach et al., Fig. 2.   Healthy control (HC, solid lines) and schizophrenia (SZ, dashed lines) group mean time-frequency data for 40 Hz (black), 30 Hz (green), and 20 Hz (orange) driving conditions are plotted for phase-locking factor (PLF) (left) and total power (right) measures on the top row. The rate of change (i.e., slope) in 20 ms increments from each measure in all conditions are plotted on the bottom row. All values are based on the group average taken in bands ±2 Hz around the stimulated frequency. Gray shading between 200 and 400 ms highlights the period of the auditory steady-state response with greatest stability across all conditions, groups, and measures.

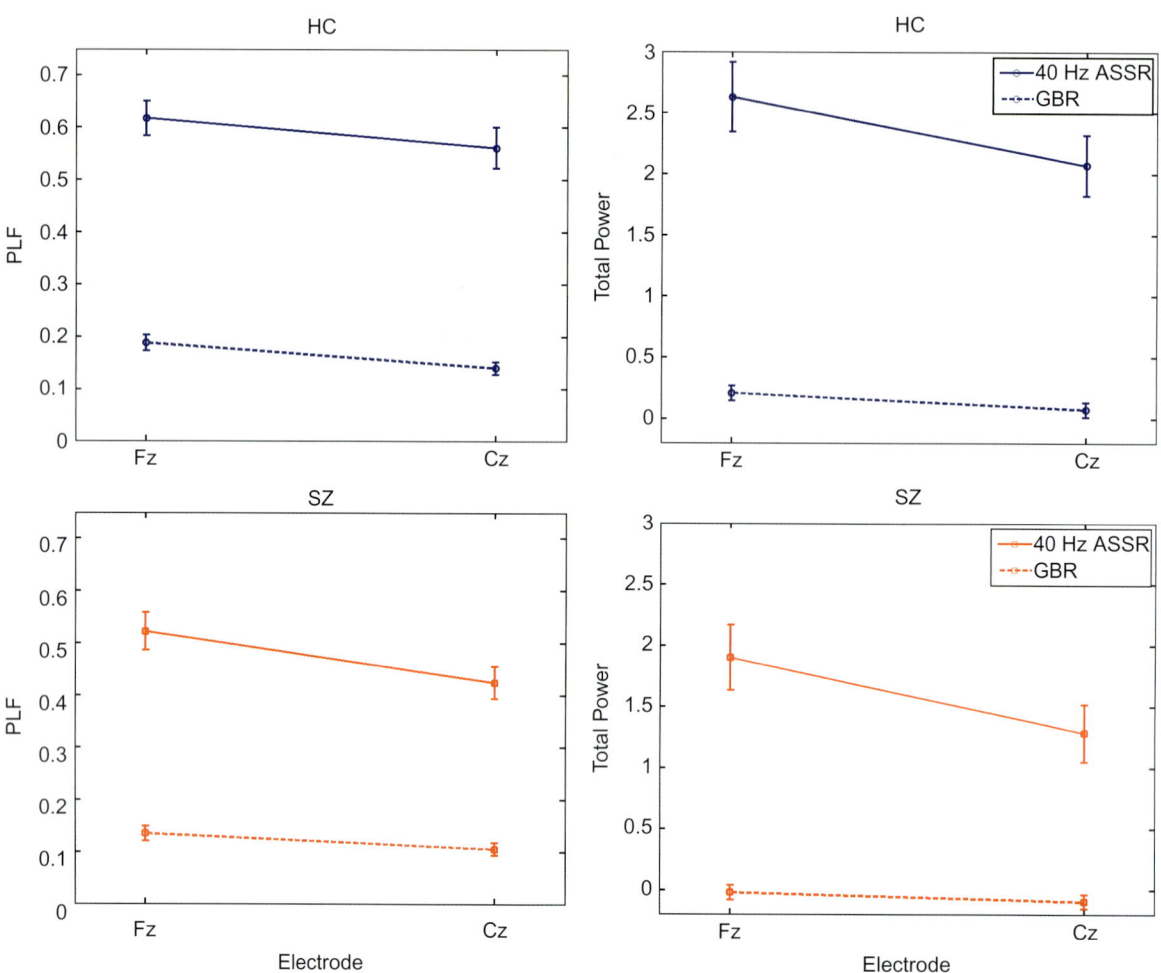

B.J. Roach et al., Fig. 3. Healthy control (HC, blue lines) and schizophrenia (SZ, red lines) group means and standard error bars from gamma-band response (GBR) and 40 Hz auditory steady-state response (ASSR) conditions at electrodes Fz and Cz are plotted for phase-locking factor (PLF) (left) and total power (right).

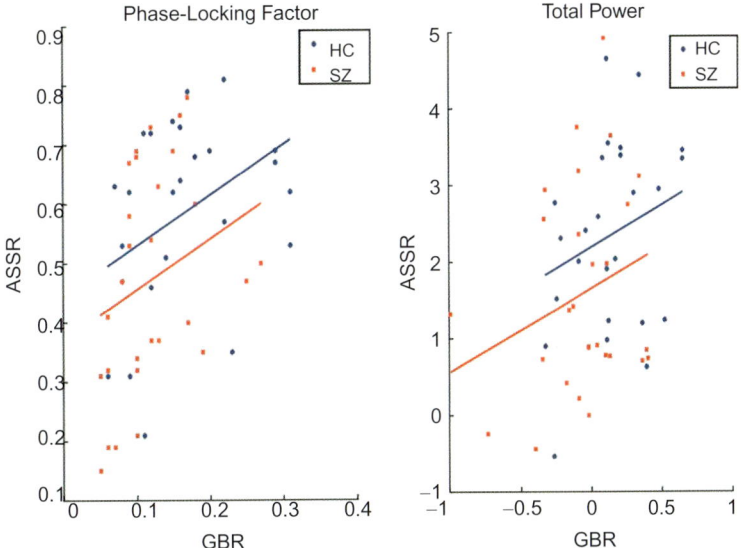

B.J. Roach et al., Fig. 4. The relationship between standard tone gamma-band response (GBR: *x*-axis) and 40 Hz auditory steady-state response (ASSR: *y*-axis) is illustrated with separate scatter plots for phase-locking factor (PLF, left) and total power (right). Each point represents single subject (schizophrenia (SZ): red square; healthy control (HC): blue circle) data, averaged across 35–50 Hz and 20–60 ms for the GBR or across 38–42 Hz and 200–400 ms for the ASSR. Regression lines are plotted separately using the common slope and separate intercepts for each group (SZ: red; HC: blue) to show the relationship between paradigms for PLF (partial *r* (controlling for group) = 0.326, *p* = 0.018) and total power (partial *r* (controlling for group) = 0.254, *p* = 0.069).

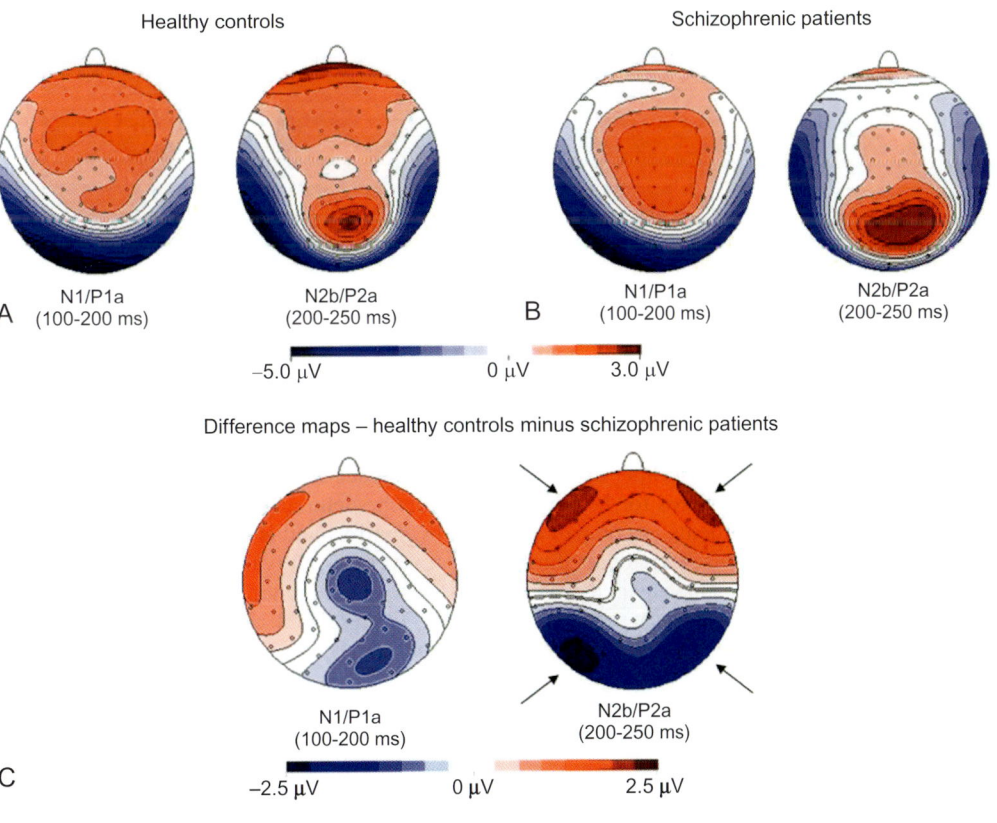

Anuradha Sharma et al., Fig. 1. Voltage topography maps for the early and late ERPs. (A) Voltage maps for healthy controls during the early (100–200 ms) and late (200–250 ms) ERP time intervals. Maps confirm the frontal positive and occipito-temporal negative distribution of brain electrical activity during the examined time intervals. (B) Voltage maps for schizophrenia patients during the same intervals which show a distribution of activity during the early interval similar to healthy controls but during the later time interval there is a reduced frontal positive and posterior negative activity as compared to healthy controls. (C) Voltage maps for difference waves (healthy controls minus schizophrenia patients). Patients show a greater reduction in the frontal positive and posterior negative activity in the later time interval.

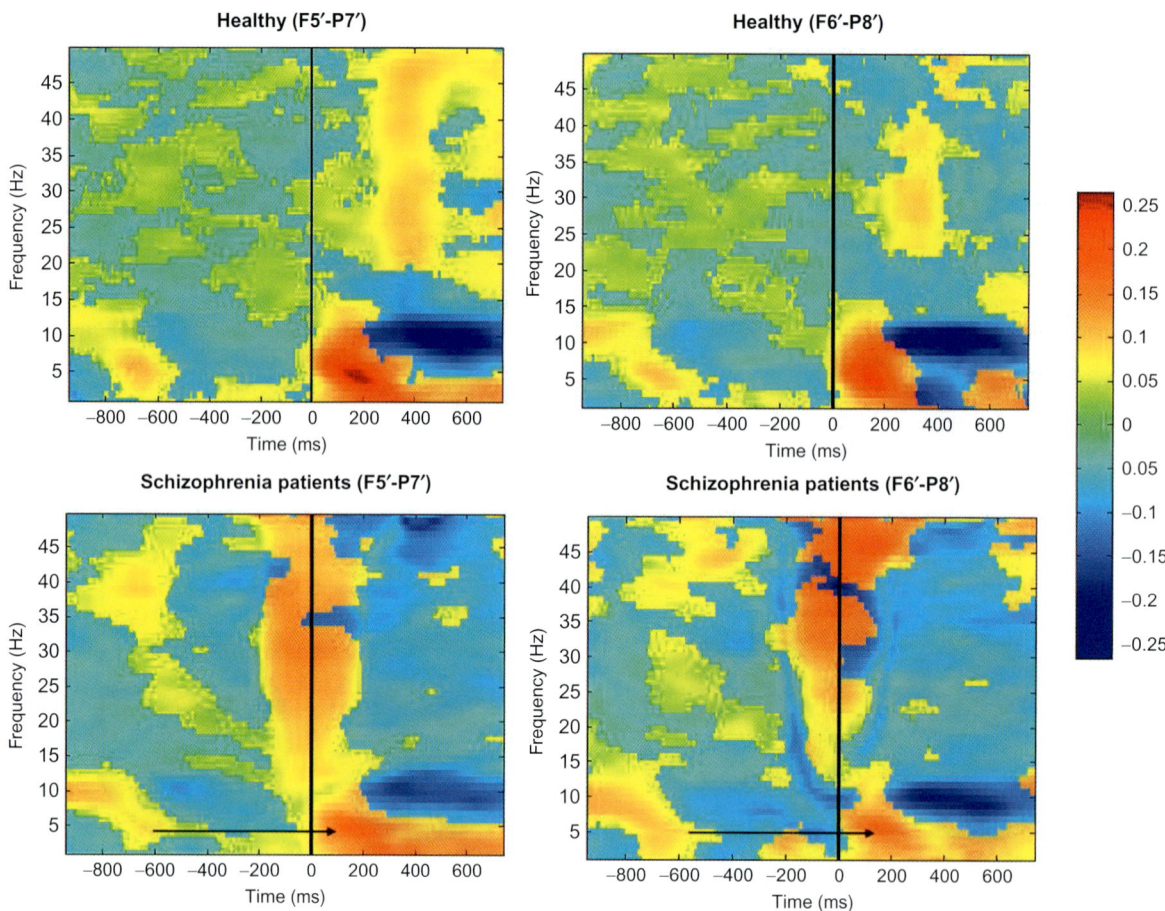

Anuradha Sharma et al., Fig. 3. Grand-averaged plots of event-related fronto-posterior coherence changes. Reproduced from Sharma et al. (2011). Time- and frequency-resolved coherence related to the task is shown for healthy controls and patients separately for the left (F5′–P7′) and right (F6′–P8′) hemispheres. 0 ms refers to the onset of the word stimulus. With respect to baseline, fronto-posterior coherence was significantly increased between 0 and 250 ms post stimulus in both hemispheres for healthy controls for the delta and theta frequencies. This coherence increase was significantly less in patients as compared to healthy controls and is indicated by arrows in the figure. The increased event-related coherence in patients during the pre-stimulus interval (–200 to –0 ms) seen in the plot, turned out to be due to one patient showing an extremely high value of coherence (30 times the standard deviation) for the beta and gamma frequencies during this time interval. Even-related coherence analysis specifically for 100–200 ms and 200–250 ms time intervals revealed group differences across both time intervals.

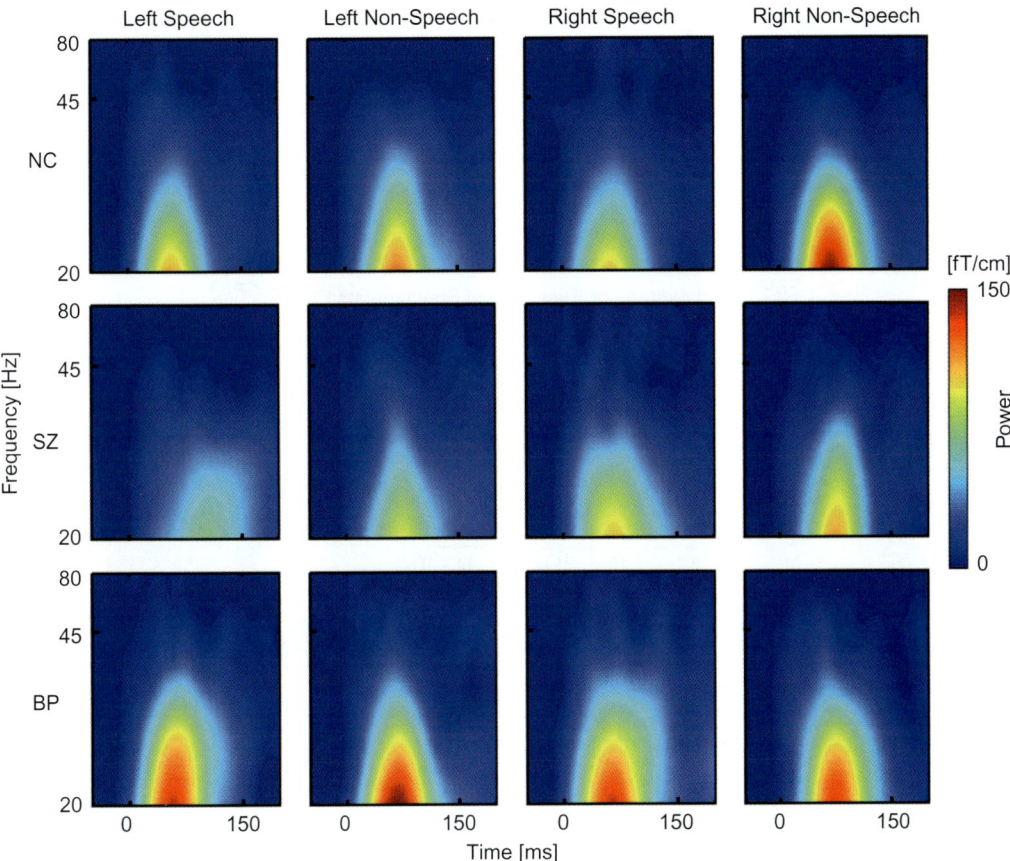

Toshiaki Onitsuka et al., Fig. 1. Overall average time–frequency maps of evoked neural oscillation power to speech sounds and pure tones in patients with bipolar disorder (BP), patients with schizophrenia (SZ), and normal controls (NC). The color scale represents the evoked neural oscillation power. (Adapted from Oribe et al., 2010.)

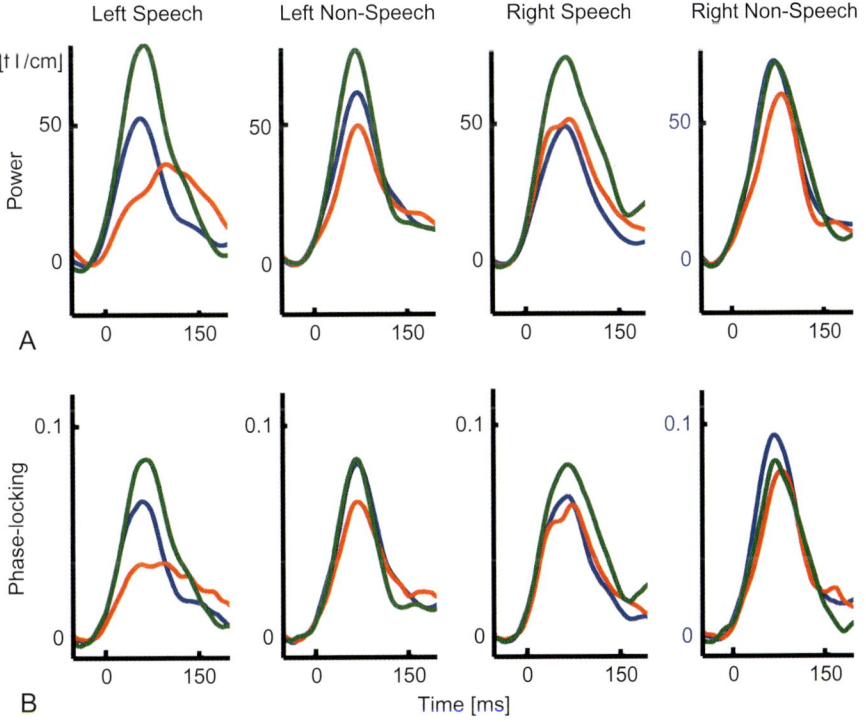

Toshiaki Onitsuka et al., Fig. 2. (A) The overall average of the evoked neural oscillation power waveforms across 20–45 Hz. (B) grand average evoked neural oscillation phase-locking waveforms of schizophrenia (red), bipolar disorder (green), and normal control subjects (blue). (Adapted from Oribe et al., 2010.)

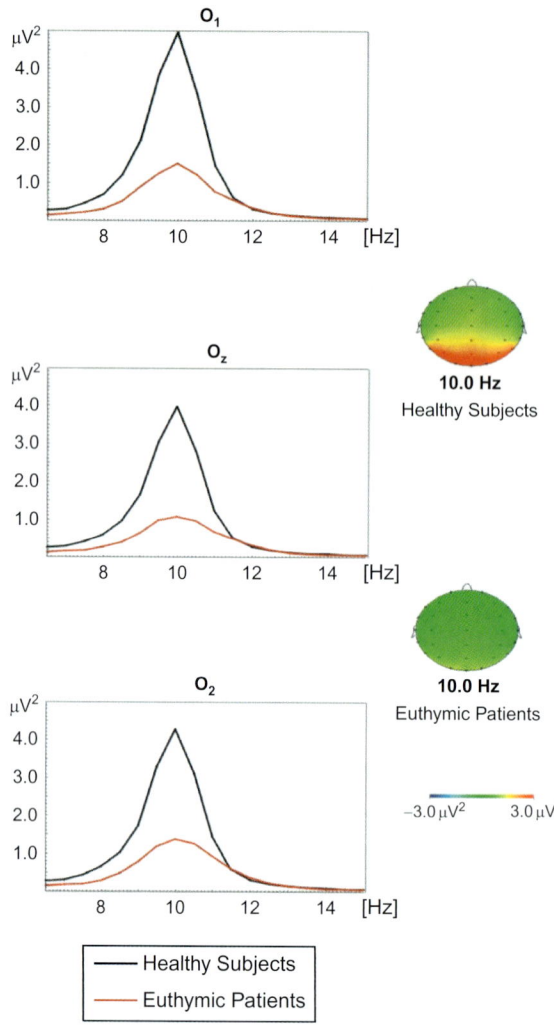

Grand Average of Eyes Closed Spontaneous EEG

Ayşegül Özerdem et al., Fig. 1. Grand averages of power spectra of 18 healthy and 18 euthymic subjects for the eyes-closed condition. The locations presented are from top to bottom: top (O_1), central (O_z), and bottom (O_2) electrodes. The black line is the grand average of power spectra of evoked response in healthy participants. The red line is the grand average of power spectra of evoked response in euthymic participants.

Visual Event Related Beta Responses Grand Averages

Target

Healthy Subjects

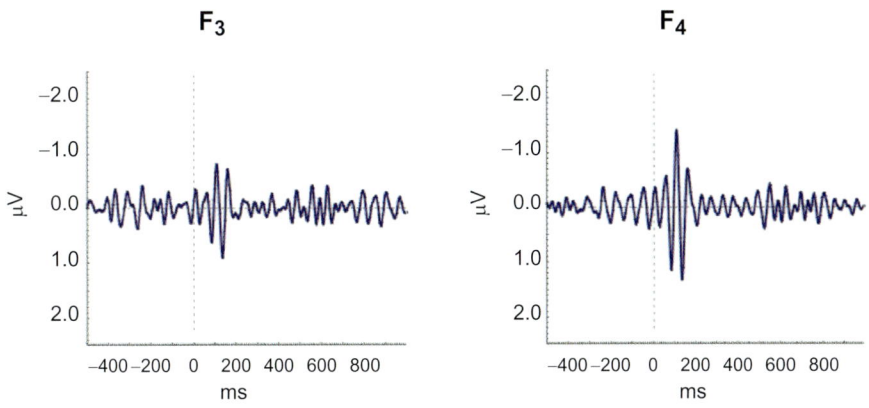

Drug-free Euthymic Patients

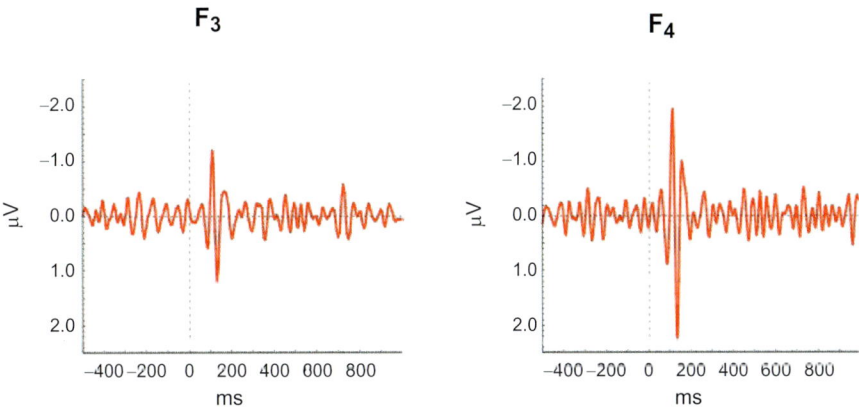

Lithium-treated Euthymic Patients

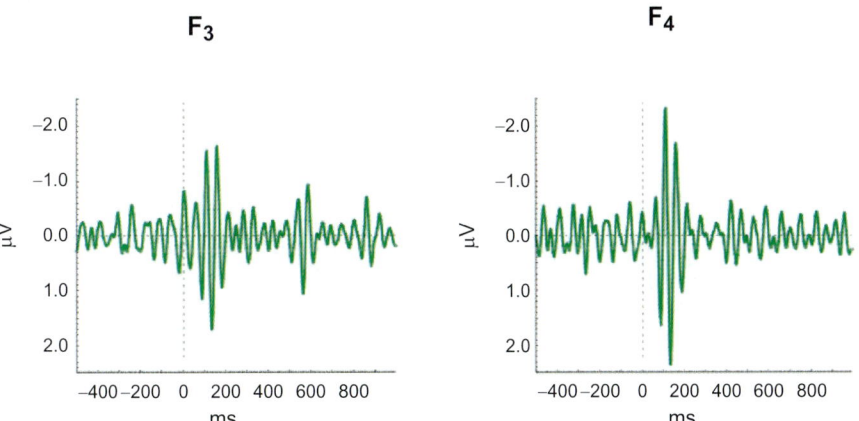

Ayşegül Özerdem et al., Fig. 2. Grand averages of event-related beta responses in left (F_3) and right (F_4) frontal electrode sites in (from top to bottom) healthy controls, untreated euthymic patients, and in patients under lithium monotherapy.

4–6 Hz

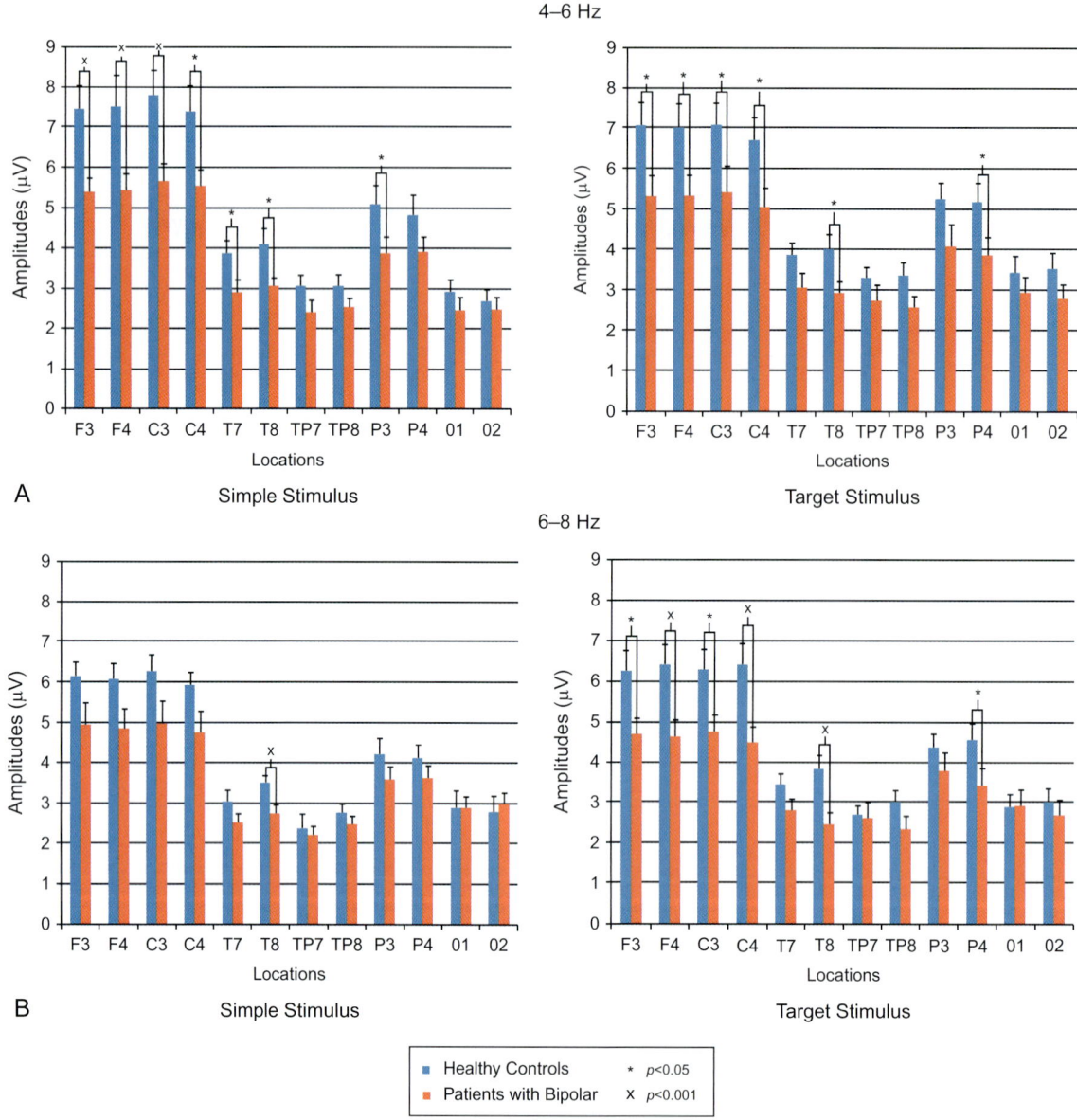

6–8 Hz

Ayşegül Özerdem et al., Fig. 3. (A) Mean amplitudes of patients with bipolar disorder and healthy controls in 4–6 Hz frequency range. Red bars represent patients with bipolar disorder and blue bars represent healthy controls. * p values lower than 0.05; $^{\times}$ p values lower than 0.001. (B) Mean amplitudes of patients with bipolar disorder and healthy controls in 6–8 Hz frequency range. Red bars represent patients with bipolar disorder and blue bars represent healthy controls. * p values lower than 0.05; $^{\times}$ p values lower than 0.001.

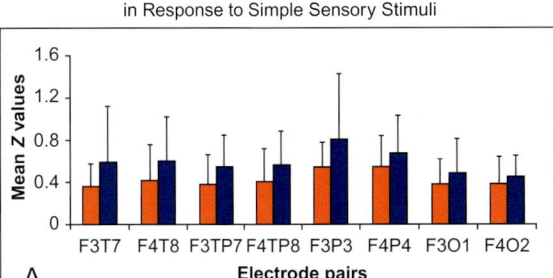

Event-related Gamma (28-48 Hz) Coherence in Response to Simple Sensory Stimuli

A

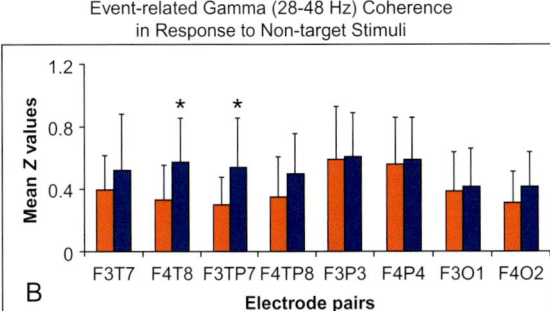

Event-related Gamma (28-48 Hz) Coherence in Response to Non-target Stimuli

B

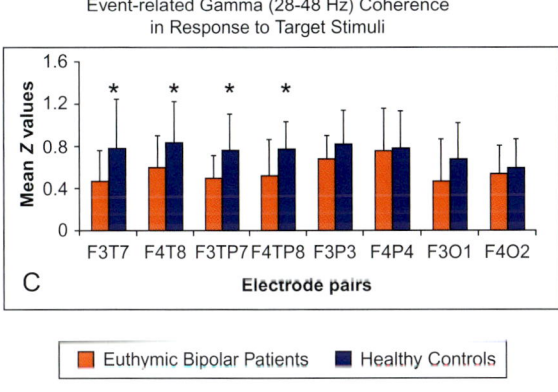

Event-related Gamma (28-48 Hz) Coherence in Response to Target Stimuli

C

Ayşegül Özerdem et al., Fig. 4. A, B, and C: mean Z values for sensory evoked (A), for event-related non-target (B), and target (C) coherence in response to visual stimuli at all electrode pairs. * $p < 0.005$.

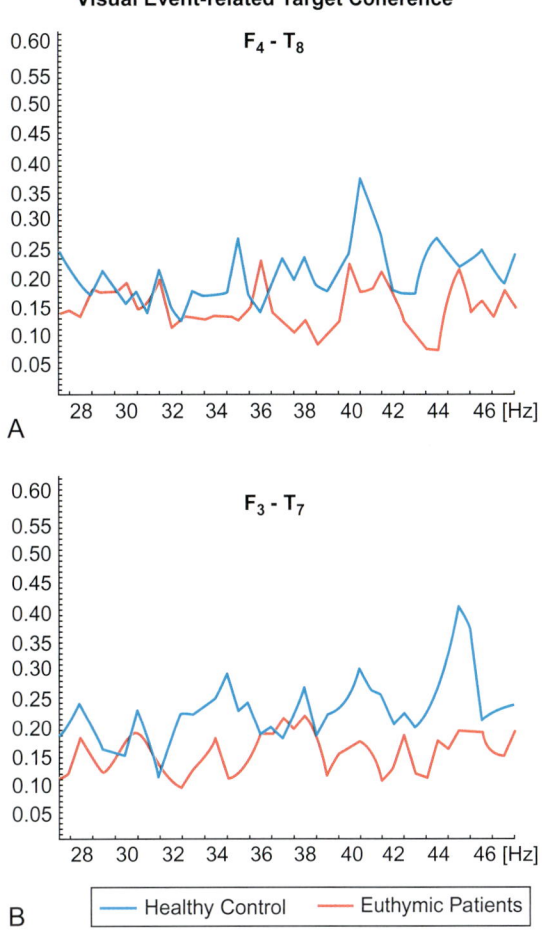

Visual Event-related Target Coherence

A

B

Ayşegül Özerdem et al., Fig. 5. Visual event-related target coherence between the right fronto-temporal (A) and left fronto-temporal (B) locations in euthymic drug-free and healthy controls. Red line represents patients and blue line represents healthy controls. The EEG coherence function is shown along the ordinate (numerical value) and the frequency (Hz) is shown along the abscissa.

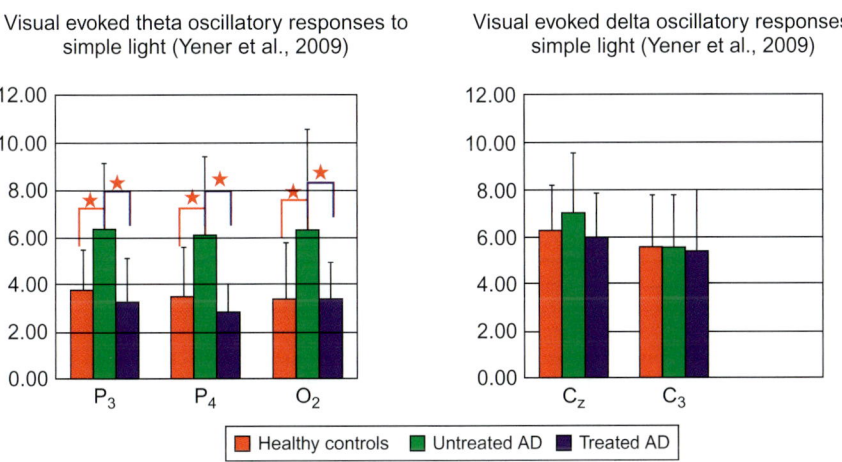

Görsev G. Yener and Erol Başar, Fig. 2. Visual SEO responses are increased contra-intuitively in AD, indicating a hyperexcitability in primary and secondary visual sensory areas. (Modified from Yener et al., 2009.)

Auditory ER delta (0.5–3.5 hz) oscillatory responses to
target stimuli

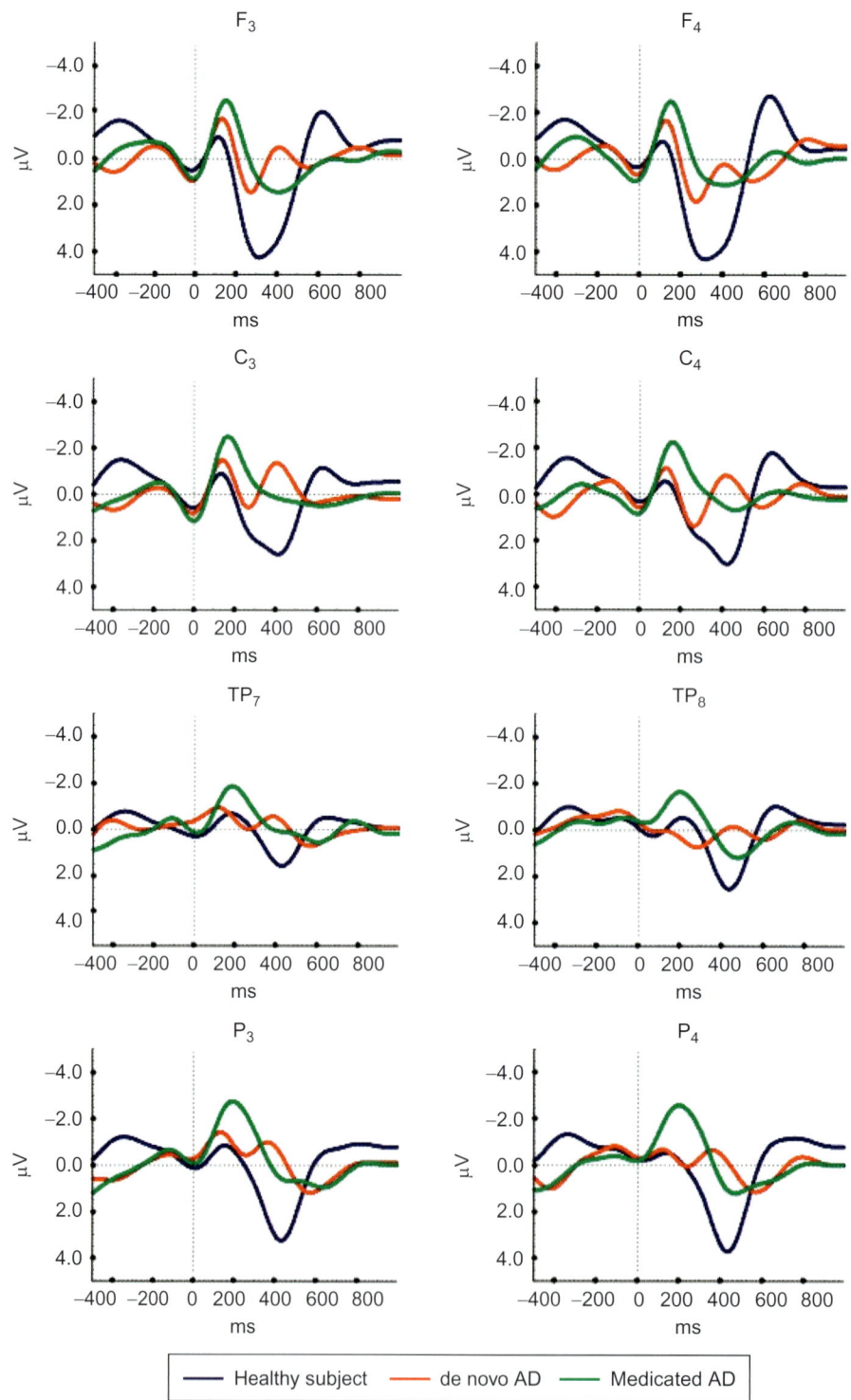

Görsev G. Yener and Erol Başar, Fig. 5. Auditory delta ERO responses are decreased in frontal regions in AD.
(Modified from Yener et al., 2012.)

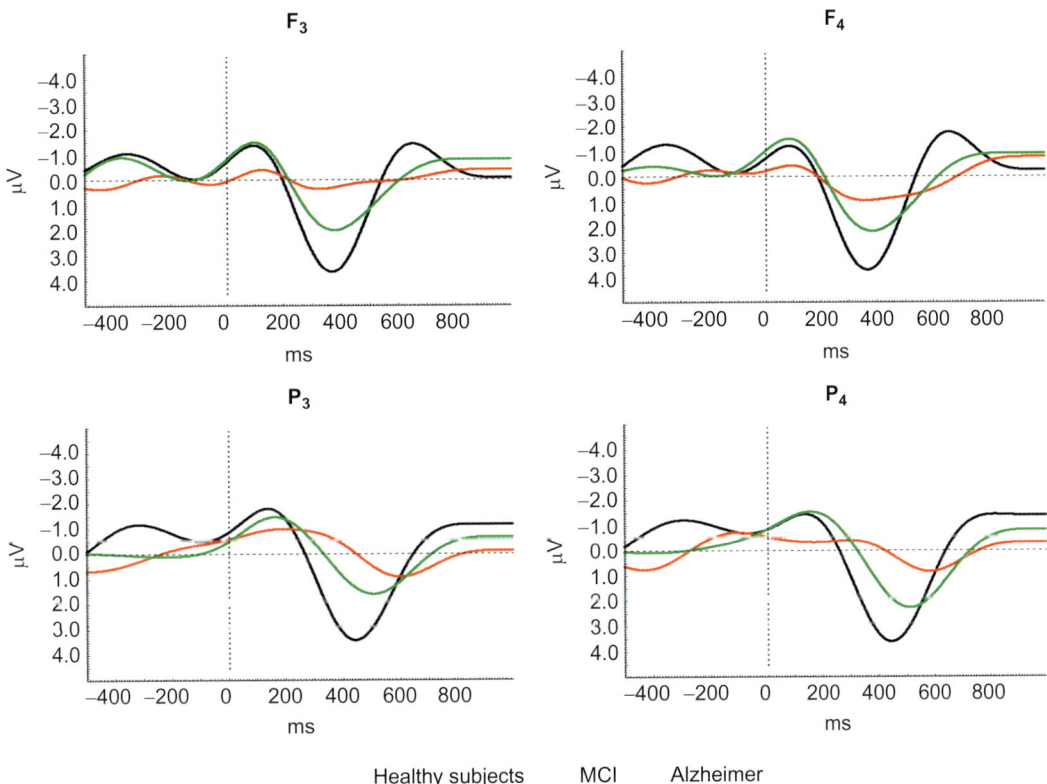

Auditory ER delta (0.5–2.2 hz) responses

Görsev G. Yener and Erol Başar, Fig. 6.   MCI and AD continuity is prominent in auditory ER delta oscillatory activity, showing gradually decreasing delta amplitudes and delayed delta peak responses among healthy subjects, MCI, and mild Alzheimer subjects. (Modified from Yener et al., 2011.)

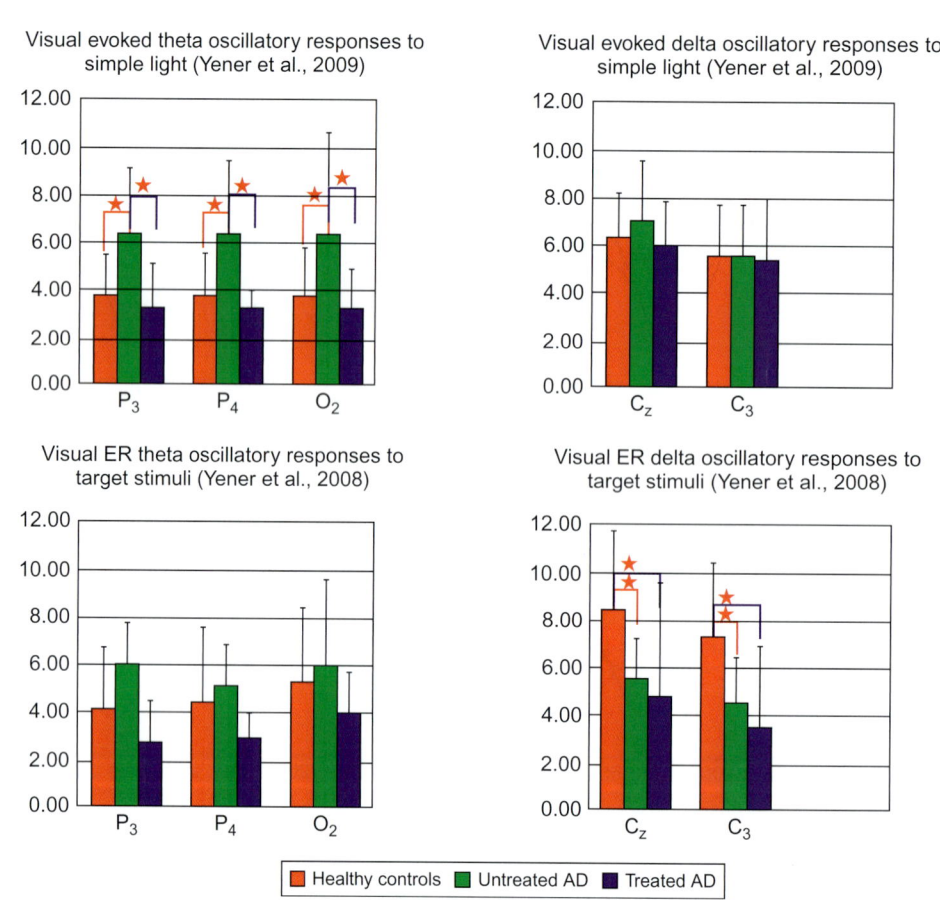

Görsev G. Yener and Erol Başar, Fig. 7.   Comparison of visual evoked and ER oscillatory activity in AD. (Modified from Yener et al., 2009.)

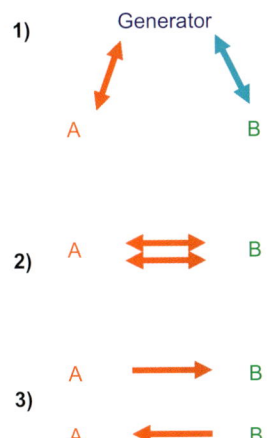

1)

Generator

A   B

2)

A ⇄ B

3)

A → B

A ← B

Görsev G. Yener and Erol Başar, Fig. 8. Bullock's electrophysiological driving sources.

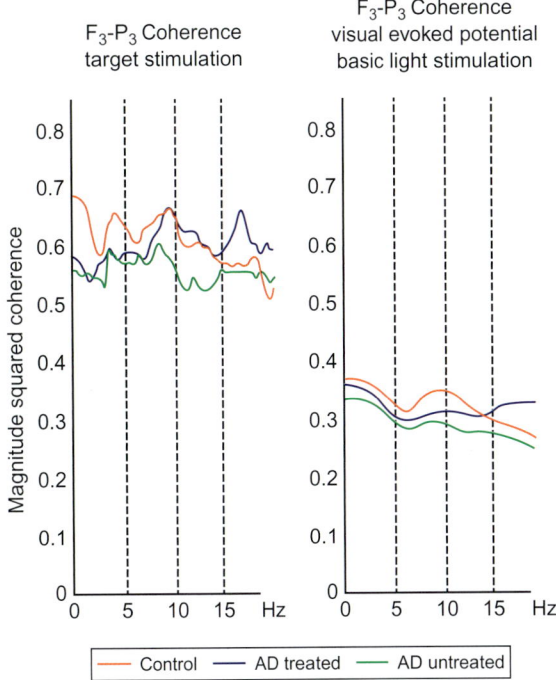

F₃-P₃ Coherence target stimulation

F₃-P₃ Coherence visual evoked potential basic light stimulation

Magnitude squared coherence

── Control ── AD treated ── AD untreated

Görsev G. Yener and Erol Başar, Fig. 10. Coherences of brain oscillations upon a cognitive task (i.e., target stimulus in classical visual oddball paradigm) reach higher values than those elicited upon simple sensory visual stimuli (i.e., basic light stimulation). Coherence, which reflects functional connectivity between fronto-parietal regions, is higher in controls than in (AD) subjects. Coherence values in alpha ranges are greater in the cholinergically treated subgroup than those with no treatment. (Modified from Yener et al., 2010.)

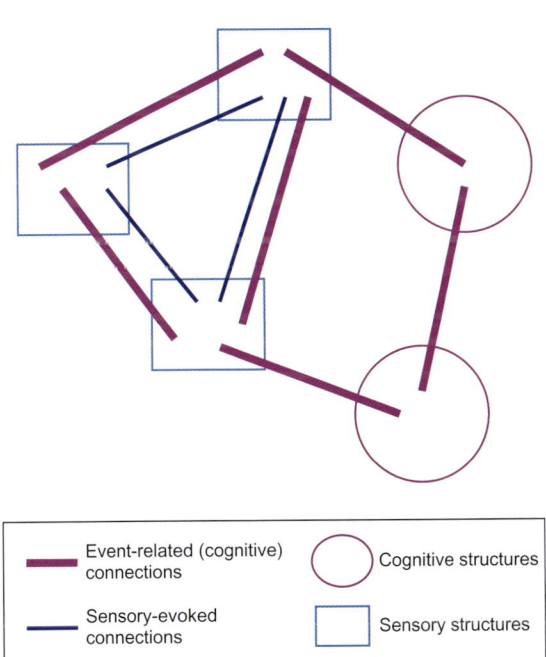

Event-related (cognitive) connections

Cognitive structures

Sensory-evoked connections

Sensory structures

Görsev G. Yener and Erol Başar, Fig. 9. Neural assemblies involved in sensory and cognitive networks. Cognitive networks (here shown by magenta lines) probably contain sensory neural elements, but also involve additional neural assemblies as shown by magenta circles. Sensory network elements are illustrated by blue squares and connections by blue lines. It is expected that sensory signals trigger activation of sensory areas, whereas cognitive stimulation would evoke both neural groups reacting to sensory and cognitive inputs.

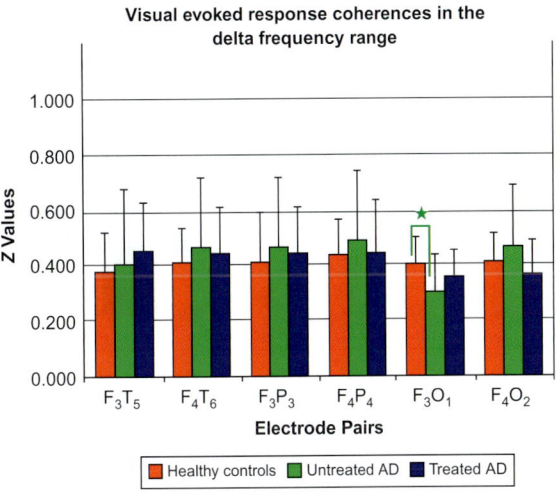

Visual evoked response coherences in the delta frequency range

Z Values

Electrode Pairs: F_3T_5 F_4T_6 F_3P_3 F_4P_4 F_3O_1 F_4O_2

■ Healthy controls ■ Untreated AD ■ Treated AD

Görsev G. Yener and Erol Başar, Fig. 11. Visual SEO responses in AD are not that different from that of controls with the exception of a mild decrease in delta band between the left frontal and occipital regions. (Modified from Başar et al., 2010.)

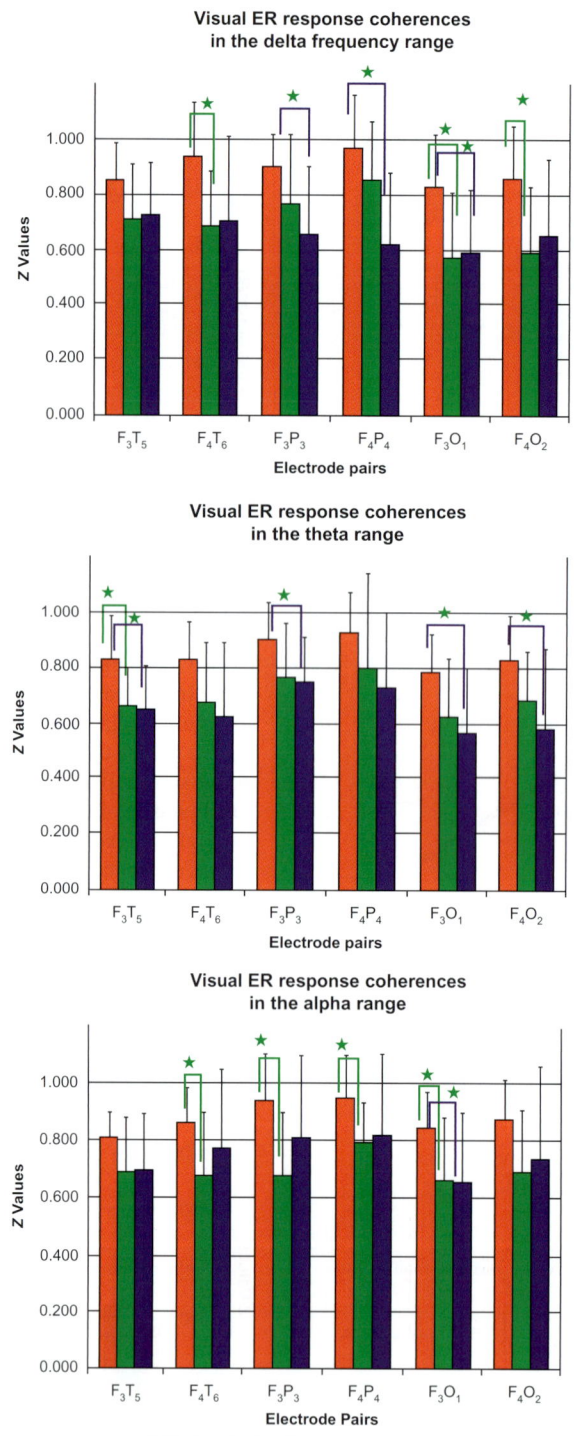

Görsev G. Yener and Erol Başar, Fig. 12.   Visual ER coherences are decreased in slower frequencies (delta, theta, alpha bands) over a wide range of connections in AD. (Modified from Başar et al., 2010.)

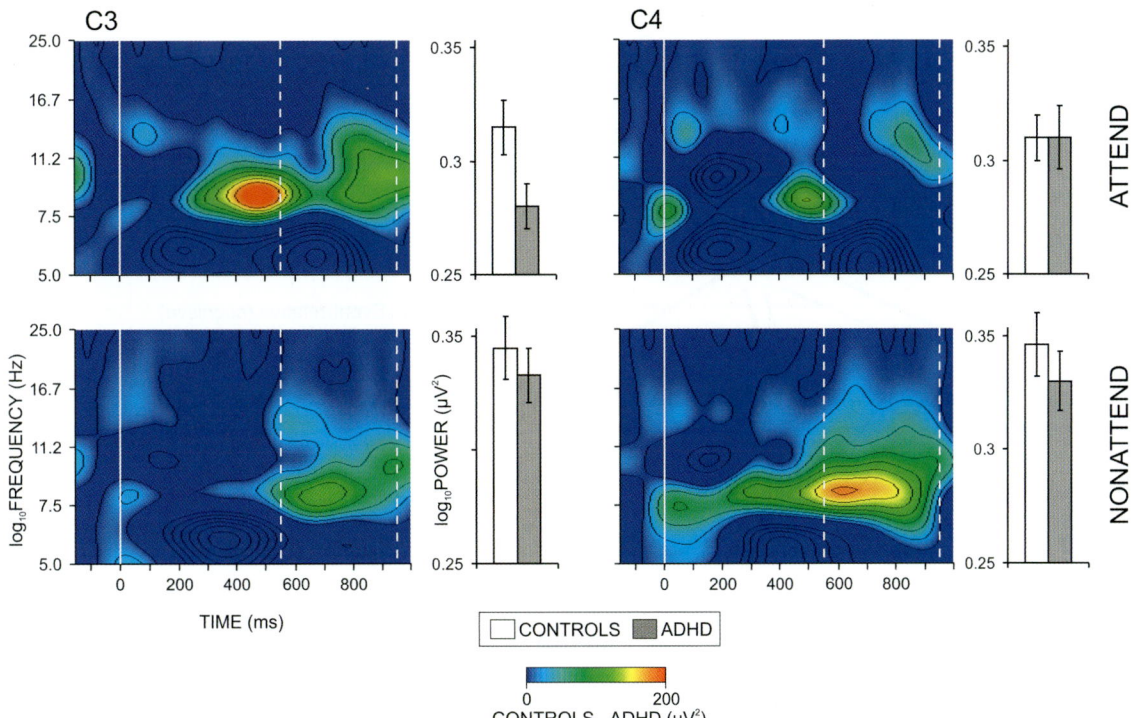

Juliana Yordanova et al., Fig. 4.   The effect of electrode position (C3, C4) on alpha band total power in selective attention task in attend and nonattend conditions for control and ADHD groups. Difference time–frequency plots show the grand average total power of ADHD children subtracted from the grand average total power of controls for attended (upper row) and nonattended (lower row) stimuli at C3 and C4. Positive values in the analyzed epoch (marked with white dash lines) indicate controls > ADHD. Bar graphs present group mean values. It is demonstrated that in contrast to controls, children with ADHD reduced alpha (mu) activity more strongly at C3 than C4 following a stimulus in the attended channel.

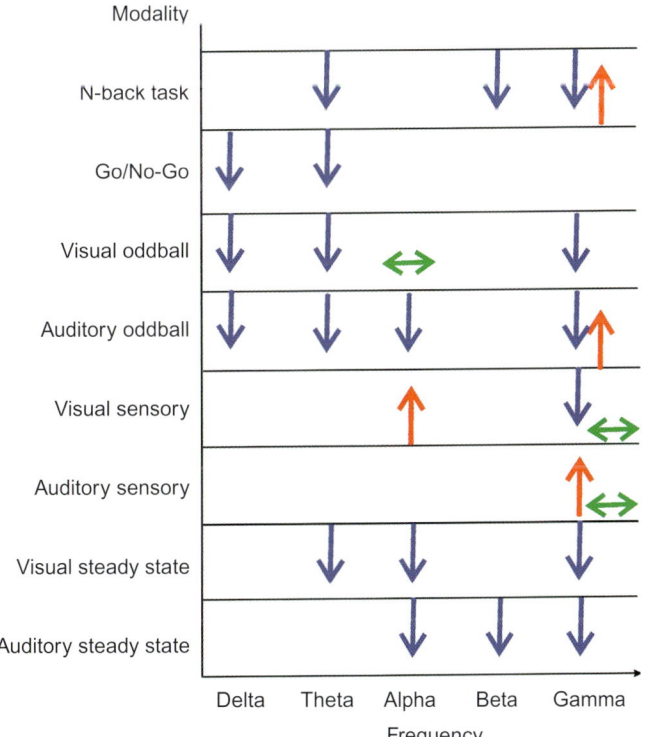

Erol Başar and Bahar Güntekin, Fig. 1.   Summary of evoked/event-related studies in schizophrenia upon application of several paradigms. The summary is based on the results described in Table 1. The "↓" and "↑" signs indicate that the evoked/ event-related oscillation is decreased or increased, respectively, in SZ patients for a given paradigm compared to healthy controls. The "↔" sign describes that there is no difference between SZ patients and healthy controls in a given paradigm.

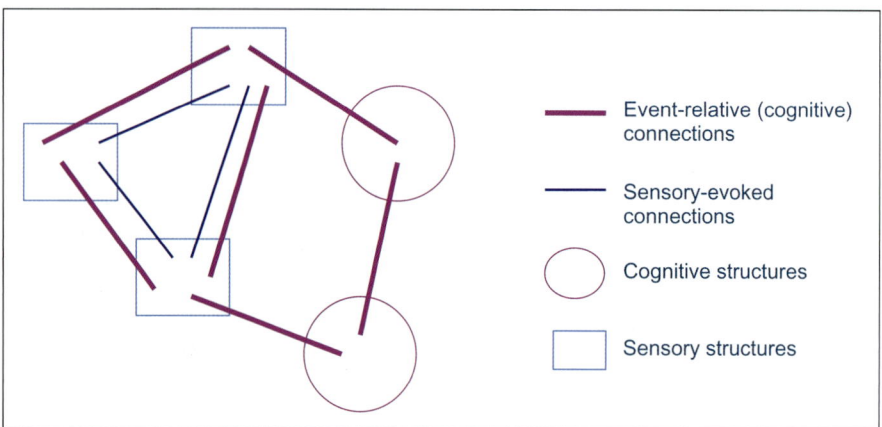

Görsev G. Yener and Erol Başar, Fig. 3. Neural assemblies involved in sensory and cognitive networks. Cognitive networks (here shown by magenta lines) probably contain sensory neural elements, but also involve additional neural assemblies, as shown by magenta circles. Sensory network elements are illustrated by blue squares and connections by blue lines. It is expected that sensory signals trigger activation of sensory areas, whereas cognitive stimulation would evoke both neural groups reacting to sensory and cognitive inputs.

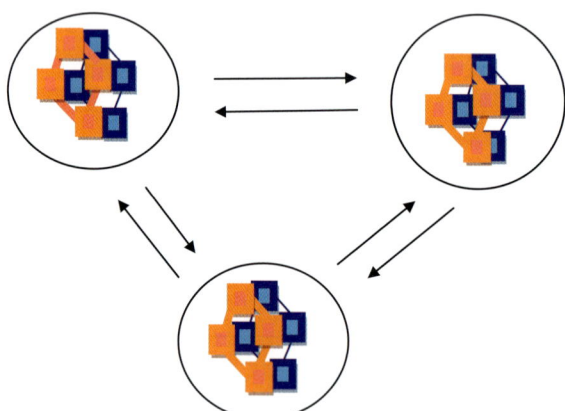

Görsev G. Yener and Erol Başar, Fig. 4. Web of sensory and cognitive networks between distant neural networks.